ISBN 978-0-483-50249-9
PIBN 10784984

The Oxford Medicine

BY VARIOUS AUTHORS

EDITED BY

HENRY A. CHRISTIAN, A.M., M.D.

Hersey Professor of the Theory and Practice of Physic, Harvard University
Physician-in-Chief to the Peter Bent Brigham Hospital,
Boston, Mass.

OXFORD UNIVERSITY PRESS

AMERICAN BRANCH, 35 WEST 32ND STREET, NEW YORK

LONDON · TORONTO · MELBOURNE · BOMBAY

Supplemented to 1926

Printed in U. S. A.

CHAPTER X

VITAMINS AND VITAMIN DEFICIENCIES

By TOM D. SPIES and HUGH R. BUTT

Table of Contents

INTRODUCTION

The advances in nutrition have received a great deal of publicity in the lay and scientific press during the last few years probably because of the most unusual and dramatic circumstances of the discovery of the vitamins. Many of the reports are correct, but others are not reliable. Consumers are being subjected to a ballyhoo that brings to mind stories of the Indian tonic days. Vitamins have been reported to cure almost every illness of man or beast. The modern science of nutrition, although it may seem to some to promise miracles, offers no elixir of life and no panaceas. It does offer specific therapy for vitamin deficiency diseases and holds promise for far-reaching results in the near future. Certain it is that vitamins are necessary for the health and vigor of the higher forms of life; yet it is equally certain that they are of no value where no deficiency exists. They are organic food substances which, in small quantities, are necessary for maintaining proper growth and continued health of the human body. The amounts required are so small that it is almost certain that they act as catalysts or help to form such in the human body. They are important in the biochemical systems of the body which govern the oxidation of carbohydrates, proteins and fats. They have functional relationships with minerals and perhaps with all other essential elements of the dietary.

Already vitamins are used widely in medicine. By prescribing them judiciously many physicians apply them successfully in their practice of medicine. Others use them injudiciously and with no success. Some refuse to use them at all. Still others prescribe them for appearance sake. The physician has been justifiably sceptical toward the introduction of each new vitamin as a therapeutic agent, but sometimes he has let his doubts give way to an attitude of complete confidence, a confidence not always warranted. The rapidity with which these advances in nutrition have come, which is shown in Fig. 1, is almost unparalleled in medicine, and there is great need for investigation by conservative physicians, who will test each new material and appraise its effect on human beings under controlled conditions.

That the present state of our knowledge of nutrition frequently is confusing and often contradictory is due largely to inadequately con-

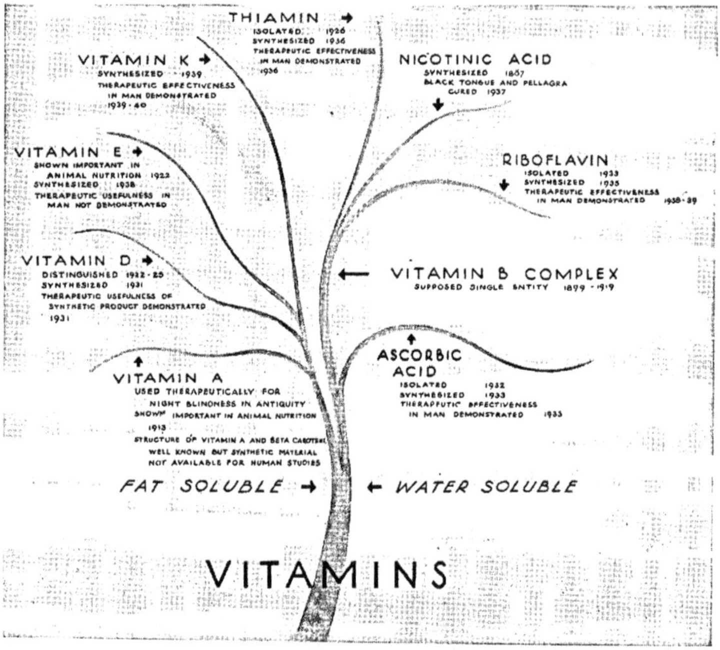

Fig. 1. Diagram showing important vitamins with important dates in their development.

trolled clinical investigations in a field that once was considered very simple. Clinical experimentation with the vitamins must continue, and at the same time we must exercise great scepticism in regard to what may be attributed to their therapeutic effect.

As physicians we abhor "polypharmacy", yet there is a logical basis for including sufficient amounts of a variety of vitamins in a single therapeutic preparation. The vitamins tend to occur together in nature, and the practice of medicine will be enriched by a full realization that the deficiency diseases occur as complexities rather than as single entities and must be treated as such. Convalescence from nutritional deficiency diseases often is shortened greatly by administering vitamins in suitable mixtures rather than by administering a single vitamin.

The use of vitamins in medicine illustrates vividly the immense surge that can be given to the biological or chemical field when it progresses to the point where it has important clinical application. Because of its great scientific and therapeutic value research on the vitamins has been of intense interest to the authors of this chapter. In writing these sections on the vitamins we have looked backward over a large experience and have eliminated all but those facts that seem essential to the physician, who would achieve his goal of full rehabilitation of every patient with nutritional deficiency diseases. It is our hope that most of the material in this chapter will be of immediate value in the practice of medicine and that much of it will interest the biochemist, the biologist, the physiologist, the pharmacologist and the student of nutrition.

In the following pages we will discuss the vitamins, in which the practicing physician will be particularly interested, the four fat-soluble vitamins A, D, E, and K, the four water-soluble vitamins, C, (ascorbic acid) and B (thiamin, nicotinic acid amide and riboflavin) and folic acid. Each of the sections has been written as a separate unit concerned only with one of these vitamins and its corresponding disease. Theories have been discussed as little as possible, and all the material is presented with as little prejudice as strong personal opinions allow.

VITAMINS A

Epidemics of xerophthalmia and keratomalacia had been reported in the medical literature some thirty or forty years before the compound termed "fat-soluble A" was recognized. These conditions were observed to appear chiefly among children; even at an early date a dietary origin was suspected, and cod liver oil was noted to be effective in ameliorating the conditions. These clinical obervations then were followed by many experimental studies, results of which suggested strongly that there was present in certain foodstuffs a fat-soluble compound which was essential for normal growth. It was not, however, until 1913 that McCollum and Davis reported the occurrence in certain foods of a compound termed "fat-soluble A". In 1922 it was shown clearly that the anti-ophthalmic factor in cod liver oil could be destroyed by oxidation without destruction of the anti-rachitic factor.

In these early experiments it was noted that swelling of the lids of one eye or both eyes developed in animals, rats, subsisting on a diet deficient in vitamin A, after which there commonly developed an inflamed and catarrhal condition of the conjunctiva with a bloody or purulent discharge. It was noted that, if this ophthalmic condition was not treated and the animals continued to live, the cornea became affected, and blindness resulted. Significantly it was noted also that without any local treatment, if the ophthalmic disease was not too far advanced, the symptoms disappeared rapidly after the ingestion of food containing an adequate amount of vitamin A. This relationship of diseases of the eye to dietary deficiency also was demonstrated experimentally in other species as well as rats, and it was shown also in these studies that certain diseases of the eye of man might be the result of deficiency of Vitamin A. Soon it was reported that xerophthalmia in man could be prevented or cured by the administration of food rich in the A vitamin[1-5].

Chemistry

Although between 1913 and 1915 McCollum and Davis and Osborne and Mendel had ascertained the presence of "fat-soluble A" in cod liver oil and in butter, it was not until 1933 that Karrer synthesized perhydrovitamin A. The structural formula of vitamin A is shown in Fig. 2.

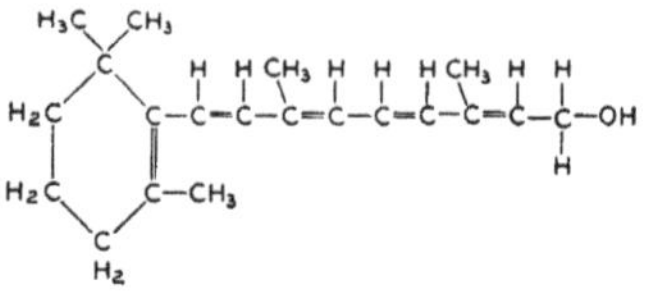

Fig. 2. The structural formula of vitamin A₁.

This primary alcoholic structure of vitamin A is important in that it allows for esterification and, therefore, the formation of compounds of vitamin A with protein, bile acids and fatty acids. These compounds of vitamin A are decomposed with liberation of the vitamin by such hydrolytic processes as occur in saponification; the vitamin is an alcohol; hence, it is not itself saponifiable. Vitamin A is a hydrogen acceptor probably because of its unsaturated form. There is some evidence to indicate that the substance readily absorbs oxygen in solution and is markedly pro-oxygenic when undergoing oxidation. However, highly oxidized vitamin A has no biological activity. Vitamin A is very sensitive to oxidation and auto-oxidizes readily. It is heat-stable but of course insoluble in water. Vitamin A does not show any absorption band in the visible region of the spectrum, but it does show a rather broad absorptive region in the ultraviolet. These properties form the basis for the spectrophotometric method for the quantitative estimation of vitamin A.

On the basis of recent reports it appears that there exists, in addition to vitamin A compound designated as "vitamin A_2". In chemical structure vitamin A_1 is related very closely to vitamin A_2, and biologically the activity is the same. Rather extensive investigations of the distribution of these two forms of vitamin A have led definitely to the conclusion that vitamin A_1 predominates in the tissues of salt-water fishes and that vitamin A_2 predominates in the tissues of fresh-water fishes. The absence of vitamin A_2 from the liver of mammals and other land animals probably can be explained by the absence of vitamin A_2 from their food. Vitamin A_2 has not been isolated in pure crystalline form. There is no evidence that vitamin A_2 plays any significant rôle in mammalian nutrition.

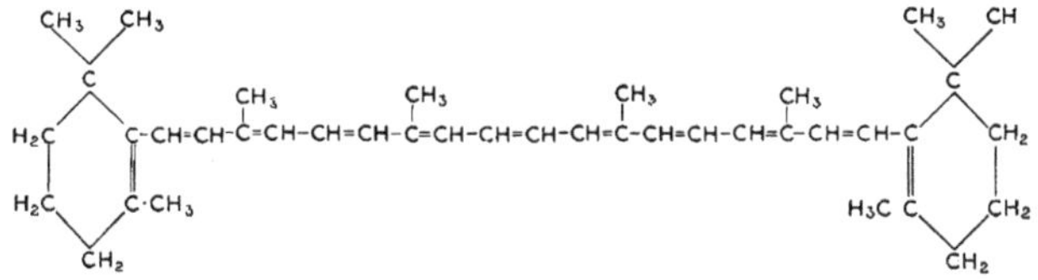

Fig. 3. The structural formula for beta carotene.

There are many reasons for assuming that some other types of vitamin A exist. Recently[6] a geometric isomer of vitamin A_1 has been reported, which has biological potency nearly the same in kind and magnitude as that of vitamin A_1.

Most of the vitamin A available to man in his diet is in the form of its precursors, the yellow and red carotenoid pigments, provitamins. For this reason the chemical properties of these compounds are rather important. There are nine different naturally occurring compounds known as "provitamins A". These are alpha, beta and gamma carotene, cryptoxanthene, echinenone, myxoxanthin, leprotene, aphanin and aphanicin. These provitamins A belong chemically to a special class called "carotenoids". They are extremely sensitive to oxidation, auto-oxidation and light but are stable to heat. Little is known of the biogenesis of provitamins A, and none have yet been synthesized. Of this large group of pigments, however, the beta form yields two molecules of the vitamin, whereas each of the other produces only one molecule. This can be seen easily in the formula of beta carotene shown in Fig. 3. Theoretically, if the splitting ocurrs in the middle, one molecule may give rise to two molecules of vitamin A. It was the ingenious research of Karrer which first proved that beta carotene contains two beta-ionone rings. It was shown also by these investigations that the beta-ionone ring is an essential component of the molecular structure of vitamin A. All the carotenoids that yield vitamin A exhibit characteristic absorption bands in the visible region of the spectrum.

Although its exact function is unknown, carotene obviously is of great importance in the physiological processes of plants. It constitutes a family associated closely with chlorophyll, although it is not lost when the chlorophyll disappears at the time of the yellowing of leaves. However, it is destroyed completely in dry dead leaves. Rapid drying by artificial heat also destroys the provitamin. All these facts are important because carotene of green leaves is brought indirectly into human nutrition through milk and eggs.

The conversion of the precursors into vitamin A apparently takes place in the animal liver, and it is of clinical significance that this transformation is retarded in the presence of phosphorus poisoning and in other forms of hepatic injury. It is thought that the conversion of carotene into vitamin A takes place by the aid of an enzyme in the liver called "carotenase". Although there is much evidence that the liver is the site of conversion, there is also some evidence that the human pancreas is involved[7].

Physiology

The absorption and utilization of vitamin A and carotene depend on many factors, and because of the differences in absorption and utilization of these two compounds, both of them must be described.

Vitamin A is a fat-soluble compound, and its absorption apparently is facilitated greatly by the simultaneous absorption of a certain amount of fat. Most observers believe that the presence of bile is not necessary for proper absorption of vitamin A, although it is still perhaps good therapeutic medicine to administer bile salts with concentrates of vitamin A in the treatment of patients who have obstruction of the biliary tract.

Absorption of the vitamin reaches the maximum in three to five hours after administration. Although there apparently is some loss of vitamin A in the stool, nothing is known of the degree of destruction of vitamin A in the gastrointestinal tract under either normal or pathological conditions. Studies on a person who had a fistula of the thoracic duct, after the administration of vitamin A or carotene by mouth, revealed that very little of the carotene passes through the chylous fluid, whereas nearly all of the vitamin A can be recovered.

Carotene is absorbed less readily than vitamin A, and absorption itself is subject to several more hazards. Proper absorption of carotene requires the presence of bile in the intestinal tract and in those conditions, in which bile is completely or partially excluded from the intestinal tract, or in those instances, in which bile salts of good quality are excreted poorly, bile must be given as a supplement to insure proper absorption. Chronic diarrhea, pancreatic dysfunction, celiac disease or sprue also may inhibit the absorption of carotene. As with vitamin A a certain amount of normal absorption of fat also seems necessary for proper transportation of carotene across the intestinal wall. It has been shown, further, that mineral oil may inhibit seriously the absorption of carotene. For this reason mineral oil should not be given soon after meals. Absorption of carotene reaches a maximal level in the blood in from 7 to 8 hours after administration, and the amount excreted in the feces accounts for only a small portion of the unutilized excess. The rest of it apparently finds other channels of excretion or is destroyed in the intestine or elsewhere. The kidney apparently does not play any part in the disposition of either vitamin A or its precursors, unless the body is flooded with either carotene or vitamin A.

The capacity to store vitamin A varies widely among different species of animals. The rat has a remarkable capacity for the storage of vitamin A, whereas the rabbit and guinea pig retain little of this substance, even when they subsist on diets rich in carotene. In these particular animals a large part of the total content of vitamin A in the body is present in the liver, although small amounts appear in the lungs and kidneys. However, in other animals, for instance fish, greater amounts of vitamin A are deposited in the tunica propria of the mucosa of the intestine than in the liver.

After absorption a greater portion of the carotene is held in the liver, where it gradually disappears from the Kupffer cells as the concentration of vitamin A in the liver increases. Vitamin A itself also is stored properly in the liver in the Kupffer cells. In human beings the vitamin A content, as in all animals, is much lower in the liver at birth than in the liver of the normal adult, irrespective of the diet of the mother. The liver probably stores about 95 per cent. of the vitamin A reserve of the body, and the amount stored is, as a rule, smallest in the liver during childhood and increases gradually with advance in age. Examination of the livers of healthy persons, who died suddenly from accidental causes, shows them to average 331 U.S.P. units of vitamin A per gram of liver tissue.

The exact mechanism by which vitamin A is called forth from its reserve stores is not known, but from several sources it appears that the distribution of vitamin A in the circulating blood and tissues is controlled in part by the nervous system. Evidence has been presented to indicate the existence of compounds of carotene and vitamin A with protein, probably albumin[8].

The excretion of vitamin A appears to be highly selective. Neither vitamin A nor the provitamins are excreted by the kidneys unless the organism is given an excessive dose of these substances. It has been reported[9], however, that in human urine vitamin A is absent in health but present in association with some pathological conditions, particularly pneumonia and chronic nephritis.

Using fluorescence microscopy as a method of visualization of vitamin A in tissue cells, Steigmann and Popper[10] found that the concentration of vitamin A in the human liver varies even under normal conditions. Among young infants there was very little storage, but in the embryo of about five months' development considerable amounts appeared, although these depots of vitamin were reduced later, and at birth only traces were distinct. The human adrenal tissue and lactating breast tissue were found to be rich in vitamin A, but the normal tissues of the human kidney, brain, cornea, bronchi and urinary tract and the inactive breast were found to be free of the vitamin. It is interesting that by this method it was found that the retinas of rats, dying of avitaminosis A with ulceration of the cornea, contained vitamin A[11].

Only extremely small quantities of these compounds can be found in the feces, and it is assumed for this reason that unutilized excesses find other channels of excretion or are destroyed in the intestine or elsewhere.

Human milk contains both carotene and vitamin A. The colostrum from the human breast has from two to three times the biological vitamin A activity of early milk, and early human milk has from five to ten times the biological vitamin A activity of cow's milk. The administration of vitamin A in large doses effectively increases the vitamin A content in the milk of the lactating human subject in the same way as in the cow. Doses of 100,000 I.U. daily more than doubled the vitamin A content of the milk[12].

Food Sources

Vitamin A occurs only in the animal organism. Fish liver oils are the richest source of vitamin A. Milk (3 U.S.P. units per gram), butter (50 U.S.P. units per gram) and egg yolks all are rich sources of vitamin A of animal origin. Margarine, when fortified with vitamin A, can be substituted for butter in the ordinary diet[13]. Vitamin A is fairly stable to heat and not appreciably soluble in water; it is, however, destroyed by oxidation, and foods which are heated for long periods show an appreciable loss of vitamin A potency. Since the vitamin activity is not affected at the temperature of boiling water, foods cooked in this manner retain their vitamin A potency. Canned foods have practically the same vitamin A value as the corresponding fresh foods, and foods, which are stored in the frozen state, maintain their maximal vitamin A value, but dried and dehydrated foods show considerable loss of vitamin A content.

The provitamins A occur in plants and generally are absent from the animal organism. There are, however, a few exceptions. Almost pure betacarotene has been found in the corpus luteum, in the human placenta and in the adrenal gland.

Human beings depend almost entirely on provitamins for their source of vitamin A. Fortunately vitamin A is widespread in nature in the form of the precursors, the yellow and red carotenoid pigments. These pigments are found in the plant world, being distributed from bacteria to garden fruits and vegetables. The pigments are found chiefly in association with chlorophyll and in the green leaves of plants, but this is not invariably true, since carrots and sweet potatoes with their yellow color also are rich in these substances.

Apparently there is a direct parallel between greenness (chlorophyll content) and vitamin A activity in foods of plant origin. Among the best sources of vitamin A are thin green leaves. The exact relationship between the degree of greenness and vitamin A activity is not understood, but it is well known that the outer green leaves of iceberg lettuce or cabbage are much more potent in vitamin A than are the inner leaves. Peas, green beans, green peppers, parsley stocks, asparagus and green celery all are known to have a high content of vitamin A. Carrots, sweet potatoes, apricots, yellow peaches and yellow tomatoes, all of which possess a yellowish color, are rich sources of vitamin A. Nuts and cereal grains, with the exception of those having considerable green and yellow color, are very poor sources of vitamin A. Yellow corn is the most important vitamin A food in this group.

Experimental Pathological Physiology

The observations of Wolbach and Bessey, Mellanby, and Moore have established growth of bone and the nature of such growth as important aspects of vitamin A deficiency. Wolbach and Bessey consider that deficiency of vitamin A retards bone growth, but Mellanby, on the contrary, believes that lack of the vitamin leads to increased activity of both the osteoblasts and osteoclasts of the bone with proliferation of cancellous bone at the expense of compact bone[14, 15, 16]. Formerly it was believed that vitamin A produced a profound effect on the nervous system. Wolbach and Bessey[14], however, have shown that in deficiency of vitamin A in rats skeletal growth is retarded earlier than that of the soft tissues in general, including growth of the central nervous system, and that in the white rat at least the nervous manifestations are due to pressure effects caused by relative overgrowth of the central nervous system.

Epithelium. – No definite changes in the skin of experimental animals have been described as following deficiency of vitamin A.

Relationship to Infection. – Since McCollum in 1917 first pointed out that severe spontâneous infection develops in rats suffering from deficiency of vitamin A, there has been a bulk of literature on this subjecr, and for many years it was believed that vitamin A did aid in some manner in combating the tendency toward infection in man. It is believed by some that the frequency of occurrence and high fatality rate of pneumonia in infants, who suffer from deficiency of vitamin A, result from disturbance of function of the mucosa of all parts of the lung. Others believe that the provision of vitamin A in large amounts is beneficial in preventing the common cold, but this whole subject is, in general, very controversial. Undoubtedly severe deficiency of vitamin A in man will lower the resistance to infection; yet administration of vitamin A during the course of an infection apparently does not have any beneficial effect on the outcome of the infection unless a severe deficiency of vitamin A also is present. Certainly there is enough evidence to indicate that there are many other factors, which have an influence on infection equal to that of vitamin A, and that some factors have a greater influence.

Hence, there is no justification for calling vitamin A "the anti-infective vitamin".

Eye. – Decreased facility for adaptation to dark is one of the earliest functional changes associated with deficiency of vitamin A. Evidence has been reported which suggests that the visual purple of the retina is a conjugated protein in which vitamin A is a prosthetic group. Exposure of the retina to light leads to a chemical change with bleaching of the visual purple, and before sensitivity can be restored, the pigment must be reconstructed. This process perhaps is reversible, but it is not always efficient, and, therefore, direct supplies of vitamin A must be constantly available. The selection of color and other visual functions depend on light of high intensity associated with the cones of the retina, whereas the rods are sensitive only to light and are especially adapted to function in dim light. Visual purple is found only in the rods and apparently serves to transform the energy of dim light into nerve impulses which, within limits, vary according to intensity of the light. Although it was believed formerly that the cone played no part in the metabolism of vitamin A, it has been demonstrated recently that the formation of visual violet or iodopsin in the cone takes place in much the same manner as does formation of visual purple in the rods. In the experimental animal as in man pathological changes in the eye occur late. Changes in both animals and man are essentially the same. Metaplasia of the epithelium of the conjunctiva and cornea is the earliest change followed by vascularization of the cornea with edema and perhaps, necrosis. Accumulation of keratin itself favors infection of the cornea, which may lead ultimately to ulceration and hypopyon keratitis.

Liver. – It has been well established that the liver enacts a major rôle in the metabolism of vitamin A, but the exact manner in which this is accomplished is still unknown. As early as 1895 Hori had made the clinical observation that night blindness and keratomalacia frequently accompany disease of the liver. Later it was shown that in patients, who have alcoholic cirrhosis without jaundice, there are subnormal powers of adaptation to darkness which improve on the adequate administration of vitamin A. Others have demonstrated repeatedly that the content of vitamin A in the liver and blood of patients, who have severe hepatic injury, nearly always is decreased markedly.

Low values for vitamin A in the blood have been reported to be associated with severe hepatic damage. Clinical improvement was accompanied by the gradual return to normal of the content of vitamin A in the blood[17].

Human Requirements

Vitamin A is essential to normal metabolism. Although the exact minimal requirement of vitamin A for man still is unknown, considerable work has been carried out in an effort to settle this point. Since the recommended daily allowances for definite nutrients as defined by the Food and Nutrition Board of the National Research Council and later adopted by the Council on Foods and Nutrition of the American Medical Association represents the thoughts of the leaders in these particular fields, it would seem well that these should be accepted.

For the average man and woman, who weighs 70 and 56 kg., respectively, the daily allowance is 5.000 international units. In the latter half of pregnancy 6,000 international units are required, and during lactation the requirement is 8,000 international units. For children aged less than a year 1,500 units are required; for those aged one year to three years, 2,000; for those four to six years old, 2,500; for those seven to nine years old, 3,500 and for those ten to twelve years old, 4,500. For children more than twelve but not more than fifteen years of age 5,000 units are required, and for those sixteen to twenty years of age, 6,000 units. Allowances in all these instances may be less, if the substance provided is vitamin A, and greater, if it is chiefly the provitamin, carotene.

Deficiency of Vitamin A in Man

Apparently deficiency of vitamin A in man is not common in this country. Normal subjects placed on a diet deficient in vitamin A appear to have sufficient stores to maintain vitamin A in the blood and tissues, such as the retina, at an adequate level for many months. Many investigators have established that deficiency of vitamin A is an uncommon disturbance even among the ill and poorly nourished[18,19]. However, follicular hyperkeratosis, pityriasis rubra pilaris and cirrhosis of the liver all are diseases, in which the thresholds of adaptation to dark have been found to be abnormal, and in which these thresholds have been improved materially through the administration of vitamin A.

Epithelium. — Cutaneous lesions (Figs. 4, 5, 6 and 7) associated with deficiency of vitamin A and analogous to those occurring in other epithelial structures have been reported by several investigators. The skin contains, however, no appreciable vitamin A in spite of the fact that the vitamin has an important influence on cutaneous and structural growth.

There is little evidence to show that dermatological conditions are influenced by, or influence, the content of vitamin A of the plasma[20].

In the skin vitamin A apparently is concerned with the process of keratinization. In conditions of long-standing deficiency of vitamin A the skin becomes dry and hyperkeratotic. These changes are evident

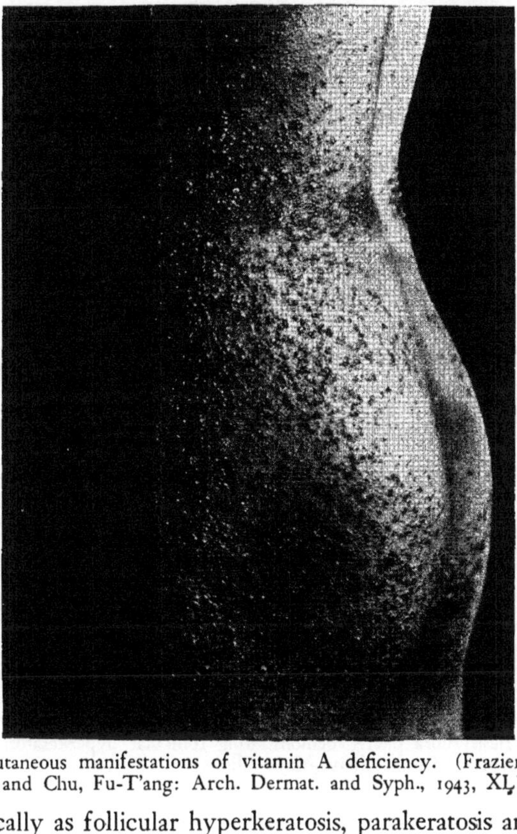

Fig. 4. Cutaneous manifestations of vitamin A deficiency. (Frazier, C. N., Hu, Ch'uan-K'uei and Chu, Fu-T'ang: Arch. Dermat. and Syph., 1943, XLVIII, 1.)

microscopically as follicular hyperkeratosis, parakeratosis and dyskeratosis. Steffens as reported by him and his associates[21] eliminated vitamin A from his diet for a period of 6 months, and although his capacity for adaptation to dark remained within normal limits, his skin became dry, and there were microscopic changes in the skin similar to those just mentioned.

The severe dermatoses of deficiency of vitamin A are found in the same geographical distribution as the advanced ocular manifestations[22]. The lesions consist of epidermal hyperplasia and glandular atrophy and are represented by papular eruptions around the pilosebaceous follicles.

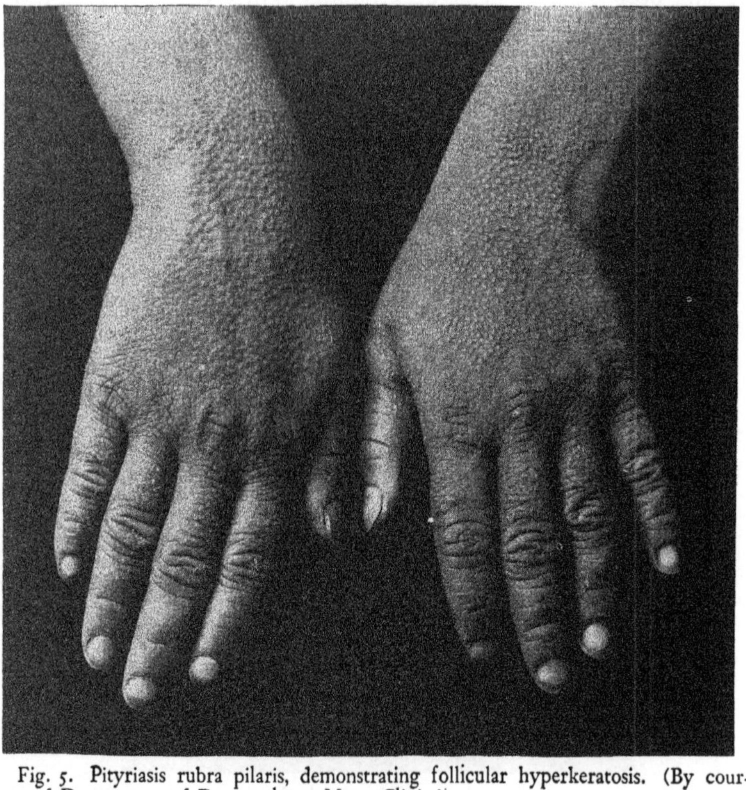

Fig. 5. Pityriasis rubra pilaris, demonstrating follicular hyperkeratosis. (By courtesy of Department of Dermatology, Mayo Clinic.)

These usually occur among persons between the ages of 16 and 30 years and not among infants. The condition is common among men, and nearly all, who have the dermatosis, also have obvious ocular manifestations of deficiency of vitamin A. Reports from the East indicate that the incidence of this symptom is as high as, or higher than, that of the ocular symptoms[23].

Eye. – In the United States xerophthalmia, keratomalacia and nyctalopia caused by deficiency of vitamin A are rare. The early pathological changes are the same as those described previously for animals. Xerophthalmia is most common in infancy, although it may be seen at all ages.

The loss of visual acuity in dim light is one of the first symptoms of deficiency of vitamin A in man. Definite pathological changes in the eye, however, occur late in man when diets deficient in vitamin A are employed[21]. Night blindness usually develops in adult persons before any

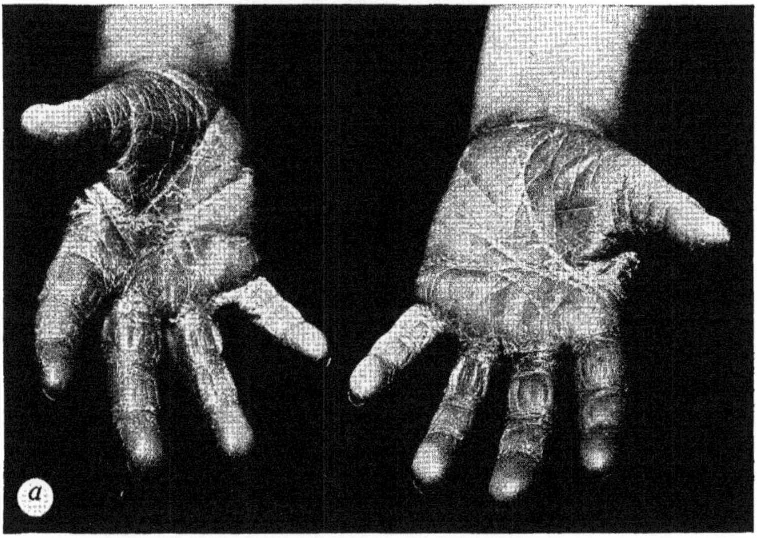

Fig. 6. Pityriasis rubra pilaris, demonstrating keratoderma palmaris. (By courtesy of Department of Dermatology, Mayo Clinic.)

types of ophthalmia develop, but usually the disease is ushered in by small triangular white patches, which appear on the outer and inner sides of the cornea, covered by white, foamlike spots consisting of corneal epithelium, which has been shed and accumulates in this position, Bitot's spots. Photophobia and conjunctivitis appear early followed by light brown pigmentation of the conjunctiva. The keratinization of the conjunctiva may extend to the cornea and lead to extreme softness and degeneration of the cornea and to ulceration, perforation and total destruction of the eye, keratomalacia. This disease may destroy the eye rapidly, and its prompt recognition, therefore, is very important.

For a number of years Spies and associates have studied the ocular symptoms occurring as a result of malnutrition among human beings. Asche and Spies have observed that Bitot's spots frequently are observed among these patients, and that they disappear soon after large doses of vitamin A have been administered. Follicular conjunctivitis is observed frequently, particularly among children, and it also often disappears after

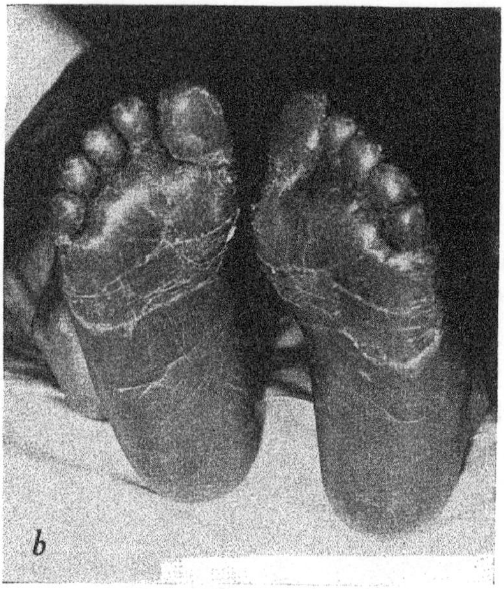

Fig. 7. Pityriasis rubra pilaris, demonstrating keratoderma plantaris. (By courtesy of Department of Dermatology, Mayo Clinic.)

the administration of large amounts of vitamin A. Mild conjunctival xerosis also has been attributed to deficiency of vitamin A[24,25,26].

Methods for Measuring Deficiency of Vitamin A

The fact that night blindness is an early symptom of deficiency of vitamin A led to the development of visual adaptation in dim light as a method for the diagnosis of deficiency of this vitamin. Whether deficiency of vitamin A can be measured by testing adaptation to dark continues to be a most controversial subject. Some contend that this method is satisfactory for measuring deficiency of vitamin A. Others contend that, although some relationship exists between readings of the biophotometer and the status of nutrition of vitamin A, yet the relationship is not close enough to warrant use of the test as a means of diagnosis of subclinical deficiency of vitamin A. It has been pointed out that the method is time-consuming, and that for this reason alone its routine clinical use practically is ruled out. Certainly minor fluctuations in adaptation to dark in terms of deficiency of vitamin A should receive little emphasis unless physical methods are used to test the reliability of the differences. It is true that a majority of workers believe that the study of adaptation to dark can be used as a test for deficiency of vitamin A, but until differences in technic and in interpretation of results have been resolved, it is impossible to be certain how far recorded observations represent physiological facts. In fact, by having human beings subsist on a diet deficient in vitamin A over long periods some investigators have been unable to produce clinical night blindness or even changes in adaptation to dark[27]. It may be, as stated by Josephs[28], that all this discrepancy is the result of lack of knowledge of methods for determining storage of vitamin A. Certainly at present there is no single simple formula for computing the needs of the body for vitamin A. Measurements of dark adaptation provide only one approach to the subject.

No definite correlation between biophotometer readings and the content of vitamin A in the blood has been observed. Although it has been demonstrated that the amount of vitamin A in the blood is dependent on the amount provided in the diet, yet evidence as to whether determination of vitamin A in the blood is of value in judging the nutritional status still is contradictory. Recently evidence has been presented, which suggests that the concentration of vitamin A in the blood plasma is a considerably more sensitive indicator of deficiency of vitamin A than is the test for adaptation to dark.

The same contradictory evidence is presented for the measurement of vitamin A by examination of scrapings from the eye and vagina. On the basis of results of all of these studies it would be judged that the methods for measuring deficiency of vitamin A of man still are somewhat unreliable and demand further study. Among some physicists and chemists there still is doubt as to whether the small quantities of vitamin A present in the blood stream of man can be measured with the chemical methods available.

Toxicity

If large amounts of vegetables containing carotene are ingested by normal persons and persons suffering from certain diseases such as diabetes, carotene may accumulate in the skin in amounts sufficient to cause a deep yellow color. Such a condition is known as carotenemia. This condition, so far as is known, is compatible with good health.

It is difficult to evaluate the reports concerning the injurious effects on man which follow the ingestion of cod liver oil. Some observers, when administering large doses, 80 c.c., of cod liver oil, have noticed the appearance of dermatitis of the face and scalp. Sensitivity to cod liver oil resulting in eczema also has been reported. However, on the basis of the general favorable clinical results of the use of cod liver oil and other preparations containing vitamin A the physician should be extremely certain that it is harmful before he discontinues its use. Certainly, when the average therapeutic dose is employed, no such toxic effect will be observed.

It has been reported recently that in growing rats, given the purest available form of vitamin A in excess, skeletal fractures and hemorrhage develop rather characteristically[25].

Diagnosis of Vitamin A Deficiency

Undoubtedly the incidence of marked deficiency of vitamin A in the United States is very small. Of course the supposition that states of partial deficiency may be common has received repeated emphasis, but as yet no definite methods have been developed by which these subnutritional states can be diagnosed.

Night Blindness. – The first symptom of this syndrome is loss of visual acuity in dim light. This particular symptom may occur in the presence of various diseases of the eye such as toxic amblyopia, detachment of the retina or retinitis pigmentosa, but these conditions usually are excluded easily. The patient may complain of dancing lights before his eyes or similar visual disturbances, and of course, by means of testing for adaptation to dark he will exhibit a pathological condition. This condition must be suspected in cirrhosis of the liver, instances of severe and prolonged pyloric obstruction, severe chronic diarrhea and any other condition which may produce a generalized nutritional deficiency.

Xerophthalmia. – The symptoms of xerophthalmia have been given already under the heading, "Deficiency of Vitamin A in Man–*Eye*".

Lesions of the Skin. – Within the past few years several groups of investigators have reported on patients who had cutaneous lesions which were considered to be the result of a deficiency of vitamin A. These lesions are shown best in Figs. 4, 5, 6 and 7. Many investigators believe that this manifestation of deficiency of vitamin A is overlooked frequently.

Subclinical Form.–It is practically impossible to clinically diagnose subclinical deficiency of vitamin A. These forms probably are frequent, however, and must be considered under various conditions in which inability to carry out proper absorption or proper intake or utilization of vitamin A is suspected.

Differential Diagnosis

Although various laboratory procedures, such as measurement of the content of vitamin A in the blood and testing for adaptation to dark, in time may be very helpful in diagnosis of deficiency of vitamin A, the best method of differential diagnosis still depends on close clinical observation. Night blindness, xerophthalmia and keratomalacia are not confused easily with any other conditions and should be recognized readily. Treatment should be instituted at once.

Treatment of Vitamin A Deficiency

The use of vitamin A in treatment is indicated in those syndromes, which result from deficiency of vitamin A in the diet or from deficiency of vitamin A resulting from improper absorption or utilization. The best treatment with vitamin A still involves prophylactic therapy. In general the response to treatment with vitamin A of specific syndromes resulting from the deficiency is slow, and recovery may involve weeks and months of time.

Persons, who possess normal powers of absorption of carotene and vitamin A and who have night blindness, may be treated by diet alone or diet plus vitamin A supplement. In those cases, in which night blindness results from faulty absorption such as is caused by gastrocolic fistula, gastrointestinal continuity first must be re-established before treatment, unless the compounds are administered intramuscularly.

Xerophthalmia and keratomalacia require the same treatment as night blindness, but it is perhaps wise to administer doses of from 50,000 to

100,000 units in the form of potent fish liver oil by the oral or parenteral route.

In the presence of lesions of the skin the best results have been obtained from doses of 100,000 to 300,000 international units of vitamin A administered daily over a period of two to three months. It must be remembered that results of treatment of lesions of the skin require periods of 2 to 3 months, and the physician should not become discouraged because there is not a dramatic response.

When patients who have chronic diarrhea are being treated, it should be borne in mind that these patients require more vitamin A than is necessary for normal persons. Patients, who have hepatic disease, likewise require rather large doses of the vitamin. In such instances from 10,000 to 20,000 international units of vitamin A administered daily is considered to be an adequate dose. A person, from whose intestinal tract bile is excluded completely or partially, should be given supplements of bile salts with vitamin A supplement.

Obviously in the treatment of any of these conditions diets rich in vitamin A and its precursors should be prescribed in addition to the potent supplement containing vitamin A.

VITAMINS D

There is little doubt that rickets has been prevalent for many centuries. It was not, however, until about 1882 that cod liver oil was suggested as a remedy for the condition[29]. Hopkins[30] suggested that rickets was caused by the absence of an accessory foodstuff, and in 1913 the beneficial influence of sunlight on the assimilation of calcium was reported.

It was Mellanby[31], however, who in 1918 discovered the nutritional importance of animal fats in the normal calcification of bones, and who concluded that the antirachitic factor was similar in distribution to fat-soluble A. Later rickets was induced in rats by special diet, and Steenbock and Black[32] as well as Hess[33] found that antirachitic potency could be induced in foods by ultraviolet irradiation. McCollum named the antirachitic material "vitamin D".

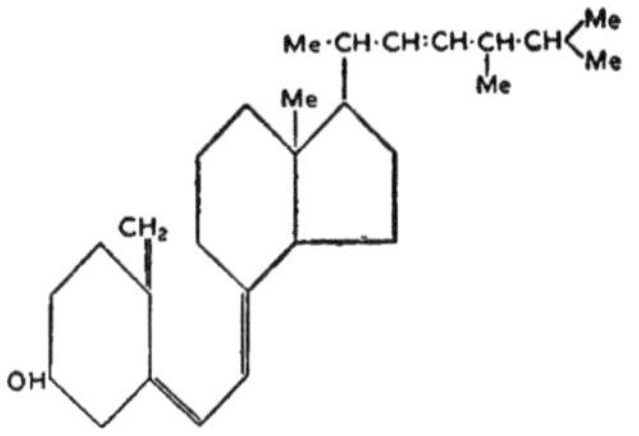

Calciferol (Vitamin D_2)

Fig. 8

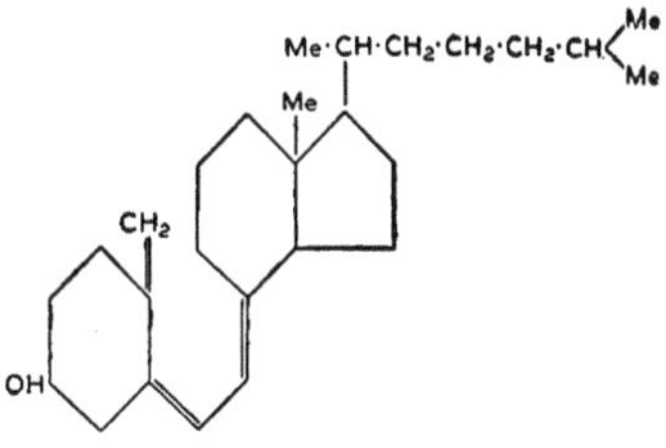

Activated 7-dehydro-cholesterol (Vitamin D_3)

Fig. 9

Fig. 8. The structural formula for calciferol (vitamin D_2).
Fig. 9. The structural formula for activated 7-dehydrocholesterol (vitamin D_3).

CHEMISTRY

A compound, which can be activated to a vitamin D, is known as a "provitamin D". These compounds belong to the sterol family and are distributed widely over the animal and plant kingdoms. The most prevalent provitamin D in higher animals and in human beings is 7-dehydrocholesterol, whereas ergosterol is predominant in yeast, molds and plants. Activated ergosterol, viosterol or calciferol is known as "vitamin D_2" (Fig. 8) and activated 7-dehydrocholesterol is known as "vitamin D_3" (Fig. 9). There is no vitamin D_1, this term having been used for a lumisterol-calciferol mixture originally mistaken for a pure vitamin. "Vitamin D_4" is the term sometimes applied to activated 22-dihydroergosterol, and "vitamin D_5" sometimes is referred to as 7-dehydrositosterol.

Ergosterol has the empirical formula, $C_{28}H_{44}O$. The conversion of this provitamin to vitamin D is not a simple process but involves a series of photochemical changes which are initiated when ergosterol is exposed to ultraviolet light. During this reaction several substances are formed, lumisterol, pro-tachysterol, tachysterol and finally, calciferol (vitamin D_2). Further irradiation of vitamin D_2 produces a toxic compound, which has no antirachitic activity and is known as "toxisterol".

Inactive 7-dehydrocholesterol is the principal provitamin occurring with the cholesterol of animal fat. Ultraviolet irradiation of the skin, feathers and fur of animals, therefore, produces activated 7-dehydrocholesterol. For this reason the principal antirachitic agent present in natural fat oils, eggs and irradiated milk is activated 7-dehydrocholesterol. Just as in the case of ergosterol the changes produced by the activation of 7-dehydrocholesterol are entirely photochemical. The physical and chemical properties of 7-dehydrocholesterol resemble those of calciferol. Both of these substances have been isolated in crystalline form, but attempts at synthesis have been unsuccessful.

Dihydro-tachysterol is a sterol of considerable practical importance. It is prepared from the acid ester of tachysterol and, when administered to human beings, causes an increase of the concentration of calcium in the blood. In therapeutic circles it is known as "A.T.10", and it is useful in infantile and postoperative hypoparathyroid tetany.

The isolation and identification of the pure vitamins D have been most difficult tasks. The exact number of naturally occurring vitamins D is unknown, but only four vitamins designated "D_2, D_3, D_4" and "D_5" have been prepared in essentially pure form. Only vitamin D_2 and vitamin D_3 have been isolated in the pure form from fish liver oils. These vitamins are fat soluble, and in the pure state are white, odorless crystals. Vitamin D_2 (Fig. 8) is an isomer of ergosterol, from which it is derived, and it has the empirical formula, $C_{28}H_{44}O$. Vitamin D_3 (Fig. 9) can be derived from 7-dehydrocholesterol.

Physiology

Absorption and Storage.—The various forms of vitamin D are absorbed readily from the intestinal tract and especially from the small bowel. This absorption is facilitated by the presence of fat, but bile salts also are necessary for proper absorption. Recent investigations indicate that the salts of desoxycholic acid may be concerned particularly with the absorption of the liposoluble vitamins. The factor of absorption also enters into such diseases as celiac disease, sprue and other fatty diarrheas which are attended commonly by deficiency of vitamin D.

From the intestines vitamin D is said to be absorbed into the blood. There is also some evidence to show that most of the vitamin D is absorbed first into the lymph of the thoracic duct, and that its rate of absorption is comparable to that of vitamin A[34]. Normal human blood contains about 50 to 135 international units per 100 c.c. of serum. The human being apparently has no special place for storage of vitamin D, although substantial amounts can be found in organs such as the liver, spleen, brain and lungs. The heart has been found consistently to be devoid of any stored amounts of vitamin D. Failure of this storage mechanism, coupled with defective secretion of bile salts, may lead to secondary avitaminosis D in cases of hepatobiliary disease. This possibility has been emphasized further by the observation that in animals normal hepatic function is necessary to promote the antirachitic action of vitamins.

Apparently vitamin D can pass only in limited amounts through the placental walls. Newborn babies have practically no vitamin D in their tissues, even though their mothers had an abundant supply during gestation. Recent data clearly indicate that the ability to increase the vitamin D content of human milk or cow's milk by large oral doses of vitamin D is very limited. Even when massive doses were ingested daily by a mother, the antirachitic potency of the milk was insufficient completely to prevent rickets in the breast-fed infant[35].

No results of quantitative studies are available which would indicate how much destruction of vitamin D occurs in the organism. Obviously some is destroyed, and some is excreted mainly through the bile and intestinal tract but not through the kidneys.

The concentration of vitamin D in the blood of human beings has been studied inadequately. Observations indicate that there is a wide zone of so-called normal concentration varying from 66 to 165 U.S.P. units per 100 c.c. of blood.

Calcium and Phosphorus Metabolism. — Vitamin D is concerned chiefly with the regulation of calcium and phosphorus in the body, but the exact chemical nature of this mechanism is not understood clearly. No one yet has demonstrated whether vitamin D enters directly into the combination with these elements or their salts or merely assumes the rôle of catalyst. However, it can be demonstrated easily that the growth of bones is related to the action of vitamin D. An early symptom of deficiency of vitamin D is a lowered content of phosphorus in the blood serum and later, a lowering of the blood level of calcium.

In general the concentrations of calcium and phosphorus in the blood serum reflect the amounts of these elements ingested. The ratio of these elements seems to be important in the rachitogenic diet, since a high-calcium and low-phosphorus diet is associated with a low content of inorganic phosphate in the blood serum and vice versa. The absolute amount as well as the ratio determines the content of calcium and phosphorus in the body fluids, and these values increase as the amounts given are increased. However, in the presence of an adequate amount of vitamin D the values for calcium and phosphorus in the serum tend to become normal regardless of the type of diet employed.

Although secondary in importance to the calcium-phosphorus ratio the acid-base ratio of the diet may be a factor in the production of rickets or tetany. There is some evidence to show that rickets is associated with an acid metabolism and tetany with an alkaline one. In neither of these conditions, whether it occurs clinically or is produced experimentally in animals, is there a definite alteration of the acid-base equilibrium of the blood.

The action of vitamin D on calcium and phosphorus metabolism seems to be concerned chiefly with the absorption of the elements from the intestinal tract. The normal infant excretes about 90 per cent. of his calcium intake in the feces and usually excretes a small amount in the urine. When vitamin D is not given, the calcium in the urine disappears. This is an attempt on the part of the body at conservation of minerals. The concentration of calcium in the feces increases, and the retention of calcium becomes subnormal. If the intake of calcium is low or the deficiency severe, the fecal calcium actually may exceed the intake, and thus the condition known as "negative calcium balance" ensues. A similar sequence of events occurs in the case of phosphorus, except that the amount of phosphate contained in the urine usually is increased[36,37].

The effect of vitamin D in producing a reversal of these conditions is striking. The intestinal excretion of calcium and phosphorus is decreased, calcium appears in the urine, and the calcium balance is restored to normal. The changes in the concentration of calcium and phosphorus in the serum are reflectors of this calcium balance.

In recent years it has been shown that there exists in the body an enzyme, phosphatase, which is intimately related to phosphorus metabolism. The exact function of phosphatase in the serum is not known, but whatever it may be, there is no question that in diseases of the bone, and especially resorptive ones in which osteoblastic activity is increased, the concentration of phosphatase in the serum is increased. Such is the case in rickets. An increase in the concentration of phosphatase in the serum is perhaps the first definite evidence of development of the rachitic condition; it precedes roentgenological changes and diminution of the amount of serum phosphate. The concentration of serum phosphatase is high in cases of active rickets, and the administration of vitamin D decreases the concentration toward normal but more slowly than it decreases the concentration of calcium and phosphorus. The concentration of phosphatase may not reach normal for several months after there is evidence of healing. The increase of the concentration of serum phosphatase in cases of rickets apparently acts as a protective mechanism.

The difference in action between vitamin D and parathyroid extract is often the source of confusion, and it is important to the clinician that this distinction be clear. Although both preparations increase the concentrations of calcium and phosphorus in the serum, parathyroid extract acts specifically on the serum calcium, and in parathyroid tetany it may even decrease the concentration of serum phosphate. In cases of rickets the principal action of vitamin D is in raising the low concentration of serum phosphate; only when administered in very large doses does it raise the concentration of serum calcium to more than normal. Parathyroid extract increases the concentration of serum calcium by withdrawing the element from the bone; vitamin D exerts this effect by increasing the intestinal absorption of calcium or by diminishing its re-excretion from the intestinal mucosa. The distinction may be clearer, if the reader remembers that the toxic effect of parathyroid extract is decalcification but that that of vitamin D is hypercalcification.

Although the parathyroid glands have been shown to undergo hypertrophy in cases of rickets, this is a result, rather than the cause, of rickets. Indeed, injections of parathyroid extract have been shown to retard the healing of rickets, and removal of the parathyroid glands from animals makes the production of rickets more difficult.

Food Sources

Vitamin D occurs in nature only in small amounts. Only in small quantities, likewise, does it occur in most members of the animal kingdom. The living plant and fresh vegetables contain no detectable amount of this vitamin.

Although the fat from fish contains relatively large amounts of vitamin D, the fat of other animals contains little or none of it. A very small amount of the vitamin is present in milk and milk products and in the yolk of hen's eggs. Sardines, tuna, herring and salmon, either fresh or canned, are fairly good sources of the vitamin. The average diet, however, contains relatively small amounts of vitamin D.

The accepted standard unit for expressing the strength of vitamin D as adopted by the League of Nations Health Organisation and by the United States Pharmacopoeia is defined as "The vitamin D activity of 1 mgm. of the international standard solution of irradiated ergosterol found equal to 0.025 micrograms of crystalline vitamin D". This is the international unit (I.U.) accepted as the U.S.P. unit. In administering antirachitic agents the physician should think in terms of units of vitamin D, since this is the only way in which the doses of the various substances containing vitamin D, which differ greatly in volume, can be reduced to a common denominator. For example, 1 teaspoonful, 4 c.c., of cod liver oil contains approximately 350 units, 1 quart of reinforced milk, 400 units and 1 mgm. of calciferol, 400,000 units.

The most satisfactory sources of vitamin D are fish liver oils. The vitamin D in cod liver oil probably is chiefly activated 7-dehydrocholesterol. Cod liver oil is universally obtainable and is effective in the prevention and treatment of any deficiency of vitamin D. There is great variation in the concentration of vitamins A and D in the oils obtained from different species of fish. The oil of the *Percomorphi* exhibits the greatest concentration of vitamin D. Fish oils are prepared by the manufacturer by combining oils from various species in such a way that the final mixture has a concentration of vitamin D equal to that of viosterol in oil. These preparations have the merit of providing vitamins D and A in high concentrations, so that both can be administered in doses measured in drops. The disadvantage of unpleasant taste is again encountered, but the quantity required is small, so that the disagreeable taste is not a serious disadvantage. Vitamin D in these preparations has chiefly the form of activated 7-dehydrocholesterol.

According to the United States Pharmacopoeia, cod liver oil must contain at least 100 units of vitamin D per gram. When large dosage of vitamin D is required, more concentrated sources of vitamin D usually are employed. One gram of viosterol in oil contains "at least 10,000 units of vitamin A" to meet the requirements of the United States Pharmacopoeia, twelfth revision. The special dropper accompanying commercial preparations is designed to deliver a drop containing 222 units. The vitamin D content of viosterol is 100 times that of standard cod liver oil. Viosterol owes its vitamin D activity to activated ergosterol.

Viosterol in oil is tasteless, which obviates the difficulty of administration encountered in the case of cod liver oil. Viosterol suffers one disadvantage as compared with cod liver oil and other fish oils, that is, it does not contain vitamin A. However, its tastelessness makes it one of the best vehicles for administering vitamin D to adults and older children.

Irradiated vitamin D milk is also a source of vitamin D. Vitamin D activity is added to milk of this type by exposure to active ultraviolet rays from artificial sources. The irradiation is accomplished in such a manner that standardization is fixed at 135 international units per quart. It has been found impracticable to irradiate the milk further because of the production of an unpleasant taste. In irradiated milk the vitamin occurs chiefly in the form of activated 7-dehydrocholesterol.

The various sources of vitamin D vary in potency but may be substituted for each other on the basis of unitage. Much work has been done to determine whether there is any difference in the antirachitic activity of the various chemical forms of vitamin D. The only conclusion that has been reached at present is that there is no essential difference.

In spite of the numerous claims for various preparations of vitamin D in oil, cod liver oil is still the most economical form in which to obtain the vitamin. Cod liver oil or one of the concentrated fish oils seems preferable to the preparations containing viosterol, if for no other reason than that it seems advisable to prescribe a preparation of vitamin D, which is also rich in vitamin A. rather than one which contains only vitamin D.

Experimental Pathological Physiology

According to Wolbach and Bessey[38] experimental rickets in animals duplicates completely the spontaneous disease in man and in animals. To understand better the changes in bone, which occur in a deficiency of vitamin D, the normal sequence in the growth of bones must be understood. Long bones increase in length by the endochondral formation of bone. The narrow place of epiphyseal cartilage is supported by bone on the epiphyseal surface, and its diaphyseal side is penetrated uniformly by capillaries. During growth continuous proliferation of cartilage cells occurs on the epiphyseal side, and there is degeneration of matured cells on the diaphyseal surface. These degenerating cells are replaced by capillaries and osteoblasts, which affect the deposition of bony matrix.

Wolbach said that the growth of bone by endochondral formation of bone is achieved "by a continuously retreating gap in the continuity of tissues maintained on the epiphyseal side by continuous renewal of cartilage cells and on the diaphyseal side repaired by vascular outgrowth comparable to repair of any defect of tissues by the process of organization or granulation tissue formation. In normal growth there presents on the diaphyseal side of the narrow cartilage a continuous layer of clear or empty cartilage cells forming an almost straight line."

The cessation of the formation of osteoblasts is the first sign of deficiency of vitamin D in the bone. The growth of the cartilage, however, continues. The epiphyseal cartilage increases in width because of continued proliferative activity, and this thickening is irregular, since the cessation of degeneration does not occur simultaneously in all portions of the plate. In the absence of the ingrowth of capillaries and osteoblasts there is a failure of calcification of the cartilaginous matrix, and newly formed bones during the active stage of the disease have an osteoid structure. The basic structural alteration in rickets is not the failure of formation of bone but the failure of calcification.

The disturbance manifests itself most markedly where the most rapid growth occurs, for example, at the lower epiphysis of the femur. Longitudinal sections of a rachitic bone will reveal a wide, irregular zone of ossification at the junction of the epiphysis and diaphysis. This region is known as the "rachitic zone". Microscopically a large amount of osteoid tissue is found adjacent to the shaft, and irregular columns of cartilage cells project into this osteoid tissue. Growth of the bone is delayed or stopped completely in proportion to the severity of the process. On microscopic examination of sections of the shaft osteoid lamellae are found under the periosteum and lining the haversian canals and marrow spaces. The structural changes in the bone are not identical in every case. In one type of the disease there is a large medullary cavity with a thin, porous cortex, a form approaching osteomalacia. In another type the cortex is thick but porous, and the medullary cavity is small.

The bony deformities resulting from these alterations vary according to the amount of stress to which the individual bones are subjected. Before the infant walks there may be flattening of the occiput resulting from the weight of the head, since the excess of osteoid tissue in the occipitoparietal bones makes them soft and yielding, craniotabes. There is enlargement of the costochondral junctions, rickety rosary, and alterations in the bony thorax may give rise to various deformities, Harrison's groove, pigeon breast, funnel breast. The weight of the body produces deformities of the lower extremities from the bending of the bones in children who have assumed the erect posture (Fig. 10). Growth of the long bones, particularly the femur, may be greatly delayed, and the adult may be of short stature as a result. The epiphyses are enlarged, and it is not uncommon for genu valgum or genu varum to develop. Occasional instances of dwarfism have a rachitic basis. Deformities of the spinal column are not common.

In late rickets the changes are similar to those of early rickets except that the osteoid tissue develops in the subperiosteal and endosteal portions rather than at the epiphysis. Osteomalacia presents a similar picture.

The effect of vitamin D in reversing these changes has been demonstrated clearly with experimental animals. After it has been administered, the cartilage cells generally appear along the diaphyseal border at the end of 24 hours, and extensive vascular penetration is visible within 48 hours; this permits the deposition of bone-forming salts. The mass of irregular cartilage cells becomes arranged into short, orderly columns of a few cells, and osteoid material is no longer formed. This is the basis of the line test as used in assay of vitamin D.

It must be remembered that the fundamental defect in rickets is not in the bone. It has been shown that slices of rachitic bone and cartilage become calcified when placed in normal blood serum. The primary fault in rickets resides in the body fluids, which do not make bone salts available to the bone. The action of vitamin D is to bring about alteration of the calcium and phosphorus in the body fluids so that they may be available to the bone. It has been suggested recently that vitamin D probably does not exert its therapeutic effects through improvement in intestinal absorption of phosphorus but rather by intensification of phosphorus turnover in bone. This results in hyperphosphatemia and a decreased visceral phosphorus turnover[39].

Human Requirement

The exact human requirements for vitamin D are unknown. The requirement of vitamin D varies greatly among individuals and among persons of various ages. Since the average diet furnishes so little vitamin D, it must be assumed either that the requirement of vitamin D for man is extremely low or that his needs usually are provided by exposure to sunshine. The requirement of vitamin D during adult life has not been determined, but undoubtedly the vitamin is necessary for older children and for adult persons. The minimal amounts recommended for infants should be sufficient for those of this age group. During pregnancy and lactation and for children less than a year old 400 to 800 international units of vitamin D constitute the daily requirement as recommended by the Food and Nutrition Board of the National Research Council. In administering antirachitic agents, as emphasized previously in this chapter, the physician should think in terms of units of vitamin D, since this is the only way in which the doses of the various substances containing vitamin D, which differ greatly in volume, can be reduced to a common denominator.

Methods for Measurement of Vitamin D

When almost pure, crystalline vitamin D is used, it can be determined by measurement of the characteristic absorption spectrum in the ultraviolet. There is no chemical method by which the presence or amount of vitamins D can be determined accurately. Two methods generally are employed for the biological assay of vitamin D_3. A simple and convenient method[40] which concerns the growth response of chicks has been described recently.

Clinically roentgenological examination of the bones of the forearm and wrist is recommended both for the diagnosis of rickets and for determining the healing process. Determination of the amounts of calcium and phosphorus in the blood also may be helpful in following the course of rickets in human beings. According to some recent reports phosphatase activity is a valuable and probably the most sensitive index of active rickets[41].

Toxicity

When extremely large doses of vitamin D are administered to animal or man, certain pathological changes are noted[42,43]. Hypervitaminosis D is an exaggerated form of the physiological effect of the vitamin. The concentration of calcium and phosphorus in the serum is increased, and calcification occurs at an increased rate. Metastatic calcification may occur in the renal tubules, heart, blood vessels, bronchi and stomach[44]. In advanced degrees of h e .tam.nos.s D resorption of bone is the most prominent feature[45]. The animals lose weight rapidly, an intense diarrhea develops, and death occurs in 5 to 14 days. If smaller doses are administered, the animal may survive and the described lesions will remain for at least 6 months. Diets low in calcium and phosphorus may prevent the calcification process, but the degenerative changes occur.

Some adult persons treated with large doses of vitamin D may complain of nausea, headache, diarrhea, anorexia, urinary frequency or lassitude. Adults treated with large doses of vitamin D for arthritis have exhibited various manifestations of toxicity; the susceptibility of an individual will vary at different times[46,47]. Danowski and his associates[48] have reported two instances of dangerous complications resulting from the promiscuous and protracted treatment of arthritis with large quantities of vitamin D without medical supervision. The patients concerned took from 150,000 to 500,000 international units daily for 6 years in one case

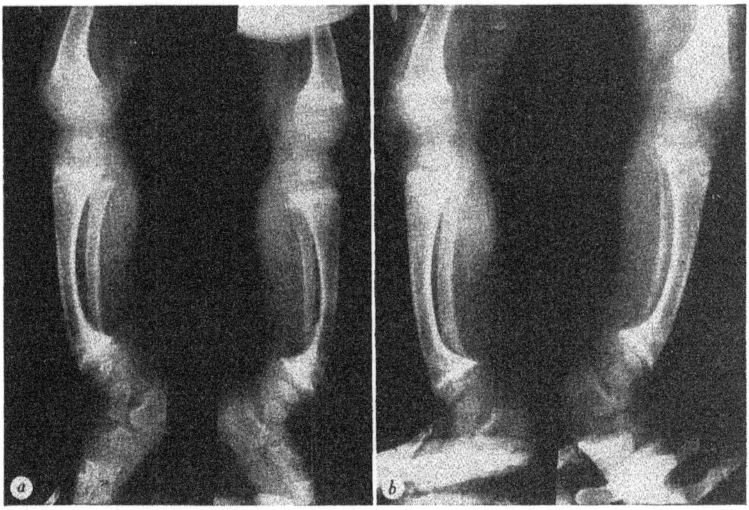

Fig. 10. Florid rickets in young twins (*a*) and (*b*), illustrating deformities, wide, irregular epiphyseal lines and characteristic cupping of the metaphyses. (By courtesy of Department of Pediatrics, Mayo Clinic.)

and for 13 months in the other. Both patients experienced osteoporosis, anemia, elevated values for blood nonprotein nitrogen, hypercalcemia and albuminuria. Extensive deposits of calcium in the soft tissue developed in one patient. One had hypertension with retinal vascular changes. After the administration of vitamin D had been discontinued, there was gradual clinical improvement in these two patients. However, no serious toxic effects have been reported in cases in which doses up to 1,000,000 units have been administered to rachitic children.

In spite of the aforementioned possible effects, the physician need not, in general, fear toxicity as an effect of vitamin D. If renal insufficiency exists, the physician should use caution; repeated urinalyses should be conducted while vitamin D therapy is being employed.

Diagnosis of Vitamin D Deficiency

Although some report that the incidence of undiagnosed rickets in certain sections of the United States may be as high as 75 per cent., yet the presence of this disease is extremely difficult to determine with reasonable certainty except when the condition is severe. Several recent reports tend to affirm this fact[49]. The clinical diagnosis hinges on the finding of the various deformities described in the consideration of the pathological changes. Among the more important of these are craniotabes and the rachitic rosary. In the early or mild stage the physician may encounter difficulty in distinguishing this condition from the normal softness of the baby's skull. The rachitic rosary is one of the most constant signs of rickets, but much skill is required to distinguish it from the normal enlargement of the costochondral junction. An enlarged fontanelle may be evidence of rickets, but in many cases there is premature closure. Bowlegs (Fig. 10*a* and *b*) and deformities of the thorax, chicken breast and funnel breast, Harrison's groove, are of common occurrence, but their presence alone is not pathognomonic, since they occur also in many other conditions.

To one acquainted with the intricacies of this sort of diagnosis the roentgenogram offers invaluable aid in the recognition of rickets, but there are many pitfalls in differential diagnosis. A description of the changes revealed by the roentgenogram (Fig. 11) is out of place here; the reader can find them in textbooks of radiology. Since rickets is not primarily a disease of bone, roentgenological evidence may be lacking early in the course of the disease.

The concentration of calcium and phosphorus in the serum usually is altered in the presence of rickets. The concentration of inorganic phosphate is more constantly lower than that of calcium; the product of the concentration of these two minerals is of more constant value. In the acute stage of deficiency of vitamin D there is an elevation in serum phosphatase. With few exceptions this appears to be a satisfactory measure for the detection of early acute rickets[50].

Rachitic tetany also is a derangement in calcium and phosphorus metabolism which results from deficiency of vitamin D. The latent and manifest forms are the two types of infantile tetany encountered clinically. In the former there are no apparent symptoms, and the hyperirritability of the nervous system must be elicited by artificial excitation of the peripheral nerves. The manifest form gives rise to tonic states and generalized convulsions.

The most reliable and delicate sign in the diagnosis of latent tetany is Erb's phenomenon. A galvanic current is employed to distinguish irri-

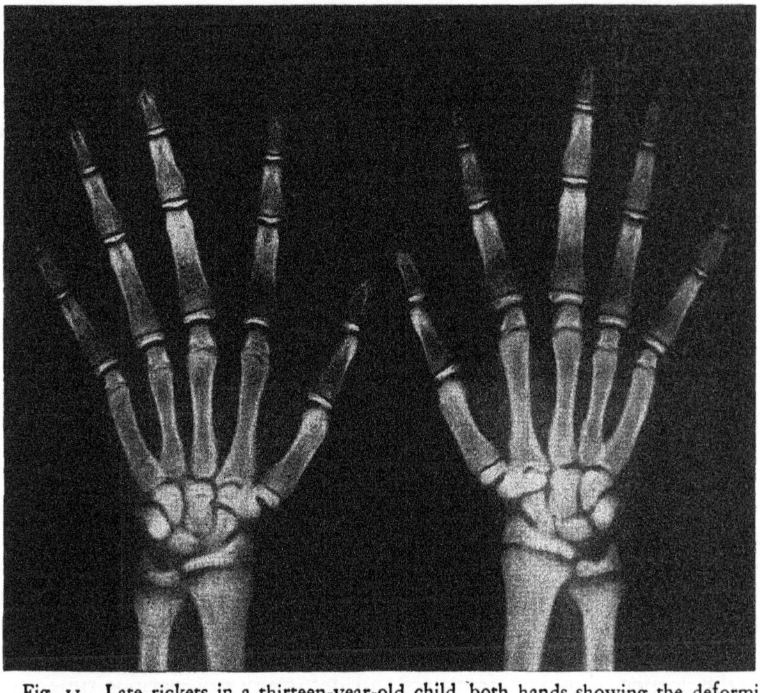

Fig. 11. Late rickets in a thirteen-year-old child, both hands showing the deformities, wide, irregular epiphyseal lines and characteristic cupping. (By courtesy of Department of Pediatrics, Mayo Clinic.)

tability of the nervous system. The Chvostek sign is another rather reliable method of diagnosis. The Trousseau phenomenon is described often as diagnostic of infantile tetany, but it probably is not so reliable as the other two mentioned. Among laboratory observations the presence of a low concentration of serum calcium is of extreme importance in the diagnosis of tetany. In latent tetany the value for the serum calcium usually is in the neighborhood of 7 to 8 mgm. per 100 c.c., and it may decrease to 5 to 6 mgm. in cases of manifest tetany.

The outstanding manifestations of tetany are the typical carpopedal spasms, the characteristic "tetany facies", laryngospasm and of course, the convulsive seizures. The diagnosis of manifest rachitic tetany is, as a rule, not difficult. In the differential diagnosis the physician must consider laryngitis, congenital laryngeal stridor, nervous holding of the breath and meningitis.

In osteomalacia as in rickets the essential abnormality is deficient calcification of the osteoid tissue. It is seen occasionally in men, but is encountered most often in women, especially among those who are pregnant. Usually numerous causative factors are operative in any single case of osteomalacia, but in all cases there is presumably a deficiency of vitamin D. In most cases osteomalacia as observed in the United States is associated with chronic steatorrhea. As a result of the faulty digestion and absorption of fat, insoluble calcium salts are formed, and the fat-soluble vitamin D is excreted in the excess fat. This has been well demonstrated by various investigations carried out in cases of osteomalacia.

In the mild form of osteomalacia the patient may complain only of weakness or of pains in the bones of the legs or in the lower part of the back while standing or walking. In cases of severe osteomalacia the patient may seek medical aid because of the distressing symptoms of severe tetany. Another patient may suffer from a crushed vertebra resulting from moderate lifting or a minor fall. In cases of advanced disease severe backache is the most common symptom. This pain is aching in character, often is generalized and is worse in the winter, when there is greater deficiency of vitamin D than at other times. Muscular weakness may be marked, and a waddling gait is not uncommon. Often there is marked sensitivity of the bones to light pressure. The skeletal deformities are numerous. In the roentgenogram generalized osteoporosis, thinning of the cortices, bowing, fractures and deformities of various types are evident.

The diagnosis of osteomalacia is not particularly difficult, if the physician suspects its presence. Tetany, occurring in association with chronic diarrhea, or a calcium-phosphorus deficiency always should suggest osteomalacia. Any skeletal disease characterized by generalized decalcification, such as the osteoporotic forms of hyperparathyroidism, senile osteoporosis and the like, may be mistaken for osteomalacia. The treatment of osteomalacia is essentially the same as the treatment of rickets.

Treatment of Vitamin D Deficiency

Of primary importance in the treatment of rickets is the promotion of healing of the lesion as rapidly as possible. The dose suggested as a preventive, although it is actually capable of effecting cure in simple

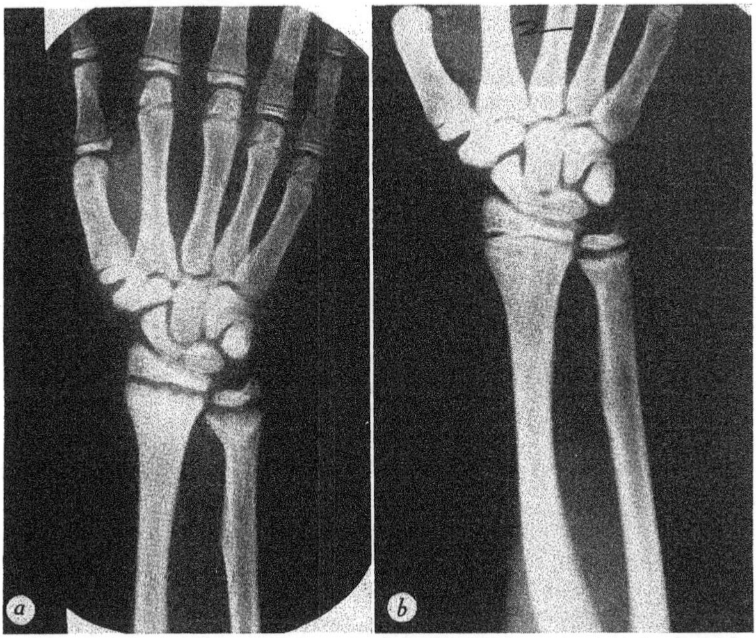

Fig. 12. Late rickets in a thirteen-year-old child. On the left (*a*) before treatment with approximately 1,000,000 units of vitamin D daily in the form of activated ergosterol, (The activated ergosterol is not on the market but was used experimentally. It was supplied by the Mead, Johnson and Company); (*b*) after treatment, some five months later. (By courtesy of Department of Pediatrics, Mayo Clinic.)

rickets, brings about this cure too slowly. A dose of 1,000 U.S.P. units, 3 teaspoonfuls of cod liver oil, daily will control advanced rickets in most cases in 3 to 4 weeks. For premature infants often it is necessary to administer 10,000 to 20,000 U.S.P. units daily to effect a cure, and the condition of some infants is so refractory to treatment as to require 60,000 units daily. Once the disturbance has been brought under control, as evidenced by determinations of blood calcium and phosphorus or by roentgenological examinations, the dose of vitamin D can be reduced to a preventive level. In cases in which older children are hypersusceptible to rickets, it may be necessary to continue the administration of large doses; the increased requirements of the premature infant usually are transitory.

The treatment of active rickets with large, single doses of vitamin D administered parenterally has received considerable attention during the past few years[51-54]. Administration of 500,000 to 1,000,000 U.S.P. units of vitamin D to children who had rickets, including premature infants, has been followed by rapid healing without clinical evidence of toxicity (Fig. 12). In these cases the value for serum phosphatase may become normal as early as the fifth or sixth day, and roentgenographical evidence of healing also may be noted.

Many have believed that infants can be protected successfully from rickets for the whole of one winter by the ingestion of a single large dose of vitamin D. Recently Krestin[55] made a clinical trial of the procedure, using full-term infants and children from 2 months to 3 years of age, who showed no radiological or clinical evidence of rickets. On the basis of results of his study, he suggested that, when a child is first seen in late winter or spring, one dose of 7.5 mgm. of calciferol, vitamin D_2, having an activity of 300,000 international units, probably is sufficient for protection until the next winter. When the child is seen for the first time in fall or early winter, the dose should be repeated after three months. For premature infants and those recovering from marasmus or acute illnesses larger and more frequently administered doses may be necessary.

There are occasional cases in which rickets does not respond to treatment with the usual amounts of vitamin D[56,57]. In some cases rickets is due to a disturbance of the acid-base balance and has been treated successfully by the administration of sodium bicarbonate or by the use of massive doses of vitamin D. The quantity of vitamin D needed may be so large that it approaches dosages that are definitely toxic. While the maintenance dose is being established, it is desirable to examine the urine every 1 to 3 days for albumin, erythrocytes and calcium casts. The blood calcium should be determined weekly and should not be allowed to rise above 12 mgm. per 100 c.c., if the dosage exceeds 20,000 units daily for an infant or 50,000 units for a child. Administration of the vitamin should be discontinued, if anorexia or nausea appears.

In the treatment of rachitic tetany it is important that the effects be produced rapidly. It has been pointed out that the primary derangement in tetany is in the concentration of serum calcium, and it is necessary that this be remedied rapidly by the administration of calcium salts. The usual method is to administer 3 or 4 gm. of calcium chloride intravenously as an initial dose. This should be followed by a dose of 1 gm. 4 times daily for 2 or 3 days, and then by 1 gm. twice a day for 5 to 7 days. In the administration of vitamin D a program similar to that described for the treatment of rickets may be followed.

Having made a diagnosis of rickets, determined which method of treatment to use and used it, the physician now is confronted with the problem of how to ascertain if this therapy is accomplishing the desired results. The best way to do this is to determine the concentration of calcium and phosphorus in the serum. If the concentration of calcium is within normal limits, and the concentration of inorganic phosphate rises to 5 mgm. per 100 c.c., vitamin D therapy is succeeding. In ordinary cases, in which the usual doses are administered, the concentration of the serum phosphates may be expected to reach normal on about the tenth day of treatment. In the absence of chemical and roentgenological examinations appraisal of treatment becomes very difficult; bony deformities disappear very slowly. Perhaps the best clinical indication that therapy with vitamin D is succeeding is improvement in muscle function as evidenced by efforts on the part of the child to walk or to sit up. He seems to gain strength and becomes more active. The bony deformities gradually disappear, and the bones acquire an increased degree of rigidity.

Methods of preventing the occurrence of rickets should be common knowledge to every physician. For preventive measures the importance of commencing administration of the vitamin early and reaching the full dose by the end of the second month of the infant's life cannot be repeated too often[58]. It is best to begin with a dose of a half teaspoonful, 2 c.c., of cod liver oil, 175 units; after a few days this may be increased to 1 teaspoonful, 4 c.c. or 350 units, and in the next 2 weeks raised to 2 teaspoonfuls, 8 c.c. or 700 units. Use of this dose should be continued until the child is 2 years of age. If there is any reason to suspect that the child may be susceptible to rickets, the dose should be increased during the first year so as to supply 1,000 units of vitamin D daily.

Irradiated milk does not exhibit sufficient potency in vitamin D for the prevention of rickets in cases in which a susceptibility exists. Sunlight may be relied on for the prevention of rickets in the summer months, but in the winter for all practical purposes the rays of the sun may be regarded as devoid of antirachitic rays.

VITAMIN E

CHEMISTRY

As early as 1922 a new factor, most abundantly present in wheat-germ oil, was demonstrated as needed in the rat for the successful completion of pregnancy in the female and for continued fertility in the male. In 1936 this factor was identified successfully as alpha tocopherol (Evans, Emerson and Emerson)[60]. Fernholz[60] in 1938 proposed the formula for alpha tocopherol on the basis of oxidative degradation with chromic acid, and synthesis was accomplished later independently in three laboratories[61] (Fig. 13).

Three factors have been isolated from natural material, namely, alpha, beta and gamma tocopherol. Beta tocopherol and gamma tocopherol are homologues of the natural substance and have almost identical properties but slightly less biological activity. Natural gamma tocopherol

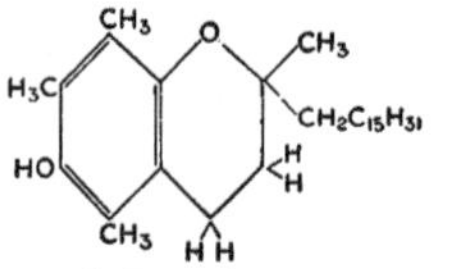

Fig. 13. Structural formula for alpha tocopherol.

is approximately 50 per cent. more potent than synthetic dl-gamma-tocopherol, and natural beta tocopherol is about 100 per cent. more active than synthetic dl-beta-tocopherol[62]. These substances are readily soluble in lipid solvents but are only slightly soluble in water. Although stable at high temperatures (200° C.), they rapidly lose their activity in the presence of ultraviolet light or mild oxidizing agents. The long-recognized resistance to rancidity of vegetable oil that contains vitamin E might be cited as an everyday example of its oxidation-inhibiting quality.

There are numerous compounds related to the tocopherols, which have been shown to exhibit vitamin E activity, but they do so in a limited manner when compared to tocopherol. Of some special interest is naphtho-tocopherol, which shows vitamin E activity in 25 mgm. doses but also shows vitamin K activity in doses of from 300 to 600 gamma[63]. The tocopherols themselves have a certain structural specificity, and the removal of a methyl group from the aromatic nucleus or the aliphatic side chain greatly diminishes the vitamin E activity of the substances. The acetate of tocopherol is equal in biological activity and possesses the added advantage of increased stability over that of tocopherol. It has been suggested that synthetic racemic tocopherol, tocopheryl acetate, be made the international standard for vitamin E, and the suggestion has been adopted. The international unit is the vitamin E activity of 1.0 mgm. of the standard preparation, racemic tocopherol acetate in olive oil. The quantity represents the average amount which prevents resorption gestation in rats deprived of vitamin E when the substance is administered orally[64,65].

Physiology and Pathology

These fat-soluble vitamins E and their esters are in the presence of bile acids easily absorbed from the intestinal tract[66], and on intake of esters the free vitamin appears in the blood. Excess doses cause the excretion of a certain amount in the feces, but only traces are found in the urine. This suggests that the vitamin is inactivated in the organism, probably by an oxidation mechanism. These vitamins are stored in very small amounts in animal body fats, in the muscles and in the anterior lobe of the pituitary gland.

In animals a lack of vitamin E manifests itself chiefly by changes in the reproductive mechanism; it was on the basis of this observation that the terms "antisterility vitamin" and "reproductive vitamin" were derived. In the presence of vitamin E deficiency conception occurs in the female rat, but it is followed by "resorptive sterility". In the male rat degeneration of the germinal epithelium and spermatozoa develops to the point of complete loss of reproductive power.

For a number of years interest was centered exclusively on the rôle which this vitamin played in reproduction. It seems that such an action was too narrow a definition of its function. In the absence of vitamin E in the diet of many animals muscular dystrophy and a characteristic paralysis of the hindquarters have been shown to develop[67, 68, 69]. Although vitamin E appears essential for the integrity of the skeletal muscle of many species, the relationship of these disturbances to human muscular dystrophies is by no means clear. It has been suggested that it is concerned in some way with the contractile phase, and increased oxygen uptake in the muscle tissue has been observed during vitamin E deficiency[70]. This possible relationship to human muscular disturbances remains an inviting subject for further investigation.

Recently another activity of vitamin E has been recognized. In a series of studies Hickman and associates[71, 72, 73] have shown that natural vitamin E enhances the growth-promoting power of vitamin A alcohol and vitamin A acetate. The vitamin A activity of carotene is markedly influenced also by the intake of tocopherol. It is suggested that this sparing action on the A vitamins is due chiefly to repression of oxidation in or near the gastrointestinal tract. Recently it has been shown also that tocopherol increases both the storage of vitamin A in the liver and the stability of carotene in the intestinal tract. It appears that the rôle of tocopherol as an intestinal antioxidant has been established[74].

We have no exact knowledge of the quantitative requirements of man for vitamin E. We lack also precise assays of the vitamin E content of foodstuffs. Apparently vitamin E occurs in most foods, and it is noteworthy that one of the greatest obstacles, which investigators encountered, was in obtaining a diet deficient in this vitamin. Wheat-germ oil is the richest source of vitamin E, but also it is found in considerable amounts in cottonseed oil, lettuce oil, rice-germ oil and other seed-germ oils.

Various authors have used wheat-germ oil in doses varying from 0.25 c.c. to 6 c.c. daily, and it may be of significance that any apparent success was the same in spite of any variation in the dose used. Toxic reactions have not been reported in cases, in which small doses were administered, and large doses of wheat-germ oil have given rise to only minor symptoms. The danger of production of neoplasms by the use of such oil appears to be nonexistent.

A chemical method for the determination of tocopherols in blood plasma has been described[75], and in a small series of cases values for tocopherol in human normal plasma were found to average 1.20 mgm. per 100 c.c.

Clinical Use of Vitamin E

Whether or not avitaminoses occur in man has not yet been definitely decided. Vitamin E has been used in the treatment of many clinical ills, but to date justifiable conclusions have been difficult to make.

There is some evidence to support the view that vitamin E may exert a beneficial influence in certain cases of habitual abortion[76], threatened abortion and abruptio placentae. In the presence of male and female sterility, menstrual disturbances, the toxemias of pregnancy, faulty lactation and vaginal pruritus the reported results are at variance and cannot be accepted until further evidence has accumulated.

In the treatment of human myoneurogenic disturbances with vitamin

E the results have been most discouraging. Recently, however, Milhorat and Bartels[77] have suggested that tocopherol forms a condensation product with inositol in the gastrointestinal tract, and that the inherited defect in muscular dystrophy is a deficiency in this reaction of condensation. These and other more recent suggestions stimulate hope that vitamin E is a factor to be reckoned with in human physiology and perhaps in human disease[78].

VITAMINS K

The introduction of vitamin K in clinical medicine came as a result of an observation of Dam and his associates[79-81] of Copenhagen, Denmark. They showed that a deficiency disease could be produced in chicks subsisting on feed washed in ether and could be cured by the administration of an antihemorrhagic material present in hog liver fat, hemp seed and certain cereals and vegetables. Later it was shown by these investigators that deficiency in this dietary factor resulted in diminuition in the amount of prothrombin in the circulating blood, which led to fatal hemorrhagic diathesis. The term "vitamin K" was proposed by Dam as an abbreviation of the name "Koagulations Vitamin" to apply to the substance that was necessary for the prevention of a nutritional deficiency disease in chicks. Soon it was suggested by Quick of the United States that deficiency of vitamin K might be present in patients who had obstructive jaundice. These suggestions now have been confirmed amply and extended, and within a relatively short time various workers in this country and abroad[79-85] have demonstrated that vitamin K under most circumstances is a specific remedy for deficiency of prothrombin.

Chemistry

In 1939 McKee and his associates reported the isolation of vitamin K_1 from alfalfa and of vitamin K_2 from putrefied fish meal and presented

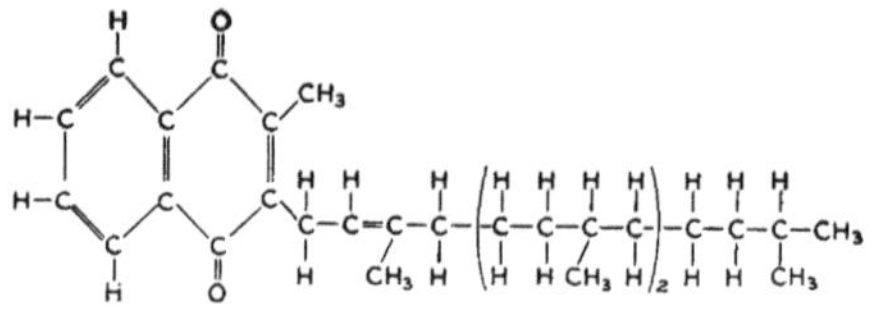

Fig. 14. The structural formula of vitamin K_1 (2-methyl-3-phytyl-1,4-naphthoquinone).

evidence to indicate a quinoid structure of these vitamins. For the final isolation and synthesis of vitamin K_1 Doisey and his associates, Almquist and Klose, Fieser and his associates, Dam, Karrer and co-workers are responsible. Independently these groups of investigators reported the structure of the vitamin K_1 molecule to be 2-methyl-3-phytyl-1, 4-naphthoquinone (Fig. 14). This vitamin is identical with 2-methyl-1,

4-naphthoquinone with the exception that vitamin K_1 has a phytyl side chain in the three position. The synthetic product also is identical with natural vitamin K_1, which is obtained from alfalfa. Exposure to sunlight destroys the vitamin activity of alfalfa within several hours, although, if artificial light is used, little destruction is observed within 24 hours. The pure preparations, however, are destroyed by both sunlight and artificial light. Under ultraviolet light rays the oxide of vitamin K_1 is about 3 times as stable as vitamin K_1 but has the same clinical effect as vitamin K_1.[86] A large part of the activity of concentrates of vitamin K is destroyed by alkali, by strong acids and by aluminum chloride. The vitamin is fat soluble and at low temperatures forms yellow crystals.

Vitamin K_2 is another natural vitamin K and was isolated first from putrefied fish meal. The structure of this vitamin still is under discussion. Some investigators believe the probable structural formula is 2-methyl-3-difarnesyl-1, 4-naphthoquinone with an empiric formula $C_{41}H_{56}O_2$. This compound is also fat-soluble and has been obtained as light yellow, crystalline flakes.

The demonstration of the quinoid structure of the vitamins K has stimulated great study of the many substances which possess a quinoid nucleus. The first report of a synthetic compound having antihemorrhagic activity was made by Almquist and Klose, who found that phthiocol (2-methyl-3-hydroxy-1, 4-naphthoquinone) possesses marked antihemorrhagic activity, but that it is only 1/500 as active as vitamin K_1. Phthiocol is the yellow pigment found in the human tubercle bacillus. Of all the naphthoquinone derivatives studied 2-methyl-1, 4-naphthoquinone has proved to be the most active. This compound can be synthesized by the oxidation of 2-methyl-naphthalene. This material is very slightly soluble in water. In solution its activity is impaired by sterilization with steam; therefore, it is rather unstable unless special precautions are taken. This compound is so active that several investigators have suggested that it be adopted as a basic standard for assay of vitamin K. By some assays this compound has been found to be about three times as potent, on a basis of weight, as vitamin K_1. Because of the great usefulness of this compound in clinical medicine the Council on Pharmacy and Chemistry of the American Medical Association on the recommendation of the Committee on Nomenclature authorized the use of "menadione" as a nonproprietary name for this substance[87].

Many other compounds have been tested for vitamin K activity. Most of those, which have such activity, are basically 1, 4-naphthoquinone or the corresponding hydroquinone; a few, however, are not. The compounds, 4-amino-2-methyl-1-naphthol hydrochloride and 2-methyl-1, 4-naphthohydroquinone-3-sodium sulfonate, are water soluble and, therefore, have proved to be of considerable use clinically. These compounds are not so active as 2-methyl-1, 4-naphthoquinone, but they are active enough to produce desired clinical results. Apparently these derivatives of the simpler quinones are utilized more efficiently than are the corresponding derivatives of the natural vitamins. A monosodium-bisulfite of menadione has been given the nonproprietary name of "menadione bisulfite"; it is also an active water-soluble derivative of menadione[88].

Physiology

Many investigators have shown that the presence of bile in the intestinal tract is essential for proper absorption of the fat-soluble vitamin K, and there is, futhermore, some evidence to suggest that these fat-soluble compounds are absorbed better, if other fats are present in the intestinal tract. Clinically it is well established that the presence of bile, or more correctly, the presence of adequate amounts of bile salts, is required for the proper absorption of vitamins K. The exact point of absorption in the intestinal tract is not known, but clinical experience indicates that concentrates of vitamin K are not absorbed through the colon or upper part of the ileum, but that they are absorbed readily through the upper part of the small intestine. Recently it has been reported that excessive amounts of liquid petrolatum administered with meals may prevent proper absorption of this vitamin.

The vitamin is not stored readily in the body, but it has been found in the livers of lower animals in relatively small amounts. Greaves has shown that in the liver of the rat vitamin K is not stored in appreciable amounts. Results of clinical work would indicate that the same observations are applicable to the human being. In so far as is known, vitamin K is not present in the urine. It can be demonstrated in the feces, but whether it is there because the feces merely hold the organisms which are known to contain vitamin K, or whether the presence of the vitamin in feces is referable to real excretion of vitamin K, remains to be established. The vitamin is not present in human bile collected under sterile conditions. In chicks subsisting on a normal diet the spleen, red muscle, gizzard, bone marrow and pancreas were found to contain relatively large amounts of vitamin K, whereas the liver and lungs were found to contain somewhat less.

It has been shown that 2-methyl-1, 4-naphthoquinone is bacteriostatic and bactericidal for both gram-positive cocci and gram-negative bacilli, and similar effects have been noted in the case of many fungi. The mode of action apparently consists of the blocking of essential enzymes through combination with sulfhydryl groups. This mode of action is similar to that suggested by other investigators for several antibiotic agents, including penicillin[89].

Little is known concerning the action of vitamin K in the animal organism. It has been well demonstrated that this vitamin and related compounds have some relationship to the blood-clotting mechanism.

Avitaminosis K produces a decrease in the prothrombin level of the blood, which increases rapidly after the administration of vitamin K. Vitamin K does not form a part of the prothrombin molecule, since orally administered prothrombin does not show vitamin K activity. The manner in which vitamin K participates in the formation of prothrombin is not known. It has been suggested that vitamin K is a reversible oxidation-reduction catalyst, the hydroquinone form of which is oxidized readily by molecular oxygen. This reversible character of the vitamin may be used to explain the fact that small quantities produce the characteristic effect[90].

More recently a hypothesis has been reported, which suggests that the antihemorrhagic effect of vitamin K and its synthetic analogues is due to biochemical degradation to phthalic acid, and that it is largely a function of their capacity to be transformed into the latter[91]. The authors[92], who advanced such a hypothesis, regard phthalic acid as the true carrier of biological activity and suggest that natural vitamin K and its synthetic analogues be regarded as provitamins. Recently these authors have isolated phthalic acid from the urine of man and of the dog after the administration of menadione. Menadione itself was not found in the urine, whereas administered phthalic acid was excreted quantitatively and unchanged. These finding have some strong suggestive supporting evidence. Dicumarol, a vitamin K antagonist, owes its activity to degradation to a simpler compound, namely, salicylic acid. The vitamin K compounds may owe their antihemorrhagic activity to their easy degradation to phthalic acid. The attractive hypothesis, which results, is that the antagonism of dicumarol to vitamin K is due to the competition in vivo of two structurally similar molecules. Phthalic acid possesses two carboxyl groups on a benzene ring; salicylic acid possesses one carboxyl and one hydroxyl group. The competition of structurally similar molecules, acting as either substrates or co-enzymes for enzyme systems, is common knowledge among chemists.

In so far as is known at present, vitamin K has no relationship to immunity, infection, pregnancy and lactation, the nervous system, gastro-intestinal tract or cardiovascular system, but it is associated intimately with normal physiological function of the liver and with proper coagulation of the blood. Its exact rôle in coagulation of the blood is not known. It is known to be necessary for proper formation of prothrombin, but the manner in which this is accomplished remains to be determined. A deficiency of vitamin K arising from any cause produces a deficiency of prothrombin in the circulating blood, and in all instances except those, in which there is severe hepatic damage, this deficiency of prothrombin can be corrected by the proper administration of vitamin K.

Sources

Among the richest sources of vitamin K_1 are the green, leafy tissues of spinach, alfalfa, kale, cauliflower, carrot tops and chestnuts. Tomatoes, hemp seed and soy bean oil also are good sources, but fruits and cereals are poor sources of the vitamin. The parts of the plant, which contain chlorophyll, usually have the largest amounts of vitamin K.

Vitamin K_2 occurs in many bacteria, whereas yeast, molds and fungi contain little or no vitamin K. The vitamin K activity of feces of the horse, cow, sheep, hog and man has been well established. Apparently during the growth of the bacteria the vitamin K is synthesized and is retained within the bacteria, since the filtrate of the culture medium, which is free of the bacteria, contains none of the vitamin. Ether extracts[83] of these bacteria, however, have vitamin K activity. Dried human feces, both normal and acholic, are rich in the vitamin, but the vitamin K activity of feces undoubtedly results from the bacterial content within them.

Most animal materials contain very little vitamin K. Milk and eggs contain small amounts, and hog liver is very rich in this vitamin.

Experimental Pathological Physiology

In the presence of deficiency of vitamin K the prothrombin content of the blood is markedly decreased, and the blood clotting time may be considerably prolonged. In animals the principal symptom to appear during deficiency of vitamin K is the occurrence of hemorrhage.

In chicks fed on material deficient in vitamin K there develop subcutaneous, intramuscular and internal hemorrhages, profuse bleeding from minor abrasions and a delayed clotting time associated with a low content of prothrombin in the plasma. Injuries in a wide sense may determine the occurrence and severity of these hemorrhages. Results of studies by many investigators of the content of prothrombin in the plasma in hemorrhagic chick disease show that hemorrhages do not occur until the content of prothrombin has declined to about 10 to 15 per cent. of normal. It has been indicated that the clotting time is delayed only if the content of prothrombin has declined to less than 30 or 40 per cent. of normal. Thus, early in the course of the disease, when deficiency of the vitamin is less severe, the content of prothrombin in the plasma may be reduced considerably, and yet the clotting time will remain normal. This is extremely important as a clinical factor. Deficiency of prothrombin also has been produced in rats, mice, ducklings, young geese, pigeons, canaries and rabbits that were subsisting on diets deficient in vitamin K.

It has been long known that in dogs, which have biliary fistulas, an abnormal tendency to bleed develops in addition to many pathological complications. Furthermore it has been pointed out that continuous subsequent feeding of bile to such animals will correct this abnormality. This tendency toward bleeding of dogs, which have biliary fistulas, was shown later to be caused by deficiency of prothrombin which could be corrected by the administration of vitamin K. In rats, which have renal biliary fistulas, there is, likewise, a diminution in the circulating prothrombin which can be corrected by the administration of vitamin K.

Deficiency of vitamin K can be produced also by alteration of the bacterial flora of the intestinal tract. It was observed first that hypoprothrombinemia developed in young rats given sulfaguanidine in purified diets, and that the effect on the content of prothrombin in the blood could be counteracted by the administration of vitamin K[93]. It was found that the hypoprothrombinemic effect of this drug could be prevented by the administration either of p-aminobenzoic acid or of a liver fraction[94]. Sulfapyrazine, sulfadiazine or sulfathiazole, when fed to rats at a 1 per cent. level in purified diets, results in the regular production of severe hypothrombinemia within 2 to 3 weeks. Sulfaguanidine, sulfanilamide and succinyl sulfathiazole are much less effective in producing this phenomenon[95]. The action of these drugs is thought to be the result of their effect on coliform organisms in the intestinal tract[96].

It has been reported that female rabbits fed a vitamin K-deficient diet for 40 days and mated with normal males aborted during the late first or early second trimester of pregnancy. Retroplacental hemorrhages were considered responsible for the abortions, and although the content of prothrombin was lowered in the rabbits, it did not reach a critical level. If the females were bred once more, while they were subsisting on the deficient diet, abortions occurred, but normal-term pregnancies resulted when vitamin K was added to the diet[97].

Human Requirements of Vitamin K

Although it has been shown experimentally that vitamin K is required by the chick, goose, duck, canary, pigeon, turkey, rat, rabbit, mouse, dog and man[98], yet the exact amount of vitamin K required by these various species is unknown. It is known, however, that pure vitamin K_1 or synthetic compounds, which exhibit vitamin K activity in doses of 1 to 2 mgm., are capable of correcting deficiency of vitamin K in most instances. In diseases, in which there is acute or chronic hepatic damage of a severe degree, even large doses of vitamin K are ineffective in correcting the deficiency of prothrombin. In deficiency of prothrombin, produced in the human being by the administration of dicumarol [3,3′-methylenebis (4-hydroxycoumarin)], as much as 40 mgm. of menadione may be needed to correct the hypoprothrombinemia.

As a rule, large doses of vitamin K, when administered to man, do not produce hyperprothrombinemia, but the oral administration of large doses of menadione to the dog, rabbit or rat induces this condition, which may persist for several days[99].

The discussion of requirements of vitamin K for the human infant is reported under the section entitled "Deficiency of prothrombin among newborn infants."

Deficiency of Vitamin K in Man

There are a number of conditions in which a deficiency of prothrombin exists or can be produced in man that can be corrected by the administration of vitamin K[100]. Such a deficiency may occur in any of the following circumstances.

First, after ingestion of a diet inadequate in vitamin K. This condition is rare, but the clinical observation is well supported by the experimental production of low values for prothrombin in the blood of rabbits and mice after they have been caused to subsist on diets deficient in vitamin K.

Second, in the presence of inadequate intestinal absorption. This may result from (1) lack of bile in the intestine because of decreased secretion of bile salts, (2) obstruction of the bile duct from any cause, or (3) inadequate absorption attributable to various intestinal lesions

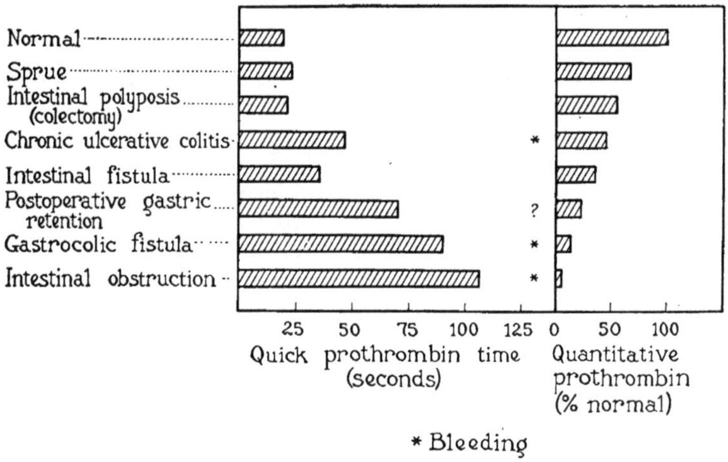

Fig. 15. The various intestinal disturbances with which may be associated a deficiency of prothrombin that can be readily corrected by the proper administration of compounds with vitamin K activity. (Butt, H. R. and Snell, A. M.: Vitamin K, W. B. Saunders Company, Philadelphia, 1941.)

such as intestinal obstruction and short-circuiting surgical procedures. It likewise has been demonstrated that severe diarrheal diseases, such as ulcerative colitis, sprue or celiac disease, may result in deficiency of prothrombin[101] (Fig. 15). A deficiency of prothrombin as a cause of bleeding in cases of various intestinal disturbances is something new in clinical medicine. Although instances of deficiency in prothrombin referable to the effect of intestinal disturbances are not often encountered, they do comprise a rather distinct group and one which warrants close observation. When patients, who have extensive disease of the intestine such as sprue, chronic ulcerative colitis, intestinal obstruction or ileitis, or who have undergone multiple short-circuiting operations on the intestinal tract experience hemorrhage either before or after surgical treatment, deficiency in prothrombin should be recognized and corrected before other forms of treatment are instituted. One of the most important points in the management of these conditions is that the physician follow the content of prothrombin in the blood closely before and after operation in all cases of abnormalities of intestinal mucosa, particularly in cases in which the postoperative condition requires continued aspiration of gas and secretions from the intestinal tract. This practice has solved the mystery of obscure intestinal bleeding, which occurs frequently in such cases, and definitely has reduced postoperative morbidity and fatality.

Third, injury to the liver. There is, of course, considerable evidence, both clinical and experimental, to indicate that the liver plays an active part in the formation of prothrombin, and that any severe injury to this organ results in a deficiency of prothrombin[102]. It has been well demonstrated clinically and experimentally that primary hepatic disease such as cirrhosis, liver atrophy or chronic hepatitis frequently is accompanied by deficiency of prothrombin. This deficiency of prothrombin is not the result of deficiency of vitamin K but apparently is the direct result of severe hepatic damage. Under these conditions the deficiency of prothrombin usually is not relieved by the administration of vitamin K in any amount. It is well to recall that instances of severe hepatic damage occur in any disease in which the liver might be involved, and although this group of cases is somewhat small, this possibility must be kept in mind.

Fourth, ingestion of salicylates. It has been reported that when salicylates are administered to man there is a reduction of prothrombin in the circulating blood[103,104,105], and that this deficiency of prothrombin can be corrected by the administration of vitamin K[106]. These facts now have been confirmed amply. The effect of salicylates, however, even in large doses, on the prothrombin content of the blood is not great, and the occurrence of hemorrhagic manifestations is unlikely[107]. If any surgical procedure is contemplated for, or arises as an emergency in, a patient, who is ingesting large amounts of salicylates, then vitamin K obviously should be given before and after operation.

Fifth, ingestion of dicumarol. When this compound is administered to animals or to man there results, after action in vivo, a decrease in the prothrombin content of the circulating blood. The mechanism, through which the content of prothrombin is reduced, still is obscure, but evidence suggests that the synthesis of prothrombin is prevented. This occurs either through the same mechanism, which prevents vitamin K from catalyzing prothrombin synthesis, or through a direct action on the prothrombin[108].

At the low levels of menadione, which ordinarily would correct a nutritional deficiency of vitamin K, the hypoprothrombinemic action of dicumarol is not prevented. Large doses of vitamin K, however, will correct the deficiency of prothrombin produced by dicumarol[109,110,111]

Deficiency of Prothrombin Among Newborn Infants

It is rather generally agreed that during the first few days of an infant's life a deficiency of prothrombin exists in the circulating blood. Waddell and Guerry and their associates [112] were the first to report the important discovery that this physiological deficiency of prothrombin of newborn infants and the bleeding tendency, which sometimes developed, could be corrected by the administration of vitamin K. Since that time numerous reports have appeared concerning the effect of the various compounds possessing vitamin K activity on the content of prothrombin of newborn infants, and the effect of such compounds on the hemorrhage which occurs frequently. The important suggestion also has been made that the deficiency of prothrombin existing at the time of birth might account in many instances for the intracranial hemorrhages, which sometimes follow protracted labor, and which result frequently in permanent paralysis of the infant.

In Fig. 16 are plotted the prothrombin levels during the first 6 days of life as reported from various laboratories which employed a variety of methods for the measurement of prothrombin in the blood. On the basis of this figure one would be justified in concluding that the clinical material studied in these various cities was different, and that each undoubtedly represents specialized classes of patients studied under special conditions. Smith and Warner[113] believed that the clue to these discrepancies lies in the fact that the vitamin K intake of the pregnant woman has much to do with the amount of the vitamin received by the infant and hence with the content of prothrombin of the latter. Waddell and Guerry[114] have shown that the content of prothrombin in the newborn infant is much higher in summer than in winter. This probably results from the large intake of green vegetables during the summer months. The results recorded in the summer are shown in curve 4A (Fig. 16) and the results obtained in winter appear in curve 4B.

The exact cause of this deficiency of vitamin is not completely known. It has been suggested that, as soon as the presence of bacterial flora of the intestinal tract is established, the infant is capable of synthe-

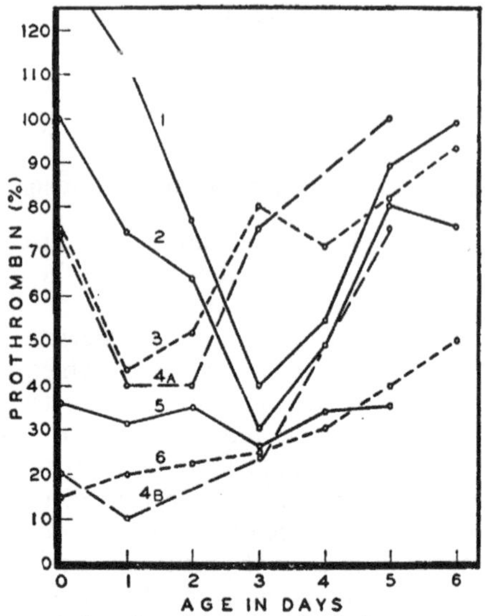

Fig. 16. The content of prothrombin in the blood of an untreated infant during the first six days of life. Curves 1 and 2 were devised by Owen, Hoffman, Ziffren and Smith in Iowa City. Curve 1 is based on the "bedside test". Curve 2 was devised according to the method of Quick. Curve 4A and 4B were prepared by Waddell and Guerry (114) in Charlottesville, Virginia; they used a microadaptation of Quick's method by Kelly and Gray. Curve 4A was charted during winter and early spring; curve 4B was computed during late spring and early summer. Waddell and Guerry expressed their results in the form of the prothrombin time (in seconds). To facilitate comparison, these values have been converted into "percentage of normal adult values" with the aid of the conversion curve of Quick. Curve 5 was prepared by Owen, Hoffman, Ziffren and Smith, in Iowa City; They employed the two-stage prothrombin method of Warner, Brinkhous and Smith. Curve 6 was computed by Kato and Poncher in Chicago; they utilized a micromethod devised by Kato. (Smith, H. P. and Warner, E. D.: Vitamin K, Clinical Aspects, in The Biological action of the vitamins; a symposium, Edited by E. A. Evans, Jr., The University of Chicago Press, Chicago, 1942.)

sizing vitamin K, a fact which has been well proved experimentally. This explanation, however, does not explain the delay in the return to normal of the value for prothrombin, a delay which occurs in many infants. To explain this phenomenon it must be recalled that the liver of the newborn infant is unable to secrete sufficient bile, that the absorption of fat is very limited and that gastrointestinal hypermotility is the rule. Thus, even though vitamin K is present, proper absorption of the vitamin would be theoretically unlikely until the digestive function approaches normal. This occurs on about the third or fourth day of life. To support the suggestion that the presence of bacterial flora in the intestinal tract is connected intimately with the return of the value for prothrombin to normal at the end of the third day, some investigators have shown that extra feeding, started within 2 hours after delivery of the infant, can prevent the subsequent development of hypoprothrombinemia. Evidence which tends to refute these theories will be discussed a little further along.

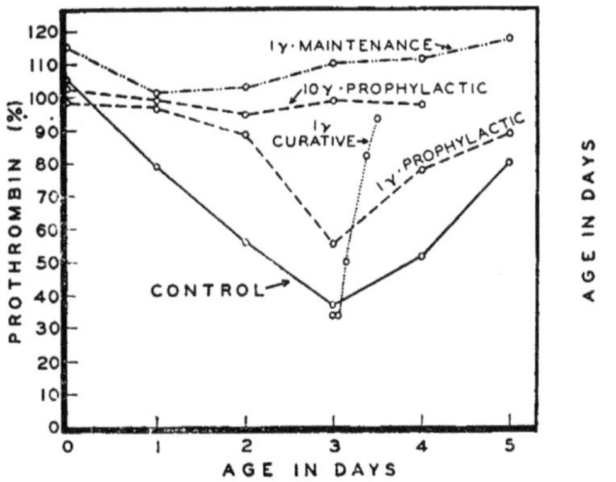

Fig. 17. The response of infants to variable doses of vitamin K. The compound used as a source of vitamin K activity was the water-soluble 4-amino-2-methyl-1-naphthol (synkamin). Administration was by intramuscular injection (Smith, H. P. and Warner, E. D.: Vitamin K, Clinical Aspects, in The biological action of the vitamins; a symposium, Edited by E. A. Evans, Jr., The Universiay of Chicago Press, Chicago, 1942.)

It has been shown by Sells, Walker and Owen[115] that the minimal vitamin K requirement of the infant is extremely low. Their results modified by Smith and Warner[113] are shown in Fig. 17. The uppermost curve in this figure shows that 1 microgram of vitamin K, given daily, is adequate to maintain the content of prothrombin at normal. It is also shown in the second curve that a dose of 10 micrograms usually would prevent the decrease shown in the untreated controls. In Fig. 17 also is seen a curve which shows that, if 1 microgram is given on the third day of life, it is followed in 10 hours by an increase in the content of prothrombin from 30 per cent. of normal to the percentage of 95.

As already mentioned, nearly all investigators have noted that the content of prothrombin increases until it has exceeded the so-called danger point as soon as the infant receives an adequate amount of milk. It always has been assumed that milk, since it was a poor source of vitamin K, served merely to introduce bacterial flora into the intestinal tract and that vitamin K was produced by these bacteria. The work of Sells, Walker and Owen[115] has shown, however, that milk does contain an amount of preformed vitamin K adequate to meet the minimal requirements of the infant.

To recapitulate, it appears that, when large amounts of vitamin K are given to the pregnant female, the vitamin is transmitted through the placenta and that some is stored in the fetus. According to Smith and Warner[113], if the diet of the mother has been adequate, the content of prothrombin in the infant is at a safe figure at birth. Frequently this is not the case, and because of the infant's lack of food intake a deficiency of vitamin K develops rather rapidly. During the critical 4 days that follow birth, a single prophylactic dose of 10 micrograms is sufficient to maintain a normal content of prothrombin. If the mother is given 1 mgm. of the vitamin, similar protection results. It seems that the vitamins may be distributed between mother and fetus almost in proportion to body weight. Apparently the infant is competent to manufacture adequate amounts of prothrombin, if vitamin K is present in sufficient amounts.

On the basis of work, reports of which are now available, it appears that a dose of from 0.5 to 1 mgm. of 2-methyl-1, 4-naphthoquinone or of any of the other synthetic quinone compounds available commercially is sufficient, in most instances, to control certain hemorrhagic disease of the newborn and that, if it is administered at the time of birth, it will prevent transitory hypoprothrombinemia. It must be remembered that failures also can occur in the treatment of infants, if sufficient hepatic damage has occurred.

It has been reported and well established by several groups of workers that the administration of vitamin K to mothers prior to delivery will prevent the usual decrease in the content of prothrombin in the blood, which is observed among newborn infants, and that the administration of vitamin K to the newborn infant also will increase the concentration of prothrombin in the plasma[116,117,118].

On the basis of results of work now available, it appears that 2 mgm.

of menadione given by mouth to a mother a half hour to forty-eight hours before delivery is effective in preventing hemorrhagic disease of the newborn infant[119]. There is good evidence to indicate that, although the feeding of vitamin K to the infant after birth increases the concentration of prothrombin, the concentrations in these instances are not so high as those achieved by antepartum administration of the vitamin to the mother.

Many workers believe that instances of cerebral hemorrhage occurring in the course of birth with minimal trauma are precipitated by small hemorrhages which endure for a number of days. For this reason many workers interested in this problem believe that the lives of some of the infants concerned might be saved, if the blood at birth exhibits better properties of coagulation. Most investigators believe that some form of vitamin K should be administered to every mother at the onset of labor. Some still insist that the vitamin also should be given to the newborn infant as an added precaution. In any event, the plan is so simple, the vitamin so cheap and the toxic reactions so minimal that this program should be adopted universally in the hope of preventing injury at birth[120].

Methods for Measuring Deficiency of Vitamin K

Since no international standard of unity has been established for vitamin K, many methods of assay and standards of unity have arisen[121]. The wide interest displayed in vitamin K and associated naphthoquinones has given rise to the need for convenient and accurate methods for their estimation. A step in this direction was made by Trenner and Bacher[122], who described a method by which many quinone-like substances can be assayed. Others recently have also reported work in this direction[123,124,125].

Of clinical importance are the methods by which deficiency of vitamin K can be recognized by simple laboratory procedures. Several excellent methods for the measurement of deficiency of prothrombin in the blood of man have been described, but in the experience of many the method developed by Quick and his associates[126,127,128,129,130,131,132] has been found adaptable for general use in the clinical laboratory. The method developed by Warner and his associates[123,124,125] also is used, with modification, in many laboratories. Details of these methods are given in several publications[126,127,128,129,130,131,132].

The so-called bedside method has come into considerable use, and is reported to be of great value for the general practitioner. Suitably compact sets for making this measurement at the bedside now are available commercially[133]. Several micromethods for the measurement of deficiency of prothrombin of infants also have been described and are used routinely in many institutions[134,135,136,137,138].

It must be admitted that all current methods for the estimation of prothrombin are, of necessity, indirect. However, certain of these methods for the measurement of prothrombin are the most nearly accurate methods available at present for estimation of the tendency of a patient to bleed in the presence of suspected deficiency of prothrombin. The information afforded by the measurement of prothrombin in the circulating blood is much more nearly accurate in the prediction of the tendency of a patient to bleed than is the measurement of the coagulation or bleeding time as formerly used in the consideration of such tendencies.

Toxicity

To date no serious untoward reaction has been observed among persons who have received reasonable therapeutic doses of natural concentrates of vitamin K, synthetic vitamin K_1 or any of the synthetic compounds exhibiting antihemorrhagic activity now available commercially. An effect has not been noted on blood pressure, respiration, permeability of capillaries or urinary excretion after the administration of any of these compounds. It has been observed, however, that doses of menadione as large as 180 mgm. administered orally to human beings result in vomiting and porphyrinuria. Other workers have noted that anemia followed the administration of large doses of vitamin K[139]. These huge doses, however, are so obviously greater than those employed for therapeutic use that at present it appears safe to continue the therapeutic administration of these synthetic compounds. Fieser wisely pointed out that some clinical consideration should be given to the possible conflict or otherwise undesirable characteristics which may be associated with conjugates resulting from administration of menadione. He pointed out that the delayed action of the administered material would appear to be subject to considerable uncertainty, and that the wide opportunity for transformation of different types would lead one to expect a variability in the response, depending on the manner of administration and the condition of the patient[140,141,142,143].

Diagnosis of Vitamin K Deficiency

The bleeding of patients, who have jaundice, occurs most frequently after surgical intervention which was calculated to relieve biliary obstruction. Hemorrhage usually is noted between the first and fourth postoperative days, but it may appear as late as the twelfth to eighteenth day after operation. As is well known, cholemic bleeding ordinarily begins as a slow oozing from the operative incision, from the gums or nose or from the gastrointestinal tract. Often, however, the first evidence of hemorrhage is afforded by the appearance of severe hematemesis or melena. Such bleeding often is controlled temporarily by the transfusion of whole blood, but all too frequently even the repeated transfusions of blood fails to control the hemorrhagic diathesis. Bleeding of this type in our experience and in the experience of many others invariably is associated with prolongation of the prothrombin clotting time.

Bleeding of patients suffering from jaundice occurs most often in the presence of those conditions in which bile is excluded completely from the gastrointestinal tract such as complete biliary obstruction produced by neoplasms of the pancreas, ampulla and gallbladder. Postoperative stricture of the common bile duct is accompanied perhaps by the second highest incidence of bleeding; intermittent obstruction caused by the presence of stones comes third. Complete external fistulas are relatively rare but often are associated with bleeding. Although bleeding is more likely to occur in those cases in which bile is excluded completely from the intestine, yet the physician must not overlook the fact that bleeding also can occur in the absence of jaundice, if the liver has been injured considerably as the result of chronic cholecystic disease. Although the foregoing facts are somewhat useful for prediction of whether or not a patient will bleed, the exceptions are so frequent that rigid clinical rules cannot be devised.

It has been well demonstrated experimentally that, if the hepatic parenchyma is injured, the amount of prothrombin in the circulating blood decreases. It has been demonstrated further by Warner and his associates and by Bollman and his associates that, if the hepatic damage in these animals is too severe, the content of prothrombin in the circulating blood does not increase after the administration of vitamin K. Likewise it has been well demonstrated clinically that patients, who have severe hepatic damage, have a decrease in the prothrombin in the circulating blood, and that occassionally they will not respond to the administration of vitamin K.

These instances of severe hepatic damage can occur in any disease in which the liver might be involved, but most frequently they are seen in cases of cirrhosis of the liver, in those in which obstruction or stricture of the common duct has existed over long periods and in those in which there is acute or subacute atrophy of the liver resulting from some primary disease or associated with acute cholecystitis. Although this group of cases is somewhat small, it is well to remember that it does exist. It is true that repeated doses of vitamin K frequently are necessary to produce the desired effect, but when the physician has doubled or tripled the usual therapeutic dose of vitamin K without producing desired effects, he can be fairly certain that, regardless of the amounts of vitamin K administered, there will be little increase of the prothrombin in the circulating blood.

A deficiency of prothrombin as the cause of bleeding in patients who have various intestinal disturbances is something new in clinical medicine, and although instances of deficiency of prothrombin referable to the effects of intestinal absorption are not encountered often, yet they do comprise a rather distinct group and one which warrants further investigation. The pathological physiology concerned in such cases has been described herein under the section on experimental pathological physiology.

The entire subject of bleeding in the newborn infant has been discussed previously in this chapter.

Obviously knowledge of the conditions in which deficiency of prothrombin may occur is a fundamental requisite for the correct diagnosis of possible deficiency of vitamin K. Although the possibility of hemorrhagic diathesis may be suspected in a particular case, measurement of the prothrombin content of the circulating blood is necessary for accurate diagnosis as well as for evaluation of proper treatment. It must be admitted that present methods for measurement of the content of prothrombin in the circulating blood of patients are subject to considerable error. The decrease in the concentration of prothrombin in the circulating blood of man seems to depend on certain unknown individual factors. Although in certain instances the concentration of prothrombin in the blood apparently depends on the degree of hepatic injury, it certainly does not have any constant relationship to the type of hepatic or biliary disease present.

On the basis of results of the various studies of Smith and his associates[123,124,125] it would appear that bleeding among animals in the experimental laboratory occurs when the value for prothrombin becomes less than 20 or 25 per cent. of normal, and that, conversely, so long as the value remains at about 20 or 25 per cent. bleeding does not occur. If this conception is understood, it is easy to see why, in certain cases, bleeding in man may occur postoperatively with little warning. Loss of blood, surgical trauma and the effects of anesthesia and trauma to the liver may reduce an already depleted supply of prothrombin to a dangerously low level; of these factors mechanical trauma is thought to be the most important. The prothrombin clotting time may, and frequently does, increase with no apparent reason within 6 to 8 hours, and with this increase free bleeding may occur without warning, and apparently normal, coagulable blood may become virtually incoagulable.

The prothrombin clotting time of the blood of patients, who have jaundice, usually increases to some extent for the first 3 or 4 days after surgical operation, but it may increase rapidly even as late as the eighteenth postoperative day. For this reason the prothrombin clotting time should be determined daily for the first 4 days after operation, and then every other day for at least 8 or 10 days longer. Any increase in the prothrombin clotting time should constitute an indication for the immediate oral or intravenous administration of vitamin K. To those patients with a high prothrombin clotting time before surgical treatment it is perhaps wise to administer the vitamin daily for several days after surgical operation, regardless of the prothrombin clotting time. A patient, whose blood has a prothrombin clotting time of more than 30 seconds, should be prepared with particular care, and one whose blood has a prothrombin clotting time of more than 45 seconds must be considered to be a potential bleeder and treated as such.

The same important diagnostic points also are applicable in those cases of various intestinal lesions in which a deficiency of prothrombin in the circulating blood may develop.

It is equally important to follow, if possible, the prothrombin clotting time of newborn infants, although it is well known that during the first few days there is a physiological deficiency of prothrombin. This caution is particularly important if any surgical procedure is contemplated during this period of life.

Unfortunately the measurement of prothrombin in the circulating blood does not always give the exact index of the tendency of the patient to bleed. Like any laboratory method this method may not give the clinical information which is always desirable. For these reasons prophylactic treatment is much better than treatment after bleeding once occurs.

Treatment of Vitamin K Deficiency

No specific remedy for the prevention and control of all instances of bleeding resulting from deficiency of prothrombin has yet been discovered. The proper administration of vitamin K or related compounds in most instances will be effective, but in addition to obtain the best results all procedures which are known to be of value in the maintenance of adequate hepatic function must be employed. Obviously the first objective in treatment of the jaundiced patient, who has a tendency to bleed, is to restore continuity of the biliary passages and protection of the hepatic parenchyma.

Regardless of the etiological factors involved in the deficiency of prothrombin in man, treatment in most instances is essentially the same. Since there are now available water-soluble synthetic compounds with

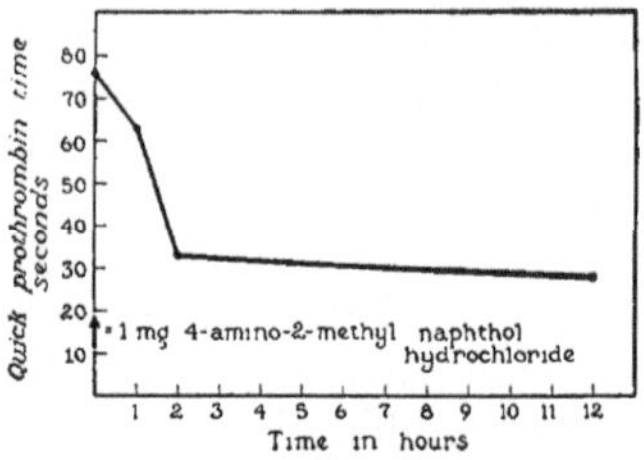

Fig. 18

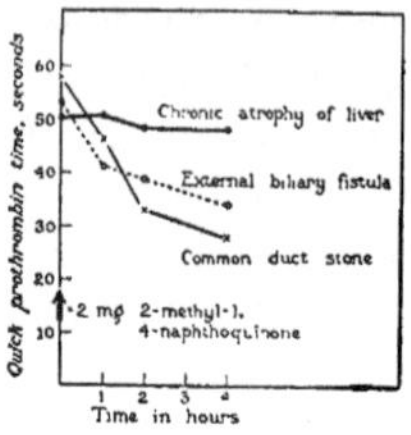

Fig. 19

Fig. 18. The effect of the intravenous injection of 1 mgm. of 4-amino-2-methyl-1-naphthol hydrochloride on the elevated prothrombin clotting time of a patient who had obstructive jaundice. (Butt, H. R. and Snell, A. M.: Vitamin K, W. B. Saunders Company, Philadelphia, 1941.)

Fig. 19. The effect and rapidity of action of the intravenous injection of 2 mgm. of 2-methyl-1,4-naphthoquinone in a case of external biliary fistula and in one of calculus of the common bile duct. The figure also shows the failure of this compound to reduce the elevated prothrombin clotting time in a case of chronic atrophy of the liver. (Butt, H. R. and Snell, A. M.: Vitamin K, W. B. Saunders Company. Philadelphia, 1941.)

vitamin K activity, the procedure of giving bile salts to insure proper absorption has been nearly discarded. These water-soluble synthetic compounds should be administered orally or intravenously in doses of from 1 to 2 mgm. daily for several days prior to, and after, surgical procedures in which deficiency of prothrombin is present or may be expected to develop. The rapidity of action of these water-soluble compounds with vitamin K activity is shown in Figs. 18 and 19[144,145,146,147].

Most investigators interested in this subject suggest that prior to operation in any of these conditions, regardless of the concentration of prothrombin in the patient's blood, vitamin K in some form should be administered for from 1 to 2 days. After operation the concentration of prothrombin in the blood should be followed carefully, and vitamin K administered as necessary. In instances, in which the level of prothrombin in the circulating blood is sharply decreased before operation, vitamin K should be administered routinely preoperatively and postoperatively for several days, and the concentration of prothrombin in the blood should be determined for at least 8 to 10 days thereafter.

Some workers[147,148] recently have felt that the change effected in a particular level of prothrombin by the administration of vitamin K may provide some index as to the nature of the disease being treated, with particular reference to intrahepatic and extrahepatic jaundice. Data now at hand do not unequivocally establish this fact.

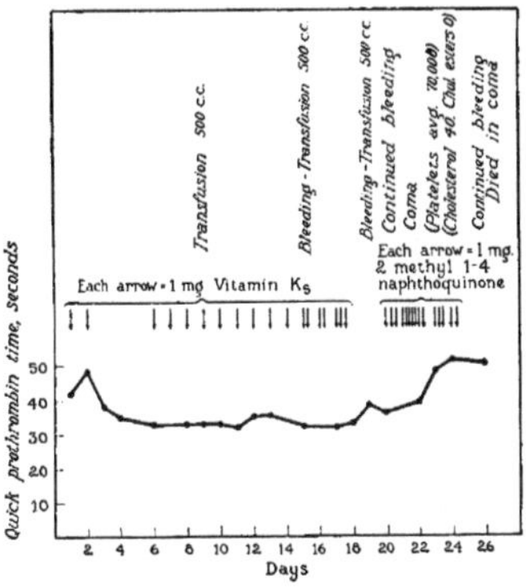

Fig. 20. The prothrombin clotting time of a patient, who had severe cirrhosis of the liver, and who received over a long period various synthetic preparations possessing marked antihemorrhagic activity. In spite of these materials, the prothrombin clotting time remained elevated. This type of case constitutes a failure of vitamin K to correct an elevated prothrombin clotting time. (Butt, H. R. and Snell, A. M.: Vitamin K, W. B. Saunders Company, Philadelphia, 1941.)

In some patients, who have severe acute or chronic hepatic damage, hemorrhage develops from deficiency of prothrombin, which cannot be corrected by the administration of even large amounts of blood or vitamin K (Fig. 20). Recently[149] it was reported that this usually uncontrollable hemorrhagic diathesis could be corrected by the giving of blood from a donor, who 24 hours previously had received a large dose of vitamin K. Results of our own work at the Mayo Clinic do not support this contention[150].

The discovery and isolation of dicumarol by Link[151] and its clinical application to the prevention of thrombosis[152] have been important steps in clinical medicine. As stated previously, the administration of dicumarol to human beings results in a decrease in the prothrombin of the blood. It is now known by means of the work of several investigators[110,153,154] that large doses of vitamin K will prevent this decrease in the content of prothrombin in the blood that follows the administration of dicumarol. Dicumarol usually is administered to patients, who have pulmonary embolism or thrombophlebitis, or who before surgery give a history of these difficulties. The doses employed vary, but as a rule a single dose of 300 mgm. of dicumarol is administered on the first day of treatment and 200 mgm. is given on the second day, followed by the administration of 200 mgm. each day, if the prothrombin time is less than 35 seconds (Quick's method of estimation of the prothrombin content). It was observed in one series of 340 patients that 27 per cent. were "sensi-

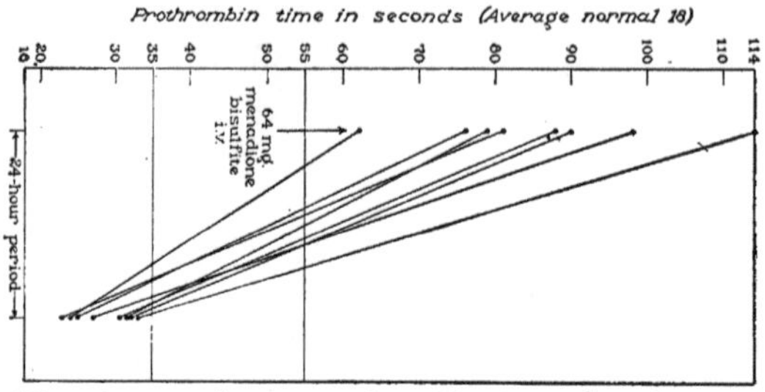

Fig. 21. Striking decrease in the prothrombin time after the adminstration of a single dose of menadione bisulfite to eight patients who had excessive hypoprothrombinemia induced by dicumarol. This was the usual response of the condition of such patients. (Cromer, H. E., Jr. and Barker, N. W.: Proceed. Staff Meet., Mayo Clin., 1944, XIX, 217.)

tive" to dicumarol[110], "sensitive" meaning that after 1 or 2 doses of dicumarol the prothrombin time increased to 60 seconds or more instead of the usual response of 35 to 55 seconds. It was considered that among these 27 per cent. bleeding might occur, and for this reason a simple and effective method of rapidly lowering the prothrombin time to the neighborhood of 45 seconds or less was needed.

The striking effect on the prothrombin time exerted by the administration of large doses of vitamin K is well shown in Fig. 21. In these cases a dose of 64 mgm. of menadione bisulfite was administered intravenously. This dosage is equivalent to 40 mgm. of 2-methyl-1,4-naphthoquinone. In an occasional case there is no response to these large doses of vitamin K. Usually, however, there is definite lowering of the prothrombin time limit within 2 hours after vitamin K has been administered, and the maximal decrease in the prothrombin time is reached in about 18 hours. Clinically these excellent responses to vitamin K indicate that another valuable safety factor has been added to dicumarol therapy.

VITAMIN C

History

In 1928, during studies on tissue respiration systems, Szent-Györgyi[155] secured from adrenal glands a preparation which he subsequently called hexuronic acid. This substance was not tested for antiscorbutic activity, however, at that time. In 1932 Waugh and King[156] succeeded in the isolation and identification of vitamin C, and subsequently it was established that their product was identical with the hexuronic acid obtained by Szent-Györgyi. One year later Reichstein, Grussner and Oppenhauer[157] synthesized vitamin C, which was named ascorbic acid.

Chemistry and Physiology

Ascorbic acid, having the formula $C_6H_8O_6$, falls into the series of hexuronic acid lactones and is closely related to the sugars. It is an

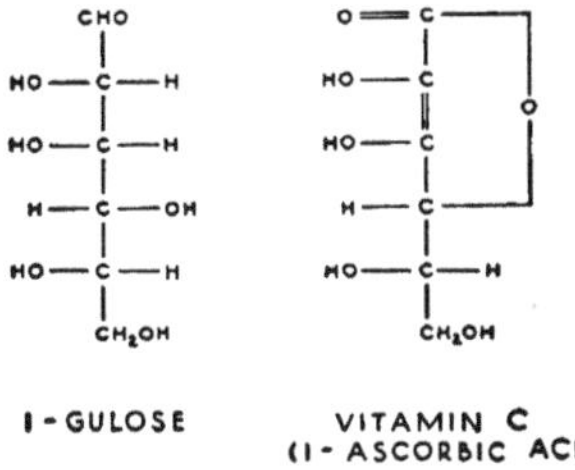

Fig. 22. Structural formula of 1-glucose and vitamin C.

enediol-lactone of an acid similar in configuration to 1-gulose. The formulae for both 1-gulose and ascorbic acid are shown in Fig. 22.

Ascorbic acid is a crystalline, colorless compound which is freely soluble in water and which has a melting point of 192° C. The crystals may form pseudo-orthorhombic or monoclinic patterns but tend to form rather dense radiation clusters (Fig. 23).

The crystals as such are very stable, but in aqueous solution rapid oxdation occurs. The oxidation-reduction reaction of ascorbic acid has been the subject of much research since 1933 because of the practical importance of possible loss of the vitamin. It is now known that many organic compounds, including indophenol notably, as well as inorganic metallic radicals such as Fe^{+++} and Cu^{+++}, will oxidize ascorbic acid. Aerobic aqueous oxidation of ascorbic acid is accelerated by ordinary as well as ultraviolet light, and in the presence of a flavin this reaction is enhanced still more. The immediate product of ascorbic acid oxidation is dehydroascorbic acid. This product is equally as potent as ascorbic acid

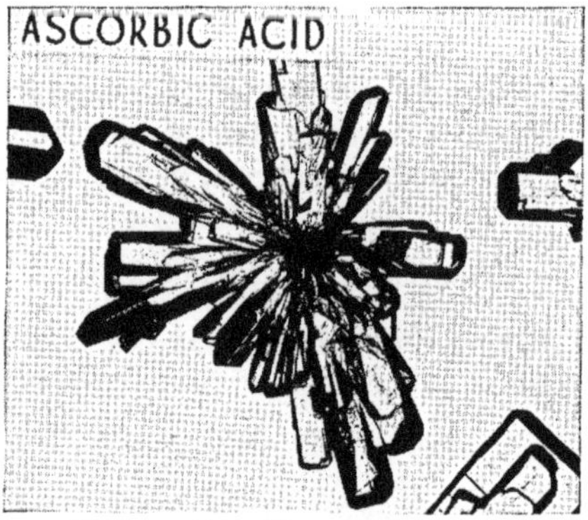

Fig. 23. Crystalline ascorbic acid.

in the treatment of scurvy. While at this level the oxidation-reduction reaction is reversible, and it is possible to reduce dehydroascorbic acid to ascorbic acid by hydrogen sulfide, cysteine and glutathione. The relationship between ascorbic acid and dehydroascorbic acid is clearly shown in Figure 24.

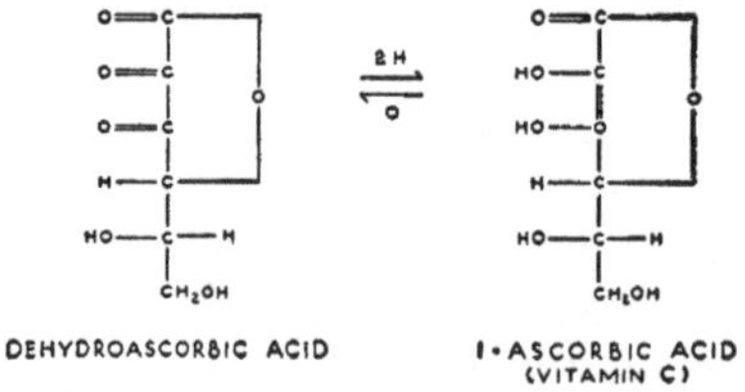

Fig. 24. Structural formula of dehydroascorbic acid and l-ascorbic acid.

Dehydroascorbic acid is fairly stable in acidic solutions of pH_4, but in solutions of a higher pH oxidation continues to an irreversible level in which there is structural rearrangement with the formation of a potent reducing substance. This substance, when oxidized, gives rise to oxalic acid and l-threonic acid, and ascorbic acid thus is destroyed.

Both the dextro- and levo-rotatory forms of ascorbic acid lend themselves to synthesis, but it is to be remembered that only the levo-rotatory form has antiscorbutic properties. The dextro-rotatory form does not protect against scurvy. Several other synthetic substances have been shown to have antiscorbutic activity but to a much lesser degree than l-ascorbic acid.

The important observations of Holst and Frölich[158] on guinea pigs and pigeons gave the first hint that the former animal required an extrinsic supply of vitamin C, whereas the latter did not. This thought was followed up, and it is now understood that of all the animals, only the primates and the guinea pig are incapable of synthesizing vitamin C. Although man is incapable of such synthesis, he is capable of storing the supplied vitamin. That this is true has been shown by many well controlled experiments, and this fact explains the latent period of three to six months or more in the development of scurvy on a vitamin C deficient diet. Ascorbic acid is widely distributed in body tissues and fluids. In general, it can be said that the younger the tissue and the higher its metabolic activity, the greater will be its ascorbic acid content. This has been well shown by the tissue titration studies of Glick and Biskind[159] on normal tissue and similar studies by Musulin and his associates[160] on rapidly growing tumor tissue. All of the glandular tissues of the body contain significant amounts of ascorbic acid, while the non-glandular body tissues and fluids contain a lesser amount. The following order approximates the decreasing concentration of ascorbic acid in the various body tissues and fluids; pituitary body, corpus luteum, adrenal cortex, young thymus, liver, brain, testes, ovaries, spleen, thyroid, pancreas, salivary glands, lung, kidney, intestinal wall, heart, muscle, spinal fluid and blood. The pituitary body contains 260 mgm. per 100 c.c., the adrenal gland 200 mgm. per 100 c.c., muscle 2 mgm. per 100 c.c. and blood plasma 1.2 mgm. per 100 c.c.

Certain of the glandular secretions and excretory products of the body also contain ascorbic acid. Human milk contains four to five times the amount of vitamin C as does cow's milk. Thus nature has provided for the relatively high vitamin C requirements of the nursing infant, who requires about 25 to 30 mgm. of ascorbic acid a day, by establishing the vitamin C content of human milk at 4 to 8 mgm. per 100 c.c. The young calf, on the other hand, is independent of its mother as far as ascorbic acid is concerned because this animal can synthesize the vitamin. Vitamin C is found normally also in the urine, feces and sweat. By far the greatest amount is excreted in the urine, the total amount excreted a day being 13 to 40 mgm. Vitamin C is a so-called "threshold" substance with a critical level of excretion at approximately 1.4 mgm. per 100 c.c. of plasma. The urinary excretion of the vitamin is enhanced by many drugs such as ammonium chloride, atropine, sodium bicarbonate, the salicylates and the barbiturates, while insulin results in a lowered excretion. An additional 6 to 10 mgm. is excreted in the feces, and another 0.55 to 0.64 mgm. per 100 c.c. is excreted in the sweat. These excretion levels obviously depend upon dietary intake and increased destruction or demand for the vitamin.

The body physiological economy of vitamin C is reflected in the concentration of the vitamin in these various excretions, fluids and tissues. Should the extrinsic supply of ascorbic acid be restricted, there is observed a disappearance of vitamin C from these elements in an order inversely proportional to their ascorbic acid content in the physiological state. Thus, urinary excretion of vitamin C ceases long before the plasma level is significantly reduced. In the same manner the plasma level may be zero, while the white cell-platelet layer is normal. This retrograde depletion, so to speak, continues until finally the pituitary body is depleted of the vitamin. The converse is true when a primate or guinea pig so depleted of vitamin C then is saturated with it. The tissues first take their share, then the body fluids, and lastly ascorbic acid appears in the body excretions. The amount of the vitamin required to induce saturation thus is a very rough estimate of the state of vitamin C nutrition. Crandon and Lund[161] and more recently Pijoan and Lozner[162] have conducted experimental studies in human scurvy which bear out this concept. One of the latter authors showed that even though the urinary excretion of vitamin C had long since ceased, and the plasma level was 0.0 to 0.2 mgm. for twenty months, the white cell-platelet layer contained 25 mgm. per 100 c.c., and clinical scurvy did not develop. These studies have been confirmed by many investigators, and there is little doubt but that the vitamin C concentration in the white cell-platelet layer of centrifuged blood correlates much better with the clinical findings than does the vitamin C concentration elsewhere. It should be remembered, however, that in the normal physiological state there is an excretion of vitamin C in the urine and that there is a concentration of ascorbic acid in the blood plasma of 1.2 mg. per 100 c.c. A deviation from these findings is not physiological and should prompt the physician to suspect a deficiency of vitamin C and guide him to an investigation of the dietary and the application of the vitamin C saturation test.

The physiological functions of vitamin C include a long list. However, the most clearly defined of these is the formation of reticulum and collagen so as to maintain the integrity of the intercellular substance[163]. It is believed that vitamin C may be the sole factor which is responsible for the cementing together of the reticulum by a translucent matrix to form collagen in between the cells of tissue. Vitamin C exerts its efforts only on tissue of mesenchymal origin. The precise mechanism of this function is unknown.

Vitamin C is concerned further with the over-all growth of the organism. It has been shown to be a powerful growth stimulant in the young plant embryos, and it is reasonable to assume that it has such a function in man. Growth and development studies are such long-term problems that only a few such observations have been made under controlled conditions in man and in the experimental animal.

As to the function of vitamin C as a hematopoietic substance there is considerable doubt. It has not been shown conclusively that deficiency of ascorbic acid itself is a direct cause of the anemia seen in association with scurvy. It is quite possible that many other factors are at work as discussed in the section on Pathological Physiology.

Accumulating evidence is appearing that vitamin C may play a rôle in resistance to infection and certain toxins. King and Menten[164] and Sigal and King[165] found that guinea pigs in the "pre-scorbutic" state were more sensitive to tissue injury by diphtheria toxin than were normal ones and that the metabolism of these animals was lowered significantly. The latter is probably a natural defense mechanism to conserve the vitamin C stores. The authors have observed that resistance to disease is lowered significantly in general nutritive failure, but how much vitamin C is directly responsible for this is not known. The function of vitamin C in certain enzyme systems still is without proof or even general agreement. That such a function may exist is not too unlikely, but this subject is so imperfectly understood that at present no concrete statements can be made.

It is evident that there is little precise knowledge concerning the physiology and metabolism of vitamin C. Studies in vitro show poor correlation with observations in vivo. A long, wide vista may lie before science with the recent advent of the capability of marking carbon atoms. By this means it may be possible to follow ascorbic acid through the body as it performs its functions in vivo.

Pathological Physiology

Deficiency in vitamin C expresses itself most characteristically in the development of scurvy. The pathological physiology of vitamin C can be understood best from a discussion of the pathological physiology of scurvy. A clearer understanding of the pathological physiology of scurvy is gained, if one recalls that the primary and most clearly defined function of vitamin C is the maintenance of the integrity of the intercellular substance. A lack or a deficiency of vitamin C results in an impairment of this function with a subsequent manifestation of the symptoms and signs of the state we recognize as scurvy. A deficiency of vitamin C may result from one or a combination of any of the several following factors; (1) a deficient dietary intake, (2) impaired intestinal absorption, (3) increased body requirements for the vitamin, (4) faulty assimilation, (5) faulty utilization and (6) increased destruction in vivo of the vitamin.

A new era in the pathogenesis of scurvy was inaugurated by S. B. Wolbach and his associates[163,166,167] from 1926 to 1937, when they showed that the intercellular substance was seriously affected in scurvy. In their scorbutic animals the ground substance and fibroblasts were present, but there was no reticulum nor collagen present. Such defective intercellular material has been found in connective tissue, bone and teeth. Within twenty-four hours after the administration of vitamin C to such scorbutic animals whole bundles of collagen were formed. Although the capillaries are believed to be involved both from the clinical and embryonic points of view, no such morphological lesions have been found.

In the formation of bone and cartilage the intercellular substance is of major importance. The lesions produced in these structures due to lack of vitamin C are similar to the scorbutic changes in other parts of the body and like them are due to a failure to form intercellular substance. The anatomical location of these lesions depends to a large extent on two factors, growth and stress. This explains why bony lesions and hematomas are seen so commonly in the child. These factors explain further the occurrence of petechiae in either usual or unusual locations. The frequently cited example of the scorbutic blacksmith, who had many petechiae over the shoulders and arms, thus is given an explanation.

Gross changes in bone in vitamin C deficiency are seen most commonly at the costochondral junctions, the distal end of the femur, the proximal end of the tibia and of the humerus and the wrist. In the scorbutic state formation of cartilage and bone matrices soon ceases. The osteoblasts are surrounded by liquid, and no collagen is to be seen. This results in the rarefied area at the ends of the diaphysis seen in x-rays (Fig. 25). The Germans aptly termed this appearance "Gerustmark", framework marrow, as the strands of apparent connective tissue seem to be surrounded by a liquid. The osteoblasts revert to their prototype in scurvy and form a fibrous rather than a bony union between the diaphysis and the epiphysis, thus permitting false motion sometimes in these areas. The cortex of the bone rarefies and becomes very thin so that

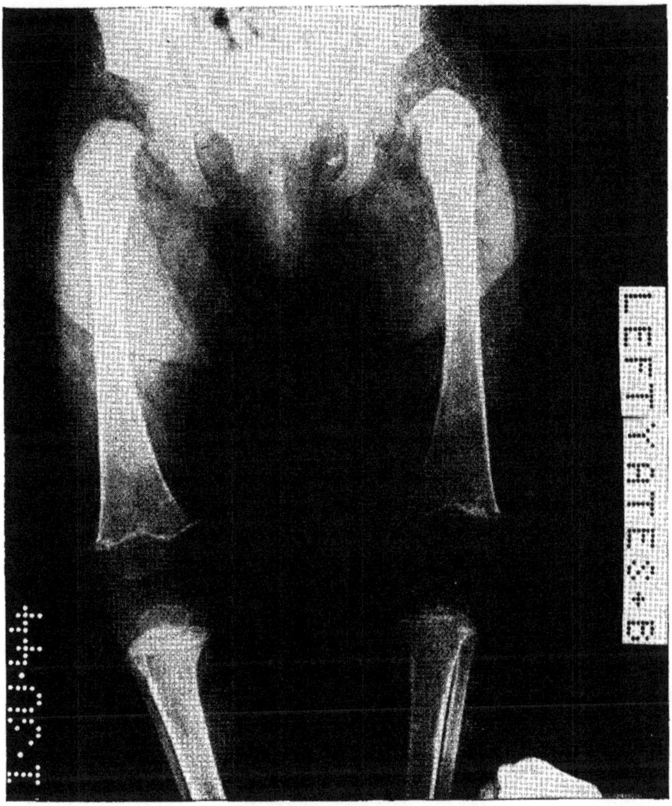

Fig. 25. X-ray of long bones in scurvy.

fractures from trivial traumata occur. The periosteum is only loosely attached to the bone and eventually becomes stripped from the shell-like cortex. Because of the unyielding nature of the cortex, subperiosteal hemorrhages occur frequently. Such hemorrhages further strip the periosteum, giving the picture so characteristic of the scorbutic state.

The response to ascorbic acid is dramatic. Within a day this sickly process is reversed, and bundles of collagen can be seen. Osteoid material appears in a few hours around the osteoblasts with the formation of trabeculae and the cessation of hemorrhages from the fragile capillaries. In short, normal bone formation starts again. Vitamin C is also essential for the callus formation necessary for the healing of fractured bones. This explains the observations made in Lind's time of the old-healed fractures breaking down when sailors developed scurvy.

Faulty formation of intercellular substance in connective tissue is of practical importance in wound healing. It has been widely observed that in the scorbutic person minor abrasions and wounds heal very slowly. Crandon[161] studied and finally settled this problem by his well controlled experiments on himself. For a period of 6 months he restricted himself to a vitamin C-free diet, supplemented by all the other known vitamins. At the end of the first 3 months on such a diet a wound was made on his back. This wound healed well, and histological examination showed ample intercellular substance and capillary formation. After he had been on the restricted diet for 6 months and had had clinical scurvy for 3 weeks, a wound similar to the first was made. The skin healed, but the wound beneath did not. Unorganized blood clots filled the wound, and histological study of the tissue showed the same lack of intercellular substance and capillary formation as was found by Wolbach in wounds of scorbutic guinea pigs. Crandon then received an intramuscular injection of 1,000 mgm. of ascorbic acid. A biopsy specimen taken from the wound 10 days later showed good healing and ample intercellular substance. This observation shows that vitamin C is an important factor in the healing of a wound, but the physician must not lose sight of the fact that wound healing is dependent on many other factors.

The lesions appearing in the mouth in vitamin C deficiency are more difficult to explain. The gingiva is involved only when teeth are present, an observation that still is without explanation. Hess[168] was of the opinion that infection played a prominent rôle in the gingival lesions, but one can observe gingival signs of scurvy before infection supervenes. Certainly there is an increase in the number of capillaries present, resulting in congestion and swelling of the gums. These vessels are of poor quality and give rise to frequent hemorrhage. The intercellular substance of the tissue itself is defective, and the gingiva becomes easily infected and subsequently breaks down to become ulcerated and even gangrenous. The teeth themselves undergo much the same change as does bone, the main defect occurring in the dentine. There is resorption of normal dentine beginning along Tome's canals and formation of an inferior type of osteodentin or of pulpstone which results from metaplasia of the dentin-forming cells. The pulp becomes hyperemic and edematous, and atrophy and degeneration of the odontoblast layer follow. There is no convincing evidence that dental decay in man is due to ascorbic acid deficiency. Falling out of the teeth in ascorbic acid deficiency is the direct result of thinning of the alveolar bone such as occurs in other bones. There still is a conspicuous lack of precise knowledge as to the relationship between vitamin C and gingival and tooth disease in man.

That the petechial and ecchymotic hemorrhages of the scorbutic state occur cannot be denied. Stress plays an important rôle in their location, and such lesions are found, where a vessel rides over a bony prominence, or where a belt has been pulled tight. The integrity of the capillary wall has been studied and morphological changes are wanting. A cement substance is believed to fuse together the endothelium of the capillaries. However, connective tissue also surrounds the capillary, and very thin collagenous fibers ensheath the endothelium. It is still undecided whether the connective tissue sheath or the endothelial cement substance is affected in scurvy. The relationship of vitamin C to so-called capillary resistance is indeed a knotty problem. Crandon[161] found that, even though he had the perifollicular hemorrhages of scurvy over his legs, the positive pressure test done in the arm was negative.

With the isolation and subsequent synthesis of vitamin C came a volume of reports that the newly available vitamin would cure many of the nonscorbutic hemorrhagic diseases. All these claims have been dispelled, and it is now established that vitamin C will have a favorable effect only on the hemorrhages of scorbutic origin. Within the past twelve years much investigation has been carried out on the permeability of capillaries. Szent-Györgyi isolated a substance, which he called citrin at first and later vitamin P. He believed this new vitamin controlled capillary permeability and resistance, and that it was responsible for the petechial hemorrhages seen in scurvy, but two years later he was unable to obtain similar results. Much has been done since then, and the reports are conflicting. Recently Shanno[169] reported on the use of rutin for the treatment of increased capillary fragility. He points out that citrin or vitamin P is an impure mixture of two flavone glucosides, hesperidin and eriodictyol. These two substances he claims are physiologically inert, and that possibly the active principle in citrin was rutin. The authors have studied the relationship of abnormal capillary fragility, ascorbic acid deficiency, vitamin P and rutin for years and have not found in their studies a sufficiently clear relationship to warrant reporting their results.

In 1930 Mettier, Minot and Townsend[170] stated that anemia is found commonly in adults with chronic vitamin C deficiency. They concluded from their studies that this anemia responded specifically when orange juice was administered but did not respond to iron or purified liver extract. They showed that the erythrocytes were normocytic, normochromic or moderately macrocytic, hyperchromic in contrast to previous teachings that the cells generally were hypochromic. They found the bone marrow to be moderately hyperplastic and normoblastic prior to therapy. After orange juice was administered, they noted an increase in cellularity of the marrow due principally to an increase in normoblasts.

Since 1930 numerous observers have reported hematological studies on persons with scurvy. Much of this work seems to indicate that scurvy and anemia do not necessarily coexist, that experimental vitamin C lack does not interfere with blood formation, and that patients with naturally occurring scurvy and anemia show erythrocyte and hemoglobin regeneration while on a vitamin C-free but otherwise adequate diet. The bone marrow has been described variously as hyperplastic with normoblastic maturation arrest, as hypoplastic and as megaloblastic. In short, the inference is that vitamin C is not essential for normal hematopoiesis, and that hemorrhage, lack of iron and some unknown vitamin B complex or other deficiency state account for scorbutic anemia. The experiment of Crandon mentioned above is worthy of note, for in spite of blood loss incurred in making various blood determinations he did not develop anemia. The hemoglobin started to fall in the third month but returned to normal values following the ingestion of ferrous sulphate daily. More recently Lozner[171] has shown that iron alone caused hemoglobin regeneration in patients with vitamin C deficiency. It is interesting that Wolbach[172] found in long-continued partial vitamin C deficiency in the guinea pig that large regions of bone marrow became devoid of blood-forming cells and the seat of a deposit of amyloid-like material. He believed that the anemia associated with the scorbutic state in the guinea pig was a secondary phenomenon. No such bone marrow deposits have been found in man, however. Hence, to state it mildly, one must say the evidence in the human being is conflicting.

The recent studies of Vilter, Woolford and Spies[173] throw light on this problem. They studied carefully 19 cases of severe scurvy admitted to a large municipal hospital. Several features worthy of special emphasis are pointed out by these investigators. The general appearance of patients with severe scurvy is distinctive. Stasis cyanosis in the extremities, sallow, dirty gray, cadaveric, skin color, somnolence, lethargy and hypotension appear insidiously and are the prodromata of peripheral vascular collapse which may occur suddenly without further warning. Cheyne-Stokes type of respiration occurs particularly in patients with arteriosclerotic cerebrovascular disease and anemia. All of these vasomotor abnormalities disappear within from 24 to 36 hours after the oral or parenteral administration of adequate amounts of vitamin C. Although

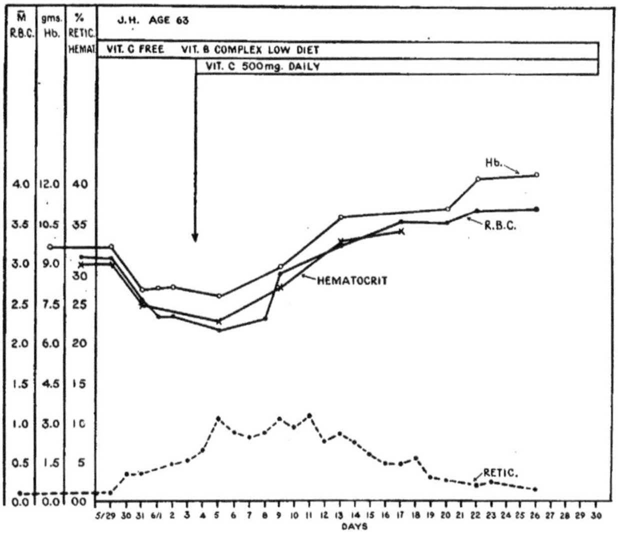

Fig. 26. Decline in erythrocytes and hemoglobin in severe scurvy as clinical course grew worse prior to vitamin C therapy (from Jour. Lab. and Clin. Med., 1946, XXXI, 609.)

the exact mechanism responsible for these changes is unknown, it should be noted that in guinea pigs and rats a direct relationship has been reported to exist between the vitamin C stored in the adrenals and the synthesis of adrenocortical steroids.

The hematological data (Fig. 26) gathered from our patients with anemia, while they are subsisting on diets very low in vitamin C and low in the vitamins of the B complex, corroborate many of the original observations of Mettier, Minot and Townsend using orange juice. Nine of the critically deficient patients either did not improve clinically or hematologically or became more anemic and debilitated on this diet. Striking hematological and clinical recovery occurred after vitamin C alone was added to the experimental régime, much the same effect previously reported for orange juice.

The authors have found other patients with mild, moderate or severe scurvy and with no anemia. In fact a normal blood picture has been found in 12 ambulatory patients with scurvy who have entered the Nutrition Clinic, Hillman Hospital. Further observations from this clinic indicate that many nutritionally deficient persons repeatedly have had negative tests for vitamin C in the plasma for as long as 5 consecutive years, and yet they did not develop clinical scurvy or anemia. The factors, which cause the development of anemia in some persons with scurvy but not in others, are not understood. Certain considerations, however, help explain this variation in patients. In the normal course of events deficiency diseases seldom occur as single entities. Deficient diets seldom are deficient in a single essential factor.

A patient with severe vitamin C depletion may have no anemia until additional strain is placed on the bone marrow by a deficiency of protein, iron or other unknown factors which may be necessary for normal hematopoiesis. Yet, after the anemia has developed, the deficiency of the latter factors may not be serious enough to prevent a remission, when large amounts of ascorbic acid are administered. In many deficient persons bed rest, which reduces metabolic requirement for all essential nutrients, may be sufficient therapy to produce a clinical and hematological remission. Depending on the interplay of multiple factors, morphological differences in blood and bone marrow and varied therapeutic responses may occur readily in patients with scurvy and other deficiency states. For these reasons observations on patients, who were critically ill with scurvy, anemia and other deficiency diseases of long-standing, cannot be compared satisfactorily with data on human subjects in whom a single deficiency state, scurvy, has been produced experimentally without the occurrence of anemia.

Symptomatology

As for its pathological physiology the symptomatology of vitamin C deficiency may be described by a summary of the symptoms of scurvy. Scurvy is encountered most frequently in the very young and the very old, but no sex, race or age group is exempt. There are certain points of difference in the scurvy seen in the young infant and that seen in the adult. For sake of clarity, therefore, an arbitrary distinction is made, and the symptomatology of these two age groups is discussed separately. The etiology and general pathology are the same, however, the manifestations in the one instance occurring in immature, rapidly growing tissue and in the other instance in mature, slow growing tissue.

Infantile Scurvy

The classical picture of acute, florid, infantile scurvy is the most widely known variety; yet it is a picture we should not allow to be seen today. In this neglected, almost terminal state the child cries out as its bed is approached. The afflicted infant lies motionless on its back with one or both thighs everted and flexed on the abdomen. The thighs are swollen and severely tender. To touch the child anywhere results in a cry of both pain and horror. This type presents a striking picture and is not easily forgotten. This form of scurvy is not the most common, nor is the practicing physician likely to see it. The most common form of the disease generally is encountered in the last half of the first year. The mother's presenting complaint may be that her child is not gaining weight properly, or that he is unusually irritable or lethargic and does not eat well. The infant appears pale and sallow, and the only physical abnormality may be very questionable tenderness over the distal end of the femur. The diagnosis of scurvy in this instance usually is based on the response to specific therapy. This is the so-called latent form of scurvy. If treatment is not instituted, manifest scurvy develops. Beading of the ribs may occur and thus complicate the picture by suggesting a diagnosis of rickets. However, vitamin D fails to correct the defect. Later, subperiosteal hemorrhages may result from trauma so trivial as not to be remembered. Such hemorrhages may occur in the adult, but it is a rare finding. The resultant swellings are very tender and usually will involve the lower end of the femur and the proximal end of the tibia, although they may involve other bones. Such hemorrhages are seen easily in the x-ray. In addition to subperiosteal hemorrhages there may be hemorrhages into the soft tissue. The hair follicles and sweat glands are particularly susceptible. Again stress is an important factor in the location of these petechiae and ecchymoses. In many instances the diaper is responsible for the production of such lesions on the inner aspect of the thigh. Gross hemorrhage may occur elsewhere as the disease progresses, giving rise to epistaxis, hemoptysis, bloody diarrhea and occasionally, hemothorax. When such hemorrhages occur in abdominal organs or in the brain, confusing and alarming symptoms ensue.

The lesions of the gums may be so mild initially as to be overlooked. They are seen only when teeth are present. The gums show a very mild, peridental hemorrhage or merely a border of increased redness about the tooth. Later the gums become swollen and purple, and as progression occurs, infection is added, and the ulcerated, fetid gum of the acute case is seen.

In addition, the infant may present early slight elevations of temperature, which become more marked as the disease continues. A similar slight increase in the respiratory rate may occur as a result of mild pain on motion of the costochondral junctions. The respiration thus may be shallow and more rapid than normal.

Adult Scurvy

The initial symptoms of vitamin C deficiency in the adult are as ill-defined as they are in the child. After a long period of deficiency of vitamin C, the adult will develop symptoms of lassitude, irritability, easy fatigability and insidious weight loss. Vague aches and pains in the muscles and about the joints appear so as to stimulate "rheumatism". The face is pale and sometimes bloated, the skin being a dirty gray, ashen color. There may be hypotension and stasis cyanosis.

In the absence of adequate therapy the symptoms and signs become more marked. The muscle and joint pains become severe and are the result of hemorrhage into and around these structures. Large ecchymoses are frequent, and their color varies greatly. The more recent ones are red, while the older ones are blue, brown or green. In addition, the well known perifollicular petechiae become evident. Again these symptoms and signs are dependent on stress and lines of force. The petechial hemorrhages may occur almost anywhere in the skin but are more common over the lower extremities. Subungual hemorrhages and splinter hemorrhages may occur. Gross hemorrhage may result in epistaxis and other manifestations as listed under infantile scurvy. Subconjunctional hemorrhages are seen occasionally.

The gum lesions follow the same pattern as in infantile scurvy. In some instances the gums become so swollen and congested as to cover the teeth completely, thereby making mastication a very painful procedure. The teeth become loose and eventually may fall out.

Anemia is not uncommon in adult scurvy, and the complaints referable to this state are the same as for any normocytic anemia. The palpitation, dyspnea and cardiac dilatation, sometimes seen, are most likely the result of the lowered erythrocyte count and consequent anoxemia.

As one follows the sequence of events from early to late scurvy, it becomes apparent that a correct and early diagnosis is very important in view of the fact that the disorder is not self-limited and that we possess specific remedies for it. The diagnosis may be difficult for those who have gleaned their information merely from the textbooks. Some persons with scurvy have been treated again and again for rheumatism. Surgeons must be alert for signs of ascorbic acid deficiency when they perform an operation for "bone tumor" or "osteomyelitis". If the treatment is inadequate, the cure may be incomplete, and the disease persist for years. At best it probably takes months or years before the tissues return to anything like their normal state after treatment.

Diagnosis

The diagnosis of vitamin C deficiency in the form of manifest scurvy in the adult or in the infant is not difficult for the well trained physician. A careful physical examination and a history of an inadequate intake of vitamin C aid in making a tentative diagnosis, and x-ray and certain laboratory tests may add confirmatory evidence.

The fundamental hemorrhagic tendency, which results from loss of tensile strength of connective tissue because of alteration in, or lack of, intercellular substance, may appear in any part of the body. Hemorrhages are most likely to occur at sites of stress due to injury, motion, growth or infection. Hemorrhages of the gums are common and painful. In the extremities, where capillary pressure is high, and at the site of the hair follicles petechiae may appear. Ecchymoses are common. Hemorrhages may occur at the joints and cause considerable pain. This may result in hyperesthesia on motion, which in infants causes fretfulness and a motionless, frog-like position of the lower limbs. In the brain, intestine or kidney gross or microscopical hemorrhages may occur.

Skeletal lesions lead to diagnostic x-ray findings. In the infant or child such lesions are likely to occur at the growing costochondral junctions and at the ends of the long bones causing a characteristic shelf-like costochondral beading. The x-ray shows a zone of diminished density which is known as the scorbutic lattice. The defective calcification at this zone predisposes to fracture with subperiosteal hemorrhage and slipping of the epiphysis. Cessation of growth allows an intensification of calcification at the zone of preparatory calcification at the epiphyseal ends of the long bones and at the periphery of the epiphyseal centers of ossification. In the x-rays these appear as "the white lines of Frankel" Eventually thinning of the cortex and trabeculae of the shaft gives the bones a "ground glass" appearance in the x-ray. In the infant or in the adult these clinical or x-ray signs of scurvy become apparent only after some three months or more on a deficient diet.

Some physicians are misinformed as to the value of laboratory tests in making a diagnosis of scurvy as an evidence of vitamin deficiency. Among investigators there is considerable difference of opinion as to the value of the urinary excretion test and the measurement of the whole blood or plasma levels of ascorbic acid in determining the state of ascorbic acid nutrition. The authors use these laboratory tests only to gain more information, never to make a diagnosis. It is certain, however, that the tissues are not adequately filled with vitamin C for months before clinical evidence of scurvy appears. Following the administration of a parenteral test dose of ascorbic acid normal persons excrete approximately 80 per cent. of the total 24 hour excretion during the first 3 to 5 hours, whereas persons deficient in ascorbic acid excrete much less. Youmans[174] is of the opinion that plasma values below 0.4 mgm. per 100 c.c. represent a state of deficiency in which clinical signs may appear. Crandon, Lund and Dill[175] found that low or even zero findings may not be critically dangerous unless maintained over a long period of time. We have observed patients who have had zero values for over 5 years without the appearance of a diagnostic lesion of scurvy. Nevertheless we are of the opinion that important information in respect to vitamin C metabolism can be gained by determination of the ascorbic acid content of the plasma. Harris, Hickman, Jensen and Spies[176] have conducted extensive studies on normal persons and on patients in the Nutrition Clinic in Birmingham. They found that the ascorbic acid of the plasma of the patients was 51 per cent. of that of the normal persons. The authors believe that a level of ascorbic acid below 0.4 mgm. per 100 c.c. indicates that the reserve supply of ascorbic acid is at a danger point, that levels of from 0.4 to 0.7 mgm. per 100 c.c. indicate that the reserve supply is low, and that values ranging from 0.7 to 1.2 mgm. per 100 c.c. indicate an adequate reserve supply.

A positive capillary resistance test suggests a depletion of vitamin C, but false positives frequently occur in the presence of severe anemia or blood dyscrasia. Even in severe scurvy a negative capillary test sometimes occurs so that this test, in itself, cannot be considered as diagnostic of scurvy.

If a diagnosis of scurvy is in doubt, a therapeutic test is recommended; 250 mgm. of ascorbic acid should be administered parenterally, while the patient is kept on his usual routine. Then, he should be watched carefully for any alteration of symptoms.

Prevention and Treatment

That fresh fruits and vegetables are of great value in the protection against, and in the cure of, vitamin C deficiency is every day knowledge. Vitamin C is present in all living tissue, but fresh fruits and plants are the best sources (Fig. 27). Rose hips, haws, currants, strawberries, cabbage, tomatoes and the citrus fruits are the richest sources. Potatoes, spinach and turnips are good sources. Many people depend on the potato for their quota of ascorbic acid by eating it daily in large amounts. One half pound of potatoes supplies about 30 mgm. of ascorbic acid, an amount which is considered adequate to protect against scurvy. The amount of vitamin C in fresh fruits or vegetables varies widely depending on maturity, time of picking, variety, season and soil.

Beginning in the second week of life the infant should be given 1 to 2 teaspoons of fresh orange juice daily or 25 mgm. of ascorbic acid. The amount should be increased to 2 ounces by the time the child is 3 months of age and to 3 ounces by the age of 5 months. Other citrus fruits may be substituted for oranges, but when tomato juice is used, large amounts should be given. If fruit juices are not tolerated, 25 to 50 mgm. of ascorbic acid should be given daily. At least 3 ounces of orange juice, comparable amounts of citrus fruits or tomato juice or 50 to 100 mgm. of ascorbic acid should be taken daily by the average adult. Larger amounts of these materials are indicated during pregnancy and lactation.

Scurvy which is due to vitamin C deficiency may be treated by administering ascorbic acid orally or by injection. Parenteral administration is about twice as effective per unit of weight as is oral administration and is indicated always in stupor or coma, or where there is difficulty in absorption from the alimentary tract. Ascorbic acid is readily soluble and may be added to sterile saline solution or to 5 per cent. glucose solution. Because it is too strong an acid to be injected intramuscularly, sodium bicarbonate should be added as a neutralizing agent to solutions for intramuscular injection. For intravenous injections neutralization is unnecessary. It should be mentioned that ascorbic acid is excreted more rapidly following intravenous than intramuscular injection. Ascorbic

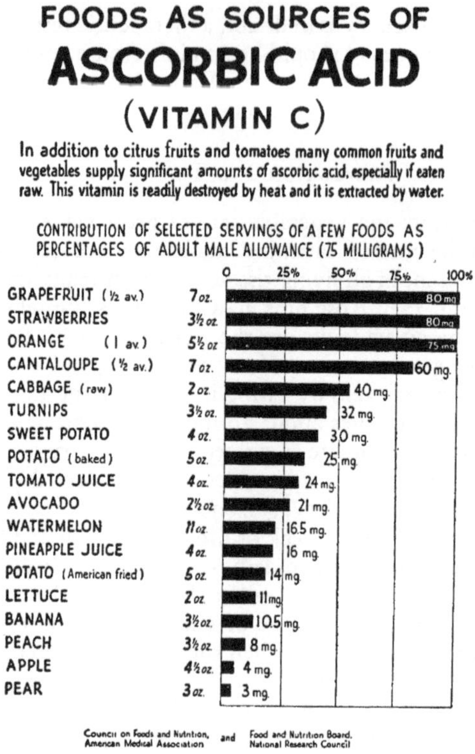

FIG. 27. Foods as sources of ascorbic acid (Vitamin C).

acid has a very low toxicity. The authors frequently have injected 1,000 mgm. or given 5,000 mgm. by mouth without any ill effects. It is very important to continue intensive therapy until all the lesions are healed and then give a daily maintenance dose of 50 to 100 mgm. orally.

It should be emphasized that the present knowledge is so meager that a precise statement of what constitutes proper dosage is not practicable. Since vitamin C deficiency is frequently a part of mixed deficiency diseases, it is not enough to insure an adequate intake of vitamin C alone. In Figure 28, showing the contrast between the nutrients supplied by dietaries of children with deficiency diseases and the allowance recommended, the degree of deficiency of other essential nutrients which remain after the deficiency of vitamin C is shown clearly.

The other vitamin deficiencies associated with many cases of scurvy should be searched for and treated. An excellent diet should be given always, and additional specific therapy should be given also and continued until all evidence of vitamin C deficiency has disappeared. When

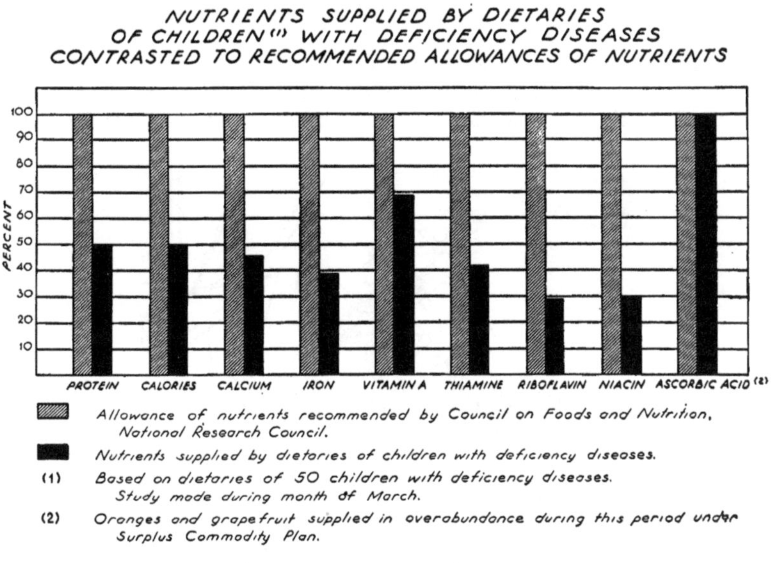

Fig. 28. Nutrients supplied by dietaries of children with deficiency diseases contrasted to recommended allowances of nutrients.

gingivitis is present, mouth washes should be prescribed, and splints for the legs should be applied when indicated.

The response to adequate therapy with ascorbic acid is dramatic. Bone tenderness decreases, purpura begins to fade, gums improve, appetite increases and loss of apprehension occurs within 24 hours after sufficient amounts are administered by the parenteral route. A similar striking improvement follows adequate oral therapy. The general treatment should be directed toward restoring the patient to a state of perfect nutrition.

VITAMIN B_1
(THIAMINE)

History

The modern era of the study of vitamin B_1 was initiated by Eijkman[177], who induced polyneuritic symptoms in fowls fed a diet of polished rice. When they were fed unpolished rice, they did not develop the disease, and rice polishings relieved the afflicted birds. Grijns[178] concluded that human beriberi and avian polyneuritis resulted from a lack of the same substances in the rice bran, but physicians and other scientists still were not impressed. It was not until Fletcher[179] and Fraser and Stanton[180] established the fact that unpolished grain would aid in pre-

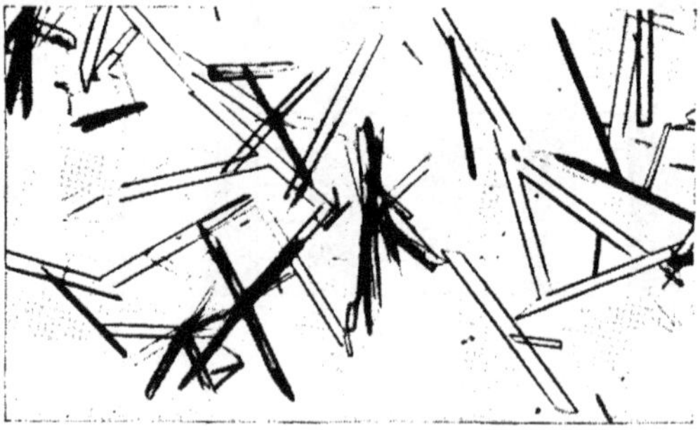

Fig. 29. Crystalline thiamine chloride hydrochloride (courtesy of Merck and Co.)

venting beriberi that serious consideration was given to these theories. Funk[181] made a concentrate of the active principle in rice polishings and thought he had isolated the antiberiberi vitamin. His coinage of the word "vitamine" was very fortunate in that it caught the imagination of many for the first time. In 1913 Vedder and Williams[182] concentrated the factor from rice polishings and showed that it was dialyzable and absorbed it on charcoal. Seidell[183] made the important contribution that it could be adsorbed on fuller's earth and removed with alkali, and Peters[184] introduced still more refinements. A milestone in the isolation was passed in 1926 when Jansen and Donath[185] successfully isolated the pure vitamin for the first time. The final word in the chapter was written brilliantly by Williams and his school[186] when they synthesized the vitamin in 1936. Throughout the scientific world the names of Takaki,

Eijkman, Funk, Vedder, Grijns, Williams, Peters, Cline, Westenbrink, Jansen, Seidell, Sinclair, Waterman and many others are held in reverent esteem as contributors of important knowledge of vitamin B$_1$.

Chemistry and Physiology

Vitamin B$_1$ (thiamine) is a white crystalline compound (Fig. 29) which is prepared synthetically as the hydrochloride (Fig. 30). The properties of the natural and the synthetic compound are identical. The

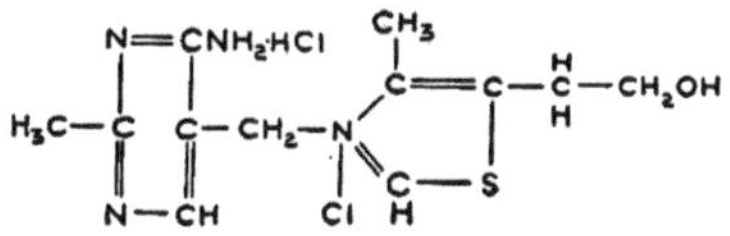

Fig. 30. Structural formula of thiamine chloride hydrochloride.

hydrochloride melts at 248 to 250° C. and is very soluble in water. It is stable at 100° C. in acid solution but is destroyed at 100° C. in neutral or alkaline solution.

Vitamin B$_1$ is important in tissue oxidation of carbohydrate compounds. Apparently it acts as a compound capable of reversing oxidation and reduction. Vitamin B$_1$ represents the reduced form and can be oxidized to a disulfide, the oxidation occurring under physiological con-

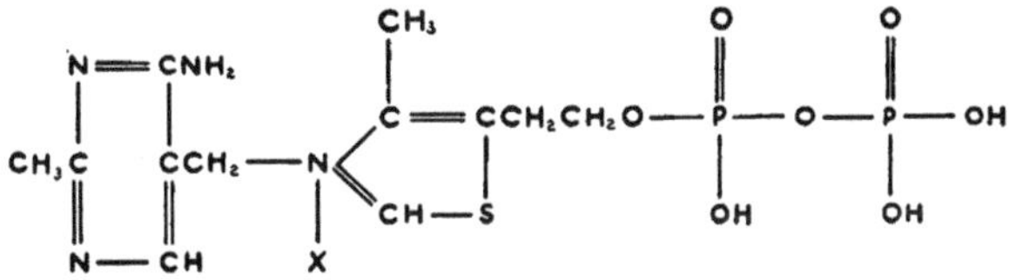

PHOSPHORIC ACID ESTER OF THIAMINE (COCARBOXYLASE)

Fig. 31. Structural formula of phosphoric acid ester of thiamine (cocarboxylase).

ditions. The disulfide shows full vitamin activity. The disulfide can be reduced to the thiol form by hydrogen, hydrogen sulfide, glutathione and other substances.

Yeast contains a specific catalyst called carboxylase, which decarboxylates pyruvic acid as is shown below.

$$CH_3.CO.\ COOH \xrightarrow{\text{Vitamin } B_1\text{–pyrophosphate}} CH_3.\ CHO + CO_2$$

The coenzyme of this reaction is the phosphoric acid enzyme of thiamine, cocarboxylase. It has been synthesized enzymatically and by chemical methods, and Lohman and Schuster[187] proved that it was the pyrophosphate of vitamin B_1. The action of vitamin B_1 in the body is due partly or mainly to the action of cocarboxylase (Fig. 31). The liver transforms much of the vitamin B_1 into cocarboxylase, and it also can hydrolyze cocarboxylase to form vitamin B_1. The kidney phosphorylates thiamine.

It appears then that vitamin B_1 in the body acts as an acceptor for such substances as adenosin-triphosphoric acid. The carboxylase system consists of a specific protein and the coenzyme, the cocarboxylase, and the metal ions. Manganese, magnesium and iron are stimulants, and zinc, calcium, nickel and cobalt retard in small concentration. Presumably the metal element in the enzyme acts as a cement substance binding protein to cocarboxylase. The chemical reactions of cocarboxylase resemble closely those of vitamin B_1. The molecular weight of the protein particle of cocarboxylase is not known, but it is estimated to be 150,000. The vitamin action occurs as a result of the specific structure of the molecule. The different salts of the vitamin have a corresponding activity. Structural alterations are followed by a disappearance of vitamin actions. The pyrimidine ring, the thiazole ring and the methylene bridge between them, an unsubstituted amino-group in 4-position of the pyrimidine ring, the 5-hydroxy-alkyl-group and free 2-4-position in the thiazole nucleus are necessary for the vitamin action.

Vitamin B_1 is widely distributed in raw foodstuffs. The richest sources are whole cereals, yeast and pork. Yet even these foods do not contain a great abundance of the vitamin. During the preparation of food for consumption much of the vitamin is lost. Heat destroys some, and since the vitamin is water-soluble, considerable is lost in discarding the water in which food is cooked. Discarding the bones of meat and the peelings and cores of fruit also accounts for some of the loss which occurs during the preparation of food. Vegetables are not rich in thiamine, but they are important sources because they are inexpensive. In the average diet approximately 25 per cent. of the total thiamine is obtained from cereals or cereal products. Unenriched white flour contains little thiamine as contrasted with whole wheat flour, only about one-tenth of the amount originally present in the whole wheat. Legumes, nuts, sugar cane, molasses and whole cornmeal are all rich in vitamin B_1.

Man cannot synthesize thiamine, nor can he store it to any great degree. The highest concentration is in the liver, kidney, heart and brain. The greater part of the total body store is in the liver and muscles. On a diet deficient in thiamine the amount stored declines rapidly at first, then more slowly, and the last traces are held most persistently. Much work is being done on the excretion of thiamine, and there is a great need to know more of its distribution in tissues.

An excess intake of thiamine is wasted chiefly by excretion from, or destruction in, the body. Only a small percentage of the intake from a diet rich in vitamin B_1 is excreted in the urine, but the kidney concentrates it from the plasma to a marked degree, twenty times or more. The fecal output is relatively small but fairly constant. At the present time our knowledge of the importance of thiamine excretion in the sweat rests on evidence too slender to be interpreted. We can be certain that in human beings and in animals the total amount excreted decreases with restriction of the vitamin in the diet.

Platt and Lu[188] have shown that the bisulfite-binding power of the blood is increased in human beings with thiamine deficiency. This determination is not entirely specific for pyruvic acid, since any aldehyde or ketone group also would give positive tests. Nevertheless, in vitamin B_1 deficiency a part of the bisulfite-binding substance has been identified definitely as pyruvic acid. In addition to lactic acid, methyl glyoxal has been found in the blood of persons with beriberi. Glyoxal is pyruvic aldehyde and is a stage of oxidation of the terminal carbon atom, whereas lactic acid is the result of incomplete oxidation of the central carbon atom.

Lewy, Spies and Aring[189] gave by injection 50 mgm. of synthetic cocarboxylase to patients with nutritional peripheral neuritis and observed that the under-excitable nerve-muscle apparatus was restored to normal excitability within one to four hours. This finding indicates that a great number of the nerve fibers were anatomically intact, although they were unable to respond properly due to the altered metabolism. In all the patients, who received only a single injection, and who continued to eat a diet deficient in thiamine, the nerve-muscle mechanism returned to its poorly functioning state within a few days. Another injection of either cocarboxylase or thiamine again relieved these patients. The more severely affected muscles remained underexcitable following a single injection, which probably means that too many of their fibers were morphologically damaged to permit prompt restoration of function. These observations support the concept that the early stage of the clinical deficiency state is characterized by a biochemical rather than an anatomical lesion. These investigators studied the thiamine excretion in the urine of these patients. It was learned that the patients retained much more of the injected cocarboxylase than did the normal controls. The bisulfite-binding substance decreased in the patients, who retained the cocarboxylase, and the same patients showed electrical and clinical improvement, which suggests an association between these factors. It may be well to stress that the degree of neuropathy seen in the south of the United States, where Lewy, Spies and Aring were working, cannot be compared to the severe forms of neuropathy seen in many clinics in association with long-standing and heavy addiction to alcohol.

Vitamin B_1 plays an important part in carbohydrate metabolism. Glucose is not oxidized directly in the body but is transformed into CO_2 and H_2O in a number of stages. Two of the intermediate products are lactic acid and pyruvic acid. It is thought that vitamin B_1 in its phosphorylated form, cocarboxylase, acts as a specific catalyst in breaking down pyruvic acid. Pyruvic acid and lactic acid are increased in the blood and in the urine of vitamin B_1 deficient patients and animals. Peters[190] has shown that the brains and kidneys of avitaminotic pigeons have a diminished oxygen uptake. Himwich, Spies, Fazekas and Nesin[191] have shown that the neurological lesions probably are due to an inability of the vitamin B_1 deficient patient to oxidize glucose efficiently. These investigators were concerned about the cerebral metabolism of patients who had pellagra with or without clinical vitamin B_1 deficiency. They reasoned that because the brain oxidized carbohydrate chiefly, any alteration in carbohydrate metabolism resulting from a deficiency of thiamine should be observed more readily in the brain than in any other organ which was capable of oxidizing fat as well as carbohydrate. The carbohydrate metabolism was studied by measuring the differences between the oxygen, glucose and lactic acid of the arterial blood and that of the internal jugular vein. They found that the average oxygen utilization for the pellagrin free of any evidence of clinical thiamine deficiency was 6.16 volumes per cent. The average for those pellagrins with clinical thiamine deficiency was 4.6 volumes per cent. The average for the entire group was 5.8 volumes per cent. The normal subjects had excellent health with no evidence of pellagra, beriberi or any deficiency, and they had a value of 7.4 volumes per cent. It seemed that a diminution of brain metabolism would best explain these findings. Correlated with this diminished oxygen uptake is the average glucose utilization of 6 mgm. per 100 c.c. No difference in utilization of lactic acid was noted between arterial and venous blood going to, and coming from, the brain. These observations afford a basis for the explanation of the mental changes observed in patients subsisting on an unbalanced high carbohydrate diet.

It is known that vitamin B_1 is essential for the normal functioning of the alimentary tract, but as yet we do not understand the exact mechanism by which it functions in predisposing to gastrointestinal disturbances. In experimental animals and in human beings anorexia, which is an early symptom of a deficiency of thiamine, disappears promptly following the administration of thiamine. Both the thiamine deficient animal and man, following the administration of thiamine, will eat food which they previously have refused. Controlled studies with thiamine have shown that the normal tone of the alimentary tract is altered in persons with thiamine deficiency. It has been observed that persons with early thiamine deficiency usually have little appetite and often are constipated. Gastrointestinal series frequently show "puddling" of the barium in the small intestine. Some of these persons improve impressively following the administration of vitamin B_1. It is certain, however, that neither lack of appetite nor constipation are in any way specific manifestations of vitamin B_1 deficiency in human beings. The breakdown in metabolism is primary and has a widespread effect on all the cells, and the effects are not equally distributed in the body. Eventually this failure to metabolize nutrients by the tissue cells halts many processes, and we then find loss of appetite while, as Peters graphically states, there is internal hunger in the tissues.

Vitamin B_1 is an essential factor for the normal growth of the young and for the maintenance of normal health for the adult. It is particularly important, however, for the physician to realize that several factors operate concomitantly and that thiamine alone is not adequate to insure proper growth. Vitamin B_1 deficiency often is associated with loss of libido in human beings and experimental animals. There is a great need for vitamin B_1 during pregnancy and lactation. The vomiting of pregnancy is common, and this in itself may be associated with a deficiency of vitamin B_1, or it may lead to further vitamin B_1 deficiency. Mothers, who have vitamin B_1 deficiency, predispose their nursing infants to thiamine deficiency.

Pathological Physiology

Vitamin B_1 deficiency affects the cardiovascular system, and the most common cause of sudden death from thiamine deficiency is acute cardiac failure. The heart is dilated and enlarged in the classical case.

It is of great interest that experimental deficiencies rarely result in serous effusions and cardiac enlargement, whereas in human beings they are not uncommon in the acute case of beriberi. There is little doubt that cases of beriberi disease and cases of serous effusion have developed on a diet low in thiamine and that the administration of thiamine will relieve the symptoms. Still, investigators have been unable to place this on an experimental basis whereby the experimental subject eats a vitamin B_1 deficiency diet and an inevitable sequence of cardiovascular disturbances occurs.

The lesions of experimental vitamin B_1 deficiency appear identical with those occurring in vitamin B_1 deficiency in man, and the majority of investigators regard experimental vitamin B_1 deficiency in animals as a disease analogous to this deficiency in man. Degeneration of the nervous system occurs in most, if not all, species with prolonged thiamine deficiency. Experimental polyneuritis in fowls is very similar to dry beriberi in man, most of the degeneration occurring in the peripheral nerves. The sciatic nerves are especially involved. Vedder and Clark[192] have shown that in both man and animals there is evidence of involvement of every fiber, although the extent of degeneration is tremendously variable in the fibers of the same nerves. The myelin degeneration may affect the peripheral nerves, the ventral and dorsal nerve roots and the tracts of the spinal cord, the medulla, pons, midbrain and the internal capsule.

Symptomatology

Various clinical forms of vitamin B_1 deficiency are described. Each case, however, presents great individual variations. In the adult the onset usually is insidious. The symptoms are characterized by cardiovascular disturbances, neuritis and edema, and these forms sometimes are termed "cardiac," "neuritic" or "wet" according to the prevailing symptoms.

The clinical picture is one of symmetrical peripheral neuritis, which is the most common finding and is associated with weakness, cramps in the legs and paresthesias and burning sensations over the soles, dorsum of the foot and ankle. The Achilles and patellar reflexes in the typical case are hyperactive early in the disease and later are absent. The weakness spreads up the legs, and the affected muscles become tender and numb. Atrophy of the muscles and skin follows. (Fig. 32) The upper extremities frequently become involved in the very severe cases, the hands and arms being affected first. Burning, numbness and weakness may be followed by wrist drop. The muscles of the trunk and diaphragm may become involved. When edema is present, it begins in the feet and legs and ascends up the body and may mask the muscle wasting. Anorexia, diarrhea and vomiting may be associated with it. Aphonia sometimes is seen in the adult, and in infantile vitamin B_1 deficiency it is a common finding.

Although severe mental symptoms usually do not develop, memory difficulties and anxiety states are common and frequently are distressing

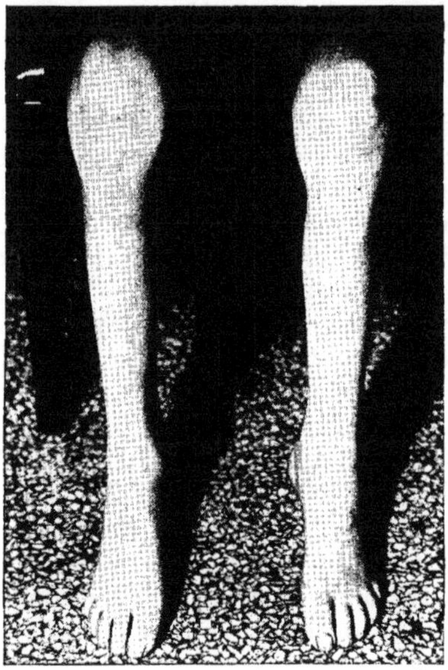

Fig. 32. Bilateral marked atrophy of muscles of leg and feet; foot drop is evident. Case of vitamin B_1 deficiency.

to the patient and his relatives. Investigators[193] have learned that there is an amazing uniformity of the mental symptoms which have little connection with the personality. The symptoms may be grouped as follows:

A. The Elementary Syndrome:
   1. Psycho-sensory disturbances
   2. Psycho-motor disturbances
   3. Emotional disturbances
B. General Symptoms of the Central Nervous System:
   1. Weakness and increased fatigability
   2. Sleeplessness
   3. Headache

The first group of symptoms resembles those which may be found in diseases of the basal ganglia and thalamus, while the second group represents general symptoms which usually accompany any disturbance of the central nervous system. The complaints and responses to therapy are practically identical, whether the personality is simple or complicated, or whether the patient is illiterate or educated. Often there is a "breakdown of personality" during the early stages of developing deficiency.

Detailed studies[194] of the emotional disturbances in persons with vitamin B_1 deficiency confirmed the findings that, in addition to the disturbed emotional reactions, there was some impairment of the intellectual and cognitive functions. Patients "jumped at the slightest sound" or "cried over the least little thing". No alteration in the electroencephalograms has been demonstrated despite the fact that within a short time after the injection of thiamine the symptoms subsided. Injections of saline given in a similar manner did not produce any relief. These emotional symptoms may occur in patients without deficiency disease, however, and the authors recommend thiamine therapy only when such symptoms are associated with a deficiency state.

Cardiovascular symptoms frequently are associated with fulminating acute types of thiamine deficiency known as "acute pernicious beriberi heart". If associated with edema it is called "wet" beriberi. Many patients die suddenly from "beriberi heart". The original cases described by Wenckenbach and other clinicians in the Orient are characterized chiefly by right-sided failure. Weiss and Wilkins[195] and the clinicians at the University of Cincinnati have examined a considerable number of patients with beriberi heart disease, and the majority did not have right-sided failure.

Infantile vitamin B_1 deficiency usually occurs among infants in the first three months of life, and the onset is rapid. The very early symptoms usually are vomiting and a distaste for food. Attacks of pain frequently occur and result in the body's being held rigid although true convulsions do not appear. The baby frets, is constipated and often has edema, considerable enlargement of the heart and cyanosis. The blood pressure is low, the liver enlarged and the pulse rapid and irregular. This form of the disease occurs chiefly in breast-fed infants whose mothers have a highly deficient diet. Unless they are treated promptly, death occurs within a day or so.

Diagnosis

Until a simple, specific, laboratory test becomes available, a tentative diagnosis must depend upon the interpretation of a reliable medical and dietary history and a careful physical examination. It is helpful to the physician to bear in mind that vitamin B_1 deficiency occurs chiefly among the following groups:

1. The indigent and persons who have erroneous dietary habits and idiosyncrasies. Such persons often subsist on a diet relatively abundant in overmilled rice, wheat or corn. Their diets rarely contain lean meat, eggs, milk, fish, fresh fruits or vegetables in sufficient amounts.
2. Persons who have any organic disease that may interfere with the ingestion or absorption of an adequate diet, the deficiency or metabolic diseases such as pellagra, pernicious anemia, sprue, alcoholic neuritis, Korsakoff's psychosis, diabetes and myxedema. Vitamin B_1 deficiency frequently is found in association with pregnancy and lactation, hunger edema, chronic colitis and cachexia from any cause. Thiamine deficiency also is found frequently in association with diarrhea from any cause. There is great danger of the physician's not recognizing isolated cases as true thiamine deficiency.
3. Persons in whom the vitamin B_1 requirement is distinctly above the average because of growth, pregnancy and lactation, hard physical exertion, hyperthyroidism and fevers.

A diagnosis of uncomplicated thiamine deficiency can be made by excluding all other causes of peripheral neuritis, organic heart disease, edema and psycho-neurosis. The mild case is much more common than acute case, but it may be recognized only with difficulty. Keeping in mind the following points noted by Vedder[196] is helpful in making an early diagnosis of the disease:

1. Slight pressure over the muscles of the calf causes pain.
2. Patients with beriberi often have areas of anesthesia over the anterior surface of the tibia.
3. Any modification of the patellar reflexes is suspicious.
4. If a patient with beriberi squats upon his heels after the Oriental manner of sitting, he may experience pain and inability to rise without using his hands.

In making a diagnosis of cardiovascular disturbances due to thiamine deficiency the big problem is to rule out heart disease of another etiology. The studies at the University of Cincinnati should be very helpful in this respect. Blankenhorn, Vilter, Scheinker and Austin[197] have pointed out that the clinical picture of the failing heart with exceedingly rapid circulation is not likely to be overlooked, and such cases are more readily remembered than the less dramatic cases. The first thought of thiamine deficiency in this type of heart disease is when the physician realizes that the etiological nature of the heart condition is obscure. The elimination of coronary arteriosclerosis as a cause is difficult. If the patient has no angina or precordial oppression, no fever, no leukocytosis, one is a little less likely to think of coronary disease or Fieldler's isolated myocarditis. Since Williams, Mason and Smith[198] and Williams, Mason Power and Wilder[199], after inducing thiamine deficiency in man, suggest that three months is about the development time of thiamine deficiency, Blankenhorn and his associates arbitrarily selected that point to aid in the evaluation of the clinical problem. Williams, Mason and Smith observed electrocardiographic changes which they induced in subjects on thiamine deficient diets and abolished by thiamine administration. Physicians in the field of nutrition, however, find that the electrocardiographic findings are non-specific, although they may aid in the final diagnosis.

Heart disease caused by thiamine deficiency is uncommon in America, but it does occur, and it is curable. The first suggestion that the heart disease may be the result of a deficiency of thiamine may come from one of a number of sources, and the value of correlating the information obtained by the physician, the roentgenologist and the nutritionist cannot be overstressed. The vivid description by Wenckenbach[200] of the acute pernicious type of heart failure, which is a valuable aid in making a diagnosis, may be summarized as follows:

1. Enlargement of the heart by percussion, auscultation and x-ray examination.
2. The presence of murmurs, chiefly systolic but also presystolic with a resonant first sound. The murmurs are increased disproportionately by exercise.
3. Visible and palpable throbbing pulsations over the heart, best felt just to the left of the sternum.
4. Bounding pulse and thrill over the great arteries.
5. Over-distended neck and arm veins and without exception a painful, swollen liver. In the most severe cases, liver pulsation.

A patient with the more common type of heart failure due to vitamin B_1 deficiency resembles any other case with degenerative heart disease. Usually, however, it is associated with edema and serous effusions.

Prevention and Treatment

The Council on Foods and Nutrition of the National Research Council has made recommendations in regard to man's requirements for the various dietary factors necessary for normal physiological function. In the chapter on riboflavin the table of the allowances for the various vitamins, including vitamin B_1, is shown. Beriberi and subclinical thiamine deficiency can be decreased greatly by the application of the following principles which will go far toward supplying these recommended allowances:

1. Fresh foods such as potatoes, native vegetables, pork, liver, eggs, milk, fruits, beans and whole grain cereals should be included in the diet whenever possible.
2. Since vitamin B_1 is water-soluble, a large amount of it is lost, when water, in which foods are cooked, is thrown away. It is recommended that the water, in which foods are cooked, be used for broths and gravies. Whole grain, barley or other grains, which are rich in thiamine, may be added to broths to afford additional protection.
3. The use of undermilled or enriched flour, cereals and cereal products is the greatest single improvement that can be made in the diet of the average person in respect to his thiamine intake, and their use should be universal. This is true particularly in low cost diets in which a preponderance of cereal foods is included necessarily because of their relatively low cost.
4. Persons chronically addicted to alcohol and persons with sprue, pellagra, pernicious anemia, colitis, diabetes mellitus, tuberculosis, senility, malignancy, cirrhosis and many other diseases are prone to develop thiamine deficiency. The incidence is high in persons with chronic debilitating diseases and increased metabolism. Accordingly, particular attention should be directed toward making the diet of such persons adequate.
5. The diets of pregnant and lactating women should be especially rich in vitamin B_1. Whenever there is any doubt as to the adequacy or utilization of food either in the mother or in the child, supplements should be given. The supplements should be continued until the proper diet is assured. The nursing mother should receive at least 5 mgm. of thiamine or its equivalent daily; the infant should receive 0.5 mgm. or its equivalent daily.

6. In persons with fever, severe gastrointestinal symptoms, hyperthyroidism and other conditions the requirement for vitamin B_1 may be distinctly above the average. It is essential for the physician to prescribe amounts above the average for such persons. For such a maintenance dose the authors suggest 5 mgm. to 10 mgm. of synthetic thiamine daily or its equivalent except when the patient is unable to absorb from the gastrointestinal tract. In such instances it is essential that vitamin B_1 be given parenterally in order to protect the person from a deficiency of this vitamin.

In the treatment of thiamine deficiency the problem is simply one of administering adequate amounts of thiamine in the way in which it can be utilized. In the adult and infant the physician should direct therapy along three lines:

1. There should be elimination of conditions causing excessive requirement for vitamin B_1 whenever possible.
2. Synthetic thiamine or its equivalent should be administered in amounts sufficient to correct the deficiency.
3. There should be symptomatic treatment and treatment for coexisting diseases.

The essence of successful treatment lies in the administration of adequate amounts of foods rich in thiamine, supplemented with large amounts of a specific therapeutic agent. The diet should contain liberal amounts of liver, pork, lean meats, eggs, whole grain or enriched bread and cereals, beans, peas and native vegetables and fruits. It should be supplemented with the following curative therapeutic substances; 6 ounces of dried brewers' yeast daily, 6 ounces of wheat germ daily or 10 mgm. of synthetic thiamine twice daily. In cases of severe thiamine deficiency even larger doses of synthetic thiamine may be indicated. In such cases it seems wise to administer 10 to 20 mgm. twice daily until the signs of thiamine deficiency have disappeared. In cases of mild deficiency doses of 10 mgm. daily are adequate. There is no question, but that the oral administration of thiamine in adequate doses is efficacious in the average case. Parenteral administration of 25 mgm. twice daily is recommended, however, when the deficiency is associated with severe cardiac failure, severe peripheral neuritis or severe gastrointestinal disturbances, or when the patient is refractory to oral therapy.

Infantile thiamine deficiency is treated most satisfactorily by giving intramuscularly or intravenously 5 to 10 mgm. of thiamine in sterile physiological solution of sodium chloride twice daily. As in the adult the action is more prompt and more efficacious, when it is administered parenterally than when it is given by mouth. When injections cannot be given conveniently, or when the infant is convalescent, 10 mgm. of chrystalline vitamine B_1 may be given orally every day. Obviously, satisfactory treatment of the mother will aid greatly in the treatment of the nursing child.

Toxicity

The practicing physician should have in mind that there is a great difference between the therapeutic and the toxic dose of thiamine. The authors, who have been studying this vitamin for ten years, have seen no evidence of cumulative toxicity in human beings. We have given as much as 500 mgm. daily to patients for a period of sixty days without any evidence of toxic effects. Since the therapeutic dose in man is only a few milligrams a day, we consider it a remarkably safe therapeutic agent. We have reported that large amounts of synthetic crystalline material, when injected intravenously, frequently cause the patient to volunteer that he experiences a yeast-like taste. There is no doubt that some persons have an indiosyncrasy to this substance, just as they may have other drug idiosyncrasies, and patients may become hypersensitive in the course of treatment.

NICOTINIC ACID AMIDE

History

Nicotinic acid was first prepared from nicotine by Huber in 1867[201], but its significance in nutrition was not discovered for many years. Between 1912 and 1916 it was isolated from rice polishings by Susuke, Shimamuri and Odake[202], Funk[203] and Williams[204,205] and in 1926 Vickery[206] found it in yeast. The amide of nicotinic acid was shown to be the active group of the coenzyme now known as coenzyme II by Warburg and Christian[207] in 1935, and at the same time Kuhn and Vetter[208] isolated it from the red blood cells of the horse and from mamma-

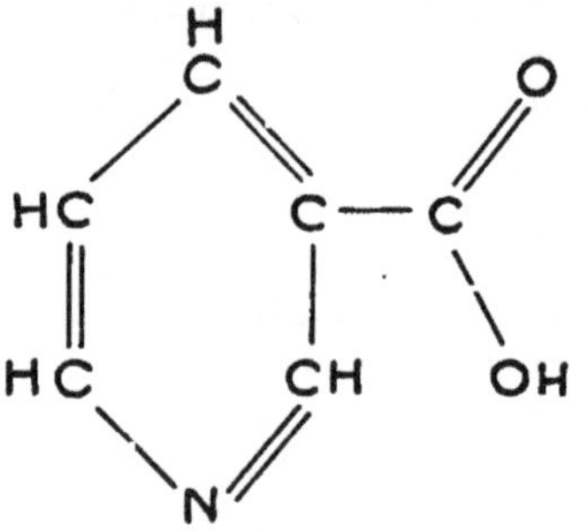

Fig. 33. Structural formula of nicotinic acid (3-pyridine carbolic acid.)

lian heart muscle. As a result of this work the interest of many investigators was directed toward discovering the rôle of nicotinic acid in nutrition. In 1937 Elvehjem, Madden, Strong and Wooley[209] isolated it from liver and showed that it was curative in canine blacktongue. Independently and almost simultaneously excellent results in treating human pellagra were reported by several investigators[210,211,212,213].

Chemistry and Physiology

There are several ways of preparing nicotinic acid, one of which is the strong acid oxidation of nicotine. It was from this method of preparation that nicotinic acid received its name. The formula for nicotinic acid is shown in Fig. 33, that for its amide in Fig. 34. Its properties, however, differ widely from the parent compound. Nicotinic acid, the beta-carboxylic acid of pyridine, is a white crystalline compound (Fig. 35) which melts at 230 to 232° C. It is moderately soluble in hot water but only slightly soluble in cold water. The sodium salt and the amide are more soluble. For parenteral administration the amide is preferable because it does not cause the flushing produced by nicotinic acid.

Nicotinic acid is very stable and is not oxidized or destroyed by ordinary cooking processes or by exposure to light.

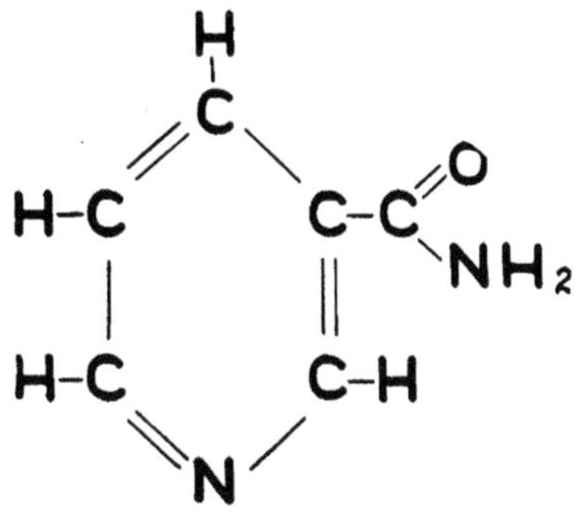

Nicotinic Acid Amide
3-pyridine carboxylic acid amide

Fig. 34. Structural formula of nicotinic acid amide.

It is widely distributed in foodstuffs, but even the richest sources, such as liver, eggs, salmon, and whole cereals, contain relatively little of this substance.

Relationship between Co-enzymes I and II and Nicotinic Acid Amide Deficiency

The spectacular clinical improvement, which follows the administration of nicotinic acid or nicotinic acid amide to pellagrins, led to increased interest in the respiratory co-enzymes I and II, cozymase and coferment, respectively, which are known to contain nicotinic acid amide. By definition these co-enzymes are relatively heat-stable, dialysable, organic catalysts which retain activity even when separated from the living cell. They are necessary for the function of specific protein enzymes. Each is produced by living cells from a combination of nicotinic acid amide, ribose, adenylic acid and phosphoric acid. The present knowledge of the chemical constitution of co-enzymes I and II indicates that they are similar in that both are pyridine nucleotides, differing only in their content of phosphoric acid. The authors of this chapter consider that the formation of enzymes governing respiration and growth of cells involves the synthesis of complex substances from simple compounds.

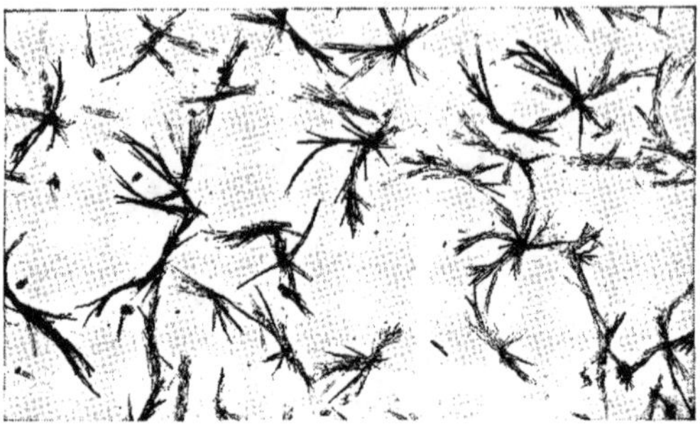

Fig. 35. Crystalline nicotinic acid (courtesy of Merck and Co.).

The methods for studying the enzymes are tedious and are not recommended for the practicing physician. Nevertheless they offer important information concerning certain aspects of the pathogenesis of pellagra and other diseases. Vilter, Vilter and Spies[214] found that the concentration of co-enzymes I and II in the whole blood of persons with deficiency diseases is slightly lower than in normal persons on optimal diets. Low values for the co-enzyme concentration of whole blood may be observed also in some persons with diabetes mellitus, roentgen sickness, leukemia and pneumococcal pneumonia. Infections, fever and excessive physical exercise tend to lower the concentration in the blood, whereas rest in bed and an increased intake of nicotinic acid or related pyridine compounds tend to increase the concentration.

Axelrod, Spies and Elvehjem[215] studied a large series of pellagrins admitted to the Nutrition Clinic at the Hillman Hospital in Birmingham, Alabama. Using a yeast growth method, which is specific for co-enzyme I, they found that there was only a slight lowering of this substance in the erythrocytes. There was a great decrease in the co-enzyme content of the striated muscle, and it continued to decrease as the pellagra became more severe, whereas it increased following the administration of nicotinic acid or nicotinic acid amide. It should be emphasized that in these studies a method specific for co-enzyme I was used, and it had no bearing on the co-enzyme II content of the tissues. The precise significance of this lowering in the co-enzyme I content of the pellagrin's muscles cannot be fully stated. Unpublished observations by Lu and Spies[216] indicate that the changes in the oxidative metabolism of the striated muscle taken from the pellagrin are less than those found in normal controls. These investigators observed that, following therapy, normal values in the muscles of pellagrins soon were restored. The anti-pellagric value of a substance, however, is not necessarily associated with its ability to affect the co-enzyme I content of the blood and other tissues. For example nicotinic acid has a profound effect upon the co-enzyme I content of human blood both in vivo and in vitro, while coramine, the diethylamide of nicotinic acid, which is also anti-pellagric, does not produce a significant increase in the co-enzyme I content of erythrocytes and muscles.

The fact that the very ill pellagrin may have only 60 per cent. of the normal concentration of co-enzyme I in his muscles offers a marvelous explanation of the long, lingering weakness which characterizes the period of development of dietary deficiency disease. Spies, von Euler, Vilter, Bean and Schlenk in unpublished observations have shown that the intravenous injection of from 10 to 50 mgm. of co-enzyme I of the highest activity is followed by dramatic clinical improvement in the acute manifestations of pellagra; yet, this amount, when distributed throughout the body, is not detectable by their highly sensitive laboratory methods.

Absorption, Distribution, Excretion and Effects

Unpublished observations by Bean, Dexter and Spies showed that nicotinic acid is absorbed from the stomach and from the small and large bowel. Absorption is more rapid from an empty stomach than it is after meals. If the absorption is sufficienty rapid, the concentration of nicotinic acid is increased in the blood, and the skin temperature of the upper part of the body is elevated. Over 80 per cent. of the persons to whom 100 to 300 mgm. of nicotinic acid is administered orally feel temporary prickly or burning sensations of the skin. A few persons complain of nausea and cramping pains in the stomach. These symptoms are transitory and are not associated with changes in general body temperature, pulse, respiration or blood pressure. All persons to whom 20 mgm. of nicotinic acid is administered rapidly by the intravenous route have transitory vasodilation. It should be remembered, however, that nicotinic acid amide is the more physiological form of the compound, and it does not produce these vasodilating reactions. There is some tendency for the blood vessels of the lower extremities to constrict following the administration of nicotinic acid, and the amounts and methods of administration have a profound effect on the skin temperature rise as is shown in Fig. 36.

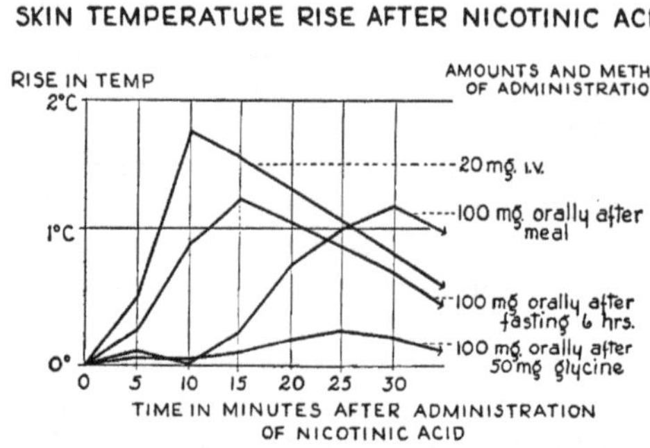

Fig. 36. Skin temperature rise after nicotinic acid (from Duncan Graham: Disease of Metabolism, W. B. Saunders Co., Phila., 1942).

Nicotinic acid amide and co-enzymes I and II are present in the blood and are excreted in the urine. These substances are so essential that the body does not allow the blood levels to be lowered greatly. The amount excreted in the urine is dependent upon many factors, including the richness of the diet and the concentration in the body tissues. When they are administered in pure form, the amount excreted depends on the size of the dose and the mode of administration. Excretion is more rapid when the material is administered parenterally than when it is given orally. When large doses of nicotinamide are injected into human beings, the material cannot be accounted for either unchanged or as known derivatives in the urine. Even after repeated doses large amounts do not appear in the urine and, therefore, must be metabolized in ways at present unknown. The metabolic derivative of nicotinamide is N-methyl-nicotinamide. Even after repeated injections of this substance it does not, for the most part, appear in the urine. It should be emphasized that for a long time it was taken for granted that human beings excreted trigonelline, the methyl betaine of nicotinic acid, as do dogs. It is known now that N-methyl-nicotinamide is the metabolic derivative chiefly excreted. The co-enzymes I and II increase in the blood and urine after nicotinic acid is administered.

Nicotinic acid compounds have been found in nearly all animal tissue. In general the concentration is highest in tissues in which the metabolism is high. In human beings with severe nicotinic acid deficiency, the concentration of the nicotinic-acid-amide-containing substance, co-enzyme I, is decreased as much as 60 per cent. in striated muscle and may be slightly decreased in the erythrocytes. Likewise in this deficiency the content of the nicotinic acid derivatives is below normal in whole blood and urine. When such patients are treated with nicotinic acid, the content of the compounds in the muscle, blood and urine containing nicotinic-acid-amide increases.

A knowledge of the level of nicotinic acid in the body tissues and excretions of pellagrins sometimes contributes valuable information concerning the degree of nicotinic acid deficiency. It also is useful in following the rate of recovery after nicotinic acid therapy has been initiated. Several methods, both chemical and microbiological, for the determination of nicotinic acid in micro quantities have been introduced. In studying biologically derived specimens we use the microbiological technics because they possess extreme sensitivity, permitting the determination of nicotinic acid in amounts as small as a few hundredths of a microgram and may be used in analyzing for nicotinic acid in the presence of large amounts of foreign material even if this be pigmented or in a solid state. The microbiological method of Snell and Wright has been used successfully in determining minute quantities of nicotinic acid in blood, urine, feces, saliva, fresh tissues and foods. Using this method, Gross, Swain and Spies[217] have found that the average person with pellagra retains more of a 100 mgm. test dose of nicotinic acid than does the normal person of similar size.

Pigment Metabolism

In 1913 Myers and Fine observed that indicanuria was pronounced in pellagrins in the presence of low hydrochloric acid in the gastric contents. Three years later Hunter showed that the previous diet was important in the determination of the fate of additional ingested tryptophane and reported the finding of urorosein in the urine of pellagrins. Studies by the authors show that many pellagrins excrete indole, indican, urorosein and various other related compounds in the urine. A number of investigators have found porphyrin in the urine of pellagrins. At one time it was thought that the excretion of porphyrin might be useful as a diagnostic test. It now appears that porphyrinuria is a result of liver damage or at least a disturbance of liver function. Naturally the alcoholic pellagrin is more prone to have liver disease than the endemic pellagrin. Urorosein and indican frequently are excreted in large amounts in early or subclinical pellagra, so that their detection may serve as a valuable warning signal of malnutrition. The test using colorimetric methods is a simple but non-specific one. The procedure is as follows:

A measured amount of urine (3 to 10 c.c.) is acidified with glacial acetic acid to a pH of about 4.0 and shaken with 5 to 20 c.c. of ether until no more red pigments can be extracted. The ether then is washed repeatedly with water. A complete separation of the two layers is allowed to take place. To a measured fraction of the ether is added one-fifth of that amount of 25 per cent. hydrochloric acid. On shaking the pigments contained in the ether fraction are transferred completely to the hydrochloric acid, which becomes stained purple or pink, the intensity of the color depending on the pigment concentration. The colorimetric estimation is made either in a colorimeter of Dubosq type against a standard solution of porphyrin or by comparison with porphyrin solutions of known concentration. The time necessary for the complete transfer of the porphyrins from the urine into the ether and from the ether into hydrochloric acid differs in various specimens, being determined by the nature of the substance present. In most specimens the process is completed in a half an hour, but as a check the colorimetric estimations may be repeated after three hours and after twenty-four hours.

Severe cases may have a negative test.

Pathological Physiology

The most common gross pathological findings of nicotinic acid deficiency are generalized emaciation of the body and atrophy of various organs. In some cases the walls of the gastrointestinal tract may show swelling, reddening and ulceration of any portion, while in other cases the walls may be thin and atrophic. The liver occasionally contains abnormal amounts of fat. Moore, Spies and Cooper[218] made a histologic study of the active lesions and also of clinically unaffected areas of the skin in the same patient.

The microscopic picture of the lesions of pellagra is similar to that found in chronic inflammatory diseases of the skin. The skin from both clinically affected and unaffected areas in pellagrins was hyperkeratotic. Parakeratosis was found also in the actual lesions. No satisfactory explanation of the atrophy which is present both in healing pellagrous lesions and in the unaffected skin can be given. That atrophy occurs normally with aging of the skin and that it may result from either external or internal pressure has long been known, but the exact mechanism involved in the process remains unexplained, and the present study affords no new information concerning it. Both the affected and unaffected skin showed edema of the corium and a moderate infiltration of lymphocytes. Since the skin lesions tend to disappear following treatment with nicotinic acid, they are to a considerable extent reversible, so it seems that they represent a specific response on the part of the skin to a deficiency of nicotinic acid and substances that act similarly. The microscopic picture of the intestinal lesions varies from atrophy to acute inflammation characterized by fibrin formation and collections of inflammatory cells. When changes in the nervous system are demonstrable, they are characterized by irregular areas of degeneration, often involving the posterior and lateral columns of the spinal cord, the posterior spinal ganglia, and the Betz and Purkinje cells.

Symptomatology

As is shown in Fig. 37, there is a lag period between the onset of symptoms and the time the patient seeks medical aid. The time between the very first day of dietary deficiency and the appearance of lesions might well be termed the deficiency development time. This period of time may be of long duration with insidiously advancing symptoms, trivial in nature but gaining importance by their persistency rather than by their severity. Before diagnostic lesions of the mucous membranes or skin appear, there is loss of appetite which is, at least in part, responsible for weight loss. Ill-defined disturbances of the alimentary tract including "indigestion" and changes in bowel function occur. General muscular weakness, lassitude, irritability, depression, memory loss, headache and insomnia frequently develop without apparent reason. Abdominal pain, burning sensations in various parts of the body, vertigo, numbness, nervousness, palpitation, distractability, flights of ideas, apprehension, morbid fears, mental confusion and forgetfulness frequently occur. There may be intermittent diarrhea and constipation. There is much that obviously is abnormal at this stage but nothing that is pathognomonic. Since the entire syndrome often appears without objective cause, a diagnosis of neurasthenia, anxiety state, malingering or neurosis may be entertained by the physician. These symptoms are not invari-

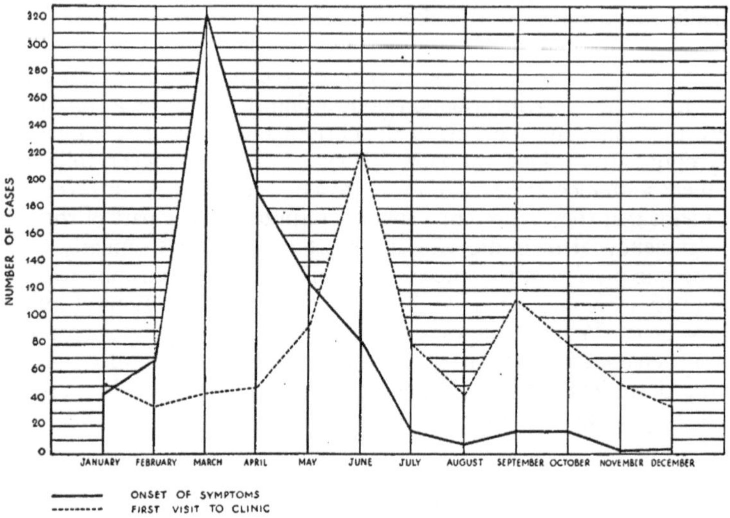

Fig. 37. Lag period between onset of symptoms and first visit to clinic.

ably present; they do not appear in any regular order, and they are not uniformly severe in every case. The individual case, however, usually repeats the same order of development of symptoms with each recurrence.

Although the identity of pellagra in children and adults is established, the clinical manifestations often are different, and for purposes of clarity it is advisable to consider them separately. It should be borne in mind, however, that from an etiological and pathological point of view such a distinction is artificial.

Endemic pellagra in infants and children has been reported by Spies, Walker and Woods[219]. These investigators find that a careful dietary history of the mother usually reveals that her diet has been inadequate during pregnancy and lactation. Frequently her milk supply is scanty, and the infant is weaned soon after birth and given food inadequate for proper nutrition, or the inadequate breast milk feedings are supplemented with such foods. From an early age most of the children have poor appetites and eat irregularly. As a rule, they prefer carbohydrate foods and often refuse all others. Usually they develop poor food habits early in life, and the parents seldom make any attempt to change them, even if a good diet becomes available. The parents frequently complain that the children are irritable, easily frightened, apprehensive, fretful and cry a great deal; that they are too tired to play but too nervous to rest; that they sleep poorly and frequently awaken crying. Few of them gain weight normally, and the few, who were robust prior to their illness, usually have lost weight rapidly. In these children soreness of the lips and tongue and burning of the stomach are common complaints as are pains in the abdomen, cramping of the legs and cramping and burning of the feet. Usually they are constipated but have occasional bouts of diarrhea during the spring and summer. These symptoms wax and wane and become more severe with each recurrence. As the children grow older, the subnormality in height and weight usually becomes more apparent as does an increasing inability to concentrate or to make normal progress in school. From the physical examination it is obvious that these children are in ill health. They appear undernourished and underdeveloped for their age. Usually their skin is dry and atrophic, making them appear much older than they are. The typical dermal and alimentary tract lesions described in adult pellagra may or may not develop. A more complete discusion of pellagra as a disease will be found in Chapter XIII, Vol. IV of Oxford Medicine.

Diagnosis

The clinical diagnosis of pellagra in adults or children depends upon identifying typical dermal lesions or characteristic mucous membrane lesions or both.

Characteristic skin lesions may appear on any part of the body. They are observed most frequently over sites of irritation, such as the dorsum of the hands, wrists, elbows, face, neck, knees, feet, under the breasts and in the perineal region. In most instances the area of dermatitis is separated sharply from the normal skin. The lesions are never static; they either advance or regress. The dermatitis begins as an erythema resembling sunburn. As the disease progresses, the area becomes reddish brown, roughened, scaly and keratotic; vesicles and bullae may form. Desquamation usually begins at the center of the lesion, and the underlying skin appears red and thickened. The intensity of the pigmentation and the thickening of the skin tend to increase with each recurrence of the disease. After repeated recurrences the skin may become either permanently pigmented, thick and roughened or thin and atrophic. In the past a diagnosis of pellagra was not ventured unless well-established bilateral lesions were evident. Such lesions are much more common than unilateral lesions. Nevertheless, Bean, Spies and Vilter[220] found 32 patients with well-advanced unilateral pellagrous dermatitis in a series of 889 cases. These investigators emphasize that in their experience the cutaneous lesions in different parts of the body often are in different phases simultaneously. One lesion may be at the stage of early erythma, another in the stage of desquamation, and still another in the stage of pigmentation. Sunlight as the exciting agent of pellagrous dermatitis has been discussed for years by many investigators. Some of the series of opinions have been discussed by Smith and Ruffin[221], Spies[222] and Stannus[223]. Suffice it to say that lesions not exposed to the sun occur, but it is generally agreed that exposure to sunlight is more detrimental to pellagrins than it is to normal persons.

Glossitis and stomatitis are early and common symptoms of pellagra, and Spies[224] has demonstrated that pellagrous glossitis is a much more sensitive gage than dermatitis in the evaluation of the severity of the disease. In the early stage of the disease only the tip or the lateral margins of the tongue are swollen and reddened. In the absence of treatment the swelling increases, redness becomes more intense, and deeply penetrating ulcers may appear along the sides and tip but rarely on top. The entire surface may be covered with a thick gray membrane filled with débris and Vincent's organisms. The tongue may be hypersensitive, although it usually is hypoesthetic. The buccal mucous membranes, the mucocutaneous surface of the lips, the gums and the palate likewise may be affected. A burning sensation of the tongue and of the mucous membranes of the pharynx, esophagus and stomach is not uncommon and usually is aggravated by hot or acid foods. Ptyalism and nausea may occur early, but, as a rule, they are advanced symptoms of the disease. Achlorhydria is present in about 50 per cent. of persons with pellagra, even after histamine stimulation; rennin and pepsinogen likewise are absent. In the majority of mild cases the bowels act normally or are constipated. Severe, persistent diarrhea with frequent watery stools tends to occur only in the more acute cases. Abdominal discomfort, pain and distention may be present at any time during the course of the disease and usually are more severe after a large meal.

Mental symptoms as a part of the pellagra syndrome have been emphasized for many years. The patient may present a train of symptoms characteristic of neurasthenia, anxiety state or other neuroses. In later stages there is loss of memory, excitement, mania, delirium, hallucinations and dementia. Even in the absence of diagnostic lesions of pellagra the patient may have central nervous system involvement.

A series of severe cases of pellagra with atypical lesions has been described by Spies, Cogswell and Vilter[225]. This type of case is difficult to diagnose and is likely to be fatal, if proper therapy is not applied promptly.

A history of prolonged subsistence on a deficient diet plus the presence of pellagra in other members of the family should lead the physician to suspect pellagra even in the absence of typical pellagrous lesions. When there is any doubt, the controlled therapeutic test should be given, since it is known that, if early pellagra is present, rapid improvement will follow specific therapy.

Prevention and Treatment

Like most nutritional deficiency states nicotinic acid deficiency is particularly prevalent among the following groups, and it is to these groups that special attention toward prevention should be directed.

1. The poor and ignorant, who subsist on an unbalanced diet, usually rich in cereals and low in meat, milk and eggs. Casal, who first described pellagra, pointed out that "mal de la rosa" occurred among people who ate corn for a staple cereal. Endemic pellagra has occurred almost exclusively among people who ingest corn or corn products. The hypothesis that corn plays a rôle in the etiology of the disease has commanded continued attention. After finding that nicotinic acid was a useful therapeutic agent, investigators have been much interested in possible antagonism between it and corn. Evidence of this antagonism has been extended by the observations of Krehl, Sarma, Teply and Elvehjem[226], who showed that cornmeal or corn grits added to a low protein diet greatly reduced the growth of young rats, and that addition of 1 mgm. of nicotinic acid per 100 grams of diet restored growth to the level observed when the diet contained no corn products. These investigators next learned that tryptophane could overcome the growth inhibitors present in the corn products. It is of considerable dietary interest that polished rice contains less nicotinic acid than corn but more tryptophane. From a clinical point of view it is of great interest that pellagra occurs

in persons who have never eaten maize (corn), but most of the endemic pellagrins of the world are heavy corn eaters. Pellagrins, who normally have a low level of vitamins in their tissues, would be most susceptible to any deleterious action of corn. Pellagrous lesions heal spectacularly, while the patient is restricted to a diet of corn products, if adequate amounts of nicotinic acid are administered.

2. Persons who because of organic diseases have difficulty in ingesting, assimilating or utilizing food. In this group are included persons whose diseases predispose them to pellagra, which usually is referred to as pellagra secondary to organic disease. More males than females have pellagra secondary to cancer and ulcer of the stomach. In pellagra following measles and whooping cough children naturally predominate. Childbearing and its associated complications predispose women from 20 to 40 years of age to pellagra, if their diets are of borderline adequacy, and the incidence is highest among women in this age group. Bean, Spies and Blankenhorn[227] have discussed the perilous burden which organic disease and surgical operations place on the undernourished.

3. Persons who are chronically addicted to alcohol and who eat very little food frequently develop pellagra which often is referred to as alcoholic pellagra or pseudo-pellagra.

4. Food faddists and persons with capricious appetites, who tend to eat little food containing anti-pellagric substances, and persons, who have subsisted on diets prescribed by physicians for certain diseases, diets which fail to supply adequate amounts of the pellagra-preventive factor.

5. Persons whose requirements for the anti-pellagric substances are increased. Pregnancy, lactation, rapid growth, hyperthyroidism, infections and increased physical exercise are all factors which increase the requirement.

It is much better for a potential pellagrin to eat sufficient amounts of lean meat, eggs, milk and vegetables and thus prevent the disease than it is for him to have to be treated for pellagra. Satisfactory diets, taking into consideration the daily allowances of nutrients recommended by the Council on Foods and Nutrition of the National Research Council, have been planned at different levels of cost by Carpenter and Stiebling[228] and will serve as an excellent guide for the physician. The liberal diet plan which they suggest provides the following variety in the course of the day or week:

Milk:

One quart daily for each child (to drink or in cooked food)
One pint daily for each adult (to drink or in cooked food)

Vegetables and Fruits:
- Six to seven servings daily
- One serving daily of tomatoes or citrus fruits
- Two and one-half to three servings daily of vegetables, at least half of which are leafy, green or yellow kinds
- Nine to ten servings a week of fruit (once a day, sometimes twice)

Eggs:
- Four to six a week; also some in cooking

Meat, fish or poultry:
- Once a day, sometimes twice

Butter:
- At every meal

Bread, cereals, and desserts:
- As needed to meet calorie requirements or as desired so long as they do not displace the protective foods

In areas, in which pellagra is endemic, the authors find that the disease usually occurs in persons whose diets have been deficient in animal proteins and relatively high in cereal foods and fats.

We have found that it is more practical to add to the existing dietary daily one-half pound of lean meat, two eggs, from one pint to one quart of milk and liberal amounts of vegetables than it is to try to change completely long-established dietary habits. When such additions are not available or practical, we have found that daily supplements of concentrates such as dried brewers' yeast or liver extract are excellent preventive agents. In such cases we recommend two ounces of dried brewers' yeast or liver extract. Persons, who do not absorb or utilize the nutrients properly or whose requirement for them is increased, are special medical problems. The authors have found that, to maintain good health in some cases, it is sufficient to give additional amounts of the foods mentioned above. In others, however, the administration of niacinamide is necessary. In these cases we usually begin with an oral dose of from 20 to 50 mgm. daily. In those rare cases, in which absorption is so meager that this oral dose is not adequate, 20 mgm. daily is given by intravenous injection. In administering niacinamide or any single synthetic substance it is important for the physician always to keep in mind that the factors which predispose to or precipitate the development of one deficiency lead to the development of others. It likewise is important for him to realize that the administration of niacinamide alone may result in improved health, but it will not restore it completely. Thus, for every pellagrin or every potential pellagrin the regular consumption of a liberal, well-balanced diet is of utmost importance.

The dietary treatment of patients with pellagra, whether they are in bed at home or in the hospital or whether they remain ambulatory, is based on the principles of good nutrition. It must be remembered, however, that the tissue stores of niacinamide as well as of the other essential nutrients are likely to be severely depleted. Accordingly the diet must supply much more than the allowances of nutrients recommended for normal persons. We recommend that the diet supply from 3,000 to 4,000 calories, 120 to 150 grams of protein and liberal amounts of minerals and vitamins. The type of food prescribed and the form in which it is given depend entirely upon the ability of the patient to ingest and retain food. Frequently the patient's desire for food is absent, and he has to be persuaded to eat. In the severely ill patient, the mouth and tongue may be so sensitive that only soft or liquid foods can be tolerated, and highly seasoned or acid foods must be avoided. In some instances only a small amount of food can be taken at one time, and it is necessary to give small feedings at frequent intervals. As the patient improves, semi-solid and solid foods can be given. In all cases with diarrhea solid foods should be added as soon as possible. In the dietary treatment of pellagra and other nutritional deficiency diseases, we have found the following diets* useful:

4,000 Calorie Liquid Diet

Suggested Hourly Feedings

7 A.M.	Cereal Gruel—1 serving (see recipe)
	Milk—1 glass
8 A.M.	Eggnogg—1 glass (see recipe)
9 A.M.	Eggnogg—1 glass (see recipe)
10 A.M.	Ice Cream
	Fruit Juice with Egg (see recipe)
11 A.M.	Eggnogg—1 glass (see recipe)
12 Noon	Cream Soup—1 serving (see recipe)
	Milk—1 glass
1 P.M.	Eggnog—1 glass
2 P.M.	Ice Cream—1 serving
3 P.M.	Eggnog—1 glass

* These diets were planned by Miss Jean M. Grant, dietitian, Nutrition Clinic, Hillman Hospital, Birmingham, Alabama.

4 P.M.	Ice Cream—1 serving
5 P.M.	Cereal Gruel—1 serving
6 P.M.	Eggnog—1 glass
7 P.M.	Cream Soup—1 serving
	Ice Cream—1 serving
8 P.M.	Eggnog—1 glass
9 P.M.	Eggnog—1 glass

Note: cup = standard 8 ounce measuring cup
glass = 8 ounce water glass

Approximate Food Value of Diet

Protein	145 gms.
Total Calories	4,134

4,000 Calorie Liquid Diet

Suggested Feedings Every Two Hours

7 A.M.	Fruit Juice with egg—1 glass (see recipe)
	Cereal Gruel—1 serving (see recipe)
9 A.M.	Eggnogg—1 glass (see recipe)
	Ice Cream—1 serving
11 A.M.	Eggnogg—1 glass
	Milk—1 glass
1 P.M.	Cream Soup—1 serving (see recipe)
	Eggnog—1 glass
	Ice Cream—1 serving
3 P.M.	Eggnog—1 glass
	Milk—1 glass
5 P.M.	Eggnog—1 glass
	Ice Cream—1 serving
7 P.M.	Cream Soup—1 serving
	Ice Cream—1 serving
	Eggnog—1 glass
9 P.M.	Cereal Gruel—1 serving
	Eggnog—1 glass
11 P.M.	Eggnog—1 glass

Note: cup = standard 8 ounce measuring cup
glass = 8 ounce water glass

Approximate Food Value of Diet:

Protein	145 gms.
Total Calories	4,134

4,000 Calorie "Soft-Solid" Diet

Suggested Meals

Breakfast, 8 A.M.
Fruit Juice—1 glass
Cooked Cereal—1 serving (½ cup)
Cream—¼ cup
Sugar—2 teaspoons
Soft Cooked Eggs—2
Milk Toast—Toast, 1 slice
Milk, ½ cup
Butter, 1 square (2 teaspoons)
Milk—1 glass
Coffee—if desired

10 A.M.
Eggnogg—1 glass (see recipe)
Ice Cream or puddings—1 serving

Lunch, 12 Noon
Cream Soup—1 serving (see recipe)
Soft Cooked Eggs
Milk Toast—Bread, 1 slice
Milk, ½ cup
Butter, 2 teaspoons
Mashed Potato or Boiled Rice – 1 serving (½ cup)
Butter – 1 pat (2 teaspoons)
Ice Cream or Pudding – 1 serving
Milk – 1 glass

2 P.M.
Eggnog – 1 glass

4 P.M.
Eggnog – 1 glass

Supper, 6 P.M.
Cream Soup – 1 serving
Cooked Cereal – ½ cup
Cream – ¼ cup
Sugar – 2 teaspoons
Soft Cooked Eggs – 2
Ice Cream or Pudding – 1 serving
Milk – 1 glass

8 P.M.
Eggnog – 1 glass

Note: cup = standard 8 ounce measuring cup
Glass = 8 ounce water glass

Approximate Food Value of Diet:

Proteins	147 gms.
Total Calories	4,153

4,000 Calorie "Solid" Diet

Suggested Meals and Between Meal Feedings

Breakfast	Fruit Juice – 1 glass Cereal – large serving Eggs – 2 Bacon or Ham – if desired Toast – 2 slices Butter – 2 pats Cream – ½ cup (for cereal and coffee) Milk – 1 glass Coffee – if desired
10 A.M.	Eggnog – 1 glass (see recipe)
Dinner	Lean Meat, Chicken or Fish – 3 ounces Potato, macaroni, spaghetti, noodles or dried beans or peas (1 serving) Vegetable – large serving (green or yellow vegetable – may be cooked or used as salad. If cooked add 1 square of butter; if used as salad, add 1 tablespoon mayonnaise.) Bread – 2 slices Butter – 2 pats Dessert – 1 serving Milk – 1 glass
2 P.M.	Eggnog – 1 glass
4 P.M.	Eggnog – 1 glass
Supper	Lean Meat, Chicken or Fish – 3 ounces Potato, macaroni, spaghetti, noodles or dried beans or peas (1 serving) Vegetable – large serving (green or yellow vegetable – may be cooked or used as salad. If cooked, add 1 square of butter; if used as salad, add 1 tablespoon mayonnaise.) Bread – 2 slices Butter – 2 pats Dessert – 1 serving Milk – 1 glass

8 P.M.	Eggnog – 1 glass
	Approximate food value of diet:
	Protein 148 Gm.
	Total Calories 3,980

Recipes

Eggnog	6 eggs; 4 tablespoons sugar; 6 cups milk. Beat eggs. Add sugar. Add milk. Beat mixture well. Chocolate syrup or vanilla may be added, if desired. *Makes 8 servings.*
Cereal Gruel	½ cup of any kind of cooked cereal thinned to desired consistency with milk and served with ¼ cup of cream and with sugar, if desired
Cream Soup	¼ cup strained vegetable or canned tomato, pea, spinach or asparagus soup. Add ½ cup cream.
Fruit Juice with Egg	Beat 1 egg well. Add 1 cup fruit juice. Add sugar as desired.

It should be pointed out, however, that in certain diseases such as allergy, diabetes and gastric ulcer, which necessitate restricting the kind or amount of food, these diets would not be suitable. Such cases require individual diet therapy, a detailed discussion of which is beyond the limits of this chapter.

Important as food is in the treatment of nutritive failure, therapy should not be restricted to food alone. Deprivation of nutrients usually has existed for years, and the average patient cannot eat enough food to supply the amount of these nutrients necessary to restore his health quickly. Accordingly supplements of the nutrients, in which the diet is deficient, are given. Until synthetic vitamins became available, dried brewers' yeast powder, wheat germ, liver concentrates and citrus fruit were given in treating deficiencies of the water-soluble vitamins. As valuable as these substances were, and still are, there are times when niacinamide is life-saving.

The amount of niacinamide or similar compounds necessary for a therapeutic response in pellagra varies tremendously from patient to patient so that no arbitrary dosage can be set. In the average case we have found that 50 mgm. administered orally 10 times a day is effective. Oral administration of niacinamide is preferable to other methods, because by this route it is absorbed more slowly, and an elevated blood concentration is maintained over a longer period of time than it is when it is administered by any other route. We have observed one patient with long-standing pellagra, however, who failed to respond to oral doses of niacinamide as high as 1,500 mgm. daily, but who improved rapidly following the intravenous administration of 50 mgm. 6 times a day.

Parenteral therapy is indicated, when a high blood concentration is desired within a short period of time, when gastrointestinal absorption is inadequate, or when the patient is in stupor or coma. In such cases 50 to 100 mgm. doses are sufficient. In order to keep the blood concentration at a high level, it should be administered in small doses at frequent intervals. The authors give 50 mgm. doses 4 times daily and inject it slowly. When parenteral administration of saline or glucose is indicated in the acutely ill patient, the vitamin can be dissolved in a physiological solution of saline or 5 per cent. glucose and administered by slow drip.

Niacinamide can be given intramuscularly in the same dosage as that suggested for intravenous injection. Intramuscular therapy is not recommended for persons with deficiency disease, however, because it is attended by some risk of abscess formation in devitalized tissues.

A satisfactory daily dose for infants is from 50 to 100 mgm. dissolved in the infant's total milk supply for the day. For parenteral administration we suggest 15 mgm. 3 times a day. If the infant is breast fed, the niacinamide can be given to the nursing mother[219]. This increases the niacinamide content of the mother's milk sufficiently to relieve the infant's deficiency. For children two or three times the dose recommended for infants is suggested and should depend upon the size of the child.

Adequate doses of niacinamide or similar substances administered to a pellagrin will (a) cause fading of the fiery redness of the mucous membrane lesions and disappearance of the associated Vincent's organisms, (b) cause disappearance of the acute mental symptoms of pellagra such as delirium, hallucinations and mental confusion, (c) relieve diarrhea, vomiting and cramping, which arise from alterations in alimentary function, (d) cause fading of the dermal erythema, (e) increase the feeling of strength and well-being, (f) result in disappearance of certain ether-soluble red pigments from the urine, (g) increase the concentration of co-enzymes I and II in whole blood and urine and, when therapy is prolonged, increase the co-enzyme content of the muscle. We wish to stress, however, that in treating pellagra or any other nutritional deficiency disease, the patient as well as his disease must be treated.

Toxicity

Nicotinic acid, in the amounts recommended for therapy, is not toxic although it and all related compounds containing the free radical produce vasodilation in the skin and an increase in skin temperature as already illustrated by Figure 36.

RIBOFLAVIN

History

The scientific world paid scant attention when Blythe[229], the English chemist, reported the presence of a fluorescent, yellow-green substance in milk in 1867. Blythe himself was interested primarily in learning something about the composition of milk, and little did he realize that the pigment, which he described, would later play a rôle in the science of nutrition. Although chemists[230] again studied this yellow material in 1925 and described some of its properties, its biochemical nature re-

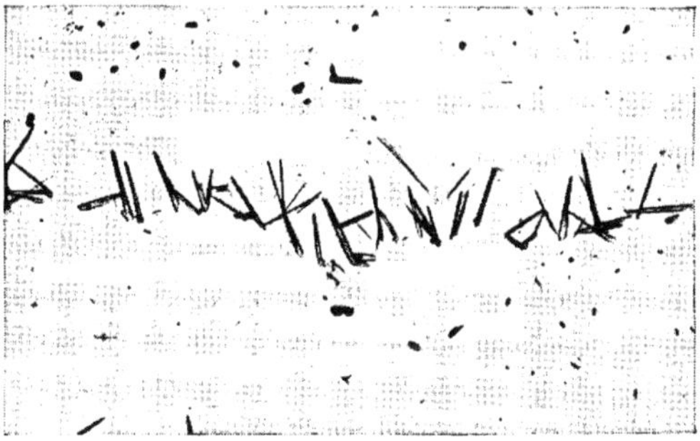

Fig. 38. Crystalline riboflavin (courtesy of Merck and Co.).

mained to be disclosed through a different source. In 1932 Warburg and Christian[231] described a new "yellow enzyme" which they obtained from the aqueous extract of bottom yeasts. It proved to be one of the most ubiquitous of the enzymes concerned in cellular respiration, and these investigators later separated this yellow enzyme into a protein component and a pigmented portion and noted that neither alone was active. In 1933 Kuhn and his co-workers isolated the pigment from natural sources[232], and in 1935 Karrer and his collaborators[233] and Kuhn and his associates[234] independently synthesized riboflavin.

Chemistry and Physiology

Riboflavin crystallizes in fine yellow needles which melt at 282° C. (Fig. 38). The structural formula of riboflavin is shown in Figure 39. The pure compound is only slightly soluble in water and ethyl alcohol and is very soluble in alkali solutions. It is insoluble in acetone, ether, benzene and choroform. The water solution is of greenish-yellow color and has an intense yellow-green fluorescence which disappears with the addition of either acids or alkalis. Light slowly destroys the vitamin activity. The decomposition is influenced also by temperature and by the hydrogen ion concentration. It has a relatively high thermostability.

Under ultra-violet light riboflavin emits a blue-green fluorescence. It is on this property that the fluorometric quantitative determination of the substance depends. A second accurate method of quantitation is based upon the conversion of riboflavin to lumiflavin by exposure to light in alkaline solution. The amount of lumiflavin then can be deter-

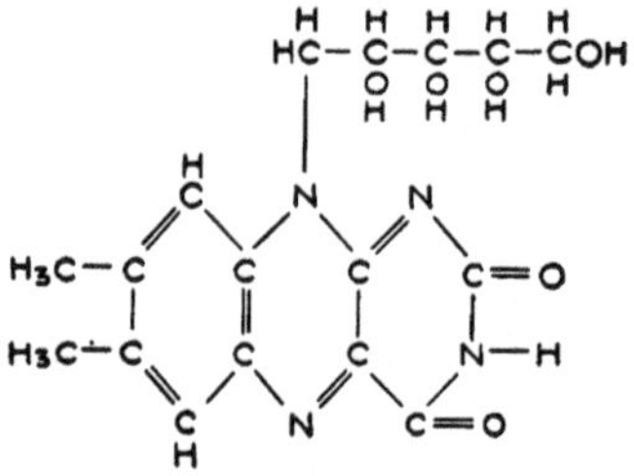

Fig. 39. Structural formula of d-riboflavin (6,7-dimethyl-9 (1'-d-ribityl)-isoalloxazine).

mined colorimetrically. A microbiological assay measures the acid production by *Lactobacillus casei;* this is proportional to the amount of riboflavin present in the system.

Riboflavin takes part in many different enzyme systems in the tissues. Each system consists of an apoenzyme and a coenzyme. The apoenzyme is a specific protein or the "Zwischenferment". The coenzyme constitutes the prosthetic group of the enzyme system, and riboflavin is an integral part of its constitution. The same coenzyme can serve as the prosthetic group of a number of different apoenzymes.

The two coenzymes containing riboflavin are (1) riboflavin-5'-phosphoric acid (riboflavin-mononucleotide) and (2) riboflavin-adenine-dinucleotide. Riboflavin acts on the various enzyme systems by reversibly accepting and donating two atoms of hydrogen. This is accomplished by the addition of the hydrogen to the one and ten positions of riboflavin. Riboflavin is the only naturally-occurring flavin with vitamin B_2 activity. Many flavin compounds have been prepared synthetically and shown to have vitamin activity. Generally speaking substitution in the six or seven position is necessary for vitamin activity, and the absence of substituents in both positions is accompanied by toxicity. An unsubstituted group in the three position also is necessary for activity.

Riboflavin is a combination of d-ribose and isoalloxazine. The phosphoric acid ester of riboflavin unites a specific, nonactive, bearer protein to form the "yellow enzyme". In the presence of an "activating enzyme" from yeast (Zwischenferment) and a thermostable coenzyme (now identified as coenzyme II, triphosphorpyridine nucleotide) the yellow enzyme is capable of oxidizing Robinson's hexose monophosphoric ester. The following scheme has been postulated for the action of this system:

(1) coenzyme + hexose monophosphoric acid $\xrightarrow{\text{Zwischenferment}}$ reduced coenzyme-phosphohexonic acid

(2) reduced coenzyme + yellow enzyme $\longrightarrow$ coenzyme + reduced yellow enzyme

(3) reduced yellow enzyme + molecular oxygen $\longrightarrow$ H_2O_2 + yellow enzyme

This system, in contrast to other well-known oxidation-reduction systems, is not poisoned by hydrocyanic acid or carbon monoxide. Since the coenzyme is alternately reduced and oxidized by the yellow enzyme, and the yellow enzyme itself is reversibly oxidized and reduced, only a very small amount of both of these substances is required for the reaction.

In similar enzyme systems the flavoprotein is concerned with oxidation of amino acids. It combines with phosphoric acid, ribose and adenine to form a d-amino oxidase. A similar dinucleotide has been described, which catalyzes the oxidation of aldehydes and lactic acid. Another flavoprotein enters the metabolism of xanthines as an oxidase. A number of flavoproteins have been described chemically; some are inactive, and the biological importance of others has not been established.

Riboflavin occurs naturally in three forms; as riboflavin per se, as riboflavin-5′-phosphoric acid and as riboflavin-adenine-dinucleotide. It may be absorbed easily by the intestine in any of these forms. The transformation of riboflavin to its phosphoric acid ester and the dinu? cleotide is a general cellular reaction. Human blood cells, for example, can make the synthesis *in vivo* or *in vitro*, but the plasma cannot. This means that riboflavin can be administered parenterally, and we often do this.

It would seem that the liver and kidney are the organs most concerned with the use of riboflavin and other substances to form specific enzyme systems. Riboflavin is excreted chiefly in the feces. When the diet is low in riboflavin, practically no riboflavin is excreted in the urine, although it is still found in the feces. An increase in the riboflavin intake of human beings is followed rapidly by an increase in the urinary output. The animal organism apparently has no special storage organ for riboflavin, although the blood level is maintained in spite of lesions in man. Larger concentrations are found in the liver and in the kidney, although a large intake of riboflavin does not increase its content to any great extent. Even when animals die from lack of this vitamin, their tissues still contain considerable amounts, often as much as one-third of the normal level. No substantial decrease of the riboflavin content of the blood and muscles could be observed in man even though they had clinical lesions[234].

If the intake from the gastrointestinal tract is increased greatly, there is only a slight increase in the amount stored. As long as the diet is adequate, riboflavin is excreted in the urine. On a low dietary intake the excretion exceeds the intake but gradually decreases. The body clings tenaciously to its stores of riboflavin. Axelrod, Spies and Elvehjem[235] could not detect a correlation between the amount of a test dose of riboflavin retained and the daily urinary riboflavin excreted in human beings. They did produce uncomplicated riboflavin deficiency in the dog, however, in which the degree of retention of a test dose of riboflavin was found to be a measure of the riboflavin deficiency.

Riboflavin is distributed so widely that it seems that each animal and plant cell contains small amounts. The amount in the seeds of plants is small but increases rapidly during germination. The richest source of riboflavin is certain fermentation bacteria. Yeast contains considerable amounts. The liver, kidney and heart contain about ten to thirty times the amount found in muscles. The retina of the eyes of many species of animal contains large quantities of riboflavin. Riboflavin tends to be found in the free form in human milk, in the urine and in the retina.

Canning processes cause the loss of from 22 to 67 per cent. of the riboflavin in foods. Ordinary cooking, however, destroys but little, and the only loss of magnitude occurs in the event that water, in which food has been boiled, is discarded. Freezing of foods for storage does not alter appreciably their riboflavin content.

Pathological Physiology

There has been so little investigation of the histological changes in human tissues in riboflavin deficiency that a pathological description is not available. Studies of gross living material, particularly the eye and tongue, have been made using the slit-lamp biomicroscope. These reveal the nonspecific changes so often accompanying inflammation and atrophy. Although our knowledge of the pathological physiology is far from complete, it is believed that the cornea and other relatively avascular tissues are dependent to a great extent on the flavoprotein for normal respiration. This may explain the vascularization around the cornea in individuals which is relieved by riboflavin.

Until recently little precise scientific knowledge has existed in regard to the assumption that congenital anomalies may occur as a result of a deficiency of riboflavin in the maternal diet. Warkany and associates[236,237] have shown that female rats on restricted diets gave birth to young with skeletal defects. Malformations occurred in the extremities, the jaw and the ribs, and there was a constant type of cleft palate. These authors have shown that the malformations could be prevented completely by giving riboflavin. One of the most interesting aspects of these studies has been the determination of the actual period of embryonic development in which the deficiency of riboflavin results in abnormal tissue differentiation. They found that the mother rat still could produce normal young, if the deficient diet was corrected on the twelfth day of gestation. The thirteenth day was the critical day; adding the supplement on the fourteenth day or any day thereafter failed to protect the young. The implications of these dramatic experiments with respect to maternal human nutrition are tremendous. It would seem that it is not enough that the mother be able to conceive; she must have adequate nutrients for normal differentiation and for normal reproduction.

It is highly probable that riboflavin may constitute a part of many enzymes other than Warburg's yellow enzyme, xanthine oxidase and d-aminoacid oxidase. This postulate might explain the all too frequent cheilosis which is not healed by riboflavin. Under such circumstances it may be that the system of hydrogen carriers and acceptors is disrupted at a point close to the active position of riboflavin and that similar pathological lesions are produced even when the supply of riboflavin is adequate or excessive. There is some suggestion that pyridoxine (vitamin B_6)[238] or iron may fit into such auxiliary systems.

The theory that the ocular lesions of riboflavin deficiency result from anoxia has been advanced[239]; the engorgement of the conjunctivae and limbal vessels may be considered an inadequate attempt to supply the tissues in this area with adequate oxygen. Thus, one might expect a deficiency of almost any enzyme to produce similar ocular signs. It is equally possible, however, that riboflavin may aid in the formation of choline esterase and through its action on acetylcholine and the autonomic nervous system effect conjunctival vasodilitation.

Since it was demonstrated that riboflavin is synthesized by bacteria in the rumens of animals, it has been suspected that this might occur in the intestinal tract of man. There has been some indirect evidence to substantiate this hypothesis[240]. The authors have been unable to determine the amount of riboflavin produced by intestinal bacterial synthesis. The type of bacterial flora and the quality of the diet are important, but it has not been determined whether or not the body can utilize the riboflavin present in viable bacteria.

Symptomatology

Perhaps the most characteristic clinical sign in riboflavin deficiency is an angular stomatitis which is called cheilosis[241]. The earliest change is a paleness of the lips, particularly at the angles but not the moist area of the buccal mucosa. The pallor usually continues for days and is followed by maceration and piling up of whitish tissue on a pink background. Superficial fissures may invade the site of the natural wrinkles at the corners of the mouth. The macerated lesions subsequently become dry, and a yellowish crust, which forms at the angles, can be removed without causing bleeding. As the disease progresses, the fissures in the corners of the mouth tend to become deeper and extend to the cheek. They may extend within the mouth so that the constantly irritated angles become raw, bleeding areas with crusts or scabs. Such lesions are sometimes very painful in the acute stage. Frequent recurrences may result in the formation of a cicatrix, giving the affected area an atrophic appearance. Cheilosis usually occurs at both angles of the mouth, but sometimes only one angle is involved (See Fig. 40). Furthermore, there may be a difference in severity of the lesions at the two angles of the mouth, and in occasional cases the lesion at one angle progresses while the other regresses. Another alteration occurs, usually in the inner surface of the lower lip; apparently with the shedding of superficial epithelium the mucous border becomes a brilliant red. On close examination one finds this to be caused by increased visibility of a myriad of minute dilated vessels. This rarely is associated with burning of the lips and tongue. The lesions of the lips and the angles of the mouth often heal spontaneously in the winter and summer and break down in the spring and fall, and persons, whose lips have undergone these changes repeatedly,

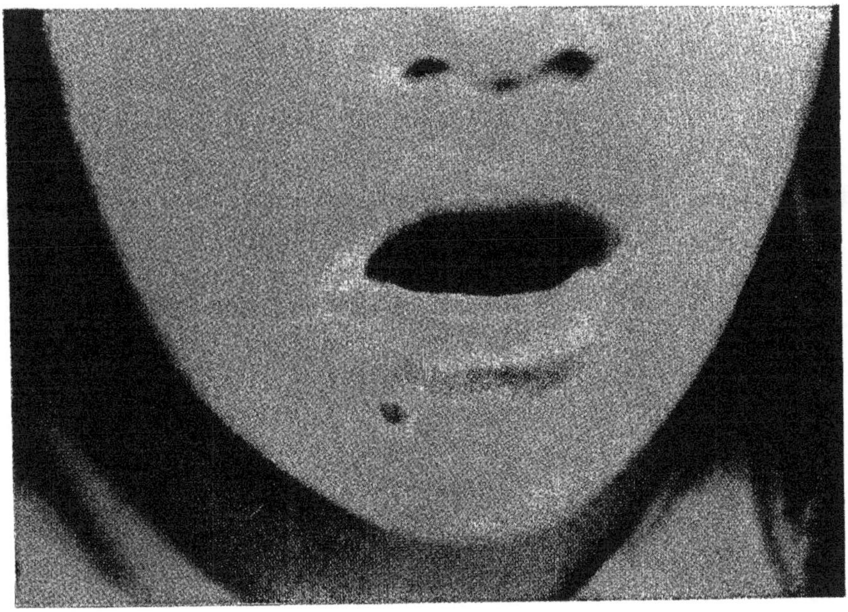

Fig. 40. Cheilosis from riboflavin deficiency.

show scarring in the angles of the mouth and mottling of the vermilion border of the lips.

Such pathological changes at the angles of the mouth have been called "perleche," which means "to lick intensively". Epidemics of perleche have been described, particularly in children's institutions. In one such epidemic Finnerud[242] called attention to a seborrhoeic dermatitis-like eruption of the face in 18 of 100 children with perleche. In 1944 he reviewed the etiology of perleche and emphasized its polyetiological nature[243]. Such lesions of the angles of the mouth, which heal with riboflavin, also yield smears and cultures positive for yeast, fungi and bacterial organisms such as staphylococci, streptococci and Vincent's organisms.

Cheilosis of a mechanical etiology must be differentiated from that caused by riboflavin deficiency. This type has been studied by Ellenberg and Pollack[244] and by Mann and Spies[245], and it has been related directly to a decrease in the vertical dimension of the face in many instances due to ill-fitting dentures, only one denture or none at all. Thus, consumption of an adequate amount of a varied diet often was impossible. When these patients were given riboflavin, there was an amelioration of the cheilosis, but the lesions did not disappear. With sagging of the facial muscles and the resultant fissures at the angles of the mouth saliva readily leaks into the intertriginous areas, and maceration and infection result. It is necessary to restore adequate dental function and a normal contour of the face in order to facilitate the healing of the lesions in these persons. It is only under such circumstances that they can ingest the foods necessary to maintain optimal nutrition.

Often the prominence of the papillae is reduced, and the tongue has a smooth appearance. It may be purplish red or magenta in color. Irregular patches of erythema may be present, but they are not as fiery red as they are in nicotinic acid amide deficiency. Frequently the glossitis of pellagra obscures that of riboflavin deficiency, and it is not until the pellagrous erythema has blanched following the administration of nicotinic acid that the underlying purplish color, characteristic of riboflavin deficiency, can be seen. Clinical trial, first with nicotinic acid and then with riboflavin, often is necessary in order to distinguish the glossitis of pellagra from the glossitis of riboflavin deficiency.

The first statement in regard to certain eye symptoms arising in persons with riboflavin deficiency is that of Spies, Bean and Ashe in 1939[246]. They described a series of symptoms which disappeared within forty-eight hours after a single injection of riboflavin and returned within ten to twenty days, if the deficient diet was continued. The syndrome was greatly amplified by Spies, Vilter and Ashe[247] the same year. They called attention to ocular manifestations of riboflavin deficiency in human beings. These manifestations included bulbar conjunctivitis, dilatation of the conjunctival vessels, burning of the eyes, lacrimation, failing vision and extreme photophobia. All the patients studied were known to have been on a riboflavin-deficient diet, and their symptoms disappeared following riboflavin therapy. Soon many investigators reported studies on riboflavin deficiency, and the next year Kruse, Sydenstriker, Sebrell and Cleckley[248] reported on nine patients and stated that the principal manifestation was keratitis. Later that year these investigators reported that by means of the slit lamp they had found vascularization of the cornea. They stressed particularly the superficial vascularization of the cornea and the finding of interstitial keratitis. Unfortunately these investigators apparently did not examine the corneas of a large number of patients, for today there is much controversy on the subject and a wide divergence of opinion. Many ophthalmologists have refused to accept the specificity of these ocular lesions.

A study of 500 patients with the ocular manifestations of riboflavin deficiency by Spies, Perry, Cogswell and Frommeyer[249] shows that these lesions frequently occurred in the absence of cheilosis or vice versa. The visual symptoms in practically all the patients were heralded by a feeling of dryness of the eyes which was followed by burning and itching and sometimes, by photophobia and lacrimation. In some cases conjunctivitis was the sole manifestation and was shown by increased visibility of the vessels of both the bulbar and palpebral conjunctivae, apparently due to congestion and dilatation. Small vessels were observed to encroach on the cornea at the scleral-corneal junction. Interstitial keratitis was observed in 60 per cent. of the patients and corneal ulceration in at least one eye in 53 per cent. In all cases an effort was made to eliminate other etiological disorders such as vernal conjunctivitis, foreign bodies in the cornea, xerophthalmia and such diseases of the uveal tract as iritis due to syphilis, tuberculosis and rheumatic fever.

Within forty-eight hours after beginning therapy there was some subjective improvement in all the patients. Improvement was volunteered in 80 per cent. of the cases. Within this period a diminution in the calibre of the dilated vessels in the eyes and a striking decrease in the photophobia and corneal ulcerations were observed. Accompanying this improvement was a decrease of hemolytic staphylococci, streptococci and xerosis bacilli in the exudate from the eyes. Relief of pain occurred and vision improved. Although 84 per cent. of the patients subsequently had recurrences, this is attributed to cessation of therapy and a return to the previous diet which was inadequate in riboflavin.

It must be emphasized that the differentiation of these superficial lesions of the eye from other types of conjunctivitis and keratitis is both difficult and uncertain. It seems that many other varieties of conjunctivitis also may be benefited by the parenteral administration of riboflavin which suggests that this vitamin may play a routine part in such inflammations.

Diagnosis

In making a diagnosis the physician should keep in mind that riboflavin deficiency may occur in either sex, at any age and in any race, that it usually occurs following subsistence for months or years on a diet deficient in riboflavin, and that it is especially common among those whose diets are inadequate. It may occur, however, as a result of a metabolic complication of some other disease state, and in such cases it is referred to as secondary riboflavin deficiency. The physiological possibilities for the induction of a secondary deficiency may be listed briefly as follows; (a) decreased intake, (b) decreased absorption, (c) increased excretion, (d) increased requirement, (e) decreased utilization, (f) increased destruction.

In a report describing observations on 500 selected cases of riboflavin deficiency Spies, Perry, Cogswell and Frommeyer[249] found that the dietaries of these patients supplied only one-third of the allowance of riboflavin recommended by the Food and Nutrition Board of the National Research Council (see Fig. 41).

What should constitute the exact criteria for the diagnosis of human riboflavin deficiency is almost impossible to estimate from the various reports. Sebrell[250] has summarized his concept as follows:

"(1) Ocular lesions, consisting usually of a vascularizing keratitis with photophobia, dimness of vision, severe injection of the vessels of the fornix and sclera, burning of the eyes, lacrimation, and in severe cases, opacities of the cornea; (2) oral lesions, consisting usually of linear fissures in the angles of the mouth, a reddened, shiny, denuded appearance of the lower lip, and a flattening of the papillae of the tongue, which becomes magenta red in color; (3) dermal lesions, consisting usually of seborrheic accumulations in the folds of the skin, especially in the nasolabial folds, around the eyelids, on the ears, and

RECOMMENDED DIETARY ALLOWANCES, REVISED 1945[1]
(Amounts Per Day)

Food and Nutrition Board, National Research Council

	Calories	Protein grams	Cal-cium grams	Iron mg.	Vitamin A I. U.[2]	Thia-mine mg.[3]	Ribo-flavin mg.[3]	Niacin (Nicoti-nic acid) mg.[3]	Ascorbic acid mg.	Vitamin D I. U.
Man (154 lb., 70 kg.)										
Sedentary	2500	70	0.8	12[4]	5000	1.2	1.6	12	75	[5]
Moderately active	3000	70	0.8	12[4]	5000	1.5	2.0	15	75	[5]
Very active	4500	70	0.8	12[4]	5000	2.0	2.6	20	75	[5]
Woman (123 lb., 56 kg.)										
Sedentary	2100	60	0.8	12	5000	1.1	1.5	11	70	[5]
Moderately active	2500	60	0.8	12	5000	1.2	1.6	12	70	[5]
Very active	3000	60	0.8	12	5000	1.5	2.0	15	70	[5]
Pregnancy (latter half)	2500[6]	85	1.5	15	6000	1.8	2.5	18	100	400 to 800
Lactation	3000	100	2.0	15	8000	2.0	3.0	20	150	400 to 800
Children up to 12 yrs.[7]:										
Under 1 yr.[8]	100/2.2 lb. (1 kg.)	3.5/2.2 lb. (1 kg.)	1.0	6	1500	0.4	0.6	4	30	400 to 800
1–3 yrs. (29 lb., 13 kg.)	1200	40	1.0	7	2000	0.6	0.9	6	35	400
4–6 yrs. (42 lb., 19 kg.)	1600	50	1.0	8	2500	0.8	1.2	8	50	400
7–9 yrs. (55 lb., 25 kg.)	2000	60	1.0	10	3500	1.0	1.5	10	60	400
10–12 yrs. (75 lb., 34 kg.)	2500	70	1.2	12	4500	1.2	1.8	12	75	400
Children over 12 yrs.[7]:										
Girls, 13–15 yrs. (108 lb., 49 kg.)	2600	80	1.3	15	5000	1.3	2.0	13	80	400
16–20 yrs. (119 lb., 54 kg.)	2400	75	1.0	15	5000	1.2	1.8	12	80	400
Boys, 13–15 yrs. (103 lb., 47 kg.)	3200	85	1.4	15	5000	1.5	2.0	15	90	400
16–20 yrs. (141 lb., 64 kg.)	3800	100	1.4	15	6000	1.8	2.5	18	100	400

[1] Tentative goal toward which to aim in planning practical dietaries; can be met by a good diet with a variety of natural foods. Such a diet will also provide other minerals and vitamins, the requirements for which are less well known.

[2] The allowance depends on the relative amounts of vitamin A and carotene. The allowances of the table are based on the premise that approximately two-thirds of the vitamin A value of the average diet in this country is contributed by carotene and that carotene has half or less than half the value of vitamin A.

[3] For adults (except pregnant and lactating women) receiving diets supplying 2,000 cal ries or less, sch as reducing diets, the allowances of thiamine, riboflavin, and min may be 1 mg., 1.5 mg., and 10 mg. 1 sly. The fat tht figures are given for different levels for thiamine, riboflavin, and min des not i ply that we an estimate the requirement of these tors within 500 calories, but they are lded merely for simplicity of calculation. Or members of the B- px also are required, thgh no values can be given. Foods supplying qe thiamine, fln, and min will tend to supply sufficient of the maining B vitamins.

[4] There is evidence that the male dult needs little or no iron.

Fig. 41. Recommended dietary allowances, revised 1945 (amount per day). Food and Nutrition Board, National Research Council.

in some cases comedones and a sharkskin-appearing lesion on the nose and over the malar eminences. In some cases the seborrheic dermal lesions may be extensive and may involve other regions of the body."

In the absence of characteristic lesions the recognition of riboflavin deficiency is difficult. An appraisal of the dietary of the patient is helpful but not an infallible guide. The scars of old cheilosis should arouse suspicion. In the prodromal period prior to the appearance of typical lesions most of the subjective symptoms result from depletion of niacinamide and thiamine stores. Neither at this period nor later, when the lesions are advanced, is there a consistently accurate laboratory test to determine the adequacy or inadequacy of the stores of riboflavin.

A tentative diagnosis is warranted in the presence of cheilosis with angular stomatitis, engorgement of pericorneal vessels and concommitant subjective symptoms of photophobia, burning and dimness of vision. Riboflavin deficiency should be suspected in the person, who presents a magenta tongue or the greasy, scaly dermatitis in-characteristic areas about the face and the "sharkskin" appearance of skin over the nose and malar prominence. In examining the tongue, however, it should be kept in mind that forceful protrusion results in compression of the ranular veins and in congestion and cyanosis. Therefore, the magenta hue should be observed in the tongue at rest within the mouth.

The therapeutic test substantiates the diagnosis. Healing of the angles of the mouth and the tongue usually is initiated after from three to six days of specific therapy. Subjective improvement in the ocular lesions usually is noticeable in 24 hours, if large doses are given, although objectively there may be little change for from two days to a week. Complete healing of the eye and skin lesions extends over a period of several weeks, and the conjunctivitis is prone to relapse when treatment is discontinued.

Prevention and Treatment

Riboflavin deficiency can be prevented either by the use of synthetic riboflavin or by the consumption of foods rich in riboflavin. The practicing physician is urged to read the sections on vitamin B_1 and nicotinic acid for the dietary management and general recommendations for the prevention and treatment of nutritional deficiencies. Single vitamin deficiencies occur rarely, and despite the fact that riboflavin deficiency may dominate the clinical picture, it is unlikely that the physician will see a patient who has uncomplicated riboflavin deficiency. There are no definite lesions which are pathognomonic of riboflavin deficiency. The cheilosis or the ocular manifestations may or may not be due to riboflavin deficiency. The authors give from 5 to 50 mgm. of riboflavin, but as a rule, they find that 10 mgm. daily is adequate for the average case. It may be given orally, intravenously or intramuscularly. Subcutaneous

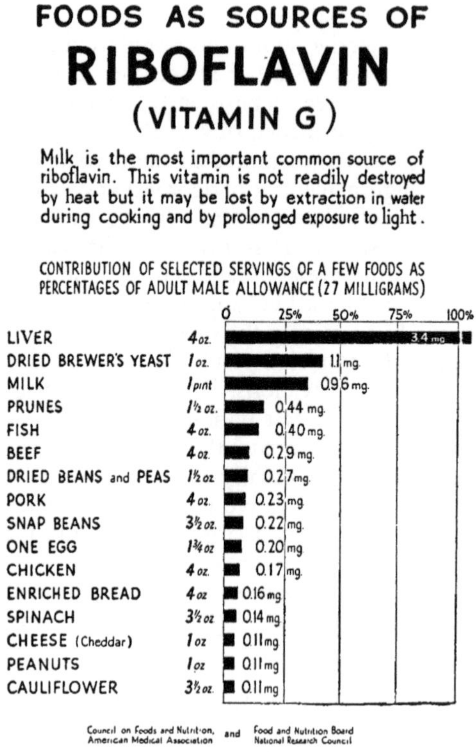

FIG. 42. Foods as sources of riboflavin (Vitamin G).

administration causes considerable pain. The symptoms are relieved much more quickly by parenteral than by oral therapy. Cheilosis, corneal ulceration, corneal vascularity, photophobia and non-infectious conjunctivitis respond rapidly to treatment with riboflavin, if they are due to a deficiency of riboflavin. The tendency of lesions to reappear after cessation of treatment is common and may occur even when the dietary is at an optimal level. Consequently frequent observation is necessary for a long period of time. Should relapse occur, the reinstatement of therapy usually affords prompt amelioration of the symptoms. The authors wish to stress, however, that neither the cheilosis nor the dilated blood vessels of the eye are pathognomonic of riboflavin deficiency. They may arise from other causes in which case riboflavin will not correct them.

Toxicity

Riboflavin is practically non-toxic. Mice fed over 5,000 times the daily requirement do not show any pathological symptoms. The authors have given 100 mgm. daily for three months to patients without any ill effects resulting.

FOLIC ACID

History

The finding of a synthetic chemical compound of known molecular structure, which is effective in treating persons with nutritional macrocytic anemia, pernicious anemia and the macrocytic anemia of sprue is a medical event of great importance. This substance, commonly called "folic acid", is the newest member of the vitamin B complex. The name folic acid originally was given to a mixture of substances obtained in nearly pure form from spinach by Mitchell, Snell and Williams[251]. Their concentrate was shown to support growth for two organisms frequently used in microbiological investigations, *Lactobacillus casei* and *Streptococcus faecalis*. Strictly speaking, the *Lactobacillus casei* factor, or pteroylglutamic acid as it properly is termed chemically, should not be called folic acid. The term has become so widely used, however, that it will be regarded as synonmous with the *Lactobacillus casei* factor or pteroylglutamic acid.

This substance gradually emerged as a separate entity as the result of the work of many investigators in many laboratories over a period of eight years. In 1938 Stokstad and Manning[252] reported that a purified diet, even when supplemented with crude concentrates containing thiamine, riboflavin, niacin, pyridoxine and pantothenic acid, would not satisfy the nutritional requirements of chicks, but that the missing factor was supplied by the addition of concentrates from yeast and alfalfa[253]. In 1940 Hogan and Parrott[254] reported that an anemia developed in chicks on a purified diet, unless they were given an unidentified factor, which could be supplied with suitable preparations obtained from liver. The same year Snell and Peterson[255] showed that an unidentified water-soluble factor, "the yeast norite eluate factor", was necessary for the growth of *L. casei*. Later Hutchings and his associates[256] observed that, when the factor was concentrated from extracts prepared from liver, the potency in promoting the growth of chicks on a purified diet was found to increase simultaneously with the potency as measured by *L. casei* factor. This proved to be similar to the "folic acid" obtained from spinach by Mitchell, Snell and Williams. Minute quantities of the *L. casei* factor were obtained in crystalline form from liver by Pfiffner and his associates[257] and from liver and yeast by Stokstad[258]. In 1945 it was synthesized by Angier and his co-workers[259] and a few months later they published its structural formula (see Fig. 43)[260]. A review of many aspects of the studies, which led to the isolation and synthesis of folic acid and studies on its clinical use, has been published recently by Berry and Spies[261] and by Spies[262].

Chemistry and Physiology

As can be seen from the formula (Fig. 43), folic acid contains a pteridine ring and one molecule each of para-aminobenzoic acid and

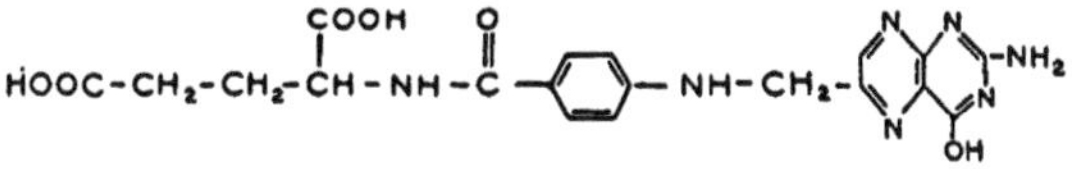

N-[4-{[(2-amino-4-hydroxy-6-pteridyl)methyl] amino} benzoyl] glutamic acid

Fig. 43. Structural formula of the liver *L. casei* factor

glutamic acid. Pteroic acid and glutamic acid are of great interest because of their chemical relationship to the folic acid molecule. As can be seen from their chemical formula in Figs. 44 and 45, pteroic acid differs from folic acid, pteroylglutamic acid, by the absence of one molecule of glutamic acid. In their studies on the synthesis of folic acid Angier and his associates found that by substituting p-aminobenzoic acid

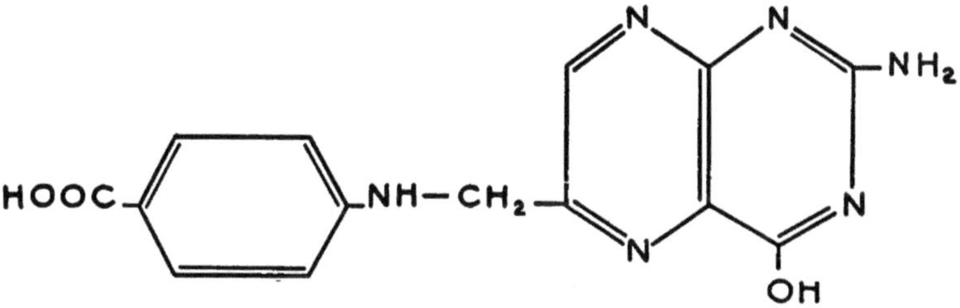

Fig. 44. Structural formula of petroic acid.

for p-aminobenzoyl-1(+)-glutamic acid in the process a compound was produced which had growth activity for *Streptococcus faecalis* but not for *L. casei* and the chick. The term assigned to this compound is pteroic acid. In contrast to pteroylglutamic acid, which is a potent hemopoietic agent, pteroic acid and glutamic acid do not show any hemopoietic activity when administered either separately or together. It must be assumed, therefore, that these substances must be prefabricated to form pteroylglutamic acid before they can be utilized by the body for blood regeneration.

Folic acid is a bright yellow substance which crystallizes as is shown in Fig. 46. It is destroyed fairly rapidly by heating with dilute mineral acids, and sunlight has a destructive effect on a solution of folic acid. It occurs in nature in a free form and also as a part of various complexes. The following substances have been isolated in crystalline form; (1) vitamin B_c, (2) *Lactobacillus casei* factor from liver, (3) *Lactobacillus*

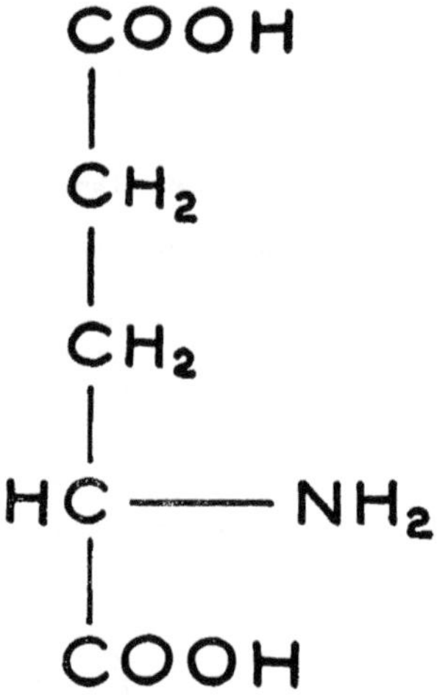

Fig. 45. Structural formula of glutamic acid.

casei factor from yeast, (4) another *Lactobacillus casei* factor isolated from a fermentation residue and (5) vitamin B_c conjugate. Vitamin B_c, the *L. casei* factor from liver and the *L. casei* factor from yeast are identical with the synthetic product described by Angier and his associates. This compound, folic acid or pteroylglutamic acid, contains one molecule of glutamic acid. In contrast, the conjugated *L. casei* factor isolated from the fermentation residue yields three molecules of glutamic acid and is called pteroyltriglutamic acid. The vitamin B_c conjugate contains 7 molecules of glutamic acid and is termed pteroylheptaglutamic acid. The structural formulas of these substances could be written as is shown in Fig. 47, although the precise structure is not known at this time. These substances are somewhat effective in producing a hemopoietic response in certain types of macrocytic anemia in relapse but less effective per unit of weight than is folic acid[263]. Within 24 hours after the administration of pteroylglutamic acid to persons with pernicious anemia there is a great increase in the urinary excretion of this substance, whereas the administration of vitamin B_c conjugate is not followed by a great increase in the amount of folic acid excreted in the urine of some patients with pernicious anemia (Fig. 48).

Whether or not most animals can synthesize folic acid has not been determined. The relative scarcity of it in animal tissues suggests that, if

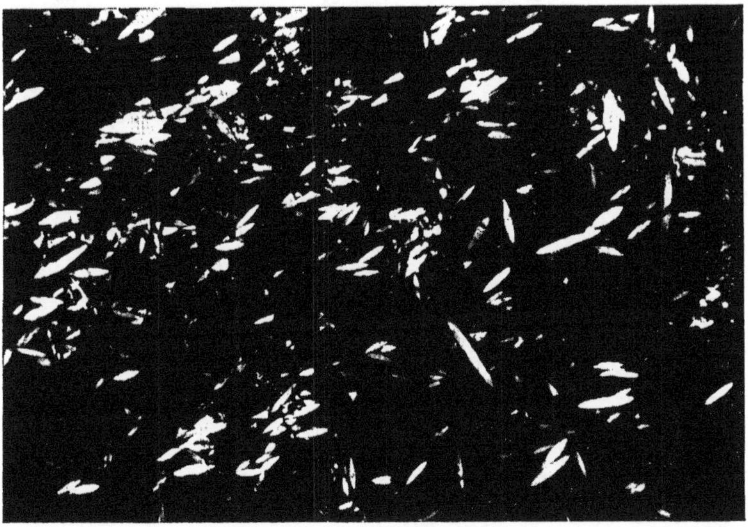

Fig. 46. Microphotograph showing crystalline folic acid (courtesy of Lederle Laboratories, Inc.).

it is synthesized, only small quantities of it are produced or only small amounts are stored. It is possible that the bacteria normally present in the intestinal tract of some animals, such as the rat, may synthesize considerable quantities. Experimentally folic acid has been found to be essential for the proper nutrition of a variety of micro-organisms and laboratory animals either as a growth-promoting or a hemopoietic-stimulating factor or both[261,262]. Although its rôle in human nutrition is not clear, its effectiveness in the treatment of macrocytic anemias in relapse has been established.

Pteroylglutamic acid is distributed widely in both plant and animal tissues. At the present time the distribution of folic acid in foods usually is studied by microbiological assays. Olson, Burris and Elvehjem[264] have classified foods assayed for their folic acid content by such methods as follows:

1. Very high in folic acid content: deep green leafy vegetables, liver

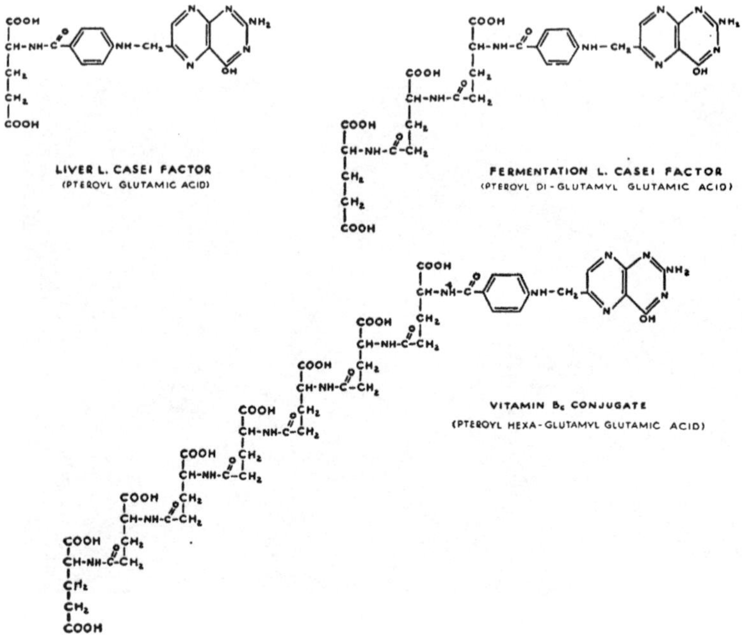

Fig. 47. Suggested structural formulae for fermentation *L. casei* factor and vitamin B$_c$ conjugate.

2. High in folic acid content: fresh green vegetables, cauliflower and kidney
3. Medium in folic acid content: beef, veal, dry breakfast cereals from wheat
4. Low in folic acid content: root vegetables, tomatoes, cucumbers, light green leafy vegetables, bananas, pork, ham, lamb, cheese, milk, dry cereals prepared from rice or corn and many canned foods

Pathological Physiology

Folic acid has a profound effect on the bone marrow of persons with certain types of macrocytic anemia in relapse. Nevertheless, it cannot

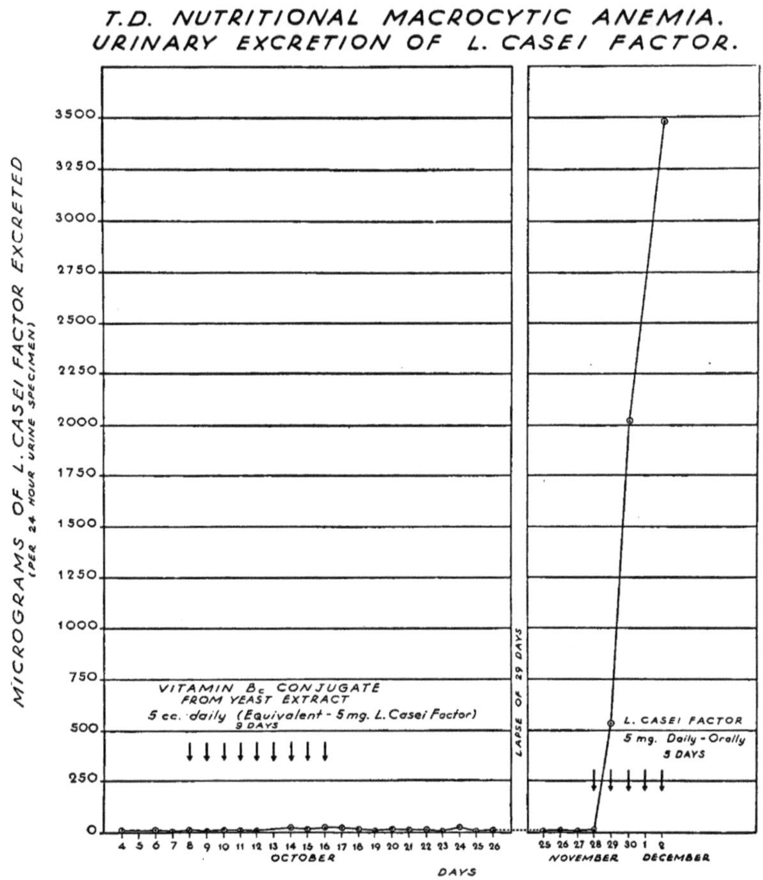

Fig. 48. Chart showing excretion in the urine of folic acid after giving to a patient with nutritional macrocytic anemia 5 c.c. of vitamin Bc conjugate daily for 9 days.

be said that the megaloblastic arrest of the bone marrow was caused by a folic acid deficiency. Liver extract and ventriculin produce a similar therapeutic effect, yet there is much reason to believe that folic acid is different from the anti-anemic factor or factors in these substances.

By using the sternal puncture in patients under investigation, it is possible to follow the action of folic acid step by step in the bone marrow. In contrast to the peripheral blood picture, where changes first become appreciable several days after the onset of treatment, profound transformations of the bone marrow occur earlier. Reticulocytosis can be detected in the bone marrow, sometimes as early as the second day. The number of megaloblasts and early erythroblasts decreases progressively, and the late erythroblasts and normoblasts increase. Eventually the normal ratio of nucleated red blood cells and white blood cells of the marrow is re-established. In the following series of studies done at the time the patient was admitted to the hospital and twice during therapy one sees a disappearance of the megaloblastic arrest, and the bone marrow becomes normal.

Bone marrow study on admission

Sternal bone marrow was obtained by means of the Turkel trephine;

200 W.B.C. were counted.

Cells	*Number*	*Percent*
PMN	120	60.
Metamyelocytes	56	28
C myelocytes	2	1
B myelocytes	0	0
A myelocytes	0	0
Basophils	2	1
Basophilic myelocytes	0	0
Eosinophils	4	2
Eosinophilic myelocytes	10	5
Plasma cells	2	1
Megakaryocytes	0	0
Primitive cells	4	2
Total	200	100
Megaloblasts	12	
Early erythroblasts	6	
Late erythroblasts	9	
Normoblasts	15	
Total	42	

Impression: Hyperplastic bone marrow with megaloblastic arrest. arrest.

Bone marrow study made on the 51st day of treatment showed:

Cells	*Number*	*Percent*
PMN	86	43.0
Metamyelocytes	50	25.0
C myelocytes	3	1.5
B myelocytes	4	2.0
A myelocytes	5	2.5
Basophils	1	0.5
Basophilic myelocytes	1	0.5
Eosinophils	9	4.5
Eosinophilic myelocytes	35	17.5
Plasma cells	2	1.0
Megakaryocytes	1	0.5
Primitive cells	3	1.5
Total	200	100
Megaloblasts	6	
Early erythroblasts	11	
Late erythroblasts	20	
Normoblasts	109	
Total	146	

Impression: A reactive bone marrow which shows a good response to therapy. There is still some evidence of megaloblastic arrest.

Bone marrow study made on the 74th day of treatment showed:

PMN	94	47.0
Metamyelocytes	54	27.0
C myelocytes	8	4.0
B myelocytes	5	2.5
A myelocytes	2	1.0
Basophilic myelocytes	1	.5
Eosinophils	6	3.0
Eosinophilic myelocytes	17	8.5
Plasma	1	.5
Megakaryocytes	1	.5
Primitive	6	3.0
Lymphocytes	5	2.5
Total	200	100

Cells	*Number*	*Percent*
Megaloblasts	0	
Early erythroblasts	3	
Late erythroblasts	24	
Normoblasts	37	
Total	64	

Impression: Essentially normal marrow except for an increased number of eosinophilic elements. There has been a definite change toward normal since the 51st day of treatment.

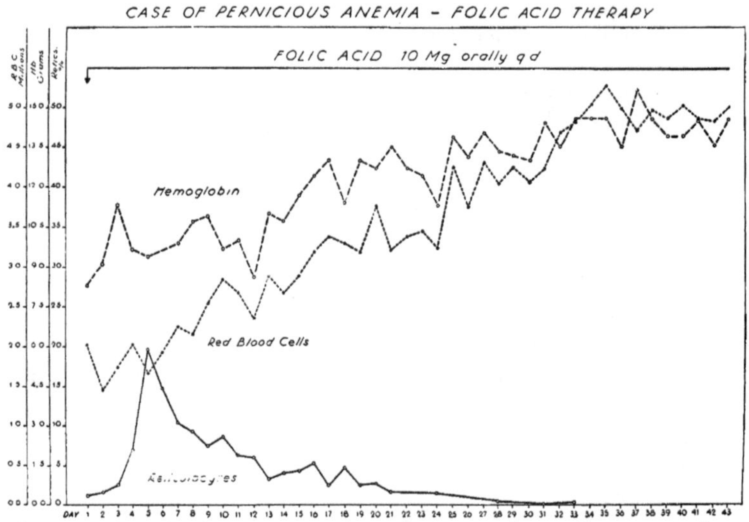

Fig. 49. Chart showing changes in hemoglobin, red blood cells and reticulocytes in patient with pernicious anemia following oral administration of folic acid.

Reticulocytosis in the peripheral blood frequently is detected from about the third to the fifth day of therapy. A peak is reached on the sixth to the tenth day. The height of the rise varies from case to case depending upon the severity of the anemia, the adequacy of the dose of folic acid and the presence or absence of complications. In addition to the reticulocytosis there is a gradual increase in the number of red blood cells and in the hemoglobin (Fig. 49). The thrombocytopenia and leukopenia, which so often are associated with macrocytic anemia, frequently are corrected by folic acid. The blood regeneration, which follows folic acid therapy, is comparable to that which follows therapy with reticulogen, concentrated liver extract. Thymine (5-methyl uracil), another anti-anemic substance, likewise produces blood regeneration[265], but the response is of a lower order than that which follows a potent liver extract or folic acid as can be seen in Fig. 50. Furthermore the large amount of thymine necessary to produce a therapeutic response, up to 15 grams daily, makes it impractical as a therapeutic substance, although it is of great scientific interest.

Symptomatology

Since it is not known that such a thing as a specific deficiency of folic acid exists in human beings, the symptomatology of a folic acid deficiency in man cannot be described. Neverthele sthe judicious administration of folic acid in suitable amounts is effective in treating Addisonian pernicious anemia, nutritional macrocytic anemia and the macrocytic anemia of pellagra, pregnancy and sprue. Some of the more pertinent findings are discussed under *Diagnosis* and *Treatment*.

Diagnosis

Although the effectiveness of folic acid as a therapeutic agent in treating Addisonian pernicious anemia, nutritional macrocytic anemia and the macrocytic anemia of pellagra, pregnancy and sprue has been established[266,267,268], it cannot be overstressed that it is of no value in treating leukemia, aplastic anemia or iron deficiency anemia. The anemia associated with liver disease usually does not respond to folic acid, but in some cases it does. Nutritional leukopenia improves following treatment with folic acid, but other types of leukopenia are not relieved. The physician, who would prescribe folic acid, should first make an accurate diagnosis.

The clinical syndromes of Addisonian pernicious anemia, nutritional macrocytic anemia, tropical sprue and the macrocytic anemia of pellagra and pregnancy are indistinguishable either from examination of the peripheral blood or from bone marrow studies. A characteristic feature of pernicious anemia is the absence of free hydrochloric acid in the gastric juice even after histamine stimulation. Many investigators agree that so-called tropical and non-tropical sprue are essentially the same

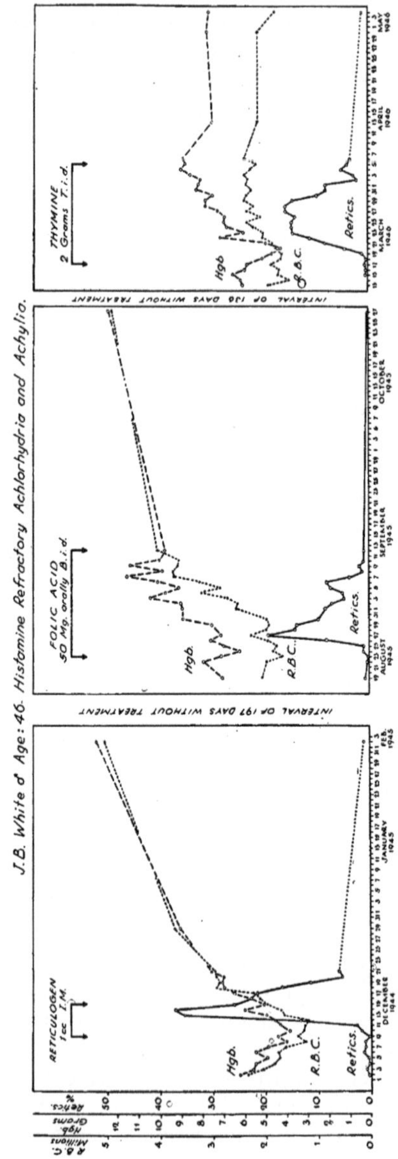

Fig. 50. Charts showing effects on blood of patient with pernicious anemia following administration in successive periods of reticulogen (concentrated liver extract), folic acid and thymine.

disease. The relationship of nutritional macrocytic anemia and sprue is more difficult to grasp. Persons with either disease may have severe diarrhea, but the characteristic diarrhea of sprue is the best differentiating feature, and it is on the presence of this type of diarrhea that the diagnosis of sprue is based. In sprue the stools usually vary in consistency from liquid to semi-solid and in color from whitish yellow to yellowish green, while in nutritional macrocytic anemia rarely are they foamy, but they are foul in odor. Bowel movements in sprue may occur from 3 to 20 or even 30 times a day, tending to occur immediately after the patient eats food of any kind, and the volume of the feces in 24 hours is greatly in excess of the normal volume. Acid steatorrhea, which almost invariably is present in sprue, does not occur in nutritional macrocytic anemia. The weight loss in sprue may be greater and less gradual than that which accompanies nutritional macrocytic anemia.

Even when a considerable number of eminently qualified physicians examine a large group of patients with anemia, a specific diagnosis is apt to be made in some cases, whereas in others opinion is divided. Frequently the physician may make a diagnosis the first time he examines the patient and observes him throughout a relapse of the disease, but during a later recurrence he may change the diagnosis. The author considers that the essential feature of the anemias, which can be expected to respond to folic acid therapy, is megaloblastic arrest of the bone marrow associated with macrocytic anemia in persons who appear to have Addisonian pernicious anemia, sprue, nutritional macrocytic anemia or the macrocytic anemia of pellagra or pregnancy.

When the physician realizes that patients with various clinical conditions respond to folic acid therapy, it might seem academic to stress the necessity of making a specific diagnosis. The prognosis and duration of therapy vary so greatly in the different types of macrocytic anemia, however, that no effort should be spared in obtaining as much precise and pertinent information as possible. The finding of the specific effect of the folic acid molecule on the cells of the bone marrow and perhaps, on other cells opens up a fresh and fertile field for the clinical investigator who must now re-define the macrocytic anemias in the light of all the various loose threads which enter into the meshwork of their pathogenesis.

Treatment

As yet no satisfactory explanation has been given for the fact that relatively large amounts of folic acid are required to produce a satisfactory hemopoietic response. Despite the many intensive clinical studies, which have been made on folic acid as a therapeutic agent, the last word

RESPONSE OF A CASE OF SPRUE TO FOLIC ACID

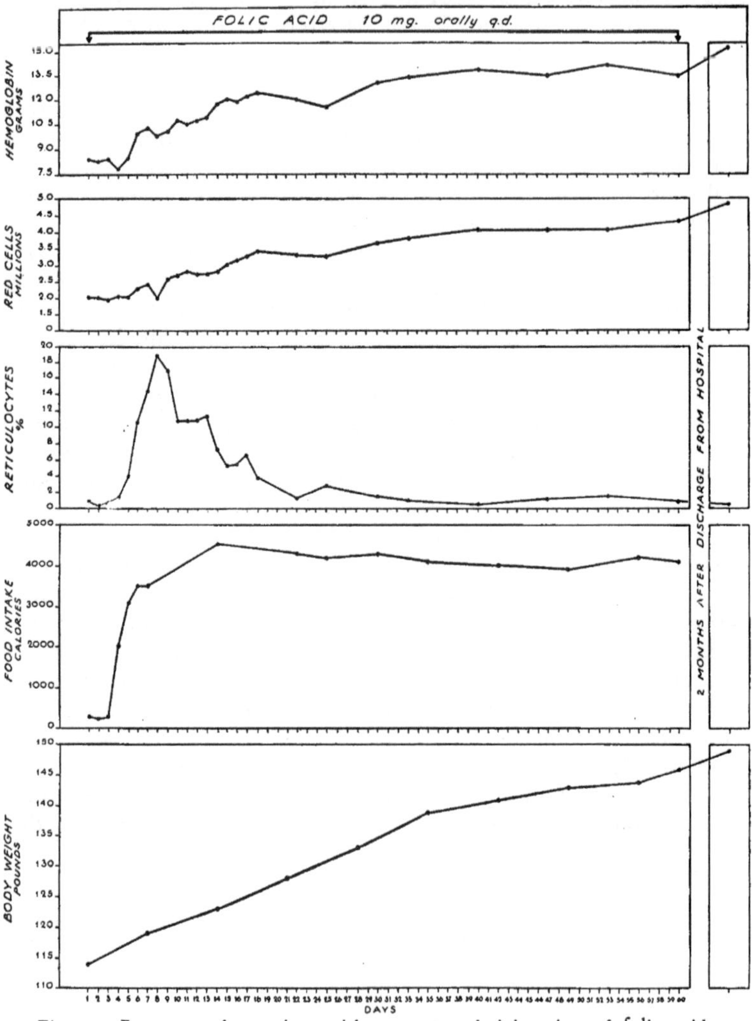

Fig. 51. Response of a patient with sprue to administration of folic acid.

on dosage cannot be stated definitely. In most cases from 10 to 20 mgm. daily in divided doses, given either orally or parenterally, is sufficient to

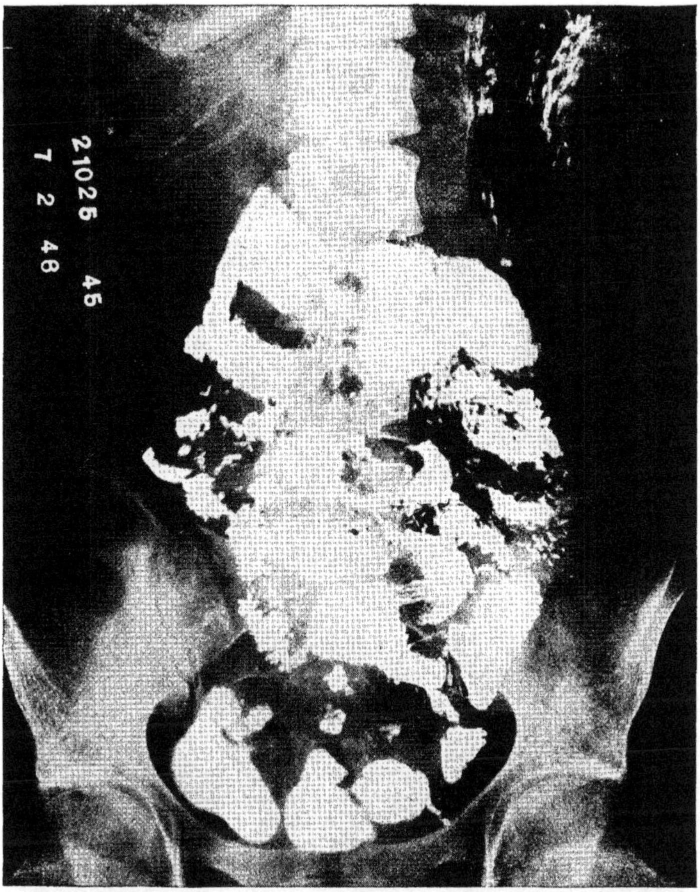

Fig. 52. X-ray showing intestinal pattern in sprue before treatment.

induce a remission in persons with nutritional macrocytic anemia, the macrocytic anemia of pregnancy, pellagra, sprue and Addisonian pernicious anemia.

The dramatic response of the bone marrow and peripheral blood to folic acid in properly selected patients with macrocytic anemia in relapse is discussed and illustrated under *Pathological Physiology*. The

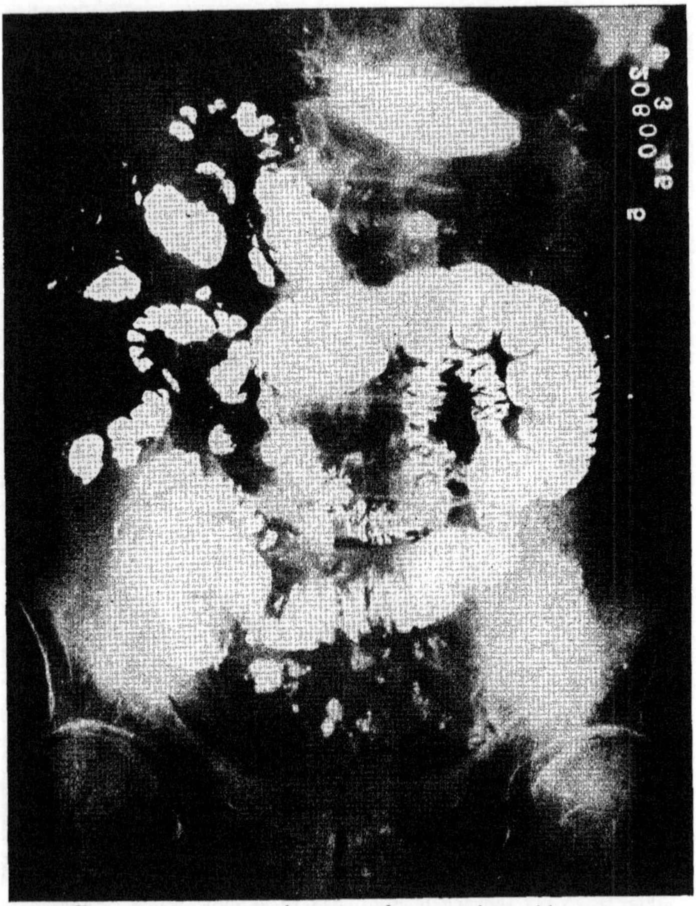

Fig. 53. X-ray showing intestinal pattern of same patient with sprue as shown in Fig. 52 before treatment.

clinical response is equally dramatic. At the time reticulocytosis begins the patients state voluntarily that they feel stronger. Those who have lost their appetites experience a great increase in the desire for food, and in many cases the food intake increases from less than 1,000 calories daily to between 3,000 and 4,000 calories within a day or two from the time reticulocytosis begins. In cases of extreme weight loss, such as that

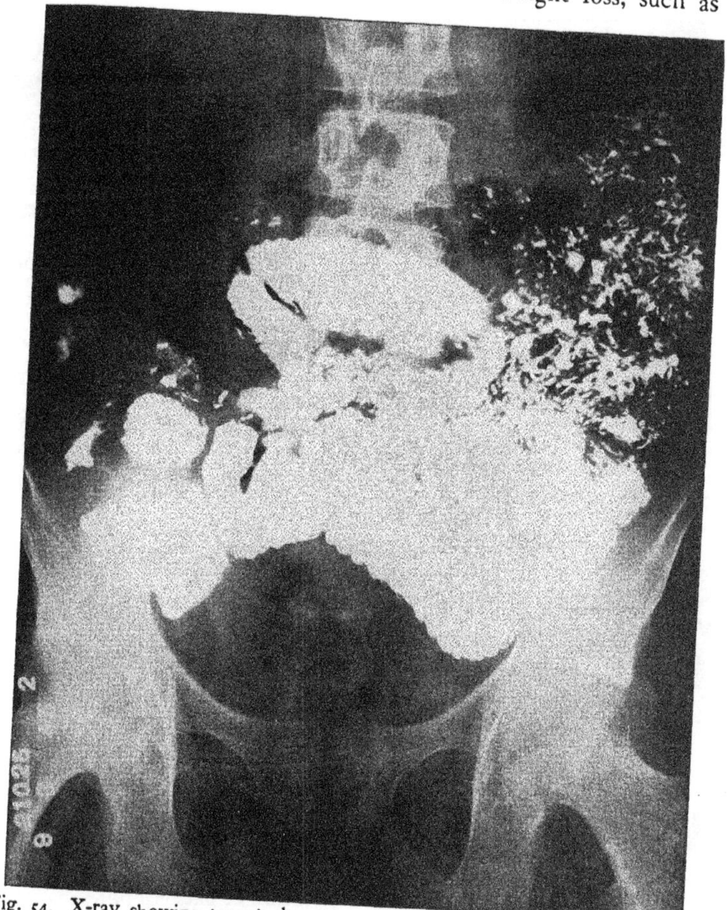

Fig. 54. X-ray showing intestinal pattern of same patient with sprue as shown in Figs. 52 and 53 before treatment.

which occurs in sprue, the gain in appetite and weight is particularly remarkable as can be seen in Fig. 51. No adequate explanation can be given for the prompt improvement in the diarrhea in nutritional macrocytic anemia. The stools may tend to become normal in frequency, color and volume.

Folic acid therapy has a striking effect on the gastrointestinal tract

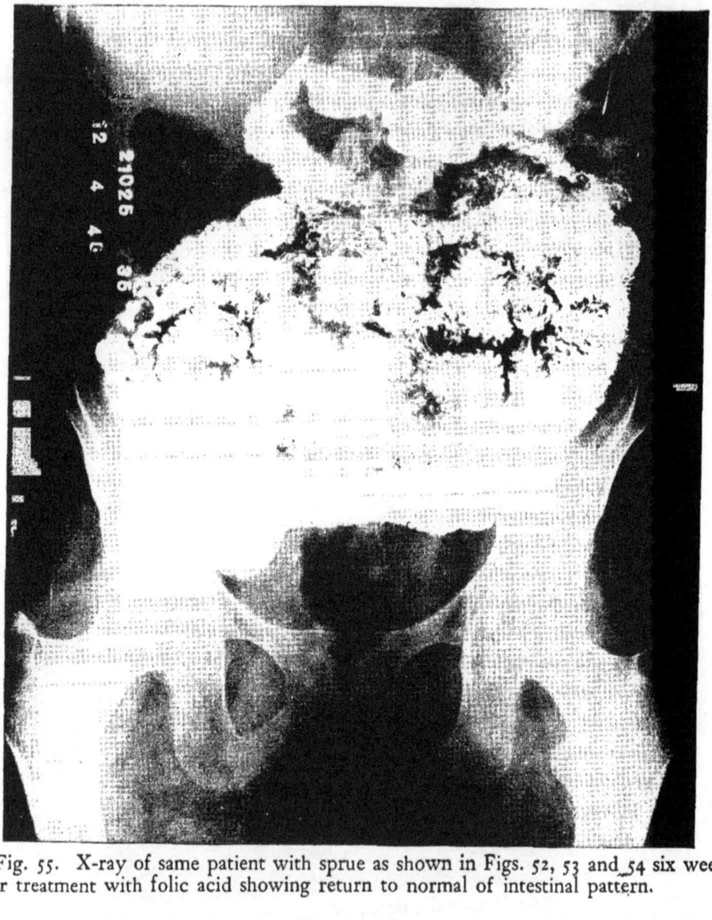

Fig. 55. X-ray of same patient with sprue as shown in Figs. 52, 53 and 54 six weeks after treatment with folic acid showing return to normal of intestinal pattern.

of persons with tropical sprue[269] as can be seen in the illustrations Figs. 52, 53, 54, 55 all made on the same patient. The first three are taken before therapy and the fourth six weeks after folic acid therapy was initiated. The abnormal dilatations and spasms seen in Figs. 52, 53 and

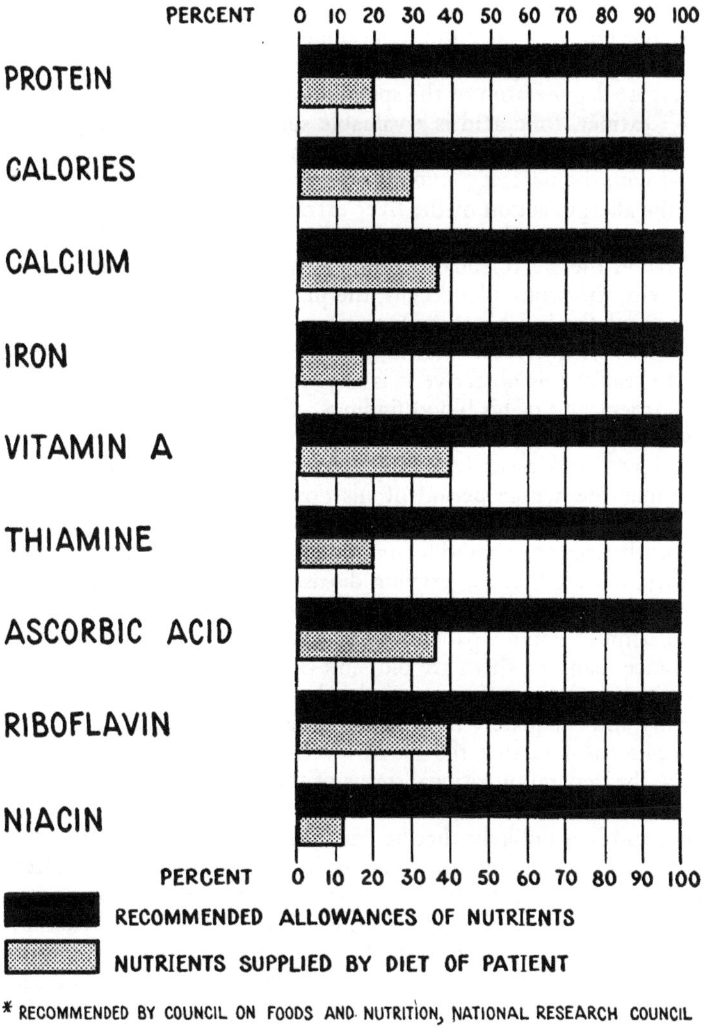

Fig. 56. Chart showing nutrients supplied by diet of patient with chronic pellagra and nutritional macryocytic anemia contrasted to recommended allowances of nutrients.

54 disappeared as can be seen in Fig. 55, which shows that the barium column is continuous and appears perfectly normal.

The chief limitation of folic acid as a therapeutic agent is that it will neither prevent the development of acute or subacute combined system disease nor relieve it once it has developed[263,270]. Liver extract along with folic acid should be given in a dosage sufficient to relieve signs of acute or subacute degeneraton of the spinal cord. In patients, who are allergic to liver extract, folic acid is a valuable substitute unless the patient has neural degeneration. In such cases folic acid therapy should be supplemented with the necesary amount of liver extract to bring steps to overcome the allergic action of the liver extract.

In the treatment of macrocytic anemia correct diagnosis is basic. The objective in the treatment of every patient is the restitution of the red blood cells, the white blood cells, the platelets and the hemoglobin, the reduction of the red blood cells to normal size and the relief of all his symptoms with the result that he becomes completely rehabilitated. In order to realize this objective it is necessary to make a thorough study of the patient and of his blood findings. Once the diagnosis is made, he should be given general therapeutic measures which will promote physical rest and mental serenity. A proper diet should be stressed throughout the whole period of his convalescence and thereafter for the remainder of his life. He should be treated with physiotherapy for any disturbances of gait and locomotion. Tranfusion should be given, if necessary, to save life. Co-existing diseases should be treated, and every effort should be made to eradicate them. During convalescence the physician must remind patients with anemia to avoid unnecessary fatigue, since many of them are old, and their heart function is impaired. Dramatic recovery can be expected, when folic acid is given promptly, efficiently and adequately to properly selected patients.

Despite the fact that the blood levels improve following folic acid therapy, the general nutritional status of the patient frequently warrants particular attention. The patient in severe relapse rarely is interested in food, and it is unlikely that he has been consuming an adequate diet (See Fig. 56). As a rule, the appetite increases tremendously after remission begins, and it is not unusual for him to consume large amounts of food. At this period it is of utmost importance to instruct every patient in regard to a proper diet. Experience has taught us that there is a great variation in the individual needs of different patients. The patient with sprue or pellagra usually is considerable underweight and has a deficiency of many nutrients. Accordingly he may need a diet that is not only high in calories but is rich in all the essential nutrients. In contrast, some persons with pernicious anemia are obese, and the caloric intake can be restricted without impairing the diet in respect to other nutrients. Some patients may have renal insufficiency, diabetes or other diseases which require special dietary control. In such cases the diet should be prescribed for the individual patient and planned with great care. In some cases macrocytic anemia is accompanied by hypochromic anemia (iron deficiency anemia). Folic acid naturally will not replenish the deficiency of iron, and in such cases optimal doses of iron should be given.

Toxicity

Apparently large amounts of folic acid can be given with impunity since one of the authors (T.D.S.) has administered 400 mgm. daily for 3 months without the patient's developing untoward symptoms.

BIBLIOGRAPHY

Vitamin A

1. SHERMAN, H. C. and SMITH, S. L.: The vitamins, Ed. 2, The Chemical Catalog Company, Inc., New York, 1931.
2. MEDICAL RESEARCH COUNCIL: Vitamins: a survey of present knowledge, His Majesty's Stationery Office, London, 1932.
3. McCOLLUM, E. V. and DAVIS, M.: The necessity of certain lipins in the diet during growth, Jour. Biol. Chem., 1913, XV, 167.
4. OSBORNE, T. B. and MENDEL, L. B.: The relation of growth to the chemical constituents of the diet, Jour. Biol. Chem., 1913, XV, 311.
5. McCOLLUM, E. V., SIMMONDS, N., BECKER, J. E. and SHIPLEY, P. G.: Studies on experimental rickets. XXI. An experimental demonstration of the existence of a vitamin which promotes calcium deposition, Jour. Biol. Chem., 1922, LIII, 293.
6. ROBESON, C. D. and BAXTER, J. G.: A new vitamin A, Nature, London, 1945, CLV, 300.
7. BRAZER, J. G. and CURTIS, A. C.: Vitamin A deficiency in diabetes mellitus, Arch. Int. Med., 1940, LXV, 90.
8. DZIALOSZYNSKI, L. M., MYSTKOWSKI, E. M. and STEWART, C. P.: The mode of occurrence of carotene and vitamin A in human blood plasma, Biochem. Jour., 1945, XXXIX, 63.

9. LAWRIE, N. R., MOORE, T. and RAJAGOPAL, K. R.: The excretion of vitamin A in urine, Biochem. Jour., 1941, XXXV, 825.
10. STEIGMANN, F. and POPPER, H.: The influence of large doses of vitamin A upon the plasma vitamin A level, Am. Jour. Med. Sci., 1944, CCVII, 468.
11. POPPER, H.: Distribution of vitamin A in tissue as visualized by fluorescence microscopy, Physiol. Rev., 1944, XXIV, 205.
12. HRUBETZ, M. C., DEUEL, H. J., Jr. and HANLEY, B. J.: Studies on carotenoid metabolism. V. The effect of high vitamin A intake on the composition of human milk, Jour. Nutrition, 1945, XXIX, 245.
13. COUNCIL ON FOODS AND NUTRITION: Margarine fortified with vitamin A, Jour. Am. Med. Assoc., 1944, CXXVI, 168.
14. WOLBACH, S. B. and BESSEY, O. A.: Vitamin A deficiency and the nervous system, Arch. Path., 1941, XXXII, 689.
15. MELLANBY, E.: Skeletal changes affecting nervous system produced in young dogs by diets deficient in vitamin A, Jour. Physiol., 1941, XCIX, 467.
16. MOORE, L. A.: Relationship between carotene, blindness due to constriction of the optic nerve, papillary edema and nyctalopia in calves, Jour. Nutrition, 1939, XVII, 443.
17. ADLERSBERG, D., SOBOTKA, H. and BOGATIN, B.: Effect of liver disease on vitamin A metabolism, Gastroenterology, 1945, IV, 164.
18. LEWIS, J. M. and HAIG, C.: Vitamin A status of children as determined by dark adaptation, Jour. Pediat., 1940, XVI, 285.
19. STEVEN, D. and WALD, G.: Vitamin A deficiency: a field study in Newfoundland and Labrador, Jour. Nutrition, 1941, XXI, 461.
20. CORNBLEET, T., POPPER, H. and STEIGMANN, F.: Blood vitamin A and cutaneous diseases, Arch. Dermat. and Syph., 1944, XLIX, 103.
21. STEFFENS, L. F., BAIR, H. L. and SHEARD, C.: Photometric measurements on visual adaptation in normal adults on diets deficient in vitamin A, Proceed. Staff Meet., Mayo Clin., 1939, XIV, 698.
22. SEBRELL, W. H.: Nutrition in preventive medicine, Jour. Am. Med. Assoc., 1943, CXXIII, 280.
23. FRAZIER, C. N. and HU, CH'UAN-K'UEI: Cutaneous lesions associated with a deficiency in vitamin A in man, Arch. Int. Med., 1931, XLVIII, 507.
24. BRUNSTING, L. A. and SHEARD, C.: Dark adaptation in pityriasis rubra pilaris, Arch. Dermat. and Syph., 1941, XLIII, 42.
25. MOORE, T. and WANG, Y. L.: Hypervitaminosis A, Biochem. Jour., 1945, XXXIX, 222.

26. WIEHL, D. G. and KRUSE, H. D.: Medical evaluation of nutritional status. V. Prevalence of deficiency diseases in their subclinical stage, Milbank Mem. Fund Quart., 1941, XIX, 241.

27. SHEARD, C.: WAGENER, H. P. and BRUNSTING, L. A.: Disturbances of visual adaptation and their clinical significance, Proceed. Staff Meet., Mayo Clin., 1944, XIX, 525.

28. JOSEPHS, H. W.: Studies in vitamin A; relation of vitamin A and carotene to serum lipids, Bull. Johns Hopkins Hosp., 1939, LXV, 112.

Vitamin D

29. TROUSSEAU, A.: Rickets, In Lectures on Clinical Medicine, The New Sydenham Society, vol. 5, lecture LXXXVI, p. 47, London, 1872.

30. HOPKINS, F. G.: Feeding experiments illustrating the importance of accessory factors in normal dietaries, Jour. Physiol., 1912, XLIV, 425.

31. MELLANBY, EDWARD: A further demonstration of the part played by accessory food factors in the aetiologly of rickets, Jour. Physiol. (Proceed.), 1918, LII, liii.

32. STEENBOCK, H. and BLACK, A.: Fat-soluble vitamins. XVII. The induction of growth-promoting and calcifying properties in a ration by exposure to ultra-violet light, Jour. Biol. Chem., 1924, LXI, 405.

33. HESS, A. F.: Experiments on the action of light in relation to rickets. Am. Jour. Dis. Child, 1924, XXVIII, 517.

34. FORBES, G. B.: Chlyothorax in infancy; observations on the absorption of vitamins A and D and on the intravenous replacement of aspirated chyle, Jour. Pediat., 1944, XXV, 191.

35. POLSKIN, L. J., KRAMER, B. and SOBEL, A. E.: Secretion of vitamin D in milks of women fed fish liver oil, Jour. Nutrition, 1945, XXX, 451.

36. LIU, S. H.: The rôle of vitamin D in the calcium metabolism in osteomalacia, Chinese Med. Jour., 1940, LVII, 101.

37. ALBRIGHT, F., SULKOWITCH, H. W. and BLOOMBERG, E.: A comparison of the effects of vitamin D, dihydrotachysterol (A.T. 10) and parathyroid extract on the disordered metabolism of rickets, Jour. Clin. Invest. 1939, XVIII, 165.

38. WOLBACH, S. B. and BESSEY, O. A.: Tissue changes in vitamin deficiencies, Physiol. Rev., 1942, XXII, 233.

39. SHIMOTORI, N. and MORGAN, A. F.: Mechanism of vitamin D action in dogs shown by radioactive phosphorus, Jour. Biol. Chem., 1943, CXLVII, 201.
40. JONES, J. I. M. and ELLIOT, J. F.: The biological assay of vitamin D_3, Biochem. Jour., 1943, XXXVII, 209.
41. KLASMER, R.: Serum phosphatase activity and clinical rickets in children in Jerusalem, Am. Jour. Dis. Child., 1944, LXVII, 348.
42. BILLS, C. E.: Physiology of the sterols, including vitamin D, Physiol. Rev., 1935, XV, 1.
43. GOLDBLATT, H.: Die neuere Richtung der experimentellen Rachitisforschung, Ergebn. d. allg. Path. u. path. Anat., 1931, XXV, 58.
44. SPIES, T. D. and GLOVER, E. C.: Renal lesions with retention of nitrogenous products produced by massive doses of irradiated ergosterol, Am. Jour. Path., 1930, VI, 485.
45. JAFFE, H. L.: Hyperparathyroidism (Recklinghausen's disease of bone), Arch. Path., 1933, XVI, 236.
46. REED, C. I., STRUCK, H. C. and STECK, I. E.: Vitamin D; Chemistry, Physiology, Pharmacology, Pathology, Experimental and Clinical Investigations, University of Chicago Press, Chicago, 1939.
47. BAUER, J. M. and FREYBERG, R. H.: Vitamin D intoxication with metastatic calcification, Jour. Am. Med. Assoc., 1946, CXXX, 1208.
48. DANOWSKI, T. S., WINKLER, A. W. and PETERS, J. P.: Tissue calcification and renal failure produced by massive dose vitamin D therapy of arthritis, Ann. Int. Med., 1945, XXIII, 22.
49. YOUMANS, J. B., PATTON, E. W., SUTTON, W. R., KERN, R. and STEINKAMP, R.: Surveys of nutrition of populations; 4. The vitamin D and calcium nutrition of a rural population in middle Tennessee, Am. Jour. Pub. Health, 1944, XXXIV, 1049.
50. REPORT OF A CONFERENCE ON METHODS AND PROCEDURES: Nutrition survey of population group, Pub. Health Rep., 1942, LVII, 189.
51. STROM, J.: The treatment of spasmophilia with a single massive dose of vitamin D_2, Acta paediat., 1939, XXV, 251.
52. VOLLMER, H.: Treatment of rickets and tetany by parenteral administration of one massive dose of vitamin D; toxicity of vitamin D, Jour. Pediat., 1940, XVI, 419.
53. ZELSON, C.: Prevention of rickets in premature infants with parenteral administration of single massive doses of vitamin D, Jour. Pediat., 1940, XVII, 73.
54. GUNNARSON, S.: Treatment of rickets with a single massive dose of vitamin D_2, Acta paediat., 1939, XXV, 69.
55. KRESTIN, D.: The prophylaxis of rickets by single massive doses of vitamin D, Brit. Med. Jour., 1945, I, 78.

56. BAKWIN, H., BODANSKY, O. and SCHORR, R.: Refractory rickets, Am. Jour. Dis. Child., 1940, LIX, 560.
57. COUNCIL ON PHARMACY AND CHEMISTRY: The use of vitamin D in the treatment of refractory rickets, Jour. Am. Med. Assoc., 1943, CXXIII, 287.
58. PARK, E. A.: The therapy of rickets, Jour. Am. Med. Assoc., 1940, CXV, 370.

Vitamin E

59. EVANS, H. M., EMERSON, O. H. and EMERSON, G. A.: The isolation from wheat germ oil of an alcohol, α-tocopherol, having the properties of vitamin E, Jour. Biol. Chem., 1936, CXIII, 319.
60. FERNHOLZ, E.: On the constitution of α-tocopherol, Jour. Am. Chem. Soc., 1938, LX, 700.
61. KARRER, P., SALOMON, H. and FRITZSCHE, H.: Zur Kenntnis des Vitamins E, Helvet. chim Acta., 1938, XXI, 309.
62. HARRIS, P. L., JENSEN, J. L., JOFFE, M. and MASON, K. E.: Biological activity of natural and synthetic tocopherols, Jour. Biol. Chem., 1944, CLVI, 491.
63. TISHLER, M., FIESER, L. F. and WENDLER, N. L.: Nature of the by-product in the synthesis of vitamin K_1, Jour. Am. Chem. Soc., 1940, LXII, 1982.
64. HUME, E. M.: Standardization of vitamin E, Nature, London, 1941, CXLVIII, 472.
65. MEMORANDUM ON THE INTERNATIONAL STANDARD FOR VITAMIN E from the Department of Biological Standards, National Institute for Medical Research, Hampstead, London, N. W. 3. League of Nations, Health Organization, Quart. Bull., 1940–1941, IX, 443.
66. GREAVES, J. D. and SCHMIDT, C. L. A.: Relation of bile to absorption of vitamin E in the rat, Proceed. Soc. Exper. Biol. and Med., 1937, XXXVII, 40.
67. MacKENZIE, C. G., LEVINE, M. D. and McCOLLUM, E. V.: The prevention and cure of nutritional muscular dystrophy in the rabbit by alpha-tocopherol in the absence of a water-soluble factor, Jour. Nutrition, 1940, XX, 399.
68. MacKENZIE, C. G., MacKENZIE, J. B. and McCOLLUM, E. V.: Uncomplicated vitamin E deficiency in the rabbit and its relation to the toxicity of cod liver oil, Jour. Nutrition, 1941, XXI, 225.
69. MacKENZIE, C. G. and McCOLLUM, E. V.: The cure of nutritional muscular dystrophy in the rabbit by alpha-tocopherol and its effect on creatine metabolism, Jour. Nutrition, 1940, XIX, 345.

70. FRIEDMAN, I. and MATTILL, H. A.: The oxygen consumption of skeletal muscle from animals deprived of vitamin E, Am. Jour. Physiol., 1941, CXXXI, 595.
71. HICKMAN, K. C. D., KALEY, M. W. and HARRIS, P. L.: Covitamin studies; I. The sparing action of natural tocopherol concentrates on vitamin A, Jour. Biol. Chem., 1944, CLII, 303.
72. HARRIS, P. L., KALEY, M. W. and HICKMAN, K. C. D.: Covitamin studies; II. The sparing action of natural tocopherol concentrates on carotene, Jour. Biol. Chem., 1944, CLII, 313.
73. HICKMAN, K. C. D., KALEY, M. W. and HARRIS, P. L.: Covitamin studies; III. The sparing equivalence of the tocopherols and mode of action, Jour. Biol. Chem., 1944, CLII, 321.
74. GUGGENHEIM, K.: The biological value of carotene from various sources and the effect of vitamin E on the utilization of carotene and of vitamin A, Biochem. Jour., 1944, XXXVIII, 260.
75. QUAIFE, M. L. and HARRIS, P. L.: The chemical estimation of tocopherols in blood plasma, Jour. Biol. Chem., 1944, CLVI, 499.
76. COUNCIL ON PHARMACY AND CHEMISTRY: The treatment of habitual abortion with vitamin E, Jour. Am. Med. Assoc., 1940, CXIV, 2214.
77. MILHORAT, A. T. and BARTELS, W. E.: The defect in utilization of tocopherol in progressive muscular dystrophy, Science, 1945, CI, 93.
78. PAPPENHEIMER, A. M.: Rôle of nutritional deficiency in nervous and chemical nature, Nature, London, 1935, CXXXV, 652.
tory animals, Assoc. Research Nerv. and Ment. Dis., Proceed., (1941), 1943, XXII, 85.

Vitamin K

79. DAM, H.: The antihaemorrhagic vitamin of the chick. Occurrence and chemical nature, Nature, London, 1935, CXXXV, 652.
80. DAM, H. and SCHONHEYDER, F.: A deficiency disease in chicks resembling scurvy, Biochem. Jour., 1934, XXVIII, 1355.
81. DAM, H., SCHONHEYDER, F. and TAGE-HANSEN, E.: Studies on the mode of action of vitamin K, Biochem. Jour., 1936, XXX, 1075.
82. BUTT, H. R., SNELL, A. M. and OSTERBERG, A. E.: The use of vitamin K and bile in treatment of the hemorrhagic diathesis in cases of jaundice, Proceed. Staff Meet., Mayo Clin., 1938, XIII, 74.
83. WARNER, E. D., BRINKHOUS, K. M. and SMITH, H. P.: Bleeding tendency of obstructive jaundice: prothrombin deficiency and dietary factors, Proceed. Soc. Exper. Biol. and Med., 1938, XXXVII, 628.

84. BUTT, H. R. and SNELL, A. M.: Vitamin K, W. B. Saunders Company, Philadelphia, 1941.
85. BRINKHOUS, K. M.: Plasma prothrombin; vitamin K, Medicine, 1940, XIX, 329.
86. DAVIS, W. A., FRANK, H. A., HURWITZ, A. and SELIGMAN, A. M.: Intravenous use of vitamin K_1 oxide, Arch. Surg., 1943, XLVI, 296.
87. COUNCIL ON PHARMACY AND CHEMISTRY: Menadione, nonproprietary term for the substance 2-methyl-1,4-naphthoquinone, Jour. Am. Med. Assoc., 1941, CXVI, 1054.
88. MENOTTI, A. R.: Water-soluble derivatives of menadione, Jour. Am. Chem. Soc., 1943, LXV, 1209.
89. COLWELL, C. A. and McCALL, M.: Studies on the mechanism of antibacterial action of 2-methyl-1,4-naphthoquinone, Science, 1945, CI, 592.
90. McCAWLEY, E. L. and GURCHOT, C.: Mechanism of action for vitamin K, Univ. California Publ., Pharmacol. (no. 27), 1940, I, 325.
91. SHEMIAKIN, M. M., SCHUKINA, L. A. and SHVEZOV, J. B.: Studies in the vitamin K group. II. The mechanism of biological action of vitamin K and of its synthetic analogs, Jour. Am. Chem. Soc., 1943, LXV, 2164.
92. SHEMIAKIN, M. M. and SCHUKINA, L. A.: Experimental corroboration of the mechanism of biological action of quinones of the type of vitamin K, Nature, London, 1944, CLIV, 513.
93. BLACK, S., OVERMAN, R. S., ELVEHJEM, C. A. and LINK, K. P.: The effect of sulfaguanidine on rat growth and plasma prothrombin, Jour. Biol. Chem., 1942, CXLV, 137.
94. BLACK, S., McKIBBIN, J. M. and ELVEHJEM, C. A.: Use of sulfaguanidine in nutrition experiments, Proceed. Soc. Exper. Biol. and Med., 1941, XLVII, 308.
95. KORNBERG, A., DAFT, F. S. and SEBRELL, W. H.: Production of vitamin K deficiency in rats by various sulfonamides, Pub. Health Rep., 1944, LIX (pt. 1), 832.
96. WHITE, H. J.: Comparative activity of sulfonamides against coliform bacteria in the intestines of mice, Bull. Johns Hopkins Hosp., 1942, LXXI, 213.
97. MOORE, R. A., BITTENGER, I., MILLER, M. L. and HELLMAN, L. M.: Abortion in rabbits fed a vitamin K deficient diet, Am. Jour. Obst. and Gynec., 1942, XLIII, 1007.
98. KARK, R. and LOZNER, E. L.: Nutritional deficiency of vitamin K in man; a study of four non-jaundiced patients with dietary deficiency, Lancet, 1939, II, 1162.

99. FIELD, J. B. and LINK, K. P.: Note on hyperprothrombinemia induced by vitamin K, Jour. Biol. Chem., 1944, CLVI, 739.
100. KARK, R. and SOUTER, A. W.: Hypoprothrombinemia and avitaminosis-K in man, Brit. Med. Jour., 1941, II, 190.
101. SHARP, E. A., KONDER HEIDE, E. C. and GOOD, W. H.: Vitamin K activity of 2-methyl-1,4-naphthoquinone and 4-amino-2-methyl-1-naphthol in hypoprothrombinemia, Jour. Lab. and Clin. Med., 1941, XXVI, 818.
102. BUTT, H. R., LEARY, W. V. and WILDER, R. M.: Diseases of nutrition; review of certain recent contributions, Arch. Int. Med., 1942, LXIX, 277.
103. MEYER, O. O. and HOWARD, B.: Production of hypoprothrombinemia and hypocoagulability of the blood with salicylates, Proceed. Soc. Exper. Biol. and Med., 1943, LIII, 234.
104. SHAPIRO, S.: Studies on prothrombin. VI. The effect of synthetic vitamin K on the prothrombinopenia induced by salicylate in man, Jour. Am. Med. Assoc., 1944, CXXV, 546.
105. SHAPIRO, S., REDISH, M. H. and CAMPBELL, H. A.: Studies on prothrombin: IV. The prothrombinopenic effect of salicylate in man, Proceed. Soc. Exper. Biol. and Med., 1943, LIII, 251.
106. SHAPIRO, S.: Studies on prothrombin. VI. The effect of synthetic vitamin K on the prothrombinopenia induced by salicylate in man, Jour. Am. Med. Assoc., 1944, CXXV, 546.
107. BUTT, H. R., LEAKE, W. H., SOLLEY, R. F., GRIFFITH, G. C., HUNTINGTON, R. W. and MONTGOMERY, H.: Studies in rheumatic fever. I. The physiologic effect of sodium salicylate on the human being, with particular reference to the prothrombin level of the blood and the effect on hepatic parenchyma, Jour. Am. Med. Assoc., 1945, CXXVIII, 1195.
108. LINK, K. P.: Anticoagulant 3,3'-methylenebis (4-hydroxycoumarin), Federation Proceed, 1945, IV, 176.
109. SHAPIRO, S., REDISH, M. H. and CAMPBELL, H. A.: Prothrombin studies: III. Effect of vitamin K upon hypoprothrombinemia induced by dicumarol in man, Proceed. Soc. Exper. Biol. and Med., 1943, LII, 12.
110. CROMER, H. E., Jr. and BARKER, N. W.: The effect of large doses of menadione bisulfite (synthetic vitamin K) on excessive hypoprothrombinemia induced by dicumarol, Proceed. Staff Meet., Mayo Clin., 1944, XIX, 217.
111. BRODIE, D. C., HIESTAND, W. A. and JENKINS, G. L.: Inhibitory effect of certain naphthoquinones on hemorrhagic action of dicumarol, Jour. Am. Pharm. Assoc., (Scient. Ed.), 1945, XXXIV, 73.

112. WADDELL, W. W., Jr., GUERRY, DuPONT, III, BRAY, W. E. and KELLEY, O. R.: Possible effects of vitamin K on prothrombin and clotting time in newly-born infants, Proceed. Soc. Exper. Biol. and Med., 1939, XL, 432.
113. SMITH, H. P. and WARNER, E. D.: Vitamin K; Clinical Aspects, p. 211; Symposium on Biological Action of Vitamins, Univ. Chicago, 1942.
114. WADDELL, W. W., Jr. and GUERRY, D., III.: The rôle of vitamin K in the etiology, prevention and treatment of hemorrhage in the newborn infant. Part II, Jour. Pediat., 1939, XV, 802.
115. SELLS, R. L., WALKER, S. W. and OWEN, C. A.: Vitamin K requirement of the newborn infant, Proceed. Soc. Exper. Biol. and Med., 1941, XLVII, 441.
116. LAWSON, R. B.: Treatment of hypoprothrombinemia (hemorrhagic disease) of the newborn infant, Jour. Pediat., 1941, XVIII, 224.
117. VALENTINE, E. H., REINHOLD, J. G. and SCHNEIDER, E.: The effectiveness of prenatal administration of 2-methyl-1,4-naphthoquinone in maintaining normal prothrombin levels in infants, Am. Jour. Med. Sci., 1941, CCII, 359.
118. ROSS, S. G. and MALLOY, H. T.: Blood prothrombin in the newborn: the effect of vitamin K upon the blood prothrombin and upon haemorrhagic disease of the new-born, Canad. Med. Assoc. Jour., 1941, XLV, 417.
119. HELLMAN, L. M. and SHETTLES, L. B.: Prophylactic use of vitamin K in obstetrics, South. Med. Jour., 1942, XXXV, 289.
120. LEHMANN, J.: Vitamin K as a prophylactic in 13,000 infants, Lancet, 1944, I, 493.
121. ANSBACHER, S.: Editorial review: The bioassay of vitamin K, Jour. Nutrition, 1941, XXI, 1.
122. TRENNER, N. R. and BACHER, F. A.: A quantitative reduction-oxidation method for the estimation of vitamin K_1 and associated quinones and naphthoquinones, Jour. Biol. Chem., 1941, CXXXVII, 745.
123. IRREVERRE, F. and SULLIVAN, M. X.: Colorimetric test for vitamin K_1, Science, 1941, XCIV, 497.
124. SCUDI, J. V. and BUHS, R. P.: Colorimetric oxidation-reduction method for determination of K vitamins, Jour. Biol. Chem., 1941, CXLI, 451.
125. WARNER, E. D., BRINKHOUS, K. M. and SMITH, H. P.: Quantitative study on blood clotting: prothrombin fluctuations under experimental conditions, Am. Jour. Physiol., 1936, CXIV, 667.
126. HERBERT, F. K.: Estimation of prothrombin in human plasma, Biochem. Jour., 1940, XXXIV, 1554.

127. SOUTER, A. W. and KARK, R.: Quick's prothrombin test simplified by the use of a stable thromboplastin, Am. Jour. Med. Sci., 1940, CC, 603.
128. QUICK, A. J., STANLEY-BROWN, M. and BANCROFT, F. W.: A study of the coagulation defect in hemophilia and in jaundice, Am. Jour. Med. Sci., 1935, CXC, 501.
129. BUTT, H. R. and SNELL, A. M.: Vitamin K, W. B. Saunders Company, Philadelphia, 1941.
130. BRINKHOUS, K. M.: Plasma prothrombin; vitamin K, Medicine, 1940, XIX, 329.
131. BAY, RICARDO: Hígado-protrombina-vitamina K; (estudio experimental y clinico), Bol. d. Inst. Clín. Quir., Buenos Aires Univ., 1941, XVII, 139.
132. KOLLER, F.: Das Vitamin K und seine klinische Bedeutung, Georg Thieme, Leipsig, 1941.
133. ZIFFREN, S. E., OWEN, C. A., HOFFMAN, G. R. and SMITH, H. P.: Control of vitamin K therapy. Compensatory mechanisms at low prothrombin levels, Proceed. Soc. Exper. Biol. and Med., 1939, XL, 595.
134. KATO, K.: Micro-prothrombin test with capillary whole blood; a modification of Quick's quantitative method, Am. Jour. Clin. Path., 1940, X, 147.
135. QUICK, A. J.: Determination of prothrombin, Proceed. Soc. Exper. Biol. and Med., 1939, XLII, 788.
136. BRAY, W. E. and KELLEY, O. R.: Prothrombin studies, especially in the newborn, Am. Jour. Clin. Path., 1940, X, 154.
137. KELLEY, O. R. and BRAY, W. E.: Prothrombin time determination, Jour. Lab. and Clin. Med., 1940, XXV, 527.
138. KATO, K. and PONCHER, H. G.: The prothrombin in the blood of newborn mature and immature infants; as determined by the micro prothrombin test, Jour. Am. Med. Assoc., 1940, CXIV, 749.
139. SHAPIRO, S. and RICHARDS, R. K.: The prothrombin response to large doses of synthetic vitamin K in liver disease, Ann. Int. Med., 1945, XXII, 841.
140. MOLITOR, H. and ROBINSON, H. J.: Oral and parenteral toxicity of vitamin K_1, phthiocol and 2-methyl-1,4-napthoquinone, Proceed. Soc. Exper. Biol. and Med., 1940, XLIII, 125.
141. SHIMKIN, M. B.: Toxicity of naphthoquinones with vitamin K activity in mice, Jour. Pharmacol. and Exper. Therap., 1941, LXXI, 210.
142. FOSTER, R. H. K.: Pharmacological observations on tetra-sodium-2-methyl-1,4-naphthohydroquinone diphosphoric acid ester, Proceed. Soc. Exper. Biol. and Med., 1940, XLV, 412.

143. STEWART, J. D.: Oral and parenteral use of synthetic vitamin K-active substances in hypoprothrombinemia, Surgery, 1941, IX, 212.

144. WEIR, J. F., BUTT, H. R. and SNELL, A. B.: Further observations on the clinical use of vitamin K, Am. Jour. Digest. Dis., 1940, VII, 485.

145. TOCANTINS, L. M. and JONES, H. W.: Hypoprothrombinemia: effect of peroral and parenteral administration of synthetic vitamin K substitute (2-methyl-1,4-naphthoquinone), Ann. Surg., 1941, CXIII, 276.

146. SELIGMAN, A. M., HURWITZ, A., FRANK, H. A. and DAVIS, W. A.: The intravenous use of synthetic vitamin K_1, Surg., Gynec. and Obst., 1941, LXXIII, 686.

147. ALLEN, J. G.: Clinical experience with water soluble vitamin K-like substance (tetrasodium 2-methyl-1, 4-naphthohydroquinone diphosphoric acid ester), Am. Jour. Med. Sci., 1943, CCV, 97.

148. STEIN, H. B.: "Prothrombin response to vitamin K test" in differentiation between intra- and extra-hepatic jaundice, South African Jour. Med. Sci., 1944, IX, 111.

149. KINSEY, R. E.: A new aid in control of hemorrhage in severe damage to the liver; transfusions of blood fortified by administration of vitamin K to donors, Arch. Int. Med., 1944, LXXIII, 131.

150. BUTT, H. R., SELDON, T. H. and MAGATH, T. B.: Hypoprothrombinemia: effect of transfusions of blood fortified by administration of vitamin K to donors, Arch. Int. Med., (in press).

151. LINK, K. P.: Anticoagulant from spoiled sweet clover hay. Harvey Lect. (1933–1944), 1944, XXXIX, 162.

152. BUTT, H. R., ALLEN, E. V. and BOLLMAN, J. L.: A preparation from spoiled sweet clover [3,3'-methylene-bis-(4-hydroxycoumarin)] which prolongs coagulation and prothrombin time of the blood: preliminary report of experimental and clinical studies, Proceed. Staff Meet., Mayo Clin., 1941, XVI, 388.

153. OVERMAN, R. S., STAHMANN, M. A. and LINK, K. P.: Studies on the hemorrhagic sweet clover disease. VIII. The effect of 2-methyl-1,4-naphthoquinone and 1-ascorbic acid upon the action of 3,3-methylenebis (4-hydroxycoumarin) on the prothrombin time of rabbits, Jour. Biol. Chem., 1942, CXLV, 155.

154. SHAPIRO, S., REDISH, M. H. and CAMPBELL, H. A.: Prothrombin studies: III. Effect of vitamin K upon hypoprothrombinemia induced by dicumarol in man, Proceed. Soc. Exper. Biol. and Med., 1943, LII, 12.

Vitamin C

155. SZENT-GYORGI, A.: Observations on the function of the peroxidase systems and chemistry of the adrenal cortex; description of a new carbohydrate derivative, Biochem. Jour., 1928, XXII, 1387.
156. WAUGH, W. A. and KING, C. G.: The isolation and identification of vitamin C, Jour. Biol. Chem., 1932, XCVII, 325.
157. REICHSTEIN, T., GRUSSNER, A. and OPPENHAUER, R.: Syntheses der **d**-und 1-ascorbinsaüre (C vitamin), Helv. Chem. Acta., 1933, XVI, 1010.
158. HOLST, A. and FROLICH, T.: Experimental studies relating to ship beriberi and scurvy, Jour. Hygiene, 1907, VII, 634.
159. GLICK, D. and BISKIND, G. R.: The concentration of vitamin C in the thymus in relation to its histologic changes at different stages of development and regression, Jour. Biol. Chem., 1936, CXIV, 1.
160. MUSULIN, R. R., SILVERBLATT, E., KING, C. G. and WOODWARD, G. E.: The titration and biological assay of vitamin C in tumor tissue, Am. Jour. Cancer, 1936, XXVII, 707.
161. CRANDON, J. H. and LUND, C. G.: Vitamin C deficiency in an otherwise normal adult, New Eng. Jour. Med., 1940, CCXXII, 748.
162. PIJOAN, M. and LOZNER, E. L.: Medical progress. The physiological significance of vitamin C in man, New Eng. Jour. Med., 1944, CCXXXI, 14.
163. WOLBACH, S. B. and HOWE, P. R.: Intercellular substance in experimental scorbutus, Arch. Path., 1926, I, 1.
164. KING, C. G. and MENTEN, M. I.: The influence of vitamin C level upon resistance to diphtheria toxin, Jour. Nutrition, 1935, X, 129.
165. SIGAL, A. and KING, C. G.: The influence of vitamin C deficiency upon the resistance of guinea pigs to diphtheria toxin, Jour. Pharmacol. and Exper. Therap., 1937, LXI, 1.
166. WOLBACH, S. B.: Controlled formation of collagen and reticulum. A study of intercellular substance in recovery from experimental scorbutus, Am. Jour. Path. (Suppl.), 1933, IX, 689.
167. WOLBACH, S. B.: Pathologic changes resulting from vitamin deficiency, Jour. Am. Med. Assoc., 1937, CVIII, 7.
168. HESS, A. F.: Scurvy, Past and Present, J. B. Lippincott, Philadelphia and London, 1920.
169. SHANNO, R. L.: Rutin. A new drug for the treatment of increased capillary fragility, Am. Jour. Med. Sci., 1946, CCXI, 539.
170. METTIER, S. R., MINOT, G. R. and TOWNSEND, W. C.: Scurvy in adults. Especially the effect of food rich in vitamin C on blood formation, Jour. Am. Med. Assoc., 1930, XCV, 1089.

171. LOZNER, E. L. Studies on hemoglobin regeneration in patients with vitamin C deficiency, New Eng. Jour. Med., 1941, CCXXIV, 265.
172. WOLBACH, S. B.: The pathological changes resulting from vitamin deficiency, Jour. Am. Med. Assoc., 1937, CVIII, 7.
173. VILTER, R. W., WOOLFORD, R. M. and SPIES, T. D.: Severe scurvy, a clinical and hematologic study, Jour. Lab. and Clin. Med., 1946, XXXI, 609.
174. YOUMANS, J. B.: Nutritional deficiencies, J. B. Lippincott (2nd ed.), Philadelphia and London, 1943.
175. CRANDON, J. H., LUND, C. C. and DILL, D. B.: Experimental human scurvy, New Eng. Jour. Med., 1940, CCXXIII, 353.
176. HARRIS, P. L., HICKMAN, K. C. D., JENSEN, L. J. and SPIES, T. D.: Survey of the blood plasma levels of vitamin A, carotene, ascorbic acid and tocopherols of persons in an area of endemic malnutrition, Am. Jour. Pub. Health, 1946, XXXVI, 155.

Vitamin B_1 (Thiamine)

177. EIJKMAN, C.: Eine beriberiähnliche Krankheit der huhner, Virchow's Archiv. f. Path. Anat., 1897, CXLVIII, 523, CXLIX, 187.
178. GRIJNS, G.: Polyneuritis gallinarum, Tijdschr. Nederland-Indië, 1901, XLI, 3.
179. FLETCHER, W.: Rice and beriberi, Jour. Trop. Med. and Hyg., 1909, XII, 127.
180. FRASER, H. and STANTON, H. T.: An inquiry concerning the etiology of beriberi, Lancet, 1909, I, 451.
181. FUNK, C.: The chemical nature of the substance which cures polyneuritis in birds induced by a diet of polished rice, Jour. Physiol., 1911, XLIII, 395.
182. VEDDER, E. B. and WILLIAMS, R. R.: Concerning the beri-beri-preventing substances or vitamins contained in rice polishings. A sixth contribution to the etiology of beri-beri, Philippine Jour. Sci., Sect. B, 1913, VIII, 175.
183. SEIDELL, A.: A stable form of vitamin efficient in the prevention and cure of certain deficiency diseases, U. S. Pub. Health Rep., 1916, XXXI, 364.
184. PETERS, R. A.: The action of nitrous acid upon the antineuritic substance in yeast, Biochem. Jour., 1924, XVIII, 858.
185. JANSEN, B. C. P. and DONATH, W. F.: Antineuritisch Vitamine, Chem. Weekblad., 1926, XXIII, 201. On the isolation of the anti-beriberi vitamin, Mededeel. v. d. dienst d. volksgezondh. in Nederland-Indië, 1926, XVI, 186.

186. WILLIAMS, R. R.: Structure of vitamin B_1, Jour. Am. Chem. Soc., 1935, LVII, 229. 1936, LVIII, 1063.
WILLIAMS, R. R. and CLINE, J. K.: Synthesis of vitamin B_1, Jour. Am. Chem. Soc., 1936, LVIII, 1504. 1937, LIX, 216.
187. LOHMANN, K. and SCHUSTER, PH.: Uber die Co-carboxylase, Naturwissenschaften, 1937, XXV, 26.
188. PLATT, B. S. and LU, G. D.: Chemical and clinical findings in beriberi with special reference to vitamin B_1 deficiency, Quart. Jour. Med., 1936, V, 355.
189. LEWY, F. H., SPIES, T. D. and ARING, C. D.: The incidence of neuropathy in pellagra, Am. Jour. Med. Sci., 1940, CXCIX, 840.
190. PETERS, R. A.: Biochemical lesion in vitamin B_1 deficiency, Biochem. Jour., 1938, XXXII, 697.
191. HIMWICH, E. E., SPIES, T. D., FAZEKAS, J. F. and NESIN, S.: Cerebral carbohydrate metabolism during deficiency of various members of the vitamin B complex, Am. Jour. Med. Sci., 1940, CXCIX, 849.
192. VEDDER, E. B. and CLARK, E.: A study of polyneuritis gallinarum. A fifth contribution to the etiology of beriberi, Philippine Jour. Sci., Sect. B, 1912, VII, 423.
193. FROSTIG, J. P. and SPIES, T. D.: The initial nervous syndrome of pellagra and associated deficiency diseases, Am. Jour. Med. Sci., 1940, CXCIX, 268.
194. SPIES, T. D., BRADLEY, J., ROSENBAUM, M. and KNOTT, J. R.: Emotional disturbances in persons with pellagra, beriberi and associated deficiency states, Research Publ. Assoc. Nerv. and Ment. Dis., 1943, XXII, 122.
195. WEISS, S. and WILKINS, R. W.: The nature of cardiovascular disturbances in nutritional deficiency states, Ann. Int. Med., 1937, XI, 104.
196. VEDDER, E. B.: Beriberi and epidemic dropsy. Tice's Practice of Medicine, Vol. IV. W. F. Prior Company, Hagerstown, Maryland, 1936.
197. BLANKENHORN, M. A., VILTER, C. F., SCHEINKER, I. M. and AUSTIN, R. S.: Occidental beriberi heart disease, Jour. Am. Med. Assoc., 1946, CXXXI, 717.
198. WILLIAMS, R. D., MASON, H. L. and SMITH, B. F.: Induced vitamin B_1 deficiency in human subjects, Proceed. Staff Meet., Mayo Clinic, 1939, XIV, 787.
199. WILLIAMS, R. D., MASON, H. L., POWER, M. H. and WILDER, R. M.: Induced thiamine (vitamine B_1) deficiency in man: Relation of depletion of thiamine to development of biochemical defect and of polyneuropathy, Arch. Int. Med., 1943, LXXI, 38.

200. WENCKEBACH, K. F.: Heart and circulation in a tropical avitaminosis (beriberi), Lancet, 1928, II, 265.

Nicotinic Acid Amide

201. HUBER, C.: Vorlaüfige Notiz uber einige Derivate des Nicotins, Ann du Chimie, 1867, CXLI, 271.

202. SUSUKI, SHIMAMURI, T. and OHDAKE, S.: Uber Oryzanin ein Bestandteil der Reishleie und seine physiologische Bedeuntung, Biochem. Zeitschr., 1912, XLIII, 89.

203. FUNK, C.: Studies on beriberi, VII. Chemistry of the vitamin fraction from yeast and rice polishings, Jour. Physiol., 1913, XLVI, 173.

204. WILLIAMS, R. R.: The chemical nature of the vitamins. Anti-neuritic properties of the hydroxypyridines, Jour. Biol. Chem., 1916, XXV, 437.

205. WILLIAMS, R. R.: Structure of anti-neuritic hydroxypyridines, Proceed. Soc. Exper. Biol. and Med., 1916, XIV, 25.

206. VICKERY, H. B.: Simplest nitrogenous constituents of yeast. 1. Choline and nicotinic acid, Jour. Biol. Chem., 1926, LXVIII, 585.

207. WARBURG, O. and CHRISTIAN, W.: Co-ferment problem, Biochem. Zeitscshr, 1935, CCLXXV, 464.

208. KUHN, R. and VETTER, H.: Isolierung von Nicotinaure Amid aus Herzmuskel, Bericht. Chem. Gessellsch., 1935, LXVIII, 2374.

209. ELVEHJEM, C. A., MADDEN, R. J., STRONG, F. M. and WOOLLEY, D. W.: Relation of nicotinic acid and nicotinic acid amide to canine blacktongue, Jour. Am. Chem. Soc., 1937, LIX, 1767.

210. SPIES, T. D., COOPER, C. and BLANKENHORN, M. A.: The use of nicotinic acid in the treatment of pellagra, Jour. Am. Med. Assoc., 1938, CX, 622.

211. FOUTS, P. J., HELMER, O. M., LEPOVSKY, S. and JUKES, T. H.: Treatment of human pellagra with nicotinic acid, Proceed. Soc. Exp. Biol. and Med., 1937, XXXVII, 405.

212. SMITH, D. T., RUFFIN, J. M. and SMITH, S. G.: Pellaga successfully treated with nicotinic acid, Jour. Am. Med. Assoc., 1937, CIX, 2054.

213. HARRIS, LESLIE: Address before the Birmingham (England) University Biological Society, Nature, 1937, CXL, 1070.

214. VILTER, R. W., VILTER, S. P. and SPIES, T. D.: Relationship between nicotinic acid and a codehydrogenase (cozymase) in blood of pellagrins and normal persons, Jour. Am. Med. Assoc., 1939, CXII, 420.

215. AXELROD, A. E., SPIES, T. D. and ELVEHJEM, C. A.: The effect of a nicotinic acid deficiency upon the coenzyme I content of the human erythrocyte and muscle, Jour. Biol. Chem., 1941, CXXXVIII, 667.
216. SPIES, T. D. and LU, G. D.: Unpublished observations.
217. GROSS, E., SWAIN, A. P. and SPIES, T. D.: Unpublished observations.
218. MOORE, R. A., SPIES, T. D. and COOPER, Z. K.: Histopathology of the skin in pellagra, Arch. Derm. and Syph., 1942, XLVI, 100.
219. SPIES, T. D., WALKER, A. A. and WOODS, A. W.: Pellagra in infancy and childhood, Jour. Am. Med. Assoc., 1939, CXIII, 1481.
220. BEAN, W. B., SPIES, T. D. and VILTER, R. W.: Asymmetric cutaneous lesions in pellagra, Arch. Derm. and Syph., 1944, XLIX, 335.
221. SMITH, D. T. and RUFFIN, J. M.: Effect of sunlight on the clinical manifestations of pellagra, Arch. Int. Med., 1937, LIX, 631.
222. SPIES, T. D. in CECIL, R. L.: Textbook of Medicine. Ed. 5, p. 624, W. B. Saunders, Philadelphia, 1940.
223. STANNUS, H. S.: Pellagra: Theories of causation, Trop. Dis. Bull., 1937, XXXIV, 183.
224. SPIES, T. D.: Relationship of pellagrous dermatitis to sunlight, Arch. Int. Med., 1935, LVI, 920.
225. SPIES, T. D., COGSWELL, R. C. and VILTER, C.: Detection and treatment of severe atypical deficiency disease, Jour. Am. Med. Assoc., 1944, CXXVI, 752.
226. KREHL, W. A., SARMA, P. S., TEPLY, L. J. and ELVEHJEM, C. A.: Factors affecting the dietary niacin and tryptophane requirement of the growing rat, Jour. Nutrition, 1946, XXXI, 85.
227. BEAN, W. B., SPIES, T. D. and BLANKENHORN, M. A.: Secondary pellagra, Medicine, 1944, XXIII, 1.
228. CARPENTER, R. S. and STIEBELING, H. K.: Diets to fit the family income, Bureau of Home Economics, Washington, D. C., Sept. 1936.

Riboflavin

229. BLYTHE, A. W.: The composition of cow's milk in health and disease, Jour. Chem. Soc., 1879, XXXV, 530.
230. WARBURG, O. and CHRISTIAN, W.: Ueber ein neues Oxydationsferment und sein Absorptionsspektrum, Biochem. Zeitschr., 1932, CCLIV, 438.
231. KUHN, R., GYORGY, P. and WAGNER-JAUREGG: Ueber Ovoflavin, den Farbstoff des Eiklars, Berichte d. deutsch. chem. Gesellsachaft, 1933, LXVI, 576.

232. KARRER, P. and ASSOCIATES: Zur synthese des Lactoflavins, Helv. Chem. Acta, 1935, XVIII, 1435.

233. KUHN, R. and STROBELE, R.: Ueber die Synthese des Lactoflavins (Vitamin B_2), Bericht. d. deutsch. chem. Gesellschaft, 1935, LXVIII, 1765.

234. AXELROD, A. E., SPIES, T. D. and ELVEHJEM, C. A.: A study of urinary riboflavin excretion in man, Jour. Clin. Invest., 1941, XX, 229.

235. AXELROD, A. E., SPIES, T. D. and ELVEHJEM, C. A.: The effect of nicotinic acid deficiency upon the coenzyme 1 content of the human erythrocyte and muscle, Jour. Biol. Chem., 1941, CXXXVIII, 667.

236. WARKANY, J. and NELSON, R. C.: Appearance of skeletal abnormalities in offspring of rats reared on a deficient diet, Science, 1940, XCII, 383.

237. WARKANY, J., NELSON, R. C. and SCHRAFFENBERGER, E.: Congenital malformations induced in rats by maternal nutritional deficiency, IV. Cleft palate, Amer. Jour. Dis. Child., 1943, LXV, 882.

238. MACHELLA, T. E.: Studies of the B vitamins in the human subject. III. The Response of cheilosis to vitamin therapy, Am. Jour. Med. Sci., 1942, CCIII, 114.

239. JOHNSON, L. V.: Clinical ocular conditions associated with vitamin B complex deficiencies, Am. Jour. Ophth., 1941, XXIV, 1233.

240. NAJJAR, V. A., JOHNS, G. A., MEDAIRY, G. C., FLEISCHMANN, G. and HOLT, L. E.: Biosynthesis of riboflavin in man, Jour. Am. Med. Assoc., 1944, CXXVII, 357.

241. SEBRELL, W. H. and BUTLER, R. E.: Riboflavin deficiency in man, Pub. Health Rep., 1938, LIII, 2282.

242. FINNERUD, C. W.: Perleche: a clinical and etiologic study of 100 cases, Arch. Derm. and Syph., 1929, XX, 454.

243. FINNERUD, C. W.: Perleche: its nosologic status, Jour. Am. Med. Assoc., 1944, CXXVI, 737.

244. ELLENBERG, M. and POLLACK, H.: Psuedo ariboflavinosis, Jour. Am. Med. Assoc., 1942, CXIX, 790.

245. MANN, A. W., MANN, J. M. and SPIES, T. D.: A clinical study of malnourished edentulous patients, Jour. Am. Dent. Assoc., 1945, XXXII, 1357.

246. SPIES, T. D., BEAN, W. B. and ASHE, W. F.: Recent advances in the treatment of pellagra and associated deficiencies, Ann. Int. Med., 1939, XII, 1830.

247. SPIES, T. D., VILTER, R. W. and ASHE, W. F.: Pellagra, beriberi, and riboflavin deficiency in human beings, diagnosis and treatment, Jour. Am. Med. Assoc., 1939, CXIII, 931.

248. KRUSE, H. D., SYNDENSTRIKER, V. P., SEBRELL, W. H. and CLECKLEY, H. M.: Ocular manifestations of ariboflavinosis, Pub. Health Rep. 1940, LV, 157.

249. SPIES, T. D., PERRY, D. J., COGSWELL, R. C. and FROMMEYER, W. B.: Ocular disturbances in riboflavin deficiency, Jour. Lab. and Clin. Med., 1945, XXX, 751.

250. SEBRELL, W. H.: Human riboflavin deficiency in The Biological Action of the Vitamins, Ed. by E. A. Evans, Jr., Univ. Chicago Press, Chicago, 1942.

Folic Acid

251. MITCHELL, H. K., SNELL, E. E. and WILLIAMS, R. J.: The concentration of folic acid, Jour. Am. Chem. Soc., 1941, LXIII, 2284.

252. STOKSTAD, E. L. R. and MANNING, P. D. V.: Evidence of a new growth factor required by chicks, Jour. Biol. Chem., 1938, CXXV, 687.

253. JUKES, T. H. and BABCOCK, S. H. Jr.: Experiments with a factor promoting growth and preventing paralysis in chicks on a simplified diet, Jour. Biol. Chem., 1938, CXXV, 169.

254. HOGAN, A. G. and PARROTT, E. M.: Anemia in chicks caused by a vitamin deficiency, Jour. Biol. Chem., 1940, CXXXII, 507.

255. SNELL, E. E. and PETERSON, W. H.: Growth factors for bacteria. X. Additional factors required by certain lactic acid bacteria, Jour. Bact., 1940, XXXIX, 273.

256. HUTCHINS, B. L., BOHONOS, N., HEGSTED, D. M., ELVEHJEM, C. A. and PETERSON, W. H.: Relation of a growth factor required by *Lactobacillus casei E* to the nutrition of the chick, Jour. Biol. Chem., 1941, CXL, 681.

257. PIFFNER, J. J., BINKLEY, S. B., BLOOM, E. S., BROWN, R. A., BIRD, O. D., EMMETT, A. D., HOGAN, A. G. and O'DELL, B. L.: Isolation of the anti-anemic factor (vitamin B_c) in crystalline form from liver, Science, 1943, XCVII, 404.

258. STOKSTAD, E. L. R.: Some properties of growth factor for *Lactobacillus casei,* Jour. Biol. Chem., 1943, CXLIX, 573.

259. ANGIER, R. B., BOOTHE, J. H., HUTCHINGS, B. L., MOWAT, J. H., SEMB, J., STOKSTAD, E. L. R., SUBBAROW, Y., WALLER, C. W., COSULICH, D. B., FARENBACH, M. J., HULTQUIST, M. F., KUH, E., NORTHEY, E. H., SEEGER, D. R., SICKELS, J. P. and SMITH, J. M., Jr.: Synthesis of a compound identical with *L. casei* factor isolated from liver, Science, 1945, CII, 227.

260. ANGER, R. B., BOOTHE, J. H., HUTCHINGS, B. L., MOWAT, J. H., SEMB, J., STOKSTAD, E. L. R., SUBBAROW, Y., WALLER, C. W., COSULICH, D. B., FARENBACH, M. J., HULTQUIST, M. E., KUH, E., NORTHEY, E. H., SEEGER, D. R., SICKELS, J. P. and SMITH, J. M., Jr.: The structure and synthesis of the liver *L. casei* factor, Science, 1946, CIII, 667.

251. BERRY, L. J. and SPIES, T. D.: The present status of folic acid, Jour. Hemat., 1946, I, 271.

262. SPIES, TOM D.: Experiences with Folic Acid, Year Book Publishers, Inc., Chicago, 1947.

263. SPIES, TOM D. and STONE, ROBERT, E.: Some recent experiences with vitamins and vitamin deficiencies, South. Med. Jour., 1947, XL, 46.

264. OLSON, OSCAR E., BURRIS, R. H. and ELVEHJEM, C. A.: A prelimnary report of the "folic acid" content of certain foods, Jour. Am. Diet. Assoc., 1947, XXIII, 200.

265. FROMMEYER, WALTER B., Jr. and SPIES, TOM D.: Relative clinical and hematologic effects of concentrated liver extract, synthetic folic acid and synthetic 5-methyl uracil in the treatment of macrocytic anemia in relapse, Am. Jour. Med. Sci., 1947, CCXIII, 135.

266. SPIES, TOM D.: Effect of folic acid on persons with macrocytic anemia in relapse, Jour. Am. Med. Assoc., 1946, CXXX, 474.

267. GARCIA LOPEZ, GUILLERMO, SPIES, TOM D., MENENDEZ, JOSE ARISTIDES and LOPEZ TOCA, RUBEN: Folic acid in the rehabilitation of persons with sprue, Jour. Am. Med. Assoc., 1946, CXXXII, 906.

268. SUAREZ, RAMON M., SPIES, TOM D. and SUAREZ, RAMON M., JR.: The use of folic acid in sprue, Ann. Int. Med., 1947, XXVI, 643.

269. HERNANDEZ BEGUERIE, R. L.: Roentgenologic studies on the effect of synthetic folic acid on the gastrointestinal tract of patients with tropical sprue, Am. Jour. Roentgenol. and Rad. Therapy, 1946, LVI, 337.

270. SPIES, TOM D. and STONE, ROBERT E.: Liver extract, folic acid and thyamine in pernicious anemia and subacute combined degeneration, Lancet, 1947, I, 174.

September 1, 1948.

CHAPTER X (CONTINUED)

VITAMINS AND VITAMIN DEFICIENCIES (CONTINUED)

VITAMIN B_{12}

By TOM D. SPIES

Table of Contents

History

The modern era in the search for vitamin B_{12} and substances that act similarly was initiated when Minot and Murphy[271] noted rapid improvement on feeding liver intensively to patients with pernicious anemia. It became evident that a potent liver extract would be more easily administered, and a number of crude extracts were developed and later used widely for treating patients with pernicious anemia. Many liver extracts were manufactured and tested, and it soon became obvious that the positive hemopoietic effect varied according to the source of the material, the method of extraction and other unknown factors. An intensive search in many laboratories and clinics in various parts of the world was initiated to determine the exact nature of the potent substance or substances. Strandell and his associates in Scandinavia, Karrer and his co-workers in Switzerland and Dakin, Ungley and West working in the United States and in Great Britain, all produced high concentrations of this material.

About three years ago it was shown that both folic acid and thymine are effective in producing blood regeneration in patients with certain macrocytic anemias in relapse[272], and it also was shown that they neither prevent nor control the symptoms arising from the degeneration of the posterior and lateral columns of the spinal cord[273]. Since neither of these substances was found in great concentration in most of the liver extracts, the search for the active principle in liver continued unabated.

All attempts to isolate the crystalline material were hindered by lack of a reliable assay method. In 1947 Shorb[274] found in liver extracts a growth factor required by *Lactobacillus lactis Dorner* in concentrations bearing a linear relationship to the potency of the extracts used in the treatment of pernicious anemia. Rickes, Brink, Koniuszy, Wood and Folkers[275], aided by this assay method, isolated small amounts of a red crystalline compound which was highly active for the growth of the *Lactobacillus lactis Dorner* and also was highly active in initiating a positive hemopoietic response in persons with pernicious anemia. They suggested the name, vitamin B_{12}, since the biological rôle of the new compound was so little understood, and since this name had only nutritional significance and connotation.

Smith[276] in Britain isolated the same type of crystals from liver eight days after the Merck publication. He and his associates used the recently introduced method of partition chromatography to prepare substances containing approximately 3 per cent. of the active principle. Then by treatment with trypsin, followed by more chromatography, they produced tremendous concentration with the final crystallization from aqueous acetone.

Biochemistry and Physiology

Vitamin B_{12} is a red crystalline compound which has not been prepared synthetically. Microphotographs of this vitamin can be seen in Fig. 67. When heated on the micro-stage, the crystals lose their red color at about 212° C. and do not melt below 300° C.

The structural formula of vitamin B_{12} is not known. Intensive and excellent studies are being made independently by Folkers and the Merck Research Laboratories group[277] and by the British investigator, E. Lester Smith[278] and his associates in the Glaxo Laboratories. Emission spectrographic analysis has shown the presence of cobalt in the vitamin B_{12} crystals. The vitamin appears to be the first cobalt complex detected in human or animal tissues. It appears to have six groups arranged about the cobalt atom, and the bright red color of vitamin B_{12} appears to be associated with this cobalt complex. X-ray crystallography suggests that the molecular weight is about 1,500 to 1,750. The results of the American and British investigators, although arrived at independently and often by different techniques, have agreed remarkably. Both groups

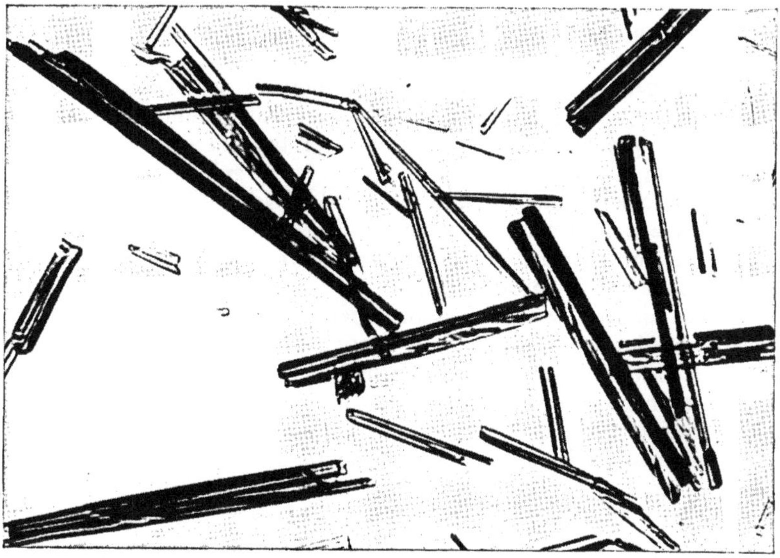

FIG. 1. Microphotograph of vitamin B_{12} crystals. (Courtesy of Dr. Hans Molitor, Merck Institute of Therapeutic Research).

not only have found the cobalt but also have reported the presence of phosphorus and nitrogen in the compound. The nutritional significance of cobalt, phosphorus and iron for animals and human beings will have to be re-evaluated when the biochemical significance of vitamin B_{12} is better understood.

Vitamin B_{12} is rather widely distributed in relatively high amounts in cow manure, fish meal, pancreatin, papain, eggs, whey, milk powder, beef extract and the cultures of a number of microorganisms. The natural vitamin then may be said to occur in a number of plant, animal and microbiological materials, yet it does not occur in abundance. Apparently man cannot synthesize the material, although the microorganisms in his alimentary tract may do so, nor can he store it to any great degree in his tissues.

Pathological Physiology

Vitamin B_{12} or substances acting similarly are required in minute amounts to maintain most, if not all, forms of life. It is necessary for the growth of certain microorganisms. It stimulates the growth of secondary-generation rats weaned from mothers that were maintained during gestation and lactation on a diet devoid of animal protein. It counteracts the growth-retarding effect of thyroid extract when fed to immature rats, and it has been found to have "animal-protein-factor" activity in chicks obtained from hens fed all-vegetable-protein rations. Thus, there is a possibility that vitamin B_{12} is identical with, or closely related to, the animal protein factor recovered from cow manure and from a number of microorganisms[279, 280].

When patients with Addisonian pernicious anemia in relapse are given vitamin B_{12}, it produces a positive hematologic response[281] and benefits strikingly the patient who has acute glossitis and acute combined degeneration of the spinal cord. It has been found to be effective in producing a hemopoietic response and great symptomatic improvement in persons with nutritional macrocytic anemia, tropical sprue and non-tropical sprue[282, 283, 284, 285, 286, 287]. When it is realized that this material can be given in microgram quantities and produce regeneration of a number of litres of blood and be followed by a great increase in appetite and body weight, it must be thought of as something affecting one of the profoundly important enzyme systems of the body.

Symptomatology

Vitamin B_{12} has been isolated so recently and exists in the pure state in such minimal quantities that vitamin B_{12} deficiency has not been described as such. The authors are of the opinion that pernicious anemia can be considered the result of vitamin B_{12} deficiency. Pernicious anemia is too well known to repeat a description of it here in detail.

The onset is characteristically insidious. The initial complaints are fatigability, weakness, numbness, tingling, stiffness, headache, nausea, lack of appetite, vomiting, dizziness, shortness of breath, palpitation, diarrhea, pallor, abdominal pain and glossitis. By the time the anemia is severe, the skin and sclerae often are lemon yellow in color. By this time complaints referable to the nervous system are present. These complaints may be associated with mental disturbances, peripheral neuritis or spinal cord degeneration. Macrocytosis is characteristic of the blood in persons with pernicious anemia, and during the relapse stage the bone marrow is hyperplastic. Failure to secrete free hydrochloric acid in gastric juice after histamine stimulation is most characteristic of persons with this disease.

Diagnosis

A clinician can easily diagnose the average case of pernicious anemia in relapse. Glossitis, numbness and tingling of the extremities, weakness, macrocytic anemia, hyperplastic bone marrow with megaloblastic arrest and achlorhydria form a clinical picture which is extremely well known. Atypical cases even in relapse are difficult to diagnose, and experts may disagree in their interpretations of the findings. The most competent physician cannot make a positive diagnosis when the patient is in full remission, irrespective of how thoroughly the physical examination and laboratory studies are made.

Prevention and Treatment

At the present time there is no known method of preventing pernicious anemia. Since it cannot be prevented, replacement therapy is essential. The hemopoietic response of patients in relapse with pernicious anemia, nutritional macrocytic anemia and tropical sprue to vitamin B_{12} is shown in Figs. 2, 3 and 4, respectively.

Vitamin B_{12} is effective in promoting regeneration of the red blood cells, hemoglobin, white blood cells and platelets in properly selected patients, but we do not have sufficient studies to recommend the average dose required either for full regeneration or for maintenance. As little as 1 microgram will produce a detectable blood response in an occasional case, whereas as much as 5 micrograms may fail to produce a response in a case that will respond well following the administration of 10 micrograms. The individual variation in the amount required can be overcome, however, by giving increased dosage. We have seen no case that did not respond somewhat to 25 microgram amounts, and we have seen no case that did not regenerate several million red blood cells when as much as 100 micrograms was injected.

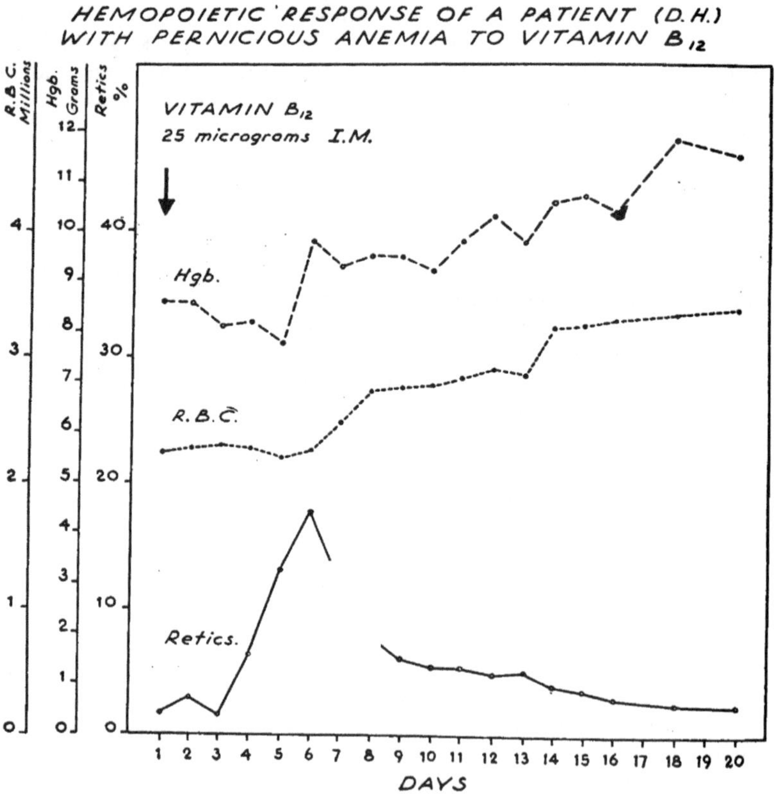

FIG. 2.

We have not had sufficient material to study properly oral therapy and cannot make any comment about it at this time. The clinical possibilities of vitamin B_{12} then are not altogether predicable, although it offers the physician a known dose of a pure compound and should thus minimize the variation in therapeutic response.

Potent doses of the new vitamin may be given without physical discomfort to the patient. A number of persons with pernicious anemia develop allergy to liver extracts, and in some parts of the world the

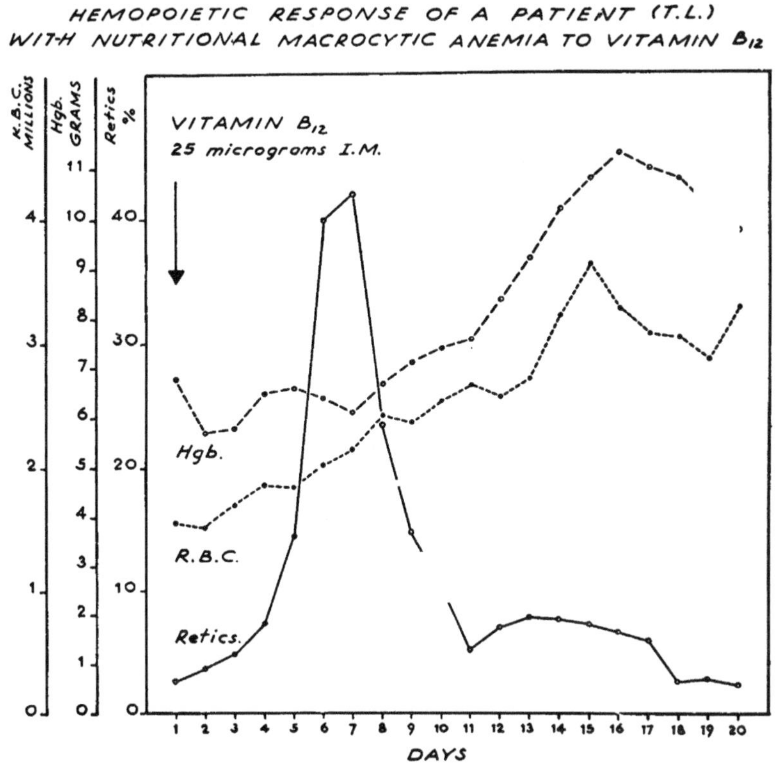

Fig. 3.

commercial liver extract preparations are not potent. Persons, who have acute manifestations of subacute combined degeneration of the spinal cord, are benefited when given vitamin B_{12}.

Suffice it to say that the limitations and therapeutic indications of vitamin B_{12} are not yet fully known, but it is by far the most potent therapeutic agent per unit of weight yet introduced into medicine. Unfortunately it is still in the experimental stage, and the supplies of vitamin B_{12} are inadequate as yet for routine treatment of pernicious anemia.

HEMOPOIETIC RESPONSE OF A PATIENT (R.L.) WITH TROPICAL SPRUE TO VITAMIN B_{12}

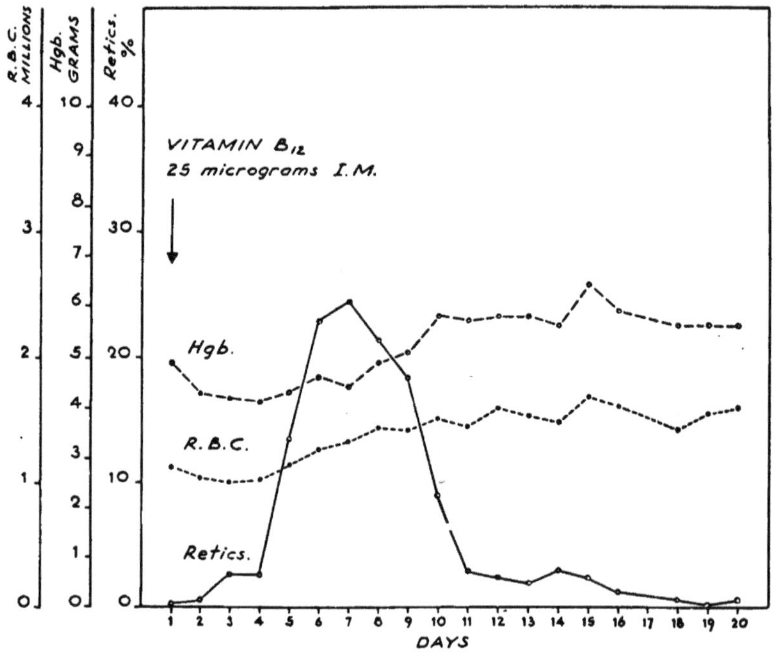

Fig. 4.

Toxicity

The practicing physician should keep in mind there is such a great difference between the therapeutic dose and any theoretical toxicity of vitamin B_{12} that there is no danger of even accumulative toxicity, and he should remember that it is a safe and effective therapeutic agent when it becomes available in sufficient amounts to use in practice.

BIBLIOGRAPHY

VITAMIN B_{12}

271. MINOT, G. R. and MURPHY, W. P.: Treatment of pernicious anemia by a special diet, Jour. Am. Med. Assoc., 1926, LXXXVII, 470.

272. SPIES, T. D.: Experiences with folic acid, The Year Book Publishers, Chicago, 1947.

273. SPIES, T. D. and STONE, R. E.: Some recent experiences with vitamins and vitamin deficiencies, South. Med. Jour., 1947, XL, 46.

274. SHORB, M. S.: Activity of vitamin B_{12} for the growth of Lactobacillus lactis, Science, 1948, CVII, 397.

275. RICKES, E. L., BRINK, N. G., KONIUSZY, F. R., WOOD, T. R. and FOLKERS, K.: Crystalline vitamin B_{12}, Science, 1948, CVII, 396.

276. SMITH, E. L.: Purification of anti-pernicious anaemia factors from liver, Nature, 1948, CLXI, 638.

277. RICKES, E. L., BRINK, N. G., KONIUSZY, F. R., WOOD, T. R. and FOLKERS, K.: Vitamin B_{12}, a cobalt complex, Science, 1948, CVIII, 134.

278. SMITH, E. L.: Presence of cobalt in the anti-pernicious anaemia factor, Nature, 1948, CLXII, 144.

279. OTT, W. H., RICKES, E. L. and WOOD, T. R.: Activity of crystalline vitamin B_{12} for chick growth, Jour. Biol. Chem., 1948, CLXXIV, 1047.

280. STOKSTAD, E. L. R., PAGE, A., JR., PIERCE, J., FRANKLIN, A. L., JUKES, T. H., HEINLE, R. W., EPSTEIN, M. and WELCH, A. D.: Activity of microbial animal protein factor concentrates in pernicious anemia, Jour. Lab. and Clin. Med., 1948, XXXIII, 860.

281. WEST, R.: Activity of vitamin B_{12} in Addisonian pernicious anemia, Science, 1948, CVII, 398.

282. SPIES, T. D., STONE, R. E. and ARAMBURU, T.: Observations on the antianemic properties of vitamin B_{12}, South. Med. Jour., 1948, XLI, 522.

283. SPIES, T. D., GARCIA LOPEZ, G., MILANES, F., LOPEZ TOCA, R. and CULVER, B.: Observations on the hemopoietic response of persons with tropical sprue to vitamin B_{12}, South. Med. Jour., 1948, XLI, 523.

284. SPIES, T. D., STONE, R. E., GARCIA LOPEZ, G., MILANES, F., ARAMBURU, T. and LOPEZ TOCA, R.: The association between gastric achlorhydria and subacute combined degeneration of the spinal cord, Postgraduate Medicine, 1948, IV, 89.

285. BERK, L., DENNY-BROWN, D., FINLAND, M. and CASTLE, W. B.: Effectiveness of vitamin B_{12} in combined system disease, New Eng. Jour. Med., 1948, CCXXXIX, 328.

286. SPIES, T. D., STONE, R. E., KARTUS, S. and ARAMBURU, T.: The treatment of subacute combined degeneration of the spinal cord with Vitamin B_{12}, South. Med. Jour., 1948, XLI, 1030.

287. SPIES, T. D. and SUAREZ, R. M.: Response of tropical sprue to Vitamin B_{12}, BLOOD, 1948, III, 1213.

June 1, 1949

CHAPTER XI

CLIMATE IN HEALTH AND DISEASE

By CLARENCE A. MILLS

Table of Contents

Introduction

Climate as a factor in the health of man is now beginning to receive the attention its importance warrants. Through its dominance of ease of body heat loss, it largely determines the energy level upon which man may exist in a given region, and we now know that much more than mere working ability is attached to this energy level of existence. All vital functions of the body are based upon the energy derived from cellular combustion of foodstuffs, but as an energy conversion machine the body is not of high efficiency. It is thus very sensitive to the ease with which its waste heat can be thrown off, and it is here that climatic dominance is exercised. Where heat loss is accomplished easily, growth is most rapid, maturity comes early, resistance to infection is highest, energy for thought and action is most plentiful, and health assumes a more positive and dynamic quality. As heat loss becomes more difficult, all these indices of vitality are depressed, and a lower, more vegetative level of existence results.

Particularly in America with its intense climatic contrasts should there be among physicians a clear understanding of these forces at work. Enlightened medical practice now goes far beyond the mere diagnosis and treatment of disease. Underlying most research into the treatment of disease has lain the ideal of disease prevention, the maintenance of unhindered health. Among the factors influencing this maintenance of health climatic environment probably will be found to be equally as important as adequate food supply or genetic background. Proper food is, of course, an essential requirement, but so too is the ability to utilize this food. With the lower combustion level of people in tropical warmth more vitamins are needed to utilize each gram of food than are required for optimal response in cooler climates. Man is less energetic in warm climates, but he is a more efficient working machine and shows less evidence of wear and tear. In cooler regions, where more dynamic and buoyant health prevails, the most acute and worrisome problems facing the medical profession arise from the wear and tear of too stressful an existence.

While mean temperature level and ease of body heat loss thus dominates the energetics of life, there is a second climatic factor which in some regions seriously disturbs the smooth flow of healthful functioning. Storminess or atmospheric turbulence with the accompanying sudden changes in temperature, pressure, humidity, etc., is now recognized as a major disturbing factor in certain regions of the earth where cyclonic storms prevail. These sudden changes in the atmosphere seriously disrupt tissue functioning in ways as yet little understood and seem closely related to the initiation of many types of acute infectious attacks. Storm changes certainly constitute a major health factor in regions where they are frequent and abrupt, but much more evidence must be accumulated before the physiology of their effects can be understood clearly. Physicians should realize that individuals differ greatly in their sensitiveness to storm changes. Some are utterly unfitted for existence in a stormy region and should be advised of the advantages of migration to a region of less turbulence.

This chapter is offered in the hope that it may help physicians to a clearer understanding of the workings of these climatic factors. Knowledge in this field still is in the stage of rapid expansion, but sufficient definite information already is at hand to warrant positive advice along several lines. Such advice will be presented in the final pages of the chapter, after the mechanism and details of climatic effects have been discussed. The newness of much of this field of knowledge necessitates, for its clear understanding, a rather comprehensive presentation of the physiological principles involved.

Physiological Considerations of Climatic Effects

Human Energetics

Since the most fundamental effects of climate are exerted upon the energetics of human existence, let us first consider the body as an energy conversion machine. At all times it lives and functions only by virtue of the cellular combustion of foodstuffs. Much of this combustion energy is wasted, however, because of low working efficiency. Man himself has designed a machine of greater working efficiency than is the human body. As high as 37 per cent. efficiency has been reached in Diesel engines, while even gasoline motors may reach the 20 to 25 per cent. efficiency exhibited by man (1), the horse (2) and the dog (3). The human body, however, is much more limited than are inanimate motors in the temperature range within which it can function well. Even a very few degrees of rise or fall from the normal body temperature level seriously interferes with efficient functioning.

To meet this handicap, the body has developed an intricate mechanism for control of rate of heat loss. Through the vasomotor control of blood supply to the skin the amount of heat reaching the body surface for heat dissipation can be altered with great rapidity. Normal heat loss from the deeper tissues by direct conduction is slow and is impeded by the insulating layers of fat encountered, but the blood with its high specific heat capacity and rapid circulation can carry internal heat to the body surface at a rapid rate. Blood flow through skin capillaries may be increased as much as 30-fold within a few minutes when a sudden need arises. When this increased blood flow through the skin proves inadequate for quick elimination of the heat of combustion, then the sweat glands become active and make possible a still greater increase in rate of heat loss by water vaporization.

This intricate heat-control mechanism functions quickly to meet sudden changes in heat production, as in bodily activity, or in the ease of

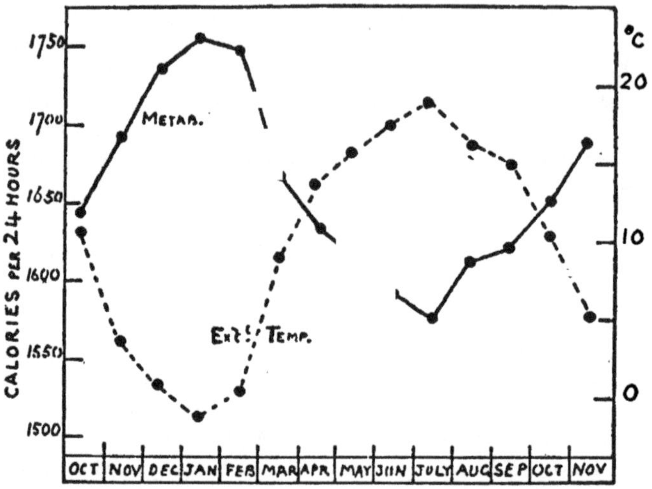

Mean monthly metabolism and mean monthly temperature. Gessler (1925), observations on himself.

FIG. 1. Seasonal variations in oxygen consumption.

heat loss, as in sudden external temperature changes. However, with more prolonged changes in the ease or difficulty of heat loss, the body adapts by an increase or decrease in its basic rate of tissue combustion. Thus, external heat that lasts only a few days calls into play only the vasomotor and sweating mechanisms, but if such heat persists for 10 days to 2 weeks, then there occurs a marked suppression in tissue combustion rate. Therein lies the chief reason why severe summer heat waves may persist for weeks but cause frequent prostration and death in the affected population only during the first 10 days or so.

It is this combustion rate response to the more prolonged changes in external temperature level and ease of body heat loss that holds greatest significance for man. Any decrease in total tissue combustion level, enforced by difficulty in heat loss, necessarily must mean a curtailment of energy available for carrying out such vital functions as growth, work performance, tissue repair and the fight against infectious invasions. Such direct linking of these vital functions to tissue combustion rate and ease of body heat loss, although logical enough, has not received the appreciation its importance warrants. Indeed there has existed among medical men in America a disbelief that any such dependence really exists. This disbelief dates back to the publication of a paper by Benedict and

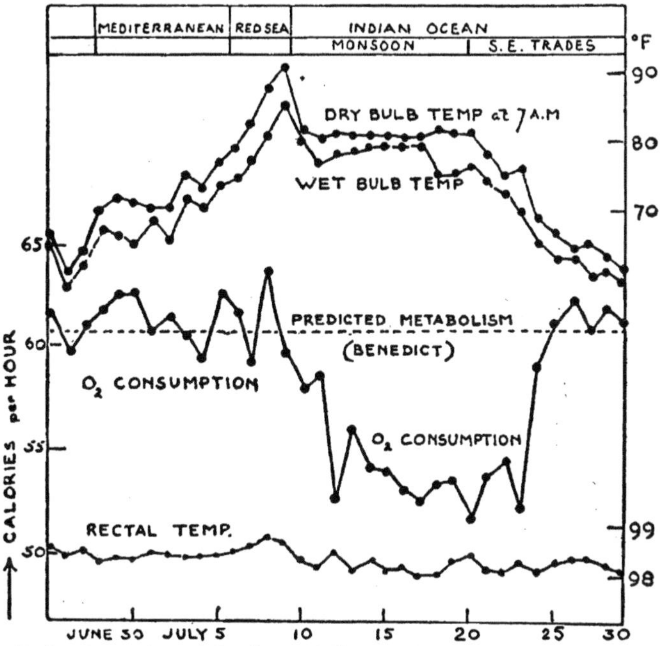

Daily observation of basal metabolism of C. J. M. during a voyage from London to Australia, June–July, 1923, and daily record of the temperatures of the dry and wet bulb thermometers at 7 A.M.

FIG. 2. Fall in oxygen consumption in tropical heat.

Cathcart[1], in which they cite oxygen consumption data on 14 subjects in Boston and claim a lack of any seasonal influence. Even though their own data presented in their article do show a strong tendency for lowest consumption rate to occur in July or August, and this in Boston where summer heat is rarely severe, this article has been extensively quoted since as indicating that tissue combustion rates are independent of external temperature levels.

This point is of such basic importance in any analysis of climatic effects that recently it was made the subject of a special article[5], in which the available evidence was presented and discussed. As set forth in that article the evidence points conclusively to a clear inverse relationship between tissue combustion rates and prevailing external temperature levels in both men and animals. Fig. 1 shows this relationship as found by Gessler[6] through all seasons of a year at Heidelberg, Germany. Fig. 2 indicates the marked suppression in resting oxygen consumption rate

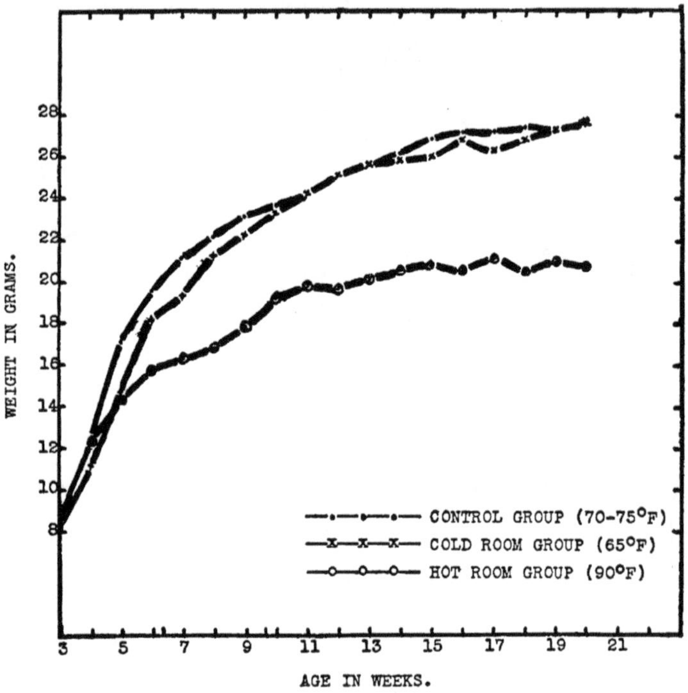

FIG. 3. Growth of white mice at different temperatures.

found by Martin[7] in himself during his passage through the zone of tropical heat on a trip from London to Melbourne. Practically all investigators, who have looked for this heat suppression of combustion rate, have found it. Let us next see what it means in terms of growth and other vital functions.

Growth Rates at Different Temperature Levels

All types of experimental animals suffer a growth retardation when heat loss becomes difficult. Fig. 3 shows the extent of this growth suppression in white mice kept at 65° F., 72° F. and 91° F. This happens even though all factors of existence other than ease of heat loss are kept constant. Animals at 91° F. eat only about half as much food as at

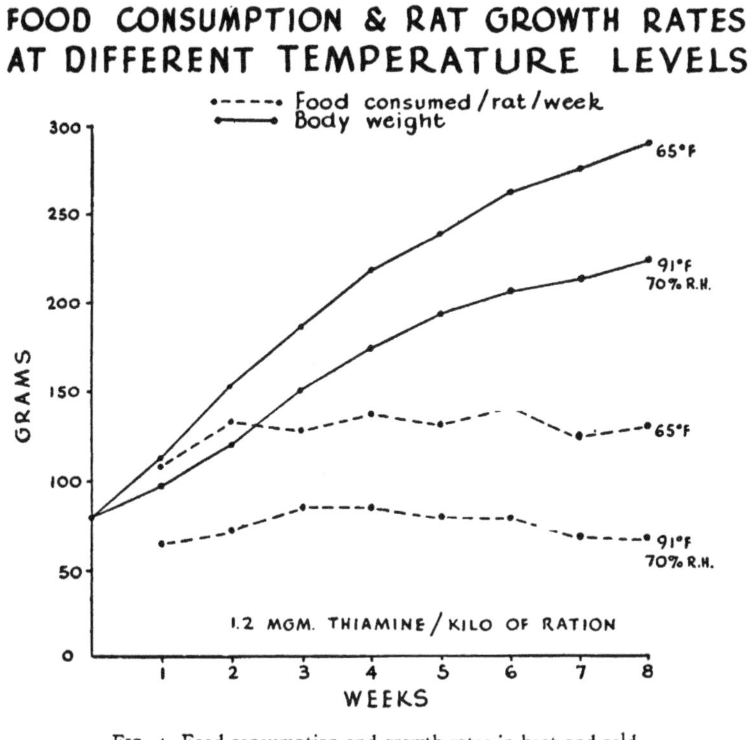

FIG. 4. Food consumption and growth rates in heat and cold.

65° F. In Fig. 4 is shown this difference in food consumption by young Wistar rats and its direct relationship to their rate of growth and final adult size. Herein lies the principal reason why domestic animals do so poorly in tropical warmth, giving lean, stringy meat of strong flavor. Coarseness of the tropical forage crops and leaching of soils under the heavy rainfall may be factors of considerable weight, but suppression of tissue combustion rate by difficulty in body heat loss probably is more important.

Children show this same retarded growth rate and inferior adult size under tropical heat conditions, while in the optimal coolness of middle temperate regions growth is most lusty and adult stature greatest[8]. The close relation of such growth differences to oxygen utilization is emphasized by the marked differences in vital lung capacity exhibited by individuals from the two types of climate. Vital capacity in Filipino college students is only a little over half as great as that of students in northern United States.

Back through human history man's stature and development has fluctuated with slow changes in earth temperatures. Middle Age warmth saw a marked decline from early Greek levels in the size of man and in his speed of development, while with the colder centuries since the time of the Renaissance the race has again shown a striking rise from the low Middle Age standards. The menarche in girls of early Greece came at 13 years of age according to Hippocrates, but with the retarded development of the Middle Ages the menses did not begin until the 16th, 17th and 18th years in European girls. A marked quickening in development has been in evidence during the last few centuries of lower world temperatures with the menses now coming 1½ years earlier than they did even 4 decades ago and the adult male height being now four inches greater than in Revolutionary days. Man was really runt-like through the warm centuries of the Middle Ages, small of stature and fine-boned. The knights, who wore the suits of armor now on display in museums, although probably the best physical specimens of the day, must have been far below the standards of today, for a well-developed American boy of 14 years would have great difficulty getting into any of the suits now on display in the Tower of London.

World temperatures have been rising quite generally again in recent decades, and the long period of improvement in racial physique seems perhaps about at an end. College youth in America, where nutritional standards have never been higher, are now showing signs of a reversal in the growth tide. The menses are now tending to begin later and the stature to be slightly less with each year's entering class of freshmen in schools of lower and middle temperate latitudes, although improvement still proceeds apace in schools of higher latitudes where depressive summer heat has not yet reached effective levels. The human race does then seem to respond to slow changes in earth temperature levels in the same manner that experimental animals respond to artificial changes in ease of body heat loss. This fact is of fundamental importance in racial welfare, for it perhaps accounts in large part for the slow undulations of advance and recession which the race has undergone through past ages and may some day give a clue to our course through the coming decades and centuries, when we shall have become able to predict future temperature trends. The matter is not just one of recession in rate of growth and development but involves also all the other factors of life dependent upon the dynamics of cellular combustion. Ability and urge to accomplish along both physical and mental lines and the positiveness of health itself seem closely bound up in this temperature dominance over human dynamics.

Development of Sexual Functions

Onset of sexual functions and degree of fertility are closely linked to ease of body heat loss and tissue combustion level. Most rapid development and highest fertility occur at environmental temperatures around 65° F. As difficulty in heat loss comes on and growth rate slackens, we regularly see also a later onset of sexual cycles in young females, both human and animal, and a lowered fertility[9]. Animals mate freely at 90° F., but conceptions are difficult to obtain and result in small litters of puny young, while at 65° F. almost every mating results in a large litter of lusty offspring. Histological changes in gonadal tissues indicate that this suppression of reproductive tissue is extensive and very real. Spermatogenic activity in the testes is almost obliterated within 10 to 14 days of application of tropical moist heat. After several weeks of adaptation some recovery of function occurs but to a much lower level of activity than is seen at lower temperature levels.

Man, living under natural climatic habitats, shows just as striking sexual variations at different levels of environmental temperature as do laboratory animals. Onset of the menses in girls occurs earliest in middle temperate latitudes and comes at a progressively later age as more and more severe tropical heat is encountered. At the present time here in North America earliest menarche is found in the upper half of the Mississippi basin. Nowhere else on earth do children grow with such lusty vigor and enter such early adolescence. Development in the Gulf States is somewhat retarded by the long summer of tropical moist heat, but most severe suppression takes place in the tropical lowlands, where depressive moist heat renders heat loss difficult at all times.

Medical literature and lay belief back through the centuries at least to the time of Hippocrates has held that earliest onset of the menses occurred in the tropics. Even though all recorded statistics contradicted this belief, still it is encountered among people of all lands, both lay and medical. Since we know it has been handed down through medical literature for two thousand years without factual support, we can well presume that it may have originated several thousand years earlier still. Only 20,000 or so years ago present middle temperate regions had polar climates, and optimal temperature conditions for man were to be found only in what are now tropical or subtropical lands. That such beliefs, perhaps once based upon real facts, can be handed down through many thousands of years without further supporting factual background is well illustrated by the ancient astrological beliefs so widely held today even among intelligent people.

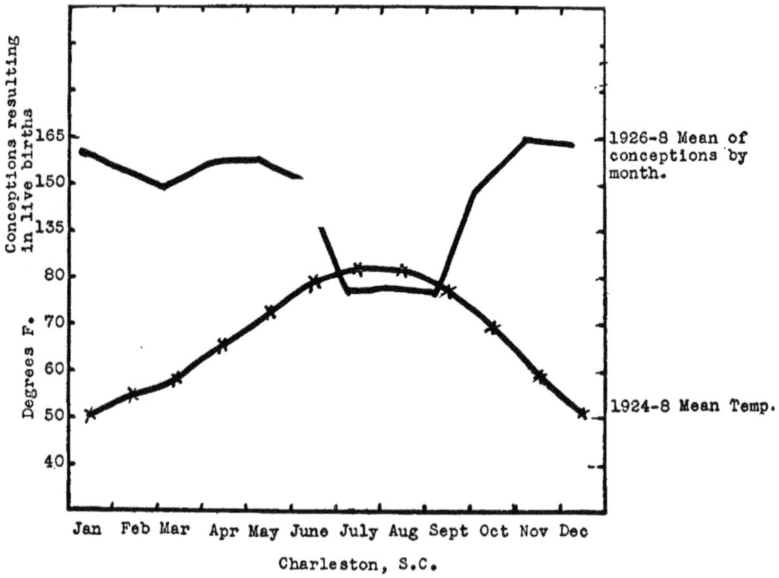

FIG. 5. Variations in conceptions, Charleston, S. C.

Fig. 5 illustrates the sharp suppression of human fertility that comes with difficulty in heat loss. Wherever human populations are exposed to seasonal swings in mean monthly temperature, highest conception rates nearly always occur when the mean temperature level is near 65° F. As mean temperatures rise above 70° F. or fall below 40° F., fertility is reduced. With really severe moist warmth, as in Japan's monsoon summer heat or in the prolonged severe heat waves of the upper Mississippi valley in North America, conceptions may be reduced as much as 50 per cent. Nor is this reduction in conceptions merely a result of less frequent intercourse in hot weather, for there occurs no significant reduction in the frequenting of houses of prostitution. Apparently both men and animals continue the mating urge in hot weather but suffer a sharp drop in biological fertility.

There has been much written about child-mothers among tropical peoples, but it is really among populations of middle temperate regions that fertility has its earliest onset. Later marriage ages of the more highly industrialized nations of the temperate zones tend to mask the early onset of fertility, but it has been brought out by a study of illegitimate first-births[10]. At Cincinnati, Ohio, the average maternal age at illegitimate first-birth was found to be 18.1 years and at Richmond, Virginia, 18.2 years for negro girls, while at Panama it was 19.3 years and in the Philippines 21.8 years. The average lag from menarche to first conception with these illegitimate first-births was 3.9 years at Cincinnati, 4.0 at Richmond, 4.5 at Panama and 6.3 in Manila. This markedly later age at first conception in the tropics occurs even in the face of a much greater promiscuity of premarital intercourse and lessened likelihood of chances for effective impregnation being missed. Maternal age at the first child-birth in Manila is the same regardless as to whether the mother be married or single.

Malnutrition from any cause tends to retard development of the sexual functions. Difficulty in body heat loss is no more effective in this respect than is inadequacy of available food supply, either in total amount or in composition, or serious childhood illnesses. The menarche usually is delayed in girls who have been subjected to any of these depressing influences through their childhood years.

Resistance to Infection

Although such factors as malnutrition, vitamin deficiency and exhaustion usually have been considered important in determining the body's ability to fight infection, there has been little apparent inclination to relate this ability to tissue combustion level. Yet such a relationship would seem logical, since all vitality factors must have their functional basis in the energy liberated from such combustion. It is infectious disease which kills people living under depressing tropical warmth, while the more energetic residents of middle temperate regions die mainly from the degenerative and breakdown ailments. In 1932 we showed that ability to survive tuberculous infection was markedly higher in Cincinnati residents who were born in the North than in those born in the Gulf States[11]. Dealing only with tuberculosis deaths among the indigent population of Cincinnati it was shown that the survival time from first symptom to death was almost twice as long in patients born in northern United States or North Central Europe than it was in those born in the Gulf States of North America or in the Mediterranean countries of Europe. Ability to survive acute appendicitis attacks also is markedly higher in the North than in the South[12]. These facts will be discussed more fully on a subsequent page.

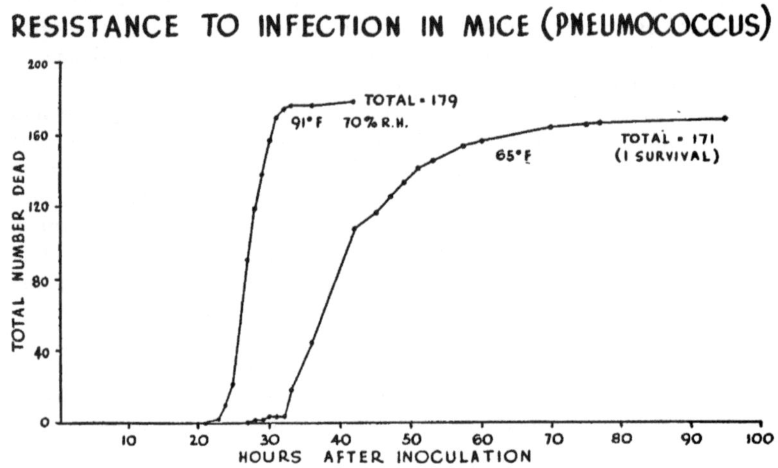

FIG. 6. Resistance to infection in heat and cold.

Human disease statistics, however, are influenced by too many extraneous factors to be of any great value in determining climatic effects, unless they can be substantiated by studies on experimental animals under carefully controlled conditions. Human data may supply indications of existing differences or trends, but conclusive proof in such a matter must come from laboratory studies. Fortunately such studies have now shown that ability to fight infection is definitely higher under conditions that facilitate body heat loss than it is where heat loss is difficult. With all other existence factors except ease of body heat loss held constant, practically all mice adapted to 90° F. will be dead after inoculation with a given dose of pneumococci organisms before those adapted to 65° F. even begin to succumb. Fig. 6 presents this fact in striking fashion, and if one uses a less lethal organism, such as a hemolytic streptococcus, then the minimum lethal dose for the 65° F. mice is found to be about four times as great as it is for those kept at 90° F. Antibody production after typhoid vaccine injection into rabbits is almost twice as great in those animals kept at the lower temperature.

Locke[13] has provided support also for the idea that combustion level is an important factor in determining resistance to infection. He found that ability of animals to survive pneumococcic inoculations or of human beings to maintain freedom from respiratory infection was related directly to their rate of oxygen utilization. The matter needs more thorough study, but in the main it would seem that man's susceptibility to infection and his chances for survival are conditioned rather markedly by his ease of body heat loss and the resulting tissue combustion level allowed him. Temperate zone man does not, then, enjoy greatest freedom from respiratory disease during the summer months because of better tissue vitality as has been so commonly supposed. Actually the fatality rate per 100 cases of acute appendicitis is almost twice as high in summer heat as in northern winter cold, and tuberculosis runs its most rapid course when symptoms of disease activity first appear in summer heat. It would now seem almost certain that the summer freedom from respiratory infection is attributable in very large part to the lessened storminess of that season and the greater freedom from body chilling. More will be said about this subject on a later page.

Vitamin and Protein Requirements

Since human vitality and energy level seem so dependent upon ease of body heat loss and tissue combustion rate, it is well to look into the combustion process itself. Perhaps tissue requirements for the combustion catalysts are higher when the combustion rate is slowed down by difficulty in heat loss. With the lowered food intake of hot climates or in summer heat it may well be that a higher dietary content of thiamine and of other combustion catalysts of the vitamin B group is needed to maintain optimal concentration for proper tissue oxidative processes. It has quite generally been considered, largely as a result of Cowgill's studies[14], that thiamine requirement is determined by the amount of glucose there is to be burned, that a more or less constant ratio exists between thiamine requirement and total non-fat calories of the diet. His studies, however, and those of others in this field were carried out at approximately optimal environmental temperatures for the animal subjects, so that there was no way of knowing whether this ratio might not vary as external temperatures were raised or lowered.

In more recent studies on this point[15] it has, in fact, been found that the optimal requirement for dietary thiamine is twice as high at 91° F. than it is at 65° F. Animals show definite inadequacy in the heat at dietary thiamine levels twice as high as those at which inadequacy ap-

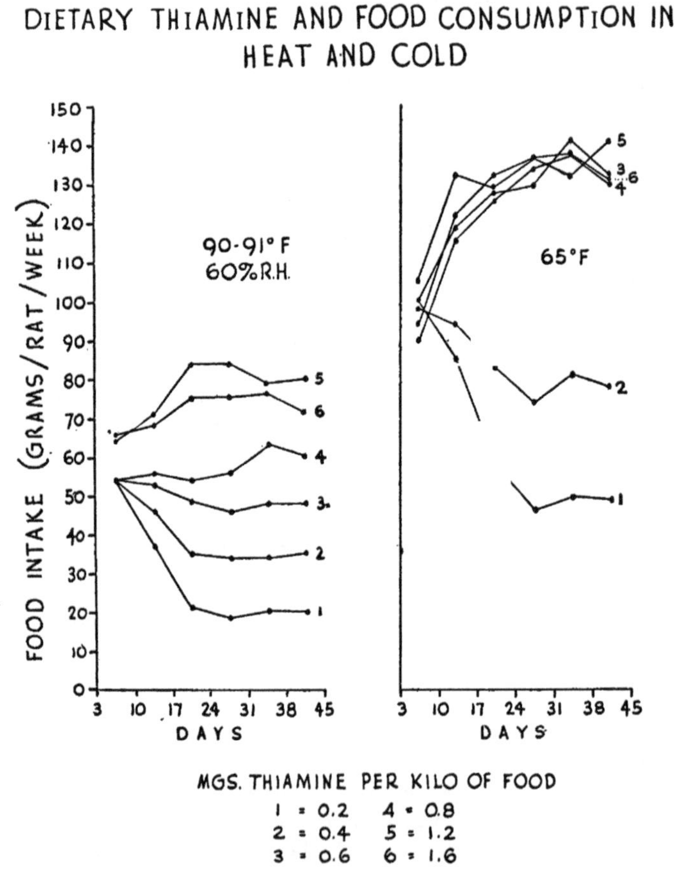

FIG. 7. Dietary thiamine and food consumption in heat and cold.

pears in a cool environment. Studies in progress indicate that somewhat similar findings will be obtained for others of the vitamin B fractions, pantothenic acid deficiency already having been found to develop with much greater rapidity at 91° F. than at 65° F.

Fig. 7 shows clearly the marked difference in optimal dietary thiamine level for Wistar rats kept in moist warmth and in a cool environ-

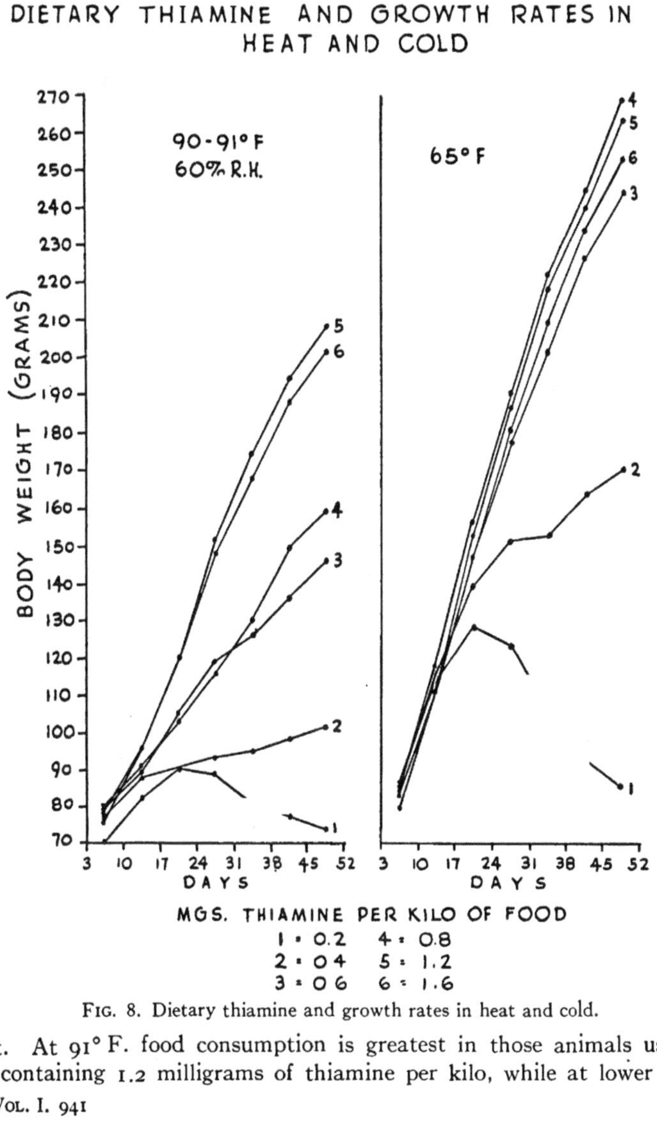

FIG. 8. Dietary thiamine and growth rates in heat and cold.

ment. At 91° F. food consumption is greatest in those animals using a diet containing 1.2 milligrams of thiamine per kilo, while at lower levels of dietary thiamine there is almost a quantitative relationship between food consumption and thiamine content. At 65° F. on the other hand food consumption is sub-optimal only at the two lowest thiamine levels, 0.2 and 0.4 milligrams per kilo of food.

In Fig. 8 these differences in dietary thiamine requirements are brought out even more quantitatively by differences in rate of growth. At 65° F. growth is almost optimal with all the groups receiving 0.6 milligrams or more per kilo of food, although the 0.8 milligram group was found to do best and usually to show the greatest gain in weight per gram of food eaten. With rats kept at 91° F. best growth was obtained at the 1.2 milligram level but with little difference at 1.6 milligrams. Best growth efficiency, grams gain in weight / grams of food eaten, was found most often at the 1.6 milligram thiamine level in the heat (90–91° F.) but at 0.8 milligrams in the cold (65° F.) as shown in the curves in Fig. 8.

These food consumption and growth differences at varying thiamine intake levels persist on through to adult life, giving at the lower thiamine levels the scrawny, stunted specimens so similar to those commonly seen among human populations living under tropical lowland heat. Many students of nutritional problems have held that a higher protein intake, particularly of animal proteins, would greatly improve the nutritional state of tropical people.

Higher cost of such protein foods has prevented any widespread trial of this idea, but unpublished results from the author's laboratory have given indications that such a step would not be beneficial in tropical heat even if it were economically feasible.

Fig. 9 illustrates in striking fashion the handicap placed upon animals living at 91° F. when their dietary protein is increased only moderately. The added difficulties in heat dissipation that result from the increased dietary protein with its higher specific dynamic action seem just as depressive to growth as do still higher external temperatures.

It is unfortunate indeed that the greater part of our dietary supply of vitamin B fractions comes in foods which are rich in protein, meats, milk products, nuts, legumes. Cereal grains provide the only exceptions, and with the two most widely used, wheat and rice, the vitamin stores are largely removed in milling processes. Tropical natives thus are doubly handicapped. Their need for vitamins of the respiratory catalyst type is sharply higher than in cooler lands, while the principal foods, through which they might meet this higher need, are more expensive and intensify their problem of difficulty in body heat loss. Fruits and starchy tubers, which supply such a large part of the tropical dietaries, are low in vitamin B fractions but can be utilized by tropical natives with least intensification of their heat loss difficulties.

Man's higher requirement for the vitamin B fractions in tropical warmth probably plays an important part in the widespread occurrence there of such deficiency states as beri beri and pellagra. The subject needs a thorough investigation, for upon this situation may hinge a considerable part of the malnutrition and low physical level seen among tropical populations. The magnitude of the problem can be appreciated only when it is remembered that half of the earth's human population

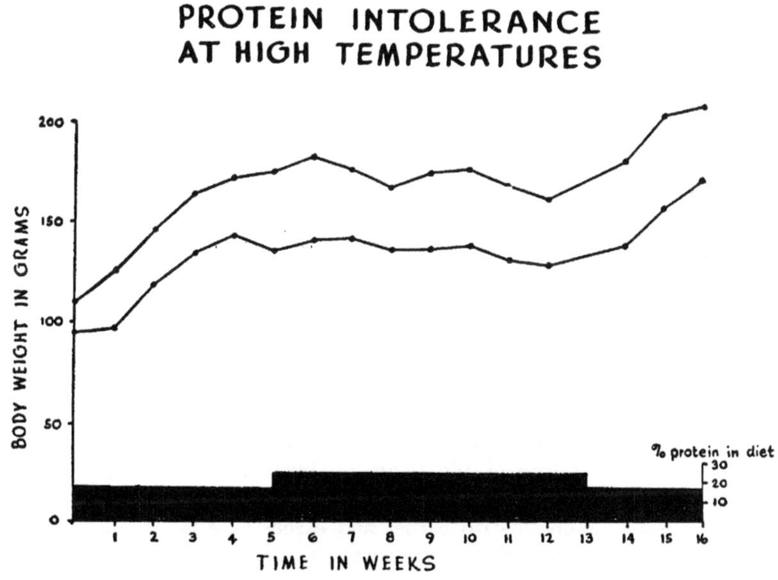

FIG. 9. Protein intolerance at high temperatures.

lives under just such depressive heat as is being discussed here. We can as yet only guess at the many bearings this variation in vitamin requirement at different temperature levels may have in the problems of human welfare. Since it affects directly cellular combustion and the source of energy for all body functions, it must, of necessity, have important bearings on all the vital processes and functions of the body. A whole new field seems to be opened up by this dynamic view of physiological response to climate.

Climate and Disease

The preceding discussion of climatic physiology provides a most useful background for an understanding of the geography of many diseases. Tropical people with their more sluggish combustion rate and lowered vitality die largely from the infectious diseases; energetic residents of cooler lands die more from the breakdown and degenerative diseases. Only with pneumococcic and streptococcic infections, largely respiratory or of the nasopharynx, is the attack frequency higher in temperate regions and then only during the seasons of great cyclonic storminess. Since these disease differences are based largely upon demonstrable differences in physiological response to living environment and are susceptible to a considerable degree of control, it seems wise that the medical profession consider them against their proper physiological background.

It is not at all surprising that clearest climatic relationships should be found for the diseases of metabolic over-stimulation or breakdown. Metabolic stress rises highest in middle temperate regions, where most nearly optimal heat loss conditions prevail, while toward tropical warmth evidences of such stress progressively decrease. Diabetes, with its breakdown in ability to metabolize the glucose upon the combustion of which depends all bodily energy, shows this climatic relationship perhaps most clearly, but the relationship is also quite evident for pernicious anemia with its exhaustion in the production of red cells to carry the oxygen from lungs to tissues. Toxic goiter and hyperthyroidism seem likely to be involved in this same environmental influence. Perhaps most worrisome to the medical profession of the stimulating regions are the growing evidences of stress and failure in the vascular system. Upon this system falls the most direct load of any tissue combustion increase, for it must transport to the tissues all the needed combustion factors. The advance of sudden heart failure toward earlier and earlier ages in American men of middle temperate latitudes is presenting the medical profession with an acute health problem to consider. Over two thirds of the American physicians dying in 1939 did so from primary failure of one sort or another in the circulatory system. Addison's disease with its adrenal failure and other exhaustion states such as myesthenia gravis and neurocirculatory asthenia also most frequently occur in these same middle temperate latitudes. And for some reason, as yet little understood, it is in these same latitudes that cancer is presenting its greatest menace to man. Leukemia, which some consider to be a form of neoplasia, is almost exclusively a cool climate disease.

Infectious diseases present the other side of the picture, for with them

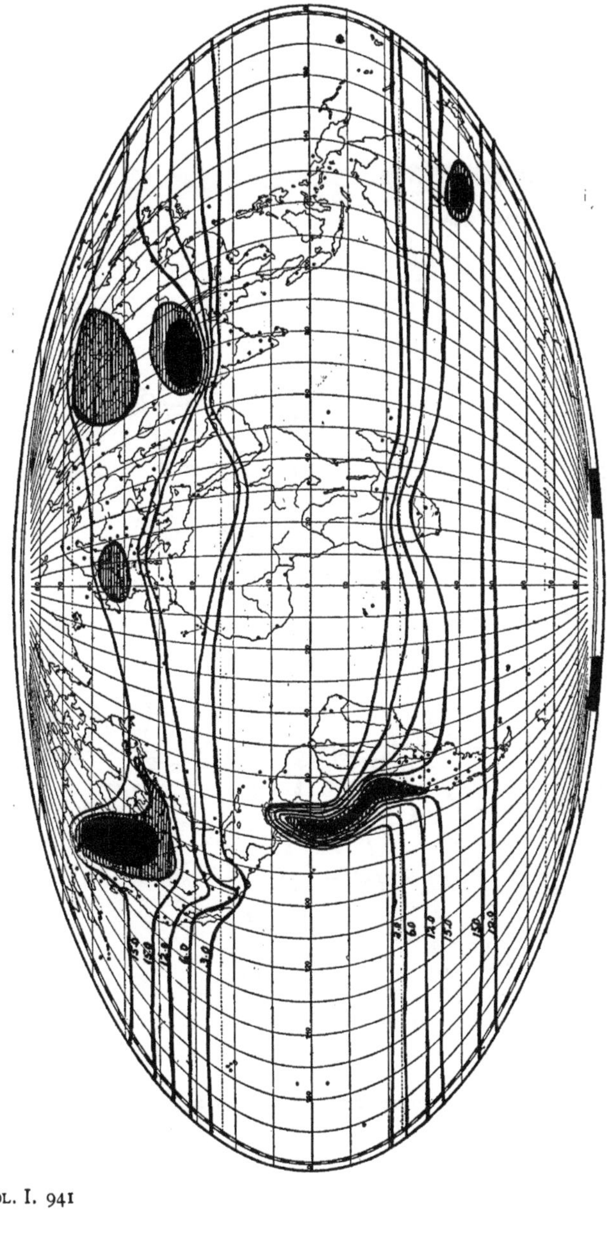

FIG. 10. Climatic stimulation over the earth.

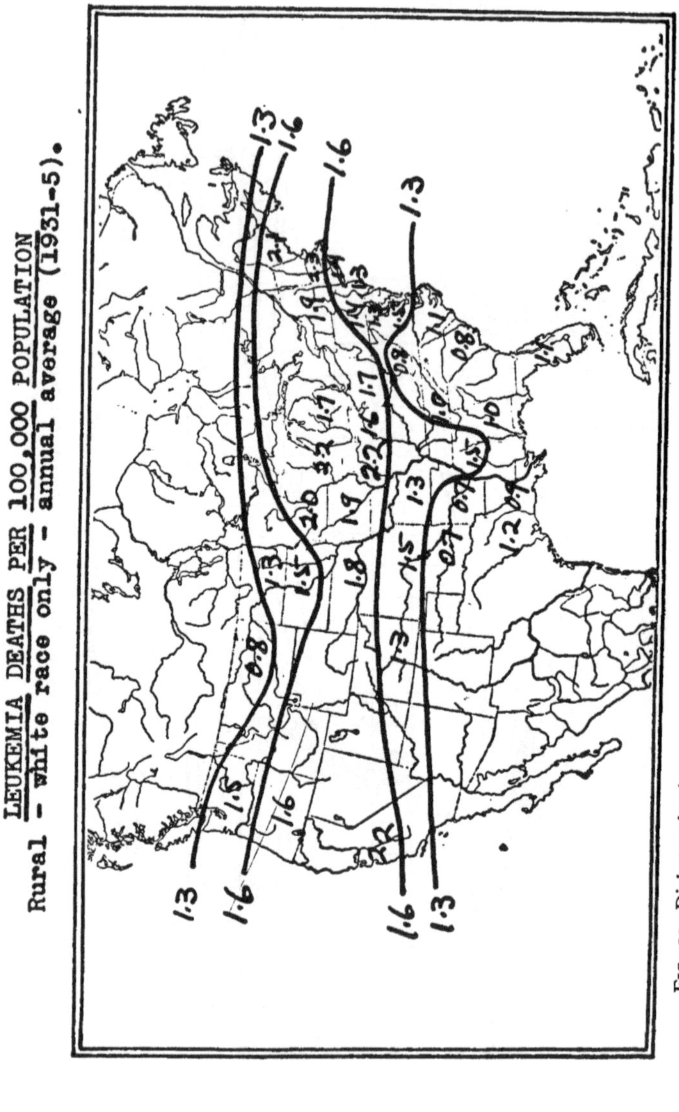

FIG. 11. Diabetes deaths per 100,000 population. Rural, White race only — annual average (1931–5).

greatest frequency and highest death rates go hand in hand with lowered tissue resistance in the debilitating warmth of tropical and sub-tropical regions. Temperatures there are more nearly optimal for parasitic and bacterial contamination of water and food supply, it is true, and added to this is the tremendous problem of insect vectors, but working beneath these major health threats in the tropics is the lowered general tissue vitality from sluggish cellular combustion. Fig. 10, showing regional differences in the intensity of climatic stimulation over the earth, is presented here so that the reader may have before him this rough idea of the metabolic driving force being exerted upon man in the different regions. The methods used in calculating the indices of climatic stimulation have been described in detail elsewhere[16]. Let us see, in greater detail in succeeding paragraphs of this section, just how important these effects of climate may be for man.

Diabetes Mellitus

With 80 per cent. of the total cellular combustion being glucose burning it is not surprising that evidences of stress should appear in the body's machinery for handling glucose under conditions that bring a prolonged and sustained increase in tissue combustion rate. No one knows as yet just what factors immediately determine which members of a population mass shall suffer this break in glucose metabolism, but the evidence is convincing that the severity of diabetes as a disease is strongly influenced in some way by climatic stimulation. While the disease occurs in tropical people, it is so mild as rarely to need attention and seldom results in severe ketosis; mild dietary management usually is sufficient for complete control. In the cooler and more energizing middle temperate latitudes, on the other hand, diabetes becomes a much more violent metabolic disturbance with ketosis a frequent and real threat to the patients' lives and with eternal and painstaking care the price to be paid for its control.

Fig. 11 shows the marked increase in recorded diabetes mortality among rural populations from the Gulf States northward in America and the decline on into Canada past middle temperate latitudes. Failure of the band of high mortality rates to continue across the upper Plains States probably is due to the younger average age of the populations of those states. The disease is now increasing in severity there as the population ages, with those states showing the most marked rise in mortality rate. In urban populations the age differences are not so great and in Fig. 12 it is seen that the band of highest urban diabetes mortality extends entirely across the continent.

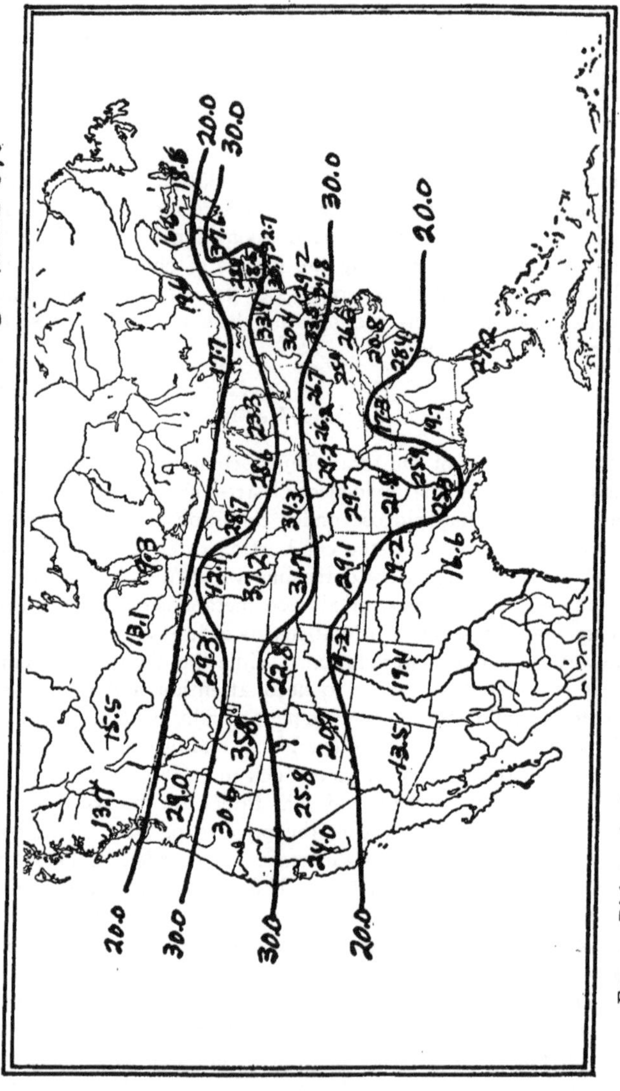

FIG. 12. Diabetes deaths per 100,000 population. Urban, white race only — annual average (1931–5).

It is not yet clear just why evidences of climatic stimulation and metabolic stress should lessen on northward into polar cold much like they do toward subtropical warmth. All metabolic and degenerative disease statistics do show a decline in severity northward from middle temperate latitudes, and the onset of the menses in girls is progressively delayed the farther north one goes. The reason may perhaps lie in the fact that in the milder winters of middle temperate regions people get outdoors more and really undergo greater exposure to increased heat loss than do people living through the prolonged winter cold of more northerly regions. Whatever the explanation may be, it does seem a fact that human vitality rises highest in middle temperate latitudes both north and south of the equator. The moderating influence of the Gulf Stream on northwestern Europe seems to cause highest vitality there to appear about 15 degrees farther north than in America. Britain, northern France, Belgium, the Netherlands, Denmark, Germany and the southern parts of Scandinavia seem to form the European counterpart of the northern half of the United States in the matter of climatic stimulation.

Fig. 13, showing the ten-fold increase in the negro diabetes death rate from south to north within the United States, gives clear indication of the price this tropical race pays for its higher energy level on migration into the stimulation of cooler regions. Vascular sclerosis in the negro is also a much more malignant disease in the northern states than it is in the south, occurring with greater frequency and running a more rapid course. Toxic goiter also becomes much more frequent, and pernicious anemia makes its appearance in a race apparently free of the disease in warmer regions.

Fig. 14 shows the European center of high diabetes mortality to cover the same west-central European countries shown in Fig. 10 to be receiving the highest degree of climatic stimulation available on that continent. Statistics for either total or urban death rates show diabetes in this area to be more severe than in other parts of the continent. In South America the disease becomes a health problem only in the temperate coolness of Argentina and Chile, while in Australia it is of low severity in the north and increases progressively toward the south.

Diabetes specialists, studying and handling the disease only in the regions where it is most frequent and severe, are inclined to doubt these statistical indications of climatic or regional differences in the disease. Less accurate diagnosis and reporting of causes of death they feel may account for most of the differences in mortality. Extensive surveys of the disease in the living populations of Massachusetts and Arizona, summarized in a recent paper entitled "The Universality of Diabetes"[17], was

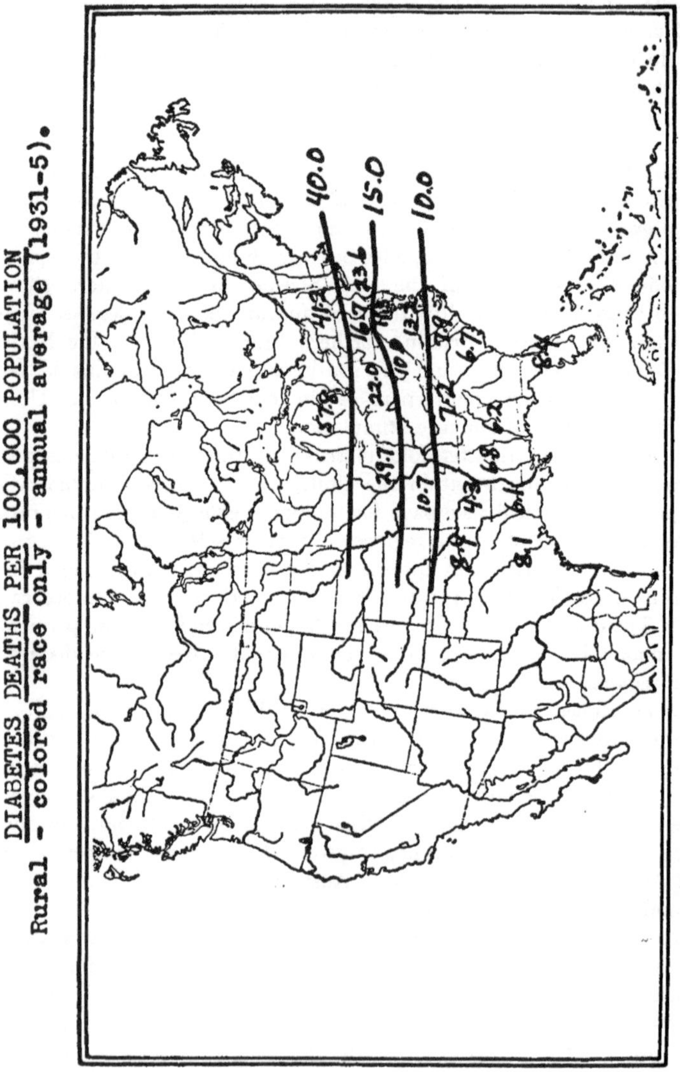

FIG. 13. Diabetes deaths per 100,000 population. Rural, colored race only — annual average (1931–5).

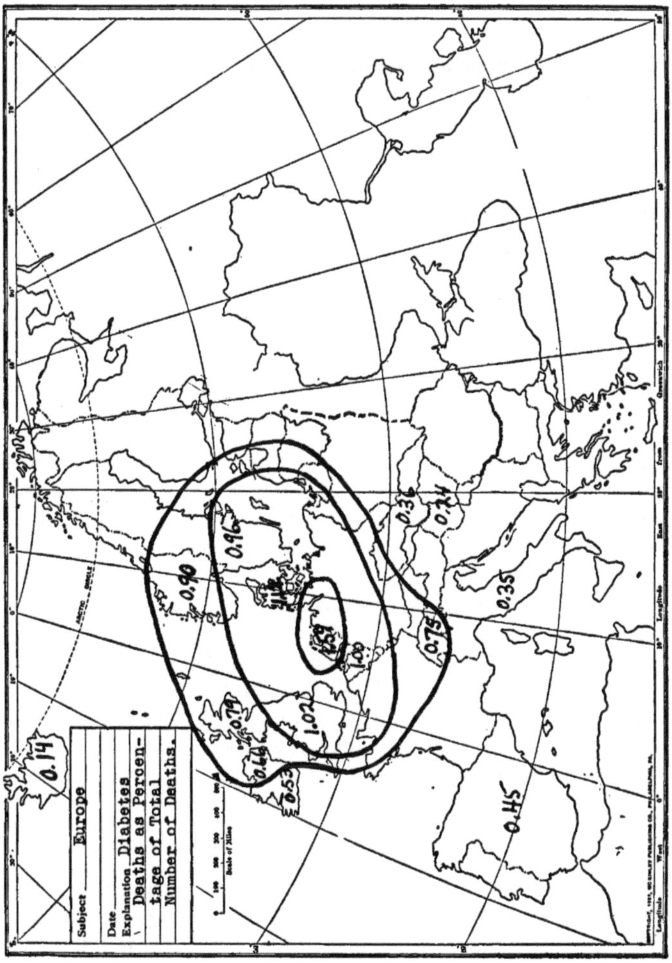

FIG. 14. Diabetes death rates in Europe.

claimed to contradict the idea that real differences do exist with such wide climatic variation as these two states show. It is unfortunate that the southern state chosen for comparison with Massachusetts should have been one so heavily populated by former migrants from northern regions, probably standing next to Florida and California in this respect. But even with this high proportion of migrants from the north the survey indicated a considerably lower diabetes death rate per 1,000 cases in Arizona than was found in Massachusetts.

The evidence for climatic differences in diabetes is being discussed in considerable detail because this disease has been studied more thoroughly than have the other metabolic disturbances, and because it bears such a direct relationship to tissue combustion rate and metabolic stress. Then too the milder course followed by the disease in warm climates is a point of great therapeutic importance for the people who must live out their remaining life span under its handicaps.

Pernicious Anemia, Toxic Goiter and Addison's Disease

Pernicious anemia shows just as clear evidences of climatic variation in severity as does diabetes. It forms a real health problem only in those same stimulating temperate regions where diabetes is so severe and is seen rarely in tropical warmth. The same holds true for *toxic goiter* and *Addison's disease.* Higher death rates from these metabolic diseases in middle temperate regions cannot be due only to the reduced infectious disease death rates there prevailing, for there is more frequent metabolic breakdown at every age throughout life. Death rates for these diseases are about twice as high for every age group in northern United States as for comparable populations along the Gulf of Mexico. A similar relationship seems to hold for other continents of the earth, although lack of uniformity in mortality records makes difficult so clear a presentation of the differences as is possible in America.

Arteriosclerosis and Heart Failure

Arteriosclerosis and *heart failure* statistics are in general still too confused and lacking in uniformity of nomenclature and diagnostic criteria to be of much value. There seems little doubt that diseases of the heart and vascular system constitute a far more serious health problem in temperate regions than in tropical warmth. The differences seem to be of about the same order as with the metabolic diseases. This would be quite in line with expectation, if circulatory failure is dependent upon stress, for the primary work load of a higher tissue combustion rate falls upon the circulatory system as the oxygen carrier. Although general mortality statistics are unsatisfactory to bring out this relationship, recently it has been demonstrated in another way[18]. Fig. 15 shows the clear inverse relationship of non-infectious heart failures to mean monthly temperature

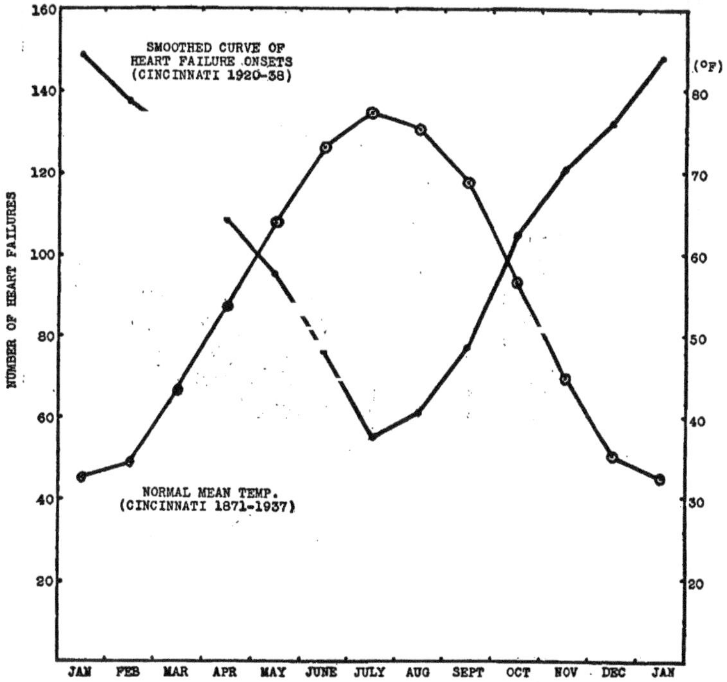

FIG. 15. Heart failure frequency and mean temperature level.

level throughout the year at Cincinnati, using only fever-free heart failure admissions to the Cincinnati General Hospital over a 20-year period. Such heart failures not only show this striking seasonal variation in frequency, but they fluctuate also with the severity of the winter cold. During certain warmer Cincinnati winters admission rates for such heart failures were only a quarter as high as during winters of normal cold. Rheumatic and arteriosclerotic types of heart failure show this relation to prevailing external temperatures, but not those due to syphilis.

Vascular sclerosis in old age might be expected in any region, but it seems that only in the more energizing regions of the earth do its devastating effects appear in the earlier decades of life. Heart failure from coronary disease is becoming entirely too frequent in the fifth decade and even in the fourth in those same energetic populations that are showing

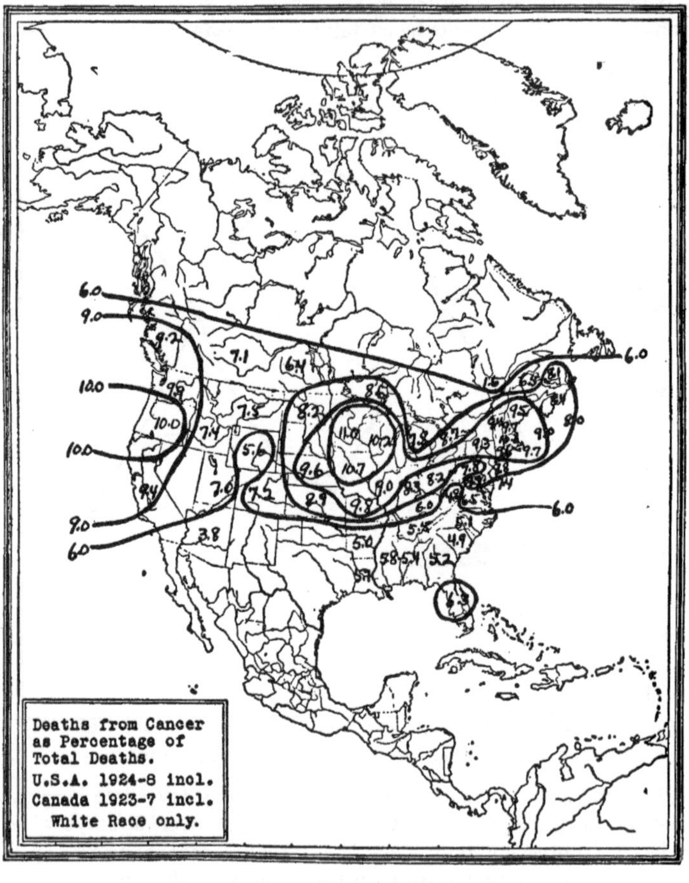

FIG. 16. Cancer death rates in America.

the highest frequency of metabolic breakdown. Negroes of the north show this vascular sclerosis problem in its most severe form, just as they suffer more severely from diabetes. With them sclerosis is most likely to assume the malignant, rapidly progressive form. Negro deaths from arteriosclerotic (non-syphilitic and non-rheumatic) causes in Cincinnati occur

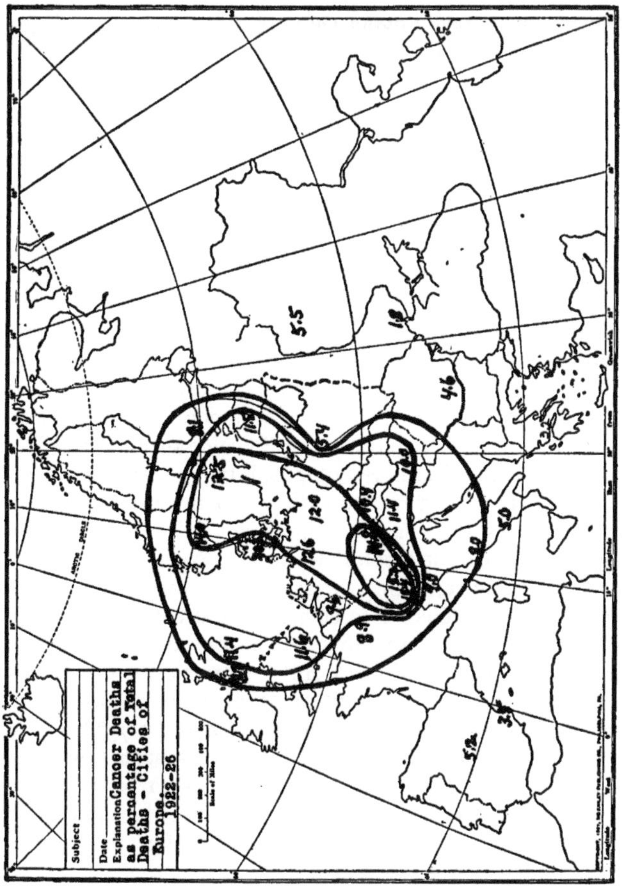

FIG. 17. Cancer death rates in Europe.

at significantly earlier ages for northern-born negroes than for those born in the Gulf States[19]. Perhaps the experimental studies, now being carried on so actively by various investigative groups, will throw valuable light on this problem of vascular sclerosis. Certainly little headway can yet be claimed by the medical profession in devising means for its control, although it constitutes a really major cause of disability and death in populations of temperate regions.

Cancer

Cancer is another major health problem against the inroads of which little headway has yet been made. New evidence is now being presented to show that here again is a type of disease showing the same climatic relationships as do the metabolic disturbances. All forms of cancer except those of the skin and buccal cavity are more frequent in populations of middle temperate regions than they are toward tropical warmth[20]. In fact cancer death rate maps for any continent show a remarkable similarity to those for diabetes (see Figs. 16 and 17 for cancer death rates in America and Europe). Use of death rates, however, is always open to the criticism that diagnostic errors or inaccuracy of death certification may mask the real disease frequency more in some regions than in others. Recent experimental proof has been obtained, though, strongly supporting the likelihood that there is a real climatic factor in cancer production.

Fig. 18 illustrates the marked suppression of cancer incidence in mice by an environment of tropical warmth. Virgin females of Little's dba strain of cancer mice, with a normal breast carcinoma incidence of over 50 per cent., were subjected to environmental temperatures of 65° F., 91° F. and 70–75° F. With all other factors of existence held constant these mice up to 20 months of age exhibited practically a normal cancer incidence in the room at 65° F., but at 91° F. there occurred a marked suppression. At ordinary laboratory temperatures, 70–75° F., there was almost the same frequency as at 65° F. but with a slight lag in time of appearance. In addition to the breast carcinomas, 11 of these mice also developed tumors of the lymphosarcomatous type in internal organs. Five of these were in the group kept at 65° F., five in the 70–75° F. group and only one in those kept at 91° F.

Tumors not only appeared less frequently and later in the heat, but their rate of growth also was markedly slower. At 91° F. they grew only half as rapidly as at 65° F., taking roughly twice as long to kill the afflicted animal. This same difference has been found for chemically-induced and transplanted tumors in mice except for those of the skin.

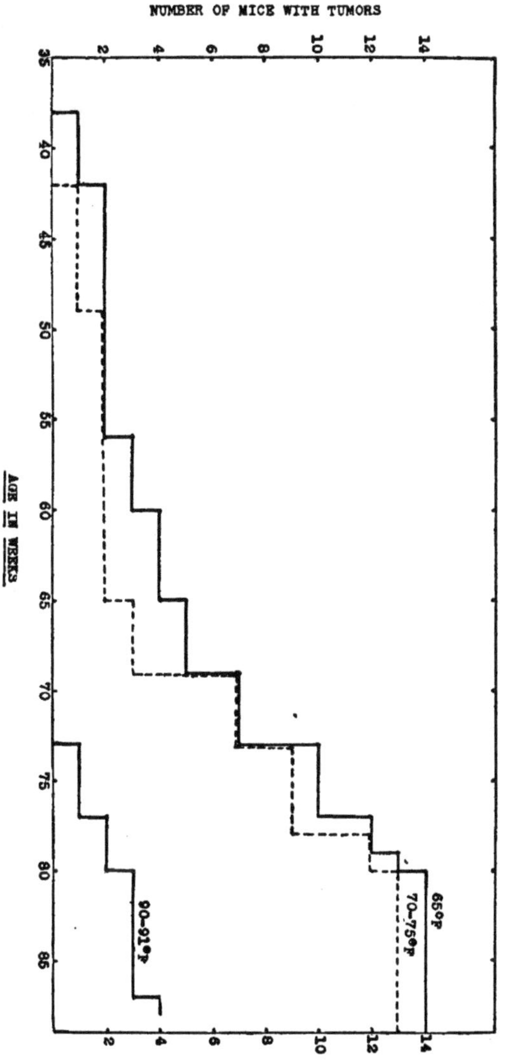

FIG. 18. Environmental temperatures and tumor incidence in mice.

Cancer masses grow most rapidly in the deeper tissues of mice kept in the cold, but in the heat they grow fastest in the skin. This is an important observation, for it would seem to indicate richness of blood supply to be a dominant factor. At 65° F. the deeper tissues need the richer blood supply to support their higher level of metabolism, while at 91° F. the difficulty of heat dissipation calls for most active circulation through the cutaneous capillaries. If the environmental temperature be raised sufficiently to produce fever in the mice and an elevation in general metabolism, then tumors of all regions grow more rapidly than in the cold.

The higher occurrence rates for skin cancers in people living in warmer climates would thus seem to be due not to greater actinic irritation from the tropical sunlight, as has been supposed, but more probably to the richer cutaneous blood supply for heat-loss purposes, and in regions of more active stimulation of the general metabolism the higher incidence of internal tumors would seem probably related to the higher combustion rate and richer blood supply in the deeper tissues.

Leukemia

Leukemia sometimes has been considered a form of neoplasia, so it is interesting to note that four tumor-free mice in the group kept at 65° F. showed post mortem evidences strongly suggestive of leukemia. Fig. 19 also shows the same band of high leukemia death rates across middle temperate latitudes of North America that was found for cancer and the metabolic diseases. All in all, it does seem that the degenerative, neoplastic and metabolic diseases are closely bound up in some way with general tissue combustion level and ease of body heat loss. The therapeutic implications of this relationship are many and varied, but their consideration will be taken up on a later page.

Infectious Diseases

As shown on an earlier page, resistance to infection and ability to produce immune bodies seem closely linked to tissue combustion rate in warm-blooded animals. Difficulty in heat loss, enforcing a lowering in tissue heat production, causes a sharp decline in ability to fight infection. This has been shown to be as true for several infectious diseases of man as for experimental infections in laboratory animals. Thus one factor of climate becomes of major importance in infectious diseases. There is, however, a second climatic factor of equally great importance. Cyclonic storminess, with the atmospheric changes that accompany passage over

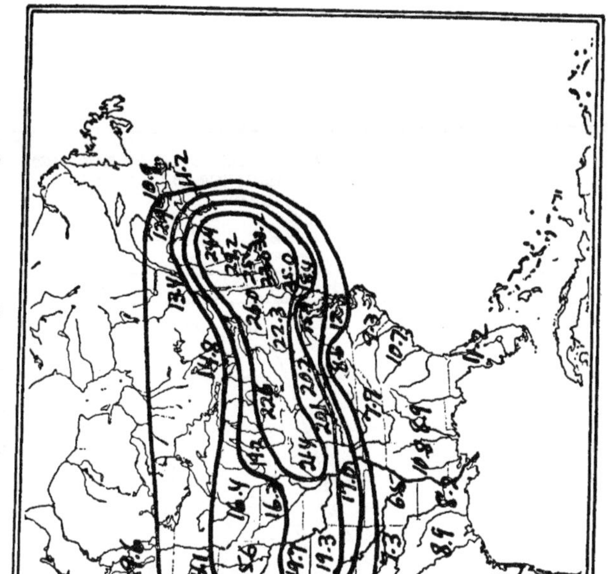

FIG. 19. Leukemia deaths per 100,000 population. Rural, white race only — annual average (1931–5).

a given region of successive "highs" and "lows", seems in some, as yet unknown, manner related to the initiation of infectious disease attacks. Respiratory and rheumatic infections are, perhaps, most closely involved in this type of climatic effect, but it also influences such other infectious attacks as acute appendicitis and puerperal septicemia.

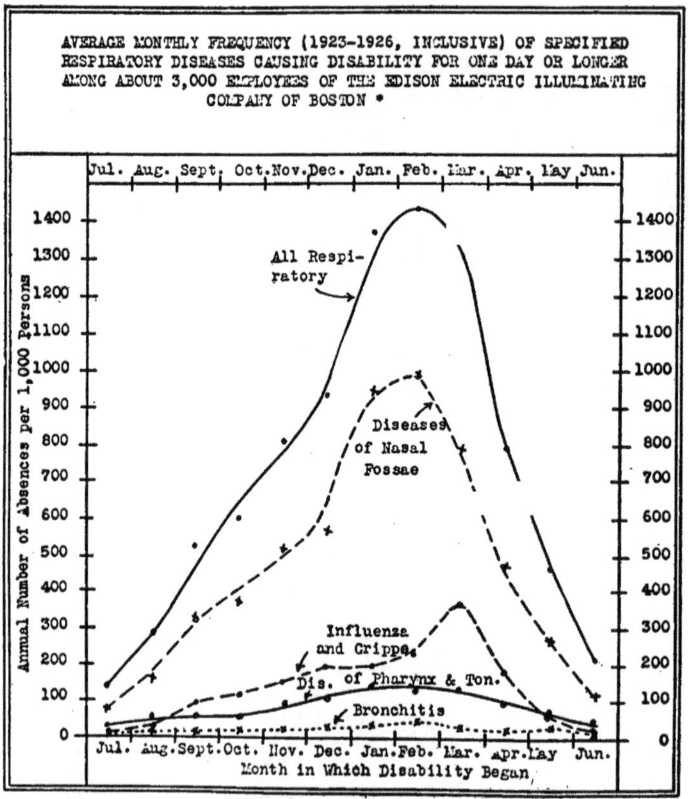

About twenty per cent of the total number of persons included in this record were women.

FIG. 20. Seasonal variations in respiratory illness.

Fig. 20 illustrates the striking degree to which respiratory infections are associated with winter cold and storminess in north temperate latitudes. Life hazards of all sorts reach a peak at this season, for to the infectious dangers of the more violent storminess is added the greater stress of an increased metabolic load. In southern hemisphere lands winter brings much less of an increase in life's hazards, for there storminess is least during mid-winter cold. The increase in mortality from respiratory infections in the United States, from summer low to mid-winter high, is almost three times as great as it is in similar latitudes of Australia. And in the United States unusually stormy winters are accompanied by much greater frequency of respiratory illness and death than are those of lesser atmospheric turbulence. Hospital admissions for acute rheumatic fever at Cincinnati show a similar parallelism with seasonal changes in storminess.

This relationship of storminess to infections is just as evident on a regional as on a seasonal basis. *Acute respiratory infections* and *acute rheumatic fever* are predominantly diseases of stormy regions, being worst in the middle temperate belt of cyclonic storms and least troublesome in calm tropical warmth. Respiratory disease in the tropics becomes a real problem only in those regions afflicted with cyclonic storms of the typhoon or hurricane type. Such regions include most of the Philippine Islands and the eastern Asiatic coast up to Japan, those parts of India around the Bay of Bengal, most of the West Indies and nearby eastern seaboard of North America and to a lesser degree the southwestern coastal region of Mexico. Low pressure storm centers passing over these regions seem to bring much the same respiratory disease problems as are faced by people living in the temperate zone storm belts. They do not have the body chilling from sudden temperature change, such as afflicts people of stormy temperate regions, but the pressure changes alone seem capable of initiating the infectious attacks. Careful physiological studies are badly needed in this field of pressure-change effects, particularly as regards disturbances in tissue water balance. Present knowledge in this field is extremely sketchy and inadequate.

In order to give a general appreciation of the storm problem over North America, there is shown in Figs. 21 and 22 the course followed by anti-cyclonic high-pressure centers affecting the United States during the four-year period, 1926–29. Each such major "high" center affects an area 1,500 to 2,000 miles in diameter, as it sweeps across the continent. From these figures one may get some idea of the relative differences in storm effects man faces in different parts of the continent during the winter and the total reduction in storminess that comes with summer warmth. In the summer storm centers cross the continent less frequently, travel more slowly and are accompanied by less abrupt and less extensive atmospheric changes. At no time of the year do major storm centers cross the southwestern part of the United States or the highland regions of Mexico. This non-stormy zone expands northeastward during

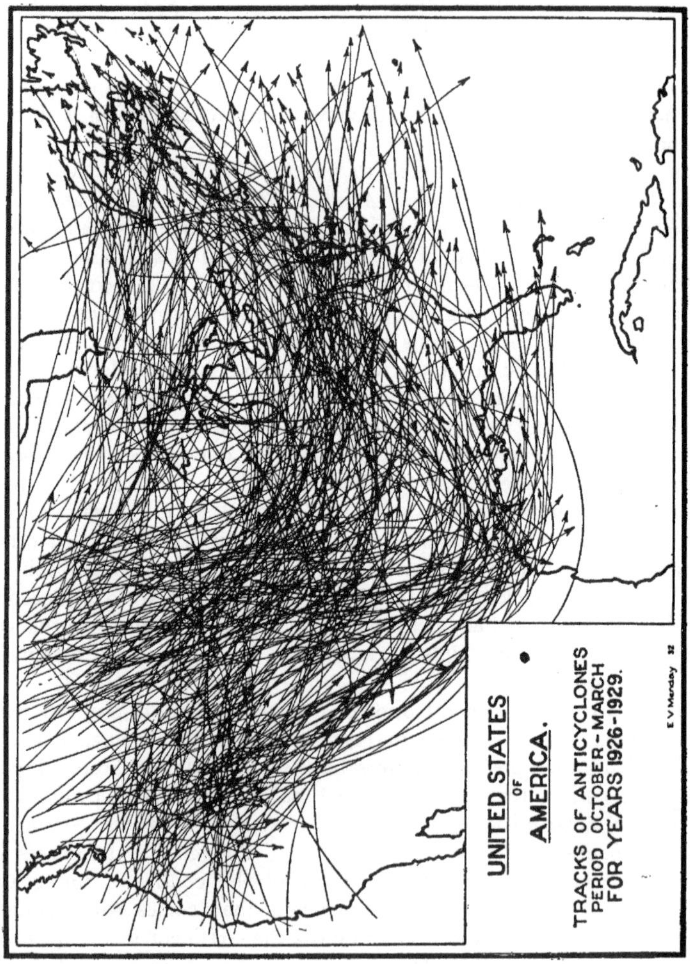

FIG. 21. American storm tracks, anticyclones, winter.

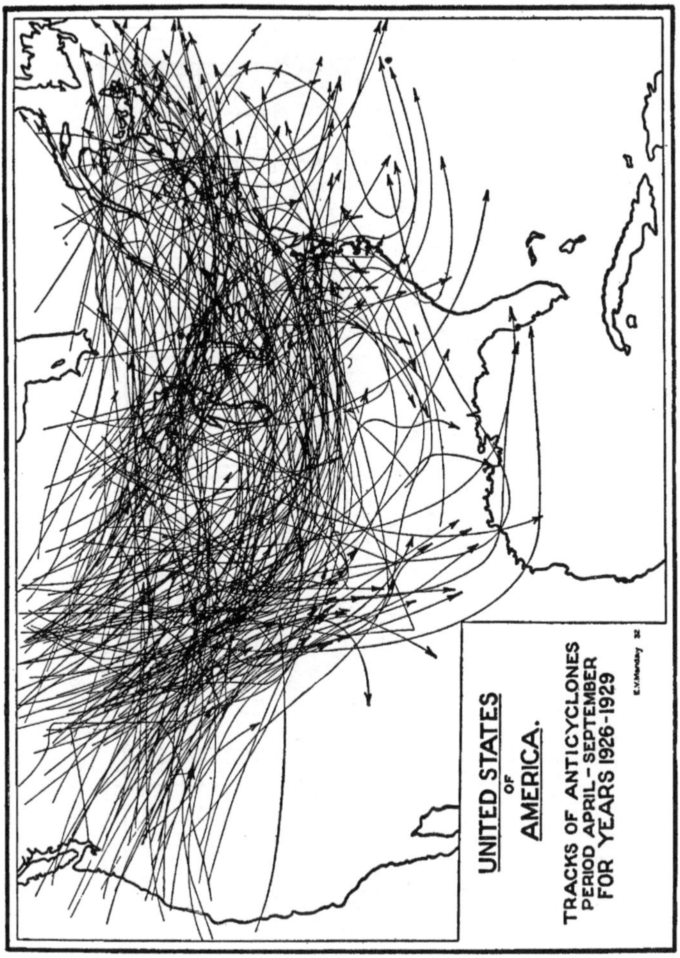

Fig. 22. American storm tracks, anticyclones, summer.

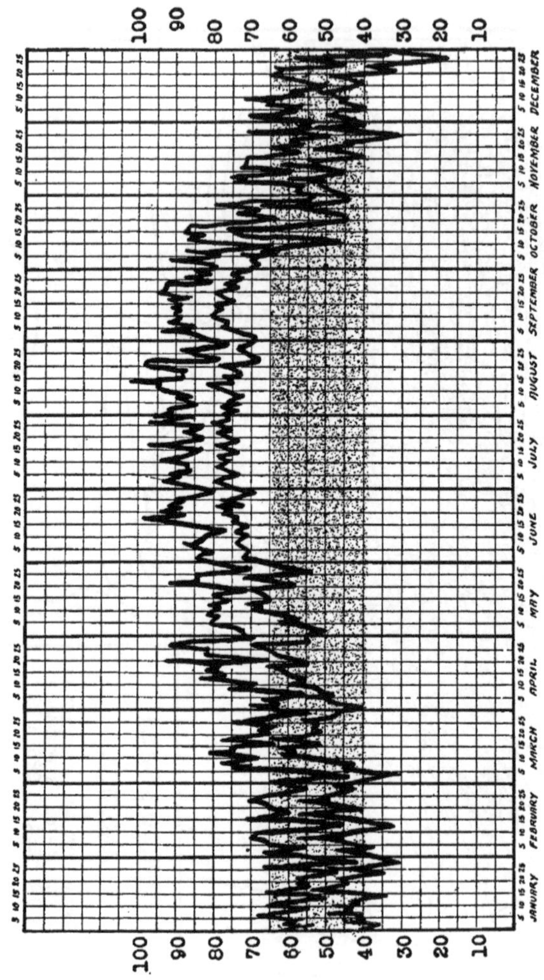

FIG. 23. Graph of daily maximum and minimum temperatures, Charleston, S. C., 1925.

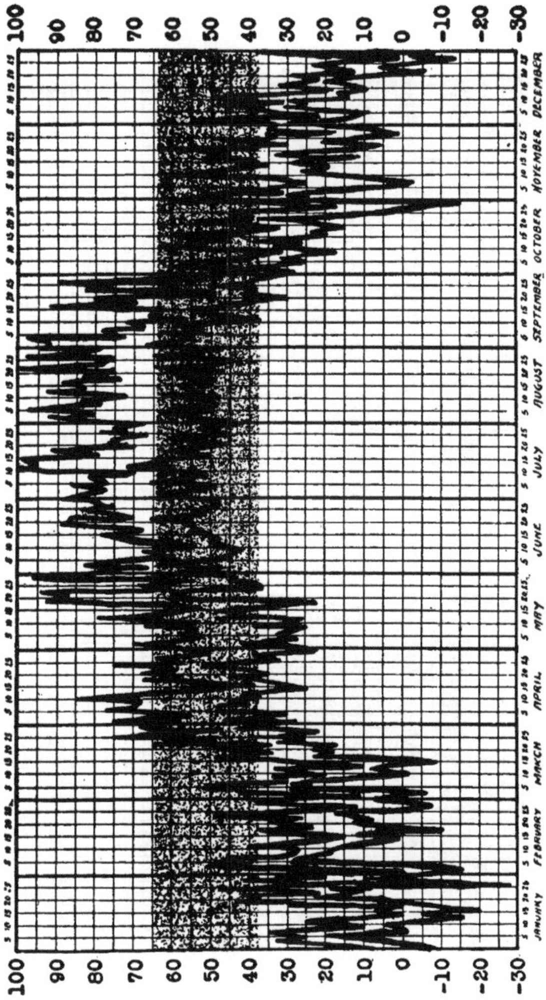

FIG. 24. Graph of daily maximum and minimum temperatures, Bismarck, 1925.

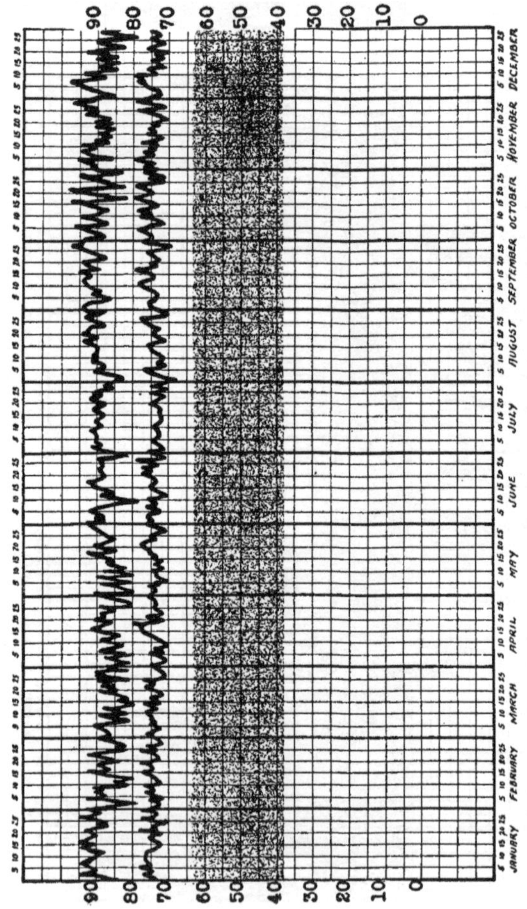

FIG. 25. Graph of daily maximum and minimum temperatures, Manaos, Brazil, 1914.

summer warmth, and at this season people of the Old South are left with the stagnant, moist heat typical of tropical regions. These two storm maps deserve considerable study, for from them can be obtained much of the storm-health story. Figs. 23 and 24, depicting the daily tempera-

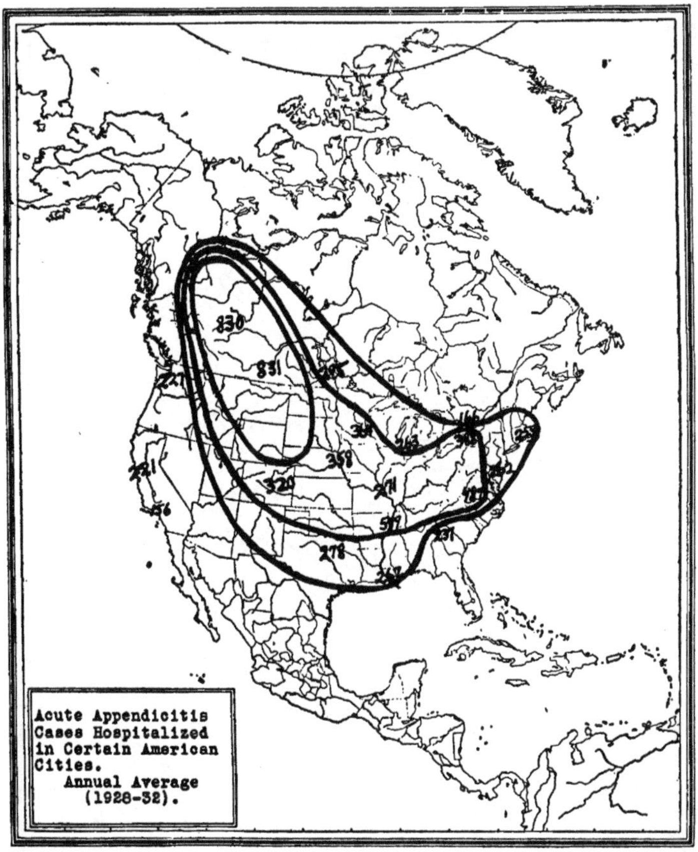

FIG. 26. Acute appendicitis cases hospitalized in certain American cities, annual average, (1928–32).

ture changes through the year at Charleston and at Bismarck, give striking emphasis to the differences in atmospheric change that these storm centers bring to the various regions over which they pass. Fig. 25 shows, for contrast, the daily temperature behavior in a non-stormy tropical region with its endless monotony of successive days of depressive moist heat.

It is in the stormy winter season and in the stormy regions of the earth that respiratory and rheumatic infections most severely afflict man-

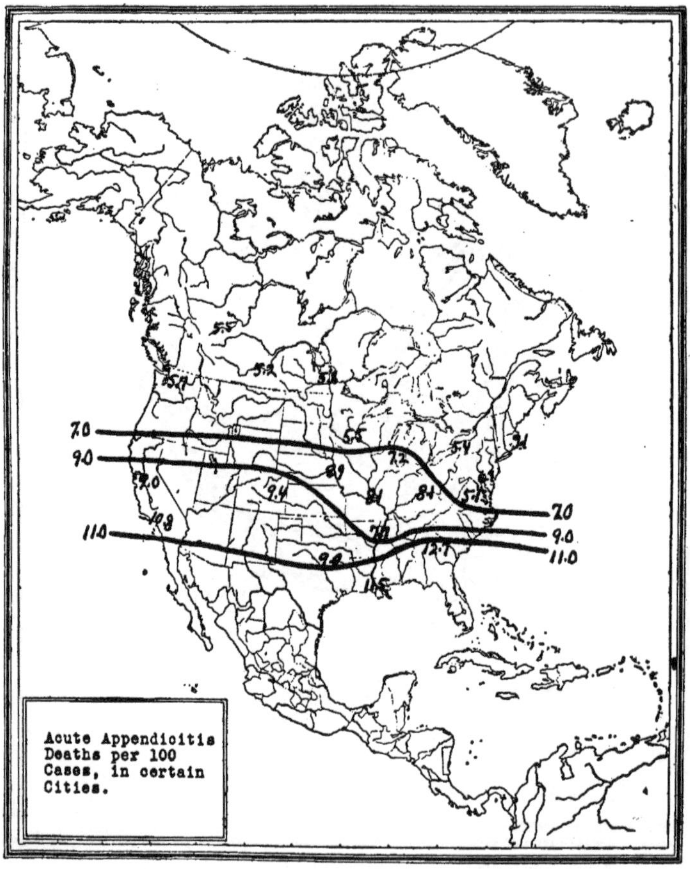

FIG. 27. Acute appendicitis deaths per 100 cases in certain cities.

kind. Benefits of migration of individuals from such regions to non-stormy areas will be discussed in the next section which deals in some detail with climatic therapy in relation to various disease conditions from which man suffers.

Acute Appendicitis

Acute appendicitis statistics, obtained in a limited survey of 25 American cities[12], illustrate well the possible relationships that might be found between climatic characteristics and infectious diseases, if morbidity statistics were more generally available. Fig. 26 hints strongly at a storm distribution of the acute appendicitis attacks with highest rates down the western plains along the major storm pathway from the Canadian Northwest. It is in this area that appendicitis becomes a rapidly fulminating disease with quick progress to perforation and spreading peritonitis, if not promptly operated upon. Nowhere else in temperate regions is it so frequent or severe. Only in the worst storm-ridden parts of the Philippines and West Indies does it compare in frequency of attacks with this central trough of North America. In non-stormy regions, either tropical or temperate, it is a much less virulent and less frequent disease. Its relationship to storminess can be shown at any given point by its tendency to occur as waves or epidemics of attacks with the approach or passing of each low-pressure center and by the sharp reduction in attack frequency as high pressure areas come along.

Regional differences in ability to survive such infectious attacks are well illustrated in Fig. 27, showing the steady fall in fatality rate per 100 attacks from the Gulf States northward. Here it is the greater ease of body heat loss and more active tissue combustion in the north that brings on better resistance to the infectious attacks. The fatality rate mounts with summer heat even in those cooler latitudes where general resistance to infection is highest.

Acute Nephritis

Acute nephritis is another infectious disease in which clear climatic relationships can be demonstrated. In both Europe and America (Figs. 28 and 29) it causes fewest deaths in regions of highest climatic stimulation, while towards either tropical warmth or polar cold its death rate rises. In the depressing moist heat of tropical lowlands it becomes a really important cause of death.

Heat Stroke, Heat Exhaustion and Heat Cramps

In addition to the profound effects upon tissue combustion rate and body functions exerted by moderate difficulties in heat dissipation, there are also more acute disturbances brought by excessively high environmental temperatures. Such disturbances are predominantly problems of human populations living in the middle temperate latitudes. This is true

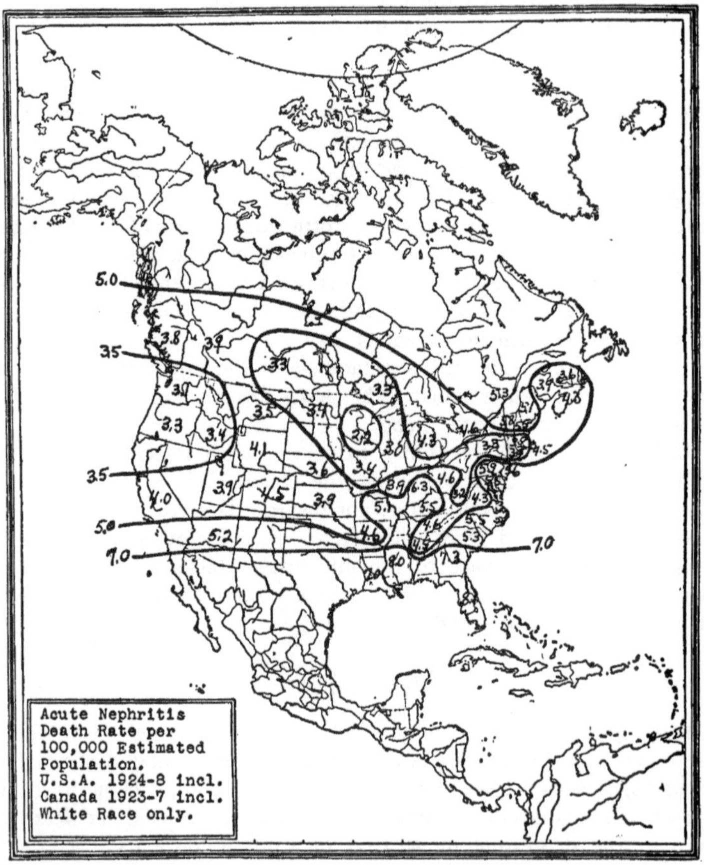

FIG. 28. Acute nephritis death rate per 100,000 estimated population, U. S. A. 1924–8 incl., Canada 1923–7 incl., white race only.

for two reasons, both of which are involved in an explanation of the physiology of these excessive heat effects.

The first reason for greatest prevalence of acute heat effects in tem-

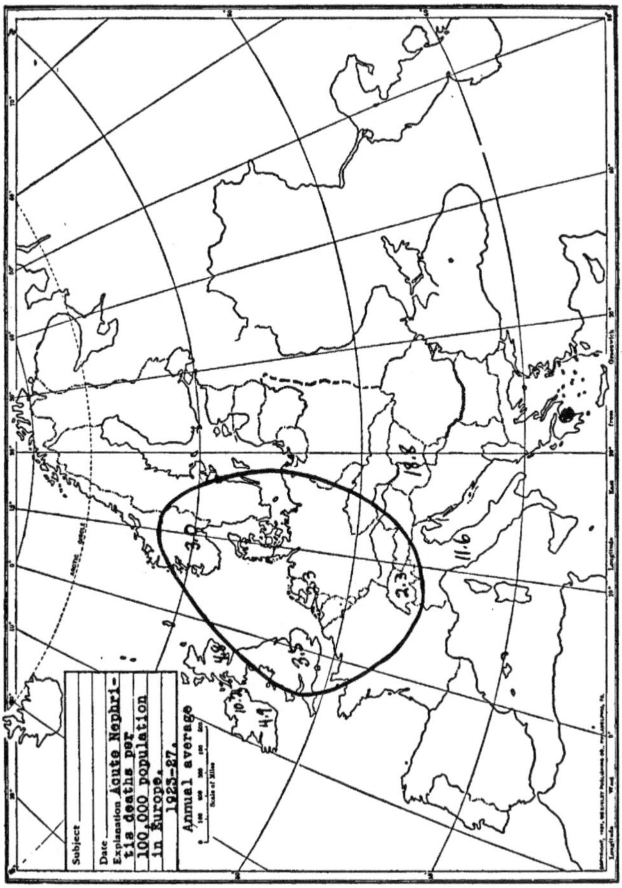

Fig. 29. Acute nephritis deaths per 100,000 population in Europe, 1923–27 annual average.

perate regions is that there man's own internal heat production is highest and his necessity for rapid heat dissipation greatest. Animal studies[21] under controlled conditions have provided a satisfactory explanation for heat sensitivity in man. Either animals or men adapted for weeks or months to cool surroundings develop a high combustion rate, and this proves embarrassing when sudden difficulty in heat loss is encountered. In regions afflicted with depressing tropical moist heat these acute heat effects are uncommon. People residing there have adapted themselves to a lower rate of internal heat production, and acute effects are seldom seen except in newcomers from cooler regions. It is in the more energetic population masses of middle temperate latitudes that acute heat effects occur in greatest profusion. Severe heat waves of summer come upon these regions suddenly, and sometimes kill thousands of people before their body heat production can be brought down within their capacity for dissipation under the difficult conditions suddenly prevailing. Particularly prone to this embarrassment from the sudden heat are the less resilient sclerotic patients and those of limited cardiac capacity. Increased peripheral circulation to facilitate the loss of internal heat throws a greater burden upon the heart, hence the heat wave dangers for those with heart trouble.

Animal and human studies have shown that 10 days to 2 weeks are required for any considerable subsidence of basic internal combustion in response to external heat. Population masses demonstrate this delay in adaptation by being able to stand considerably more severe heat in August than could be safely borne in June or early July. In fact, most heat stroke epidemics occur in early July rather than in the hotter weather of August. But if a severe July heat wave were to be inflicted upon these same populations at the height of their winter activity, its effects would be truly devastating, perhaps as much so as would a North Dakota winter, if suddenly inflicted upon the people of Manila or Singapore or Calcutta. It is, then, the prevailing internal heat production rate of man that largely determines his sensitivity to acute heat effects when faced suddenly with severe external warmth.

The second factor responsible for the greater prevalence of acute heat effects in temperate latitudes is that most severe heat actually occurs there. Dry bulb temperatures of over 100° F. are rare in tropical regions except in desert areas, while temperatures above this level are not unusual during severe summer heat waves as far north as the prairie provinces of Canada. Heat deaths and prostration occur mostly in urban and desert regions and for somewhat similar regions. With the dense vegetation of tropical lowlands, and less so in rural temperate areas, the physical surroundings of man have a high water content. Green foliage is largely water, and the high specific heat capacity of water enables it to absorb large amounts of radiant heat from the daytime sun with little rise in temperature. Baked earth, desert sands and urban building or paving materials have a very low specific heat capacity and suffer a marked temperature rise under the radiant heat load from the sun. In desert regions this daytime heat is quickly re-radiated off into space soon after sundown, but in built-up urban areas it tends to be trapped within buildings and to cause progressively higher temperatures as the heat wave persists day after day. Building construction in tropical cities takes account of this danger and provides for ample air currents to carry away any such daytime heat that gains access, but in temperate zone cities winter cold prohibits this open type of construction, and the trapping of daytime radiant heat makes the heat problem for urban dwellers worse with each added day of summer heat wave.

The exact mechanism of *heat stroke* production is not understood. Patients in a hypertherm chamber develop artificial fever but with free perspiration and without the other evidences of heat stroke. In typical heat stroke, on the other hand, cessation of perspiration seems to be one of the very early symptoms of trouble. Sufficiently severe heat will kill anyone, normal and abnormal alike, but it may well be that the previously normal individual would continue free perspiration to the end, while the abnormally heat sensitive person is so because his sweating mechanism quickly becomes deranged. Chief difficulty in studying this problem is the lack of experimental animals with a sweating mechanism at all similar to that of man. Artificial fever treatments on man have provided some valuable evidence, but even this has not been well utilized to elucidate the heat stroke mechanism. Patients who fail to perspire freely under such treatment are removed quickly as poor risks for fever therapy.

Heat exhaustion, while still a direct result of difficulty in dissipation of body heat, differs sharply from heat stroke. In the latter there is fever and delirium with full bounding pulse and elevated blood pressure, while the skin is flushed and dry. Immediately important in therapy is rapid heat removal by the best means at hand. Heat exhaustion, on the other hand, usually is characterized by subnormal body temperature, cold, pale, clammy skin, low blood pressure and a state of circulatory shock. In addition there are other symptoms of acute adrenal insufficiency, hypertonicity of the gastroenteric tract with nausea, vomiting, diarrhea, sphincter spasm and painful peristalsis. Here immediate treatment should be directed toward raising the body temperature to normal, improving the tone of the vascular system and allaying hyperactivity in the digestive musculature.

It is thus apparent that heat stroke and heat exhaustion represent radically different body responses to external warmth. Correct diagnosis is important because of the sharp difference in type of treatment indicated. Here again we are faced by a lack of knowledge as to why one individual develops the dynamic hyperpyrexia response and another the hypothermic shock reaction. Unfortunately, one experience with either type of excessive heat reaction predisposes the patient to subsequent attacks and to troublesome prodromal symptoms with external heat of relatively low order. So far no means has been discovered for overcoming this increased sensitivity induced by a preceding heat attack. Careful avoidance of exposure for the next several years remains the patient's only safe course to follow.

There exists a likely possibility that pantothenic acid deficiency may be a factor in the production of heat exhaustion. The symptoms and anatomical findings in heat exhaustion point to the adrenal cortex as the affected tissue responsible for the exhaustion state. Adrenal hemorrhage in man gives much the same clinical picture, except that it is in more acute form. In experimental animals, exposed to heat in the author's laboratory, adrenal hemorrhages were produced in few instances, but intense adrenal congestion was encountered frequently. Recent work[22, 23] has shown that such congestion and hemorrhagic necrosis of the adrenals is pathognomonic of pantothenic acid deficiency in animals, while such deficiency signs have been found much more easily produced in animals kept at high temperatures in the author's laboratory. The possibility does, therefore, exist that heat exhaustion with its attendant symptoms of adrenal failure may be based upon a pantothenic acid deficiency, and that the administration of this material would provide a useful therapeutic aid in the treatment of such exhaustion. The severe heat of coming summers will give an opportunity for trial of such therapy. Thiamine therapy, 5–10 mgm. daily, also seems to make for better heat resistance.

Heat cramps in the skeletal muscles bear little relation either to heat stroke or heat exhaustion. They are due primarily to excessive salt loss during profuse and prolonged perspiration without adequate salt intake. Relief is obtained readily by adding ordinary table salt to the drinking water or by taking it in any other convenient form. Sometimes a heat exhaustion patient will be suffering also from skeletal muscle cramps, but usually they are not associated. Laborers in desert heat and furnace rooms are particularly prone to heat cramps because of their excessive perspiration and rapid salt loss.

Sickness and Health Tides

An important point of general medical interest arises from the close association between temperature level and storminess on the one hand and infectious illnesses and metabolic breakdown on the other as set forth in the preceding pages. Definite health tides have been found[24] to accompany the periods of warmth and calm that come over the world every few years. At these times earth temperatures rise, and temperate zone storminess lessens. Winter stress is reduced greatly and summer heat increases. Human energy seems to decline during such years of warmth, for business activity falls off, and the economic machine tends to idle along until cold and storms again return. This relationship between earth weather and economic activity seems to be a true finding. More striking from a medical point of view, however, is the health improvement, which regularly comes with these years of warmth and lessened economic activity. Huntington[25] first pointed out this association between improved health and hard times, but Huntington's explanation of the relationship is no longer tenable.

Sickness and death rates do decline, and calls for medical service are lessened during years of warmth and lessened storminess, and, as falling temperatures bring increased mass energy and returning prosperity, we regularly see again a rising ill-health tide. These tides in energy and health are similar to the seasonal ones which occur in temperate regions, where winter cold and storms regularly bring greater energy but also bring higher sickness rates and death rates. Even heart failures, non-infectious, non-luetic, reflect in their course the lessened stress of these warmer years.

While there is little we can do about these tides in weather and health, it is well to appreciate their presence and significance. Periods of economic depression commonly are associated with an expectation of deterioration in health and general nutrition of the population. Even a regular repetition of health improvement in hard times, instead of health deterioration, has failed to shake the popular expectation. It is time the medical profession awakened to the fact that general health is best in those very years when the public is willing to spend least for medical services. It is not, however, that the services of the medical profession constitute a health handicap, but that powerful extraneous forces are at work altering the basic environmental factors of existence. Careful analysis of the action of these tidal forces on health has helped us toward a much clearer understanding of how environmental factors produce their effects.

Climatic Therapy

Two cardinal features of climatic effects must be kept in mind when climatic therapy is being considered. Probably of greatest importance to man in a given region is the mean temperature level and the ease with which he can get rid of his waste heat of cellular combustion. Proper ease of heat loss gives to human health a more dynamic and positive character, leading to rapid growth, early maturity, high fertility, increased resistance to infection and abundant energy for thought and action, but with the heightened cellular combustion rate necessary to support this more dynamic existence go evidences of stress and breakdown in the body machinery. Metabolic and degenerative diseases form the most troublesome health problems only in those regions where climatic stimulation is high.

With the slower combustion rate, necessitated by tropical difficulties in heat loss, existence becomes more vegetative and passive, growth and development slow down, and a sharp decline in resistance to infection allows infectious diseases to become predominant causes of death. Factors outside of man himself also contribute largely to the infectious disease problem in tropical warmth, especially better temperature conditions for the growth of bacteria and parasites outside the body and the greater abundance of insect vectors. Other important factors, while not having to do directly with lowered tissue resistance, do depend upon man's lowered combustion rate and lack of energy for thought and for work accomplishment. The low level of personal and public hygiene usually existing among tropical peoples, unless health measures are initiated and enforced by outsiders from more energizing climates, most likely is based upon the debilitating effects of the tropical warmth upon man himself. The combination of all these internal and external effects of climate makes the infectious disease problem the major one for tropical residents. People of warmer regions, who survive infectious hazards to reach more advanced ages, do so with much less evidence of metabolic stress than is seen in similar age groups of more stimulating regions. Metabolic and degenerative diseases, diabetes, toxic goiter, pernicious anemia, arteriosclerosis, cancer, are all much less prevalent in Gulf State populations than in the same age groups in middle temperate latitudes of America. Similar latitude differences are to be found in Europe.

The second climatic factor to be considered in any intelligent effort to use climatic therapy is the effect of storminess or sudden weather change. Although we as yet know little about the mechanism of its effects, weather change does seem to be an important factor in the initiation of many types of infectious attacks, particularly those of respiratory and rheumatic types. Since respiratory and rheumatic ailments bulk so large as ill health factors in stormy regions, it is necessary that this storminess factor be given proper consideration.

These are the general principles to be borne in mind when considering climatic therapy for individual cases. Physicians should help the patient come to a decision regarding permanent change of residence. For most adult people such re-location entails major economic difficulties, which tend to tie the individual to his present place of abode. It is the physician's duty, then, to help him balance the anticipated health benefits against the deterring economic factors. For younger patients not yet tied down, the problem is much more simple. But in every case it is for the physician to point out the anticipated health hazards and impairments in body function that may, reasonably, be expected from continuing on in the unfavorable environment and to detail the health advantages of the change. Each case will offer an entirely different set of difficulties and problems to be considered. And always in these considerations the physician should take an active and sympathetic part as family advisor. Let us now take up in some detail the facts upon which his advice should be based in various disease states.

Metabolic Diseases

Fairly clear indications of benefit from climatic therapy exist in the diseases of metabolic exhaustion or over-stimulation. *Diabetes* as a disease is most frequent and most severe in the energizing middle temperate regions where metabolic stress is greatest. There severe ketosis and coma are of easy occurrence and constitute major hazards for these patients. The disease exists in sub-tropical and tropical lands but as a mild, non-troublesome glycosuria with little or no tendency to severe ketosis. Mild dietary regulation usually suffices for the needed degree of control. Vascular troubles and peripheral gangrene bother diabetic patients much more in the cooler regions, where arteriosclerotic troubles are more common, and winter cold further intensifies this hazard of the disease. It seems clear, therefore, that diabetic patients should be advised of the milder course taken by their disease in warmer regions. Permanent migration into subtropical warmth should be advised whenever it is economically possible for the patient. The strong tendency of the disease to appear in children of diabetic parents makes such migration particularly advisable where there are offspring to be considered.

Migration for diabetics should consider not only transfer to subtropical warmth but also escape from cyclonic storminess. Acute infectious attacks form the most frequent cause for ketosis onset in these patients, and cyclonic storm changes seem to be a potent factor in the initiation of the infections. Migration should therefore be to a non-stormy and warm region. In North America that would mean the Southwest within 200 miles of the Mexican border from El Paso to the Pacific coast. Altitudes above 5,000 feet should be avoided because of the relief from the summer heat such elevation brings and the fair degree of metabolic stimulation brought by the wide diurnal changes in temperature. Florida and the Gulf Coast offer more depressing warmth than does the Southwest, due to the higher humidity of the air, but winter storminess and the attendant respiratory infection problem there presents a certain degree of handicap, except in the southernmost parts of Florida and Texas.

European diabetics, mostly to be found living in west central portions of the continent, would find their disease much less troublesome and easier of control, if they took up residence in some Mediterranean location. In Australia benefit would follow northward migration to more tropical portions of the continent. In Argentina similar northward migration would benefit those diabetics from the southern cool half of the country, where the disease is more frequent and troublesome.

Seasonal migration away from winter cold and storms is advisable for those diabetics who cannot make a permanent change of residence, but in such seasonal migration the dangers of too early return in the spring should always be kept clearly in mind. This point will be discussed more fully in considering respiratory disease problems.

Toxic Goiter and Hyperthyroid States

Toxic goiter and other *hyperthyroid* types of patients, except those with definite nodular goiter, benefit greatly from migration into the depressing warmth of the tropics or subtropics. Even the brief summer heat of northern latitudes tends to quiet down the symptoms resulting from a hyperactive thyroid. Definite microscopic evidence of change toward the resting type of secreting cell has been shown to result from even a few weeks' exposure of experimental animals to external warmth. Hyperthyroid patients should not expose themselves too suddenly to external heat, however, for their high rate of heat production renders them unduly susceptible to thermic fever. Application of gradually increasing external warmth gives best results. Since storminess makes little difference to these patients, and a maximal depression of internal combustion rate is desired, migration should be to regions where heat and high humidity coincide. In America that would mean the Gulf Coast, well south in Florida or Texas for the winter season. Artificial, moist warmth, if consistently and properly applied, should be just as effective in the patient's own home region, but it would necessitate an indoor existence for a considerable period at high temperatures and high humidity, 90° F. and 70 per cent. relative humidity or thereabouts.

Pernicious Anemia

Pernicious anemia likewise pursues a milder course in tropical warmth, while leukemia is almost unknown in tropical and subtropical warmth except in migrants from temperate climates. There are as yet no data available, however, regarding the benefits of climatic therapy in these conditions. For those, who can move, either seasonal or permanent migration to avoid winter cold would seem advisable. As with diabetes and toxic goiter regions of moist heat should be chosen so as to achieve the maximum of metabolic suppression and reduction in load on the hemopoietic system.

Arteriosclerosis, Hypertension and Heart Failure

Arteriosclerotic, *hypertensive* and *heart failure* patients present the clearest likelihood of benefit from climatic therapy. Blood pressures in either normal or hypertensive individuals show a decided tendency to drop with even the brief summer heat of middle temperate latitudes. This drop usually amounts to about 30 per cent. from the preceding winter level, giving marked relief from hypertensive symptoms during summer and early autumn. Both systolic and diastolic pressures of the author fall about 40 per cent. after a month spent in tropical moist heat or after a prolonged summer heat wave at Cincinnati. These falls in pressure probably are due largely to loss of vascular spasm, but the lowered general combustion rate and lessened load on the circulatory system also may play a considerable part.

Recent studies on the production of malignant hypertension and arteriosclerosis in experimental animals has suggested the possibility that vascular spasm in the renal vessels of man may be an important factor in the sclerosis picture. It may be for this reason that vascular sclerosis and failure become such dominant health threats in the most energizing and stressful climates, and that such welcome relief is brought by even the brief periods of summer heat. Fig. 15 on a preceding page indicated the marked lowering in the incidence of heart failure during summer warmth, and mention also was made of the similar reduction during certain Cincinnati winters when balmy weather largely prevailed. It does seem, therefore, that climatic and seasonal temperature levels constitute a basically important factor in determining vascular stress and likelihood of functional breakdown, and that this fact should receive serious consideration in the handling of patients with a tendency to such vascular troubles.

In this matter of cool climate or winter stress man is doubly handicapped. He not only feels the urge to be more active in cool weather, but each bit of work he does then costs him a greater expenditure of energy than would similar work accomplishment in summer warmth. It has been shown[26] that body working efficiency declines as tissue combustion rate rises, so that the climbing of a given flight of stairs carries a higher metabolic cost in winter cold than it does in summer warmth. Man in cool climates thus is faced both with the urge to be more active and to pay a higher metabolic price for such activity than does the resident of warmer regions. It may well be this combination of stresses that is at the basis of his circulatory failure problem in middle temperate regions.

At any rate it would seem clearly indicated that any individual showing evidences of the effects of such stress should be advised of these factors acting upon him and of the possible benefits of migration to a less energizing climate, and, since respiratory infections constitute a major threat to patients with limited myocardial capacity, these patients should seek particularly for freedom from winter storminess as well as for soothing warmth. Within the United States that would mean southern Florida or the Brownsville region of Texas rather than the non-stormy but slightly more stimulating Southwest. Advice regarding climatic therapy for these patients would be the same as that discussed on a preceding page for diabetics, either in America or in foreign countries, and the same precautions should be observed about returning to cool, stormy latitudes except during the milder summer months. Many people with limited cardiac capacity have died of pneumonia contracted from too early a spring return to a northern home. This danger will be discussed more fully under respiratory disease considerations.

Nervous Disturbances

For *mental* and *nervous breakdown*, *neuresthenia* and related exhaustion states there exist less clear indications for advice regarding climatic therapy. The gray matter of the brain has the highest combustion rate of all body tissues and should be expected to show most marked evidences of stress in populations living under the most stimulating climatic conditions. Such is indeed actually the case, but evidence has not yet accumulated to show whether such patients would be as much benefited by migration to more soothing climates as are the patients with metabolic and hypertensive troubles. Cerebral activity does seem to decline with prolonged external warmth, for psychological testing of college freshmen in lower temperate latitudes gives markedly lower ratings during summer heat than in winter cold, while at higher latitudes the milder summer warmth is without any such depressing effect on mental function. It would, therefore, seem desirable to try climatic sedation in cases of central nervous exhaustion, followed by the mild stimulation of such non-stormy regions as northern New Mexico or Arizona at altitudes of 5,000 to 6,000 feet. Any such climatic therapy should, of course, be accompanied by very restricted use of tobacco or alcohol and complete abstinence from all stimulants of the caffeine type. It seems advisable also to recommend a high intake of the B vitamins, particularly thiamine, during any such effort at restoration of proper cerebral function.

Infectious Diseases

So far as is known, climatic or weather conditions have little to do with the acute contagious diseases of childhood except as the indoor existence of the winter season brings greater crowding and better chance for contagion to spread. However, for respiratory and rheumatic infections climatic environment seems to be a factor of really dominant importance. Sudden stormy changes, particularly those accompanied by sharp temperature drops, initiate the infectious attacks, while the mean temperature levels under which people live largely determine ability of the body to fight the infectious invasion. Thus, rheumatic and respiratory infections occur most frequently in those stormy middle temperate regions where body resistance is highest. This is indeed fortunate, for a North Dakota winter would produce a holocaust of pneumonia deaths if suddenly visited upon a tropical population.

For *sinusitis*, *bronchitis*, *bronchiectasis* and a tendency to *repeated "colds"* climatic therapy offers very definite benefits. This is again fortunate, since only too often these conditions receive little benefit from treatment in the home climate. Epidemics of "colds" and other respiratory infections continue unabated in populations during stormy, middle temperate winters, little affected by all the claims of benefit from vaccine therapy, vitamin administration or general nutritional betterment. For most individuals susceptible to recurrent attacks of these respiratory troubles migration to a non-stormy region offers the only real hope of relief. An occasional patient with chronic bronchitis will be cured by attention to other foci of infection higher up, and a few bronchiectatic patients are helped by lobectomy. Therapy for acute sinusitis is, in the main, beneficial, but after the sinus changes have become chronic, the patient can look forward to more or less permanency of his trouble so long as he continues on in a region afflicted with frequent waves of acute upper respiratory infections. As the years pass, he may expect a spreading of the chronic changes to other nasal accessory cavities and to the bronchial tree.

An important element in this steady progression of involvement is the frequent repetition of acute flare-up with each new respiratory epidemic that comes along or with each body chilling that takes place. Persons with these chronic infections are unduly sensitive to chilling and usually make life uncomfortable for those with whom they must live. High indoor temperatures and freedom from drafts must be maintained for their comfort. Nor is this sensitivity to chilling at all psychic on their part. Degrees of chilling that do not bother normal persons in the least may result in prompt exacerbation of their troubles. For such afflicted individuals to continue living through northern winters usually means much trouble for themselves and discomfort or damage to others, who must inhabit with them the over-heated living quarters and face the sharp contrasts between indoor and outdoor air as they come and go.

Since medical science as yet has no other therapeutic answer, migration out of cold and storms should be seriously considered for such cases. If they cannot migrate, then steps should be taken to protect them from chilling without endangering the welfare of others in the household by over-heating. Warmer clothing, particularly for the extremities, should be the basis of any needed additional protection for the affected individual.

Great benefit will come to the chronically afflicted respiratory disease patient from winter migration out of northern cold and storms or from permanent change of residence to the plateau regions of the Southwest. Wintering in Florida or in the warmth along the Gulf Coast offers less relief because of two storm factors. As shown in Fig. 21, cold waves travel well southward down the Plains States during the winter months, giving the Southern States then almost as great an atmospheric turbulence as is encountered in the North. In addition, tropical low-pressure storms sweeping westward over the West Indies and Caribbean region bring added instability during the earlier winter months. These latter storms cause little temperature change, but their sharp pressure fluctuations seem to bring on many of the same body disturbances that are associated with temperate zone storm changes. Respiratory infections and deaths increase just as much from summer low to winter high in Georgia as they do in New York. Only well south in Florida or in the Brownsville district of Texas is there relative freedom from the northern type of winter storm, but even these regions remain afflicted with those of tropical origin.

Winter migration for relief from respiratory troubles should, therefore, be directed toward the southwest rather than to the south. Moderate elevations within 200 miles of the Mexican border from El Paso west will be found to offer most nearly ideal weather conditions for this purpose. Locations for permanent residence might be selected slightly farther north on account of summer heat but probably not far beyond the northern borders of New Mexico or Arizona. The point should be stressed that migration benefits soon disappear, if the patient returns to northern cold and storms, even though complete subsidence of trouble may have prevailed for a considerable period in the non-stormy climate. For those persons, severely handicapped by recurring respiratory troubles, permanent change of climate is, therefore, strongly advised, since it offers hope for a more normal existence of health and usefulness.

Tuberculosis. — This disease deserves consideration from at least two climatic angles, even though one today so often hears specialists in this field declare that change of climate offers these patients nothing that cannot be had without leaving the home region. The same two principles of climatic effect work in tuberculosis as in other chronic or semi-chronic respiratory infections, and failure to recognize their value only mitigates against the patient's chance for recovery. Acute intercurrent respiratory infections carry serious dangers for people with subacute or active tuberculosis because of their tendency to light up the tuberculosis process, and these acute infections come largely with sudden storm changes in weather. Hence, on this point, the tuberculosis patient reduces his disease hazards greatly by migration to a non-stormy climate. He may receive the same effective nutritional, rest and collapse therapy in all regions, where proper facilities are available, but only in a non-stormy climate may he achieve freedom from recurring acute infections.

The second point deserving emphasis in tuberculosis relates to those patients contracting the disease in regions of debilitating moist heat or to those with quiescent forms of the disease who contemplate any prolonged sojourn in tropical warmth. The marked lowering of tissue resistance to infection in tropical moist heat makes it imperative that patients developing the disease there be transferred at once to a more stimulating climate where a higher tissue combustion rate can be maintained. The most perfect diet cannot secure nutritional betterment in such patients so long as difficulty in body heat loss interferes with its utilization by the tissues. Transfer of these patients from debilitating tropical heat, however, should never be to a region afflicted with storms but rather to a such non-stormy, mildly stimulating climate as is offered at moderate elevations in our Southwest. Patients even with completely quiescent tuberculosis should be advised against any prolonged sojourn in tropical heat, since the sharp lowering of tissue vitality may bring on a re-lighting of the infection.

The dangers of migration into stormy temperate regions after any prolonged stay in tropical or subtropical warmth should be kept in mind always. For a northerner to make a winter visit of a week or two in the warmth of southern Florida entails no health risk, but, if he remains there for several weeks, his lowered combustion rate renders him liable to serious respiratory infection, if he return northward while winter weather still prevails. This applies particularly to the elderly winter migrant to southern warmth. Return to northern homes should be delayed until all danger of winter cold and storms is past. Movement of tropical residents to temperate regions, particularly those patients run down by debilitating disease, should be carried out during summer warmth and with careful protection against weather changes during the entire first winter.

Rheumatic Infections. — Rheumatic infections seem very closely similar to those of the respiratory system in their relationship to storminess and weather change. This similarity may well be more than coincidental, for several investigators have felt that rheumatic infections are probably secondary to those of the respiratory system. Considerable ground for this belief is provided by the great frequency with which acute rheumatic fever attacks accompany or follow those of the upper respiratory passages. Whether this relationship be real or only seemingly apparent, the strong tendency of rheumatic attacks to flare up in stormy seasons makes it imperative that these patients be protected as far as possible from weather changes. Unfortunately they seem most sensitive to barometric pressure fluctuations, against which modern housing provides no protection. Body chilling, to which they are also sensitive, is as bad for them as it is for patients with chronic upper respiratory infections.

The hazards of an active existence in stormy regions, especially during winter cold, are, therefore, even greater for patients with rheumatic infections than for those with respiratory troubles. Involvement of the heart with limitation of cardiac functional capacity by valvular lesions further complicates their winter problem. This phase of the problem was discussed in connection with sclerotic heart failure. The indications for migration of rheumatic patients to a non-stormy climate are, therefore, quite evident and emphatic. As with the respiratory infections migration should be to the Southwest rather than the South. Transportation of rheumatic patients to Florida or Puerto Rico has brought rather disappointing results, while in southern Arizona and New Mexico much more complete quiescence of the disease has been obtained. The reason for the better results in the southwest probably lies in the year-round lack of storms there as contrasted to a winter storminess from Texas eastward almost as great as afflicts the northern states.

Migration for patients with rheumatic infections should be permanent, if possible, since recrudescence is likely to follow return to northern cold and storms. If only winter migration is possible, then that should even more certainly be to the Southwest, since little storm relief will be experienced in the Gulf States at that season. For every patient developing definite rheumatic infection migration to a less stormy climate should be considered. This is particularly true with the young in whom heart lesions are so likely to develop as the infection continues through the months.

Regions of choice for migration of rheumatic patients should be to within 200 miles of the Mexican border anywhere west of El Paso. Acute rheumatic fever attacks and deaths are relatively high in frequency throughout the mountain and plateau states even as far south as the northern parts of New Mexico and Arizona[27]. Return visits of migrants to former home regions should be made during summer months when storm turbulence is at a minimum.

Leprosy. — Leprosy is another infectious disease markedly influenced by climatic differences in resistance to infection[28]. It exists as a terrible human scourge only in those tropical lowlands shown in Fig. 10 as having the lowest order of climatic stimulation. In more stimulating regions it ceases to be an active disease and becomes practically non-communicable. In tropical, moist heat it spreads easily and involves considerable percentages of population masses in some areas, while there was practically no spread from 200 cases imported into the stimulating Minnesota-Dakota region during the 19th century migration from Scandinavia. Only during the world warmth of the Dark Age centuries did leprosy become really active in temperate zone countries. In view of the disease behavior over the earth, it would seem wise to segregate patients afflicted with the disease in climatic regions where their own ability to fight the infection will be highest rather than to follow the custom now prevailing of segregation where the disease itself is worst. In America that would mean moving the National Leprosarium from Louisiana to North Dakota. In any such move great care would need to be exercised during the first winter to protect the patients against the unaccustomed vigors of northern winter, for they would be highly susceptible to respiratory infections until they had resided for some time in the more invigorating climate. This principle already is being put into practice to some degree in Australia, but the idea seems worthy of much more widespread application. Altitude stimulation in tropical highlands is never far removed from the lowland areas of debilitating moist heat.

Air Conditioning

It cannot yet be said just how far man will be able to go in overcoming natural climatic or weather effects by interior conditioning methods. It has been shown quite clearly that the biological let-down of summer warmth can be eliminated by adequate artificial cooling to facilitate body heat loss. Productivity and physical vigor of tropical workers increases in proportion as the temperature of their working environment is lowered, but if such summer cooling is done by cooling and dehumidification of the indoor air, then the sharp contrast faced by people entering and leaving such conditioned quarters tends to raise somewhat the same problems that are brought by the outdoor unstable weather conditions of winter storminess.

Indoor winter heating, if accomplished through air warming, also provides sharp contrast between indoor and outdoor air and so increases whatever health dangers reside in sudden atmospheric changes. Americans with their careful maintenance of stable indoor temperatures far above outside levels seem only to have accentuated their respiratory disease problems. Perhaps the British custom of lower indoor winter temperatures is after all better than what they have termed our over-heating.

If proper control of body heat loss to prevent winter chilling or summer depression is to be accomplished without producing contrasts between indoor and outdoor air, then it will have to be done through radiant channels. Very recent studies[29] have shown that radiant conditioning is indeed feasible both for winter heating and summer cooling. Certain difficulties remain to be overcome, but the great advantages of this type of conditioning almost certainly will bring it quickly to the fore. If heat-reflective wall coverings be used, then individuals in a room can be made comfortable in either winter cold or summer heat through radiant channels alone without regard to air temperatures or humidity. Radiant heating in the winter is easily accomplished. Adequate removal of body heat through radiant channels for summer cooling is more difficult but has operated satisfactorily under both experimental and field conditions.

Present air conditioning has brought remarkable therapeutic benefits to one class of human sufferers, the sensitization or asthma patients. To many complete relief has come by thorough filtering and condition of their indoor atmosphere, but this relief does not extend beyond the conditioned space.

Air conditioning engineers can readily bring tropical climates to temperate cities or provide temperate coolness in tropical regions. It remains for the future to show just what therapeutic use may be made of such facilities. The use of artificial moist heat for northern toxic goiter patients was suggested on an earlier page and seems well worth trying. Similar artificial depression of metabolism might be tried in other overdynamic states, both physical and mental. Summer cooling is strongly indicated for the ill during severe heat waves, while in the tropics recuperation can be greatly hastened by properly facilitating body heat loss.

* * *

It is to be hoped that the reader will see, after careful perusal of this chapter, that the therapeutic duties of a physician can no longer be concerned simply with the specific treatment of the disease at hand. He should look farther afield for the larger forces affecting his patient's welfare and future health. And among the outside forces bearing on these more general aspects of existence, climatic and weather influences are of great importance. The most perfect diet cannot lead to physical vigor and high vitality unless the heat generated in its use can be readily dissipated from the body. The physician of the future will, therefore, need to develop more deeply his interest in, and knowledge of, climatic and meteorologic influences affecting man throughout his existence in the different regions of the earth.

BIBLIOGRAPHY

1. BENEDICT, F. G. and CATHCART, E. P.: Muscular work: a metabolic study with special reference to the efficiency of the human body as a machine, Carnegie Institution of Washington, Pub. #187, 1913.
2. BRODY, S. and TROWBRIDGE, E. A.: Efficiency of horses, men and motors, Univ. of Missouri Agricultural Exper. Station Bull., #383, 1937.
3. ZUNTZ, N.: Über den Stoffverbrauch des Hundes bei Muskelarbeit, Pflüger's Arch. f. d. ges. Physiol., 1901, LXXXIII, 191.
4. BENEDICT, F. G. and CARPENTER, T. M.: "Food ingestion and energy transformation, Carnegie Inst. of Washington, Pub. #261, 1918.

5. MILLS, C. A.: Climate and metabolic stress, Am. Jour. Hygiene, 1939, XXIX, 147.
6. GESSLER, H.: Untersuchungen über die Warmeregulation. I. Mitteilung die Konstanz des Grundumsatzes, Pflüger's Arch. f. d. ges. Physiol., 1925, CCVII, 370.
7. MARTIN, C. J.: Thermal adjustments of man and animals to external conditions, Lancet, 1930, II, 617.
8. MILLS, C. A.: Geographic and time variations in body growth and age at menarche, Human Biology, 1937, IX, 43.
9. MILLS, C. A. and SENIOR, F. A.: Does climate affect the human conception rate? Arch. Int. Med., 1930, XLVI, 921.
10. MILLS, C. A. and OGLE, C.: Physiologic sterility of adolescence, Human Biology, 1936, VIII, 607.
11. MILLS, C. A.: Susceptibility to tuberculosis: race or energy level? Am. Jour. Med. Sci., 1935, CLXXXIX, 330.
12. MILLS, C. A.: Acute appendicitis and the weather, Jour. Med., Cincinnati, 1934, XV, 39.
13. LOCKE, ARTHUR: Lack of fitness as the predisposing factor in infections of the type encountered in pneumonia and in common cold, Jour. Infect. Dis., 1937, LX, 106.
14. COWGILL, G. R.: Vitamin B Requirement of Man, Yale Univ. Press, New Haven, 1934.
15. MILLS, C. A.: Unpublished findings.
16. MILLS, C. A.: Medical Climatology, Chas. C. Thomas, Springfield, 1939.
17. JOSLIN, E. P.: The universality of diabetes, Jour. Am. Med. Assoc., 1940, CXV, 2033.
18. BEAN, W. B. and MILLS, C. A.: Coronary occlusion, heart failure and environmental temperatures, Am. Heart Jour., 1938, XVI, 701.
19. MILLS, C. A.: Dangers to Southerners in northward migration, Am. Jour. Trop. Med., 1935, XV, 591.
20. MOUNTIN, J. W. and HAROLD, F. D.: Some peculiarities in the geography of cancer, Jour. Am. Med. Assoc., 1939, CXIII, 2405.
21. MILLS, C. A. and OGLE, C.: Climatic basis for susceptibility to heat stroke or exhaustion, Am. Jour. Hygiene, 1933, XVII, 686.
22. DAFT, F. S., SEBRELL, W. H., BABCOCK, S. H. and JUKES, T. H.: Effect of synthetic pantothenic acid on adrenal hemorrhage, atrophy, and necrosis in rats, Pub. Health Rep., 1940, LV, 1333.
23. MILLS, R. C., SHAW, J. H., ELVEHJEM, C. A. and PHILLIPS, P. H.: Curative effect of pantothenic acid in adrenal necrosis, Proc. Soc. Exper. Biol. and Med., 1940, XLV, 4824.
24. MILLS, C. A.: Depressions, weather and health, Human Biology, 1939, X, 383.
25. HUNTINGTON, ELLSWORTH: Civilization and Climate, Yale Univ. Press, New Haven, 1925.
26. McCLINTOCK, J. T. and PAISLEY, S.: Cost of work in relation to basal metabolism, Proc. Soc. Exper. Biol. and Med., 1932, XXX, 162.

27. MILLS, C. A.: Seasonal and regional factors in acute rheumatic fever and rheumatic heart disease, Jour. Lab. and Clin. Med., 1938, XXIV, 53.
28. MILLS, C. A.: World leprosy in relation to climatic stimulation and bodily vigor, Internat. Jour. Leprosy, 1936, IV, 295.
29. MILLS, C. A.: Control of body heat loss through radiant means, Journal Section of Heating, Piping and Air Conditioning, 1937, IX, 697.

Sept. 1, 1941.

CHAPTER XII

HEREDITY AND EUGENICS IN RELATION TO MEDICINE

By CHARLES B. DAVENPORT

Table of Contents

I. GENERAL STATEMENT ABOUT HEREDITY

In order to understand the relations of genetics, or the science of heredity, to medicine, it is necessary to be clear on the biological significance of heredity. If two fertilized eggs, one of a starfish and one of a sea urchin, are placed in a finger bowl of sea water under otherwise favorable conditions each will develop in its own way; one into a young starfish and the other into a young sea urchin. The eggs are both nearly microscopic, they look very much alike even under the microscope. The conditions surrounding them are as nearly identical as possible. Yet they develop into very different organisms, of different form and different activity. This difference in the course of development of two fertilized eggs, surrounded by identical environment, can only be due to a difference in internal factors which control their development. The internal factors which control the development of the organism are what we understand as heredity.

This property of the fertilized egg to reproduce the specific form to which it belongs is universally recognized. A child of two Scandinavian parents has at birth a trunk, two arms and two legs, a practically hairless skin and facial features of such and such form because it develops from Scandinavian protoplasm. A child of two Negro parents has a different colored skin and a different form of hair and different features because it develops from Negro protoplasm. This is heredity. Everybody believes in heredity, even those who deny its importance. The two white parents who would be appalled at having a black-skinned baby believe in heredity. The person who invests ten cents in a package of seeds marked "double, variegated petunias" has a deep faith in heredity. The only limitation to universal belief in heredity is in respect to its application to particular cases. If a man has his forefinger cut off by a hay knife, we recognize that this peculiarity which he carries through his later life is not due to heredity. If a man is born with four fingers and belongs to a family in which for generations numerous persons have been born with only four fingers instead of five, the special student of genetics will emphatically pronounce his peculiarity to be hereditary. If, however, a single case appears in a family of a child born with a finger which has been constricted, or perhaps entirely lost off before birth, we are in more doubt as to whether this is a case of uterine accident, constriction of the developing finger by adhesion to embryonic membranes, or whether there is in this case a genetic hereditary factor. We are familiar, also, with striking instances of members of the same family who have not been in close contact and who, nevertheless, show similar gestures, idiosyncrasies of speech, or special gifts. Popularly these idiosyncrasies are recognized as hereditary. But when one member of the family is feebleminded, or has epileptic fits, or shows a lack of control over actions such as makes it necessary to remove him from society, then a great difference of opinion arises as to whether these conditions are, or are not, hereditary.

Heredity is not to be regarded as a phenomenon of the same order as a particular disease entity or syndrome. It is something more fundamental and universal than that. It is the internal direction of development.

The developing egg of a particular species, if surrounded by a proper environment and if its internally directing agents are typical of the species and are without lethal factors, will develop in a predictable fashion to produce the specific form with its particular function. The egg is more or less spherical and contains somewhat unequally distributed particles of varied molecular constitution. Always in its center is the egg nucleus, formed by the union of the pronuclei of sperm and egg. The nucleus contains, floating in a fluid, a protoplasmic network in which lie granules. Before any cell division takes place the granules come together in the form of elongated chromosomes. In the act of cell division each of the chromosomes divides precisely so that each daughter cell contains the same chromosomes as the mother cell. In the chromosomes are the specific activators of development (enzymes, called "genes"), which control time and place of cell divisions and other developmental processes that eventually lead to the adult form.

Nature of Heredity and Environment

One of the commonest inquiries made of the geneticist is as to the relative importance of heredity and environment. This seems to be regarded by persons of large experience and vision and especially by those interested in social improvement as a fundamental question. It is frequently thought that those interested in human biology and sociology fall into two groups, the heriditarians and the environmentalists.

Such a division is very unfortunate and entirely unwarranted. There is in Nature no such contrast. Huxley has somewhere described life as the interaction between the internal organism and external world, and this interaction extends even to the smallest living cell.

The development of the organism and the metabolism of each cell are, it is sometimes said, determined by genes. Others stress the importance of the cytoplasm. The truth seems to be that the genes by themselves can do nothing, the cytoplasm by itself is so inert as to be ineffective. The genes act as catalysts, as enzymes, which accelerate the chemical processes going on in the cytoplasm, determine the specific chemical reaction that shall occur at any moment in the cytoplasm and thus determine the quality of the cell, whether it is a bone cell, or a muscle cell, or a nerve cell, or whatever its form and function may be. It will be noted that there are certainly hundreds, probably thousands, of different kinds of enzymes in the gene complex of the cell, that there are scores, possibly hundreds, of different kinds of molecules in the cytoplasm, that at a given moment only a particular enzyme can accelerate a particular cytoplasmic operation. Therefore, the action of the hereditary units is determined absolutely by the nature of the cell which is environmental to them, and the changes that take place in the cytoplasm are determined absolutely by the available enzymes.

Similar are the relations between the organism and its environment. The organism can do nothing without its environment; what the environment does to the organism depends upon the nature of the organism. Were 100 children to be reared from birth in an identical environment, being brought in contact with similar cultural conditions, they would still grow up to be very different, because each is highly selective in making use of what the uniform environment provides. The "best" cultural condition for one may be the worst for another. As a distinguished Frenchman once said, "The equal treatment of unequals is the greatest inequality." Though unequals may be brought in contact with the same external treatment, what use they make of that treatment is highly selective and differential. An extreme case is presented by two children one of whom is color-blind and the other has sharp color discrimination. Looking at the same painting or the same autumn foliage the two will see very different things. Similarly, if in a school room one child is deaf, while another has excellent hearing, what the two children get from the similar oral instruction of the teacher may well be very dissimilar. The deaf pupil may, indeed, secure some benefit from the instruction, but does it in a very different way from the hearing pupil. Two persons may find the taste of the same substance to be for one agreeable, for the other disagreeable.

The same principles apply in the field of medicine. During an epidemic of influenza, yellow fever, or the plague, not everybody finds the dangerous destructive agents of the epidemic to be such for him. The disease-inciting agent is destructive for those organisms which are not prepared to resist it.

This principle is illustrated in detail in the case of leukemia in mice as worked out by Dr. E. C. MacDowell with the assistance of Potter, Richter, Victor, and others. In a colony of mice which had been inbred, brother and sister, for 40 or 50 generations, there appeared several who died of leukemia. A study of their pedigree showed they were all derived from the same mother. If from a mouse about to die of leukemia, blood is taken and inoculated into another mouse of the same strain, but which has not reached the tumor age, that mouse will die from leukemia within a week or ten days. The demonstration is complete that inoculated cells carry the power of unrestricted proliferation, and this we think of as the "cause of death." But this conclusion is wrong; for if a part of the same inoculant that has resulted in the death of one mouse be put into an unrelated mouse of another strain then, apart from an erythema at the point of inoculation, there is no reaction, and the mouse continues its life unscathed. One sees then that not merely the malignant cells are the cause of leukemia, but the susceptibility of the organism, or its inability to protect itself against the leukemic cells. We are prone to divide the white blood cells into leukemic cells and normal cells. It is, on the other hand, quite as significant to divide organisms into those who are resistant to rapidly proliferating leukemic cells and those who are non-resistant. For the non-resistant organisms the environments of white blood cells, which are leukemic and those which are not, are fundamentally different, and the environment of the leukemic cell is, indeed, a fatal one. Again, for the resistant mouse the leukemic cells are no longer a worse environment than normal white blood cells. Or, looking at the matter the other way around, to the leukemic cells a non-resistant mouse is a good environment, while the resistant mouse is a bad environment; but for the normal white blood cells both types of mice constitute a good environment. Thus, we see that no environment is absolutely good or bad, but only such in relation to the particular genetical strain of organism with which it reacts. Also, the same agency may be genetical from one standpoint and environmental from another standpoint. The end result, a pathological condition, is a chemical interaction between two agents, and there is no reason for designating one as the hereditary factor rather than the other.

This point of view can be extended for the whole range of human experience. In the field of crime the question is often raised whether this is not caused by bad environment. This inquiry has no significance. Precisely the same environment, which is bad for one person and may result in that person becoming a criminal, may be good for another person and protect him from becoming a criminal. Criminal behavior results from the interaction of a particular environmental set-up and a person of particular constitution, which causes in that person a criminal reaction. On the contrary, the same environmental set-up might cause a person of different constitution to become a saint. We should speak not of bad environment but bad interactions.

Sketch of Mechanism of Heredity

General Considerations

Analysis of a chromosome shows that it is made up of a strand of more or less spherical bodies called chromomeres, and it is believed that at the center of each chromomere there lies a gene. Indeed, there are some who believe that they have seen the gene. Whether this is true, or not, the genes probably are among the largest organic molecules and are not far below the range of vision by the aid of the ultra-violet light waves.

The genes are believed to be enzyme molecules (ferments). It is the nature of each ferment that it acts only upon specific molecules to accelerate their chemical interaction. When, at any moment, there is no pair of molecules present whose interaction can be accelerated by a particular enzyme that enzyme does not function.

Starting out with a full equipment of enzymes and with appropriate equipment of building material in the cytoplasm of the egg, the catalytic action of enzymes in promoting chemical processes begins, and since in the act of cell-division the different materials of the cytoplasm are sorted out in different cells, the nature of the interaction varies in the different cells. The different forms that these cells assume must be believed to be due to a difference in the materials upon which the appropriate enzymes work. As any chemical process is completed, whether it be oxidation or dehydration or other, there is established a particular new molecular set-up upon which not the gene responsible for the particular change, but another gene, acts, a set-up such that the molecules responsible for the original particular change can not act. Thus, the essential elements of appropriate change, at proper time and place, are provided for.

From this point of view the form of man and of the twenty-six trillion cells which constitute a man are determined by the genes and cytoplasmic materials stored in the fertilized egg. If, however, the genes or cytoplasmic materials were other than they ordinarily are, then there would be produced, an organism perhaps, but not a man. Man, as we know him, is the visible expression of the interaction of human genes and human cytoplasmic materials. Man has not determined the nature of these substances, but the nature of the substances has determined man. In just the same way the substance in any fertilized egg determines its specific form, a pig, a snake, a jellyfish, or a sponge. From this point of view the history of the evolution of the animal kingdom is the history of the changes that have occurred in the materials of the germ cells; also, the anatomical and histological analysis of a man is merely a study of the visible end-result of the inter-workings of the substances that have through various spontaneous or mutative processes in the history of chromosomal evolution come to lie in the human egg.

Method of Inheritance of Particular Traits

If two individuals having precisely the same germ plasm should marry, their offspring would be exactly alike and like their parents. Ordinarily, this situation is not realized, since the germ plasm and the cytoplasm of the eggs that are produced in the same parents are not exactly alike. The dissimilarity of the genes is due to the fact that practically all human matings are hybrid matings, so that when the germ cells are formed in the body some of them are formed with genes of one kind and others with dissimilar genes. It is probable that the cytoplasmic particles are distributed somewhat differently to the different eggs. Consequently, when a union in pairs of the dissimilar egg cells and sperm cells occurs, the offspring differ from each other and are more or less unlike their parents. If one of the parents belongs to a race most of whose external characters are very dissimilar to those of the race to which the mate belongs, then a dilemma appears as to what the children will be like. Empirically we find that if the father is short in stature, has curly and black hair, deep brown eyes and swarthy skin, and belongs to a race with these characters, while the mother is tall and blond and straight-haired, blue-eyed and fair-skinned, and belongs to a race which has these characteristics, then the offspring will be in these respects much more like the father than the mother. They will be short and have curly and dark brown hair, dark eyes and swarthy skin.

The phenomenon of reappearance in the offspring of certain of the traits of the father's race and certain of the traits of the mother's race is the basis of the principle of dominance which plays a great part in modern genetics. A racial trait is said to be dominant when it appears in one of the full-blooded parents and not in the other and appears in all of the offspring. Dominance has been explained in different ways. According to one theory, the gene for the trait is present in the germ cells on one side of the house and absent in the germ cells of the other side of the house, but in the offspring it is present, though in a diluted condition. The trait that is, on this theory, absent is called "recessive." The offspring of the cited mating do not show the recessive trait though they carry it in their germ cells. If, now, two persons of this origin should marry, then one quarter of their offspring will show the recessive trait, three quarters will show the dominant trait and of those three quarters, two quarters will have it in a diluted condition again. The diluted condition is known as "heterozygosis" and the individuals of mixed origins are known as "heterozygotic." Those offspring, which show the recessive trait, are "homozygotic" for that trait, as are also those offspring that inherit double dominance of any trait.

It is to be said that the foregoing theory is not universally accepted, and there are many cases in genetics where it is not applicable. The gene responsible for a dominant trait may be opposed by a gene which is not absent, but is modified in such a way as to produce the recessive trait. The two opposing genes are sometimes spoken of as "allelomorphs" and of the allelomorphs one is dominant and the other is recessive, but neither is entirely absent. Heterozygous dominants differ from homozygous dominants in this, that the eventual trait is developed in less complete degree than in homozygous dominants. Thus in the eye color, brown pigment is dominant over the absence of brown (blue eye), but the brown pigment is deeper in the homozygous dominant than in the heterozygous dominant. Similarly, in the offspring of a Negro and a European the dark skin pigmentation is dominant, but less dark than in the full-blooded Negro. It is believed that, where there are two doses of a gene for a particular trait, the two doses work twice as fast as, and more effectively, in creating a character than a single dose.

A second principle in inheritance is that different traits are inherited independently of each other. Thus, for example, if one parent is a full-blooded

Negro and the other a Scandinavian, then the children will all have dark eyes and dark, curly hair and dark skin pigmentation. If two such children marry, then their offspring will carry the opposing traits of the ancestral races in diverse combinations. Thus, one may have a dark skin pigmentation, straight hair and narrow nose, another, light skin pigmentation with woolly hair and broad nose, or broad nose may be combined with straight hair. It has to be recognized, however, that the old idea that each gene produces only a single effect in the developing organism is not strictly correct, but each usually has a predominating effect and various minor effects. The reason for this is found in the general considerations given in the preceding section, where it is pointed out that any trait that is developed is developed because of the interaction of one or more genes responsible for this development and the cytoplasm of the egg in which these genes have come to lie, and it is clear that the chemical interaction rarely will be limited to a particular and single chemical reaction.

What determines that particular traits be dominant or recessive is not definitely explained in the second hypothesis referred to above. In general, new and recent mutations result in bringing about a recessive trait in the offspring. Most of the developmental defects in the child are due to recessive factors. Such are, for example, feeble-mindedness, epilepsy, melancholia and many others. However, not all deviations from the normal are in the nature of recessive defects. Many of the abnormalities in the development of the hand, for example, are of the dominant type.

The dissimilar nature of the genes in the germ cells of the father and the mother are, as pointed out, responsible for the dissimilarity of children. However, there is one case in which the development of two children is under the influence of precisely similar genes. This is the case of identical twins in which, it is commonly believed, two embryos arise from the same egg at an early stage of its development. These two embryos, therefore, have the same chromosomes and constituent genes and probably very similar cytoplasm. However, it is to be noted that we can not be sure that the cytoplasm of the cells from which the two embryos arise is identical, and, as a matter of fact, it not infrequently happens that the embryos which develop with a single chorion are somewhat diverse in form. Such diversity, in contrast with the ordinary identity, may be due either to dissimilarity of the cytoplasm or to differences in the intrauterine environment, among others to the stealing by the one embryo of an undue proportion of the circulating blood, thus depriving the other twin of its proper nourishment.

The genes are found in the nuclei of the germ cells, arranged in linear series along the axes of the chromosomes of the nuclei. In man there are twenty-four pairs of these chromosomes of which one member of each pair is derived from the father's germ cell and one from the mother's. Of the twenty-four pairs of chromosomes, however, there is one which has different relations in the two sexes. Thus, in the female offspring the members of this one pair are identical in their chromosomal content. In the males, on the other hand, the members of this pair have dissimilar chromosomal content. In fact, one of the chromosomes contains very few active genes. The chromosome which is inactive is known as the Y chromosome, whereas the active chromosome of the pair is known as the X chromosome. The females contain two X chromosomes, the male only one X chromosome and one Y chromosome. This difference in number of the X chromosomes determines a difference between the two sexes in the activity of the genes in their sex chromosomes, and this difference of activity is responsible for the fact that one individual develops into a female and the other into a male with differing male and female characteristics. It is true that, in vertebrates, many of the differentiating characters of male and female can be influenced by hormones early produced by the gonads, or sex glands. However, the quality of the gonads is determined by the difference in the number of X chromosomes. In the eggs of insects sex is determined only by the number of X chromosomes; there are in them no important hormones secreted by the gonads which influence the sexual characteristics.

One consequence of the existence of the sex chromosomes is a difference in inheritance of certain traits that depend upon genes which lie in them. Thus, a recessive gene of the X chromosome in a male zygote will show itself effective on the soma that develops out of that zygote, whereas a similar recessive defect in a female zygote will not show in the adult body because the recessive trait will be covered over by the normal dominant trait. There are a number of so-called sex-linked traits known in man which appear ordinarily in males, but are transferred by females over to their male offspring. Among them are color blindness, hemophilia, and optic nerve atrophy.

There are, indeed, certain characters in man which seem to be influenced not directly by genes but indirectly by the activity of the gonads; such are known as sex-limited characters. Examples are the beard in man and the large spurs and comb of the cock. The hen does not lack determiners for large spur or large comb. This may be demonstrated by grafting a testis into a young hen; large spurs and comb and male coloration soon make their appearance under the stimulus of hormones derived from the male gland.

Heretofore we have been considering characters due to a single gene whether dominant or recessive. Many traits are due to the coöperation of two or more genes which, working together, are responsible for a single trait. For example, the dark skin pigmentation of Negroes is due to the activity of two pairs of genes which probably activate the oxidation of thyrosin to form melanin. If the typical number is reduced through hybridization from four to three, two, or one, we have produced the various diluted types of pigmentation known as sambo, mulatto and quadroon. Many, if not most, human traits are due to the coöperation of two or more pairs of genes.

Thus we see that the studies of the last two or three decades upon heredity have demonstrated that it is, at the same time, much more definite and much more complex than had been anticipated. Much is still to be learned about the inheritance of traits in man. The near future will, no doubt, show that just as color blindness and sex production are linked in the sex chromosomes so other traits are linked in others of the two dozen pairs of chromosomes in the germ cells of man. The determination of the association of determiners in the twenty-four chromosomes is one of the alluring fields of research for the future.

II. INHERITANCE OF SPECIAL TRAITS,* PARTICULARLY DISEASES AND DEFECTS

Introductory Remarks

The deviations from normality that man shows fall into a number of categories. Some of them are of the nature of developmental defects, others are symptoms of disease for the production of which, in some cases, a parasitic organism has been shown to be one factor. Others are chemical peculiarities of the body due to defects in metabolism and abnormal internal secretions of various types. Without, however, attempting to classify the different causes of the abnormal conditions shown, we may consider them in groups according to the organs chiefly concerned.

One explanatory remark, however, may be ventured. Because it has been demonstrated that there is a particular parasitic microörganism responsible for the particular disease, it does not follow that the particular symptoms shown by the diseased individual are solely dependent upon that microörganism and its activities. In a great epidemic, like that of influenza, we find individuals in the same house, even in the same family, who, though they clearly harbor the germs of the disease, show very different symptoms. One can hardly think of the parasitic organisms as differing in virulence in such cases; rather the human beings in which they are developing differ in their resistance and reactions to the germ. Indeed, as every farmer knows, the harvest of his planting is determined not only by the seed put into the soil, but also by the qualities of the soil itself. Similarly, the symptoms that a microörganism will induce in the body depend not only upon the particular physiology of the microörganism, but also upon the soil in which it grows, namely, the chemical constitution of the individual. With these general remarks the different diseases and defects

* "Bibliographia Eugenica," published as a supplement to the "Eugenical News," gives fairly complete references to writings on inheritance of special traits.

found in man may be considered briefly with special reference to the part that heredity plays in inducing or modifying them.

Resistance and Longevity

When a disease or a death occurs, we are prone to assign a cause, and in all well organized states there are public mortality statistics which give the number of persons dead and "the cause of death." The "cause of death" is too narrowly conceived. A person does not die merely of typhoid fever, but dies of an inability to resist the development of the typhoid bacillus in his body. Indeed, the mortality statistics instead of being arranged under causes of death with the subdivision typhoid fever, cancer, etc., might about as properly be arranged under the rubrics "Number of persons non-resistant to typhoid fever," "Number of persons non-resistant to cancer," etc. A text book on bacteriology describes the parasitic organism which is often associated with the disease, but says nothing about the organism in which the disease-promoting germ is growing. The persons who die of a particular disease, like typhoid fever, are, however, a selected lot of the population, selected because of their physiological and bio-chemical inadequacy to meet the situation presented by germs of disease in the body.

Resistance to disease is a subject that has been studied more in plants, perhaps, than in animals. In any case, it is recognized of great, practical importance by plant and animal breeders. By proper methods of breeding there have been produced all sorts of agricultural crops which are resistant to smuts, rusts and wilts. Similarly, there are strains of domestic animals which have been bred resistant to cholera, as in hogs, to certain protozoan diseases, as in poultry and the like. In humans no attempt has been made to breed resistant strains; nevertheless there are known lines, or strains, which are highly resistant to diseases. This resistance is shown by the fact that the individuals of such lines are rarely ill and that they often live to an advanced age. Such nonagenarians are resistant not only to the ordinary germs of disease, but also to the degenerative diseases which make their appearance during the involutionary period. That longevity is inherited is clear from families that every observer can cite, and that are often described in the literature. The fact has also been repeatedly demonstrated statistically, beginning with the very full studies made by Alexander Graham Bell some twenty years ago. Besides a natural immunity and resistance there is, of course, acquired immunity, but this again is a familial trait. Persons must already have a certain amount of resistance in order to acquire immunity to possibly fatal disease; were there no such initial resistance, there would be no opportunity to build up such immunity.

The Allergies and Vitamin Insufficiencies

During the present century there has developed a clear knowledge of the anaphylactic reaction and of the allergies which are associated with it. It has also become clear that the allergic reactions are highly specific in their incidence, that while in certain families there is a wide-spread tendency toward hay fever or eczema following inhalation of certain proteins or the ingestion of particular foods, other families are quite immune to such irritating agents.

As for vitamin insufficiencies, a study that was made at the Eugenics Record Office of the incidence of pellagra in Spartansburg, S. C. showed very clearly that the disease ran a virulent course only in certain families and, indeed, in cases where severe effects followed, these were of different type in different families. There were families characterized principally by dermal symptoms, others by intestinal symptoms, others by symptoms of the central nervous system.

Similarly, the ability to resist the insufficiency of particular vitamins seems to vary in different individuals, and this difference probably has a genetical basis. There are some persons more tolerant of insufficiency of vitamins A or B, for example, than are others.

Twin Production

The number of simultaneous ovulations in a single female differs greatly in different animals running all the way from the condition in oysters where a hundred million eggs may be laid simultaneously to the condition found in many mammals and particularly in groups of primates where usually only one or two eggs are ovulated at the same time. In humans about one labor in 100 results in twins, about one in 10,000 in triplets, the higher numbers being relatively much rarer still. The tendency toward twin production depends upon the constitution of the parents. It is necessary, of course, for twin production that two eggs should be simultaneously ovulated, but of such simultaneous ovulation only a small proportion give rise to twins. This follows from some studies made many years ago by Leopold, who found that about 10 per cent. of women's ovaries showed two recent corpora lutea and, therefore, two recent double ovulations. Although, as stated, only 1 per cent. of labors are twin-producing, the discrepancy between a 10 per cent. ovulation and a 1 per cent. twin birth is to be ascribed in part to the male. Indeed, there have been published a number of observations indicating that the male is not less responsible for the production of twins than the female consort. The explanation of the deficiency is in part the failure of both eggs to be fertilized, but even more important is the failure of a certain proportion of the eggs to develop far in utero. Such intrauterine deaths, which amount to from 40 per cent. to 75 per cent. in strains of mice, seem to be due not to any pathological condition in the uterus but to the presence of lethal factors in the genes of the germ cells. If both parents carry the same lethal factors, then the egg will develop only a little way. If one parent only brings in the lethal factor, the child may develop inadequately in the organs affected, and early intrauterine death may be expected. A heavy rate of twin production is found where there is multiple ovulation and where the male is vigorous and produces sperm that is without lethal factors.

The importance of constitution in twin production is indicated by the frequent cases of particular mothers who produce twins repeatedly. One of the most striking cases (which is, moreover, very well documented) is that of Mrs. Clark of Cleveland, who by three different husbands had a total of forty-two children born over a period of less than 30 years, beginning at the age of about fourteen. During this period she averaged nearly three children at a birth, never had a single child at a time, in six instances had triplets and in four instances quadruplets. By her first husband she had only one pair of twins, by her second, two sets of twins and two sets of triplets; by her third husband the size of litter produced has averaged much higher. It is to be noted that according to the best information available her mother had only twins, triplets and quadruplets, and her grandmother in turn is stated to have had many multiple births. However, the earlier generations were not seen, since they lived in France.

The hereditary tendency to twin production has been followed not only in humans but also in sheep. Dr. Alexander Graham Bell was able by careful selection of twin breeders, both on the male and female side, to greatly increase the proportion of twins and triplets produced. From that strain, on one occasion, quadruplets developed in the uterus, but caused the death of the mother, since she was unable to give birth to them.

The Internal Secretions and Constitution

The importance of the internal secretions has become increasingly recognized during the present century. Hereditary factors have been discovered for a number of the endocrine conditions. One of the most striking has been studied in mice by Dr. E. C. MacDowell. A particular strain of highly inbred mice produced litters containing dwarfs. Investigation showed that the dwarfs had rudimentary anterior lobes of the pituitary gland. Associated with this were an inactive thyroid gland and suprarenals of which the cortex was quite inactive. The gonads of these animals also functioned inadequately. By injecting into the dwarfs the hormones from normal pituitaries the growth of the sterile dwarfs was promoted; they became nearly normal in size, and they also became sex-functional. Autopsies revealed that the thyroids and suprarenal cortex had become active, though the anterior lobes still remained rudimentary. In this strain of mice the dwarfism appeared to be due to a single recessive gene. Similar studies by Riddle and Benedict have shown that in particular strains of pigeons the activity of the thyroid gland, as measured by basal metabolism is high, in other strains it is low. In general, the developmental defects which are due to endocrine disfunction may, in turn, be ascribed to a more remote genic defect which is responsible for that disfunctioning. This genic defect passes down through the generations.

One of the most striking of the endocrine effects has to do with the build of the body. Body-build runs the whole gamut of possibilities from very slender to very fleshy and obese. These conditions of build are believed to be highly influenced, if not controlled, by endocrine conditions. To be sure, within limits, body build may be influenced by food intake. On the other hand, certain strains will not tolerate excessive food intake and, consequently, remain slender. Studies made at the Eugenics Record Office on inheritance of body-build indicate that there are two or more genes responsible for the result; that where both parents are slender the children are typically slender, that where both parents are fleshy the children are mostly fleshy, but some of them may be of intermediate or slender build. The pituitary and the thyroid both influence body build, and perhaps other endocrine glands do also. Since the anterior pituitary gland influences the growth processes and also the development of the gonads, insufficiencies in the activity of this gland result in individuals who are overweight and in whom (especially the male) the secondary sex characters are underdeveloped.

There seems to be, also, as Kretschmer pointed out many years ago, a certain relation between body build and form of psychoses. Thus, in those individuals in which the psychosis is of dementia præcox type, the individuals are prevailingly of a slender, "asthenic" type, whereas in the manic-depressive psychosis the victim has a robust, "pyknic" build. Extensive studies have been made upon body build in relation to psychoses. Kretschmer's findings have been repeatedly confirmed. However, the work which has been done has been for the most part non-quantitative. The studies of Wertheimer (1926), done in association with Dr. Adolph Meyer of Johns Hopkins University, lead to the conclusion that this relation of constitution to psychoses has been exaggerated.

The failure of the secretions from the islands of Langerhans of the pancreas is now known to be an important factor in the production of diabetes, but numerous studies have shown this to have a hereditary factor, as for example those of Gossage (1908), of Williams (1917), Pincus and White in Joslin's clinic (1933), and others.

Abnormal Growths

All vertebrates, and particularly man, are subject to extraordinary localized growths in the body, especially of the adult. While it is well known that certain families are especially apt to form these tumors, still the method of inheritance has not been definitely ascertained in the case of humans, and it is certainly particularly complicated by the random mating of humans. Light upon the factors responsible for tumor growth is thrown by studies made by Dr. E. C. MacDowell on leukemia in mice. In a strain of mice, highly inbred, brother and sister for forty generations, there appeared some individuals that died of a disease diagnosed as leukemia. These were all traced back to a single mother in a line known in the laboratory as C58. When the leukemic cells from a mouse progressed in the disease were inoculated into an unaffected mouse of this strain, even before the ordinary age of incidence of leukemia, the inoculated mouse died usually within a week. If, however, some of the same inoculant was put into mice of another strain, such as that known in the laboratory as SL, there was only a slight reaction at the point of inoculation, but no tumor was formed, or if a slight tumor appeared, it quickly vanished. It was obvious that the "soil" was different in the mice of this particular strain of C58 and in the SL strain, and that the soil of the latter did not permit the growth of the leukemic cells. If a mouse of the SL strain be mated with one of the C58 strain, then the offspring are susceptible and further studies indicate that a single factor is responsible for the susceptibility. This fairly clean-cut result was possible because of the nature of the inbreeding to which the mice had been subjected, and in consequence of which they had become genetically nearly "pure." Naturally, in the young of mice bred haphazardly one can not predict the susceptibility, and indeed all susceptible mice would probably prove to be heterozygous and produce susceptible as well as resistant individuals. This latter condition is exactly the one we find in humans where resistant and non-resistant strains have been combined for an indefinite number of generations, and two susceptible genes from the two parents will only occasionally come together in the fertilized egg, or the "zygote." It is probably on this account that statisticians have not been able to show an inheritance of a tendency toward tumor growths between parents and children. Nevertheless, the evidence is clear not only from the case of MacDowell's mice, but from other confirmatory evidence, that there is such a thing as natural resistance to tumor growth and natural susceptibility. Whatever the factor is that gives resistance, whether a particular enzyme or other factor, is not as yet known. It is, of course, quite possible that one might build up a resistance to tumor growth in an organism by appropriate technique.

Among tumors whose inheritance has been more or less well studied are the following: multiple neurofibromatosis, in which the susceptibility is dominant, also multiple telangiectases and polyadenomata of the rectum.

Skin diseases that are likewise inherited as dominant traits are epidermolysis bullosa, ichthyosis, keratosis, and persistent hereditary edema. All of these skin tumors may, on occasion, pass into malignant sarcoma, which thus shows again its hereditable basis.

Skin Diseases

A large number of skin defects and diseases, such as albinism, birth marks (nævus), keratosis, psoriasis, anonychia, hypotricosis, seborrhœa, have been shown to depend upon hereditary factors. Usually there is a dominant factor responsible for the defect. The evidence for inheritance of diseases of the skin has been presented by W. H. Siemens in a large number of papers. Heavy pigmentation in the skin was found in the negro race dominant over light pigmentation as in Europeans; apparently there are two (double) factors responsible for the deeper pigmentation. The mulattoes have only one (double) factor and quadroons only one. The tendency to early baldness, which has been regarded by many as simply an accidental disease, has been shown to be inherited as apparently a sex-limited character. The baldness tends to run in different families in particular types, and some, or all, of these types are found as specific characters in different species of primates, as Gerrit S. Miller points out. Scar tissue reacts differently in different races of mankind, forming keloid tumors in negroes.

Skeletal System

The development of bone is a complicated process that has a long phylogenetic history reflected in its complicated nature. Especially the long bones are subject to great variation depending upon the activity of certain genes that are responsible for their full development. Sometimes the bones are formed in abnormal fashion, as for example in brittle bones where the Haversian canals are improperly formed, or absent. Inheritance of this condition has been described in Bulletin 14 of the Eugenics Record Office. In other cases the long bone fails of expected linear development. The consequence is that the legs and arms are abnormally short, as one sees in achondroplastic dwarfs. Inheritance of dwarfism has been described in the "Treasury of Human Inheritance" by Rischbieth and Barrington, and reference is made to that publication for further details.

The number of digits is subject to hereditary abnormalities. Thus in poultry and the lower mammals the number may be reduced to 4 or 3, and in other cases increased to 6, or more. Always in these cases there is a dominant factor which interferes with the normally precise, definite number of digits formed on the margin of the paddle at the tip of the embryonic limb; in other cases the bones of adjacent fingers may be grown together producing the condition known as syndactylism. This is found also in poultry. The phenomenon has been treated monographically in the "Memoirs of the Galton Laboratory of Eugenics" Part 6. Even the details of forms of hand and feet are modifiable by hereditary factors. Such modifications arise as crooked fingers, double jointedness, and variations in the relative length of the first and second digits of the foot and the second and fourth of the hand.

The bones of the hand are especially liable to defects; thus ankylosis of the phalanges has been repeatedly described. A defect of this sort has been traced by Cushing through seven generations in the United States and by Drinkwater through fourteen generations. A related defect is brachydactylia, abnormalities of length of the metacarpal bones. The fourth metacarpal seems to be especially apt to develop imperfectly, possibly due to an imperfect development of the distal epiphysis. In the formation of the carpal bones hereditary factors govern, as shown by J. W. Pryor, who has traced the order of development of carpal bones in single members of various families. When the order of development of the carpal bones differ in one and the same families there is apt to be a resemblance in these sequences of development.

The form of the skull is a racial characteristic and details in size and proportions of the head are notoriously found in families. The heredity of the cephalic index has been studied by G. P. Frets.

Muscular System

While the muscular system probably has been less completely studied from a genetical point of view than the other systems of the body, yet to it have been ascribed inherited deviations from type. For example, the suppression of the palmaris longus muscle of the fore arm apparently. is inherited as a dominant. Its absence is more frequent in Europeans than in Negroes. Numerous abnormalities are due to defects in the nerves that innervate the particular muscles. Thus, peroneal atrophy has been described in extensive families as, for example, by Macklin and Bowman, 1926, in 101 descendants of an emigrant to Canada. This defect behaves as a dominant. The most extensive study of myotonic epilepsy, which shows the symptoms of spasms in various muscles, has been afforded by Lundborg, 1913, who described 2,232 individuals in seven generations. The disease is inherited as a Mendelian recessive. Myotonic distrophy, waste of muscles owing to nervous defect, takes on various forms which are apt to be found to be repeated in families where an attempt is made to trace them. Hereditary tremors have been described in animals, as for example by Riddle in pigeons, where 46 affected individuals occurred in a particular strain. Large pedigrees have been secured for human families by a number of authors. Finally small muscular deviation, such as produce face dimples, show clear dependence upon hereditary factors.

Nervous System

Above all other systems of organs, the control of the nervous system by hereditary factors is of the greatest moment to human society and to the progress of civilization, for, the constitution of the nervous system, and its reactions to internal secretions and to other bodily conditions, determines conduct, behavior, and to a large extent the interaction of man on man and race on race. These hereditary nervous factors determine emotions and aspirations, and the control or absence of control of instincts and, consequently, the individual's fitness as a social being.

That the development of the brain with its accompanying intellectual capacity is determined by the absence of one or more factors that make for normal development has been shown again and again in the innumerable studies that have been made upon the feeble-minded. A great many families have been studied in which feeble-mindedness occurs in a high percentage of cases, and the results published by Goddard (Kalikaks), Danielson and Davenport (hill folk), Estabrook (Nam family and the Jukes), Finlayson (Dack family) and many others. Such strains with mental defect are particularly apt to be found in less highly developed communities, such as occur in some mountain valleys. The isolation in these parts is apt to lead to consanguineous marriages and in consequence, in such strains, to a large proportion of feeble-mindedness due to the same factor or factors. When both parents are feeble-minded, typically all of the children are feeble-minded also, though some exceptions occur where the feeble-mindedness is due to different types of defect.

Often associated with feeble-mindedness is the tendency toward epileptic convulsions of the degenerating type, a tendency which shows itself usually at adolescence. Studies of this subject have been published in the Eugenics Record Office Bulletin, 1911, and by Römer and by Hermann. In the typical institutional cases the epileptic symptoms seem to be due to the absence of a factor that makes for nervous control. Tendency to migraine has also a clear genetic factor in many cases, and there is a remarkable concurrence of it with epilepsy in certain families.

All types of functional insanity seem to depend upon genetical defects. Of these dementia præcox has been studied most carefully from a genetical point of view by Rüdin and co-workers. This depends apparently upon the absence of a genetical factor that prevents mental deterioration and schizophrenia following the incidence of mental assaults. While for many Freudians the exogenous factor is alone to be considered, yet the high incidence of dementia præcox in particular families and its entire absence in others not less well protected from such untoward conditions demonstrates that the constitution of the individual must also be considered.

In case of depressive insanity it is probable that more than one factor is involved. There is reason for thinking that the lack of control which shows itself in great emotional output and excitability under comparatively slight stimulus is partly due to the presence of some genetical factor which inhibits self-control, while depressions are due partly to the absence of certain genetical factors that are essential to calmness under ordinary circumstances. Again, the tendency to dipsomania, nymphomania, pyromania, and the other obsessive neuroses, seem to be due to the absence of particular genetical factors responsible for control. Dipsomania seems to be dependent upon a sex-linked factor shown only by males, but transmitted through daughters. In studies on crime we are apt to look exclusively to exogenous factors, such as bad companions. A broad view of the matter requires us to consider also the constitutional factors in which certain individuals find agreeable the stimulus derived from such bad associations. In crime we must look not only at the conditions under which it was performed, but also to the nature of the individual whose behavior was so bad. In the case of the nomadic trait, which is found in vagrants, as well as sometimes in persons of wealth and culture, there is much evidence that this is inherited as a sex-linked trait (Bulletin, Eugenics Record Office, No. 12, 1915).

Among the more strictly nervous diseases the history of Huntington's chorea has been, perhaps, more completely worked out than any other. It has been possible to trace this disease in certain of our families through ten generations, and to show the way in which the germ plasm carrying the defect has migrated from Southern New England and Long Island to upper New York State, Vermont, Ohio, Michigan, Wisconsin, Kansas, Nebraska, California, Oregon, and other parts of the United States (Bulletin, Eugenics Record Office, No. 17, 1916).

It is impossible in available space to go into details concerning all of the nervous diseases which have a genetical basis. Speech defects, such as stuttering and stammering, have been shown by Bryant, Estabrook and others to recur in strikingly high incidence in particular families. Numerous paralyses of special organs, some of which have been referred to in the chapters on "Muscular System" have repeatedly been shown to have hereditary bases.

That tendency to self-destruction has a genetical basis is sufficiently demonstrated by the tendency to recurrence in particular families, and even, in them, of a particular type. This matter has been discussed by Davenport in Carnegie Institution Publication No. 236. Sometimes the tendency to suicide is a strong impulse, generally associated with manic temperament, and is thus of the type of a dominant trait. In other cases the suicide occurs in deep depression, and such depressions are associated with a recessive condition, as mentioned above.

Not only those abnormalities in the nervous system and its output which society regards as defects, but also those other nervous and mental peculiarities, which are commonly spoken of as special gifts, show the hereditary factor. Though this is not a matter primarily of medical interest, still attention may be called, in passing, to the evidence of inheritance in the factors that make great fighters, great mathematicians, great musicians, great writers, painters, explorers, missionaries, clergy, physicians and the rest.

Sense Organs

The eye is subject to scores of defects in the course of its development, and the hereditary recurrence in particular families of these defects has long attracted the attention of ophthalmologists. The most recent bibliography of these defects is that prepared by the late Lucien Howe, published as Bulletin No. 21 of the Eugenics Record Office. The list indicates which of these are inherited as dominant, which are recessive, and which are sex-linked. Of course, the method of inheritance of many of these traits is more complex, depending on two or more factors. Great advances in our knowledge of inheritance of eye defects have been made by A. Vogt of Zürich, and findings in this field have been summarized recently by P. J. Waardenburg.

Ever since Alexander Graham Bell published his "Deaf Variety of the Human Race" (Memoir of the National Academy of Sciences, 1883), it has been clear that certain forms of deafness depend upon hereditary factors. However, deafness is not a biological entity, but only a symptom. It may depend upon various genetical factors. The genetical background probably is often complex. It is necessary to distinguish sporadic congenital deafness and deafness occasioned by syphilis. The latter is of the nature of an accident, while the former depends upon genes. One type of deafness, otosclerosis, is primarily a bone defect, but functionally belongs to the present category. Otosclerosis, or progressive hereditary hardness of hearing, is due to abnormal osteogenic changes in the otic capsule and the margins of the fenestra ovalis (which is closed by the base of the stapes), so that the stapes is firmly ankylosed in such fashion that vibrations are no longer conducted by the auditory ossicles, but better directly through the bones of the head. Genetic factors in otosclerosis have been recently studied through support from the Otosclerosis Committee of the American Otological Society by C. B. Davenport, Bess Lloyd Milles, and Lillian B. Frink, whose results appear in the Archives of Otolaryngology, 1933. Heredity is complex, depending on two or possibly more pairs of factors.

Idiosyncracies of taste have been discovered recently and found to have a hereditary basis, by Snyder and by Blakeslee, (both 1931). For example, phenyl-thio-carbamide gives a bitter sensation in some human strains, in others none at all.

Alimentary System

Within the last few years evidence has accumulated of the familial basis of some of the defects in the food canal and its adnexa. Very obvious is the recurrence of inheritance of harelip and cleft palate in families. The inheritance, however, is complex. This matter has been well analyzed by J. Sanders (1934); dominant inheritance has been found through twelve or more generations.

Numerous studies have shown that there is a genetical basis for gastric and duodenal ulcers. A hypersensibility of the intestinal mucosa to chemical and mechanical irritation has been described by Jüngling (1928). The tendency to production of gall stones is also one which depends upon a hereditary chemical constitution.

Respiratory System

That there are hereditary, or racial, factors present in the mucous membranes of the nasopharynx there can be no doubt. Indeed, Undritz (1928) concludes that inheritance is the rule rather than the exception in oto-rhino-laryngological diseases. It is notorious that among colored persons there is a relative resistance to diseases that enter the body through the nasopharyngeal portals, which are so ill defended among whites. Adenoids, tonsillitis and diphtheria are much less common in our colored population than in whites, despite the superior sanitation, on the whole, of the latter race in this country.

In respect to the pneumonias it is clear that their onset is due to a reduction in bodily resistance. In different human strains there is much variation in this natural immunity, and one finds, as Pearl has demonstrated, that tendency to pneumonia is a familial tendency. To be sure, both conditions of life preceding the disease and age play an important part in the incidence of pneumonia, but back of all of these is the variability in ability to resist the multiplication of the pneumococcus germs.

Circulatory System

The heart and blood vessels, the blood itself, are all markedly under the control of hereditary factors. There have been described families where the children, at birth, are more or less cyanotic, with imperfect development of the valves of the heart. A case is described by O. Bourwinkel (1910). There is reason for believing that a tendency toward degeneration of the walls of the arteries, as well as hypertension, depend upon constitutional factors. A chapter on heredity of arteriosclerosis has been published in a book on that subject by the Josiah Macy, Jr. Foundation.

Hemophilia, which depends upon the absence of the enzyme largely responsible for the production of the clotting elements of the blood, has been shown repeatedly to run in families in a sex-linked fashion. One may conclude that the enzyme responsible for this clotting is in this sex chromosome. In affected families the males alone show the condition, but do not transmit it to their sons, as they transmit no sex chromosomes to the sons, but they do transmit the affected chromosomes to their daughters, who show no symptoms, and these daughters may transmit the defect to their sons.

Variations in the elements of the blood stream are numerous, and some of these have been shown to have a hereditary basis. The inheritance of tendency toward leukemia, or a great excess of the white blood corpuscles, has been already described. Families with pernicious anemia have been described by O. Schaumann, (1918), and other Scandinavian authors. Similarly, polycythemia has been traced through generations by E. Engelking, (1920).

Summary

The above review of diseases and defects shows sufficiently that the hereditary factors present must always be looked for, even though these diseases may never occur without the presence of a particular microörganism, for the microörganisms can not be regarded as the sole and effective cause of these diseases or defects. We must believe that the constitutional factors prepare the soil, and the nature of the soil determines the nature of the harvest, that is, the symptoms, which the seed sown upon it will produce. The medical man, who neglects in his consideration of diseases and defects the genetical factors, will never succeed completely in accounting for the phenomena with which he has to deal. Heredity is not something occasional and special. Heredity determines the very nature of the organism, both the normal organism and the organism that deviates from the normal. Only pathologists who are willing to admit that there is a disease apart from the diseased organism can decline to consider the man as well as the parasite that is one of the factors in producing disease.

III. APPLIED EUGENICS

Now that we know that the development of the physical, mental and emotional traits of man, his resistance to disease and his normal functioning are determined very largely by heredity, it follows that reasonable human beings should act in accordance with this knowledge. Our social difficulties are largely due to the presence in our population of feeble-minded, or paranoiacs, of those lacking social instincts, of those with little control over the emotions. Our present methods of dealing with these social disturbers are various. In a primitive society we may punish, scorn, or pity the individuals, according to our individual nature, but these reactions do little to solve our problem. More effective is the segregation of such persons for a longer or shorter period, but it is the custom eventually to return such segregated individuals after some years of training to the community. Since their constitution has, however, not been altered they will tend to return to their anti-social conduct. By releasing segregated individuals at a time when the reproduction urge is strong we permit the reproduction of their traits.

An appreciation of the danger of reproducing inherently defective germ plasm has led many of our states, and other countries, to attempt to exercise some control over this reproduction. All states have, indeed, recognized their right and duty to attempt to control matings. Thus we have laws against the mating of the feeble-minded, epileptic, insane, of cousins, and of inter-marriage between different races (Eugenics Record Office Bulletin No. 9). These laws have, however, primarily a legal import rather than a eugenic one, and moreover they are inadequately enforced. Something could be done to improve present conditions, if a greater control were exercised over matings by parents, or older persons, as is done more satisfactorily in other countries than in ours. In the absence of other adequate control of matings many states have found it advantageous to put on the statute books laws permitting sterilization of the genetically defective. Over one-half of the states of the Union have had such laws in the past; at present about twenty-two of the states carry them. Of all these states, California has performed more sterilizations than any other. Up to 1929, indeed, 6,225 sterilizations had been performed in the California State Hospitals, and 1,488 in institutions for the feeble-minded. In Canada, Switzerland, Denmark, Germany, and some other countries, sterilization laws are in effect. There has been some question as to the social consequences of the releasing into the general population of sterilized individuals. The evidence, however, indicates that such sterilized persons do not become the focus of immorality. The whole social aspect of sterilization is treated adequately by E. S. Gosney and Paul Popenoe in their book "Sterilization for Human Betterment," (1929). Statistics concerning sterilization in different states have been published by H. H. Laughlin in Eugenics Record Office Bulletins, and elsewhere, and sterilization is more and more becoming recognized not as a punitive but as a eugenic measure.

The prohibition of marriages between cousins has been placed upon the statute books of over one-third of the states in the Union (Eugenics Record Office Bulletin No. 9, 1913). Apparently the laws have been thus passed because of the experience of legislators with particular cases in which defective offspring have arisen from such close matings. Such legislation does not seem to be in accord with our present biological knowledge. It has now been demonstrated by geneticists, that cousin marriage per se does not lead to defective offspring. However, on the one hand it increases the incidence of defective offspring, where there is gross recessive defect in the common stock, as for example, feeble-mindedness, epilepsy and other types of insanity. On the other hand, cousin marriage is a very valuable means of perpetuating and even increasing the general developmental vigor of the children where the common stock is without such gross defect. The case of Charles Darwin, who married his first cousin, Emma Wedgwood, and produced five sons who became leaders in science, invention, and economics in Great Britain, is a case in point. The remarkable group of Walcotts and their kin, in Connecticut, which furnished a long line of Governors of the state of Connecticut, were the product of cousin marriages. To make use of our knowledge of genetics in such legislation, it were better to provide that a marriage between cousins should not be permitted without a certificate from a state Eugenics Board, after an examination of the pedigree, to make sure that there is no gross hereditary defect in the common stock.

Since the health and happiness of the United States depend so much upon the predominance of the physically, mentally and emotionally fit stock, the state may well inquire into the relative fertility of the most effective and the least effective strains. At this time throughout civilized countries, and particularly in America, through voluntary limitation of the size of families, the most successful stock is not reproducing itself in anything like the proportion of the less successful stock. The sons of Harvard University have only about 0.8 of a son, on the average, while the daughters of Wellesley have even a smaller proportion of daughters. Into a population which is strictly not reproducing itself there has entered a strong propaganda for the dissemination of "birth control" information. Were it possible through the spread of such information to diminish the relatively greater fertility of the less effective stock, the propaganda would be biologically advantageous. The birth controllist, however, early found that the less effective and thrifty stratum did not respond to the propaganda for reduction in size of families; for the parents in such stratum each child was regarded as an economic asset. The birth controllists thereupon carried their propaganda into the higher social stratum, which was already reducing the size of families to a minimum, with the idea that, were their teachings effective in the higher levels, a fashion would become established which would become adopted in the lower levels. There is, however, as yet no satisfactory evidence that the propaganda is working out in any other way than to encourage the more thrifty to diminish still further the number of their children. Thus, it may well be that the birth control propaganda in this country is diminishing the proportion of the more effective children born. It would seem desirable rather to encourage the more effective stock to have larger families than to extend more widely the principles of restriction of reproduction. Such stimulus might be given on the one hand by appealing to higher ideals and, on the other, in economic ways, by reducing taxation and inheritance levies in proportion to the number of children in the family.

A predominance of the fit will not be maintained merely by increasing the number of offspring but also by increasing the number who survive to marry, and in turn become progenitors. An intelligent society will, therefore, do its utmost to encourage the survival of its fittest strains and will be more concerned therein than in securing the survival of the children of inferior strains. The appeal sometimes made by social workers for funds to diminish the mortality rate of children of lowest social and intellectual level may well fail to arouse enthusiastic response.

Control of matings and of fertility is only part of the problem of securing the highest proportion of effective persons in the population. Until recent years the matter of immigration has been of importance in connection with this aim. In the early years of our immigration there was little selection of immigrants, and it was possible for European countries to exile to the United States those convicted of minor offenses and even sometimes of important crimes. Also, attempts were made to bring large numbers of the cheapest labor from Europe, and even from Asia, to help develop our resources. Importation from Asia was early put a stop to. Only recently has a marked restriction been made on immigration from the lowest economic stratum of Europe. Today we exclude the feeble-minded and the criminalistic. For the moment the whole problem of immigration to the United States has become less important, owing to the fact that the United States has become an old country and is already well filled. Our resources have become more than adequately exploited, so that the country offers less lure to the prospective immigrant. At the same time the opening of large areas in South America and the better economic outlook there is diverting the stream from the United States to that continent. If, and when, the immigration tide sets again towards North America, it is to be hoped that an adequate selection will be made of such immigrants to insure the highest possible quality of our future citizenship.

Recognition of the fact of heredity does not render unnecessary efforts that have been made toward education and moral and religious culture. Even plants, to yield their best fruit, must be cultivated, and the innate good traits of children may be repressed by a "bad" environment. Eugenics, however, teaches that it is as futile to try to train the feeble-minded boy to be a scholar as it is to try by cultivation to make a golden bantam variety of corn into a giant. Our efforts toward education will be more effective when we recognize first that children are all different, and when we seek, secondly, to develop to the utmost those germs of desirable traits that they possess, and, thirdly, to repress undesirable tendencies. So also in matters of health the physician must recognize that all of his patients are different, and he must urge, therefore, different hygienic training in accordance with individual needs. It is sometimes said that eugenics is a medical matter, and so it is, indeed, but it is also a social matter of the highest import. It is for physicians and those interested in social welfare and social development to unite in applying the principles of eugenics to the advancement of the State.

The facts of heredity may be well called upon to aid in certain legal procedures, especially in determination of disputed paternity. Insofar as the laws of inheritance of traits have become definitely established, they can be utilized to advantage in such disputed cases. For example, the established principle that two parents, both of whom produce no melanic pigment in their irides can have only children with the same trait, may be used to decide matters of disputed parentage, or to decide whether a given claimant for an estate, on the ground of relationship to his alleged parents, has a just claim. Valuable in this connection is the fact of inheritance of the factors that cause iso-agglutination of the blood. It appears that the red blood cells of many persons produce an enzyme called "agglutinogen," which leads to the production in the serum of the blood of corresponding "agglutinins." The commonest of the agglutinogens that are known are designated as A, B, and the corresponding agglutinins in the serum are designated as a, b. If now the blood of a person, who carries in the cells agglutinogen A, be mixed with the serum from a person with agglutinogen B and, therefore, with the agglutinin b, then the blood cells derived from this individual tend to clump in the drop. On this account it is important, in the case of blood transfusions, to secure a donor of the same blood group as the person into whose veins the blood is to be injected; otherwise agglutination will occur, and through consequent blocking of the blood vessels serious effects, and even death, may follow. Besides the two types of persons who produce agglutinogens A or B there is a third type that produces both agglutinogens A and B and corresponding agglutinins a and b. Finally, there is a fourth group which produces no agglutinogens. Such persons can receive infusion with impunity. Now, if a given child belongs to the group with agglutinogen A in the blood, and its known parent belongs to the group which produces agglutinogen B, then it must be that the other parent belongs to the group which produces agglutinogen A, or to the group that produces the two agglutinogens A and B. Similarly, a child that produces agglutinogen B and whose known parent produces only agglutinogen A, or produces no agglutinogen, must have had as its other parent one belonging to the group of B, or A B. The table describing all the possibilities for the unknown parent of disputed children with particular blood groups is given in treatises treating of the blood groups of which may be mentioned that of L. H. Snyder.

The facts of heredity may be advantageously used in other matters of social importance, such as giving advice in respect to the choice of a profession. Specifically, we may answer the question whether a given boy would probably succeed as a physician or surgeon. It is necessary before such advice can be given to consider the distribution in the family tree of high degree of success in the given profession. We do not know just how the different traits, which are responsible for success in a given profession, are inherited. We do know, however, that in some cases, as in medicine and surgery, striking cases of outstanding success in three, four, or more, generations are known. This would seem to suggest that there is at least one essential factor in such success which is inherited as a dominant trait.

To the psychiatrist a knowledge of family history of patients is of vast importance, and this fact is so generally known that family histories are now regularly taken in the best developed institutions. The late Dr. E. E. Southard, of Boston, stated that he would hardly diagnose with confidence a case of manic depressive insanity whose family history showed no other individuals who might fall into the same category. It is important, however, that the psychiatrist should not depend for knowledge of the family merely upon testimony of relatives who accompany the patient to the hospital, since for social reasons such relatives tend to minimize the importance of the genetical factor, and to cover up striking cases of similar defect in the family. Accordingly, many institutions find it advantageous to employ field workers who can be sent to the homes from which the patients come, in order to make first hand observations and inquiries concerning the traits of other members of the family.

Instead, as is so often done, of regarding heredity as a dour doctrine and one whose conclusions are fatalistic and opposed to the program of human improvement that is being promoted by sociologists and physicians, it were better to look upon heredity as a power for social regeneration of the first importance. Every farmer recognizes the incalculable value of heredity in the production of his best stocks. He controls his matings with the greatest care, since he knows that the value of the next generation will depend upon such matings. It is to be hoped that in time, in civilized countries, it will be appreciated that the future of the country depends especially on the quality of the germ-cells that are being transmitted to future generations. If these germ-cells determine the development of individuals of the highest quality, they become invaluable. One sees vast sums, amounting to even hundreds of thousands of dollars, that are spent for particular animals, such as the horse or the bull, to be used for breeding purposes. The money is not spent for muscle or bone, but for the literally microscopic enzymes that are carried in the germ cells. If all the enzymes that were used in reproduction should be brought together, they would still be beyond the limits of visibility or of weighing. For the possession of such invisible materials persons are willing to stake a fortune. If the enzymes for successful race horses, or for great milk producing cows are of such value, how much more should we treasure the germ-plasm in our population that is responsible for the most valuable social qualities.

July 1, 1934.

CHAPTER XII–A

ALBINISM

By FREDERICK R. TAYLOR

TABLE OF CONTENTS

Synonyms. — Albinismus, congenital leukopathia, congenital leukoderma, congenital leukasmus, congenital achromia, dyschroia, moon-eyes, children of the sun (Guatemala).

Definition. — Albinism is a congenital condition which, in its complete form, is characterized by a total lack of the melanin group of pigments in the body, its striking features in man being a lack of pigment in the skin, hair and eyes, with resulting photophobia, nystagmus, high-grade refractive errors and extreme susceptibility of the skin to strong sunlight and other potent sources of ultra-violet radiation. Other body pigments, not included in the melanin group, such as lipochromes, urochromes, blood and bile pigments, etc., are present. Incomplete and partial forms of albinism occur. Albinism is found widely distributed throughout the animal kingdom, and an analagous condition due to absence of plant pigments occurs in the vegetable world.

HISTORY

While albinism has doubtless existed from a very early period in the life of man, references to it in ancient literature seem surprisingly scant for such a striking condition. Lagleyze of Buenos Aires, who probably has given the most exhaustive discussion of the subject in the literature, states that a passage in the Elder Pliny's writings seems to indicate that he had seen a case of albinism, and that Hernando Cortes is said to have mentioned albinos at the court of Montezuma. There seems to have been little general scientific interest in albinism, however, before the 18th century, when many accounts of the condition by various travelers appeared, notably the early explorers in Africa, who reported albinism in Guinea, Algeria, Madagascar and along the Congo. Lagleyze tells us that in 1704 Wafer described albinos in Panama. Apparently albinism was not generally recognized in the white race until very recent times, for Lagleyze says that in 1774 DePaul stated that albinism did not exist in Europe and that it was found only within ten degrees of the equator. However, ten years later Blumenbach described some albinos at Chamonix in the Alps and apparently was the first to attribute the red light in the pupil and the apparent color of the iris to their true cause. During the past century albinism has been reported in all races from practically all parts of the world, though its frequency varies greatly in different localities.

Of special interest to the ethnologist are the varying attitudes of primitive peoples towards albinos. Often persecuted or killed, albinos have been objects of veneration in some places, especially where they are rare. Certain negro tribes represent the devil as having a white skin. In Guinea albinos have been considered sacred and invulnerable, in Senegambia, as possessed of evil spirits, in Uganda they were wondered at as curiosities and kept about the kings. According to Lagleyze on the island of Parrot in the mouth of the Calabar River in West Africa, the natives sacrificed an albino child to the god of the whites when no European merchant ship had called in a long time.

Among many interesting primitive beliefs regarding albinos may be noted the following: that they are born of women impregnated by gorillas; that they are born of women who, while asleep in the forest, were impregnated by meteors; that the morning star is the father of all albinos; that the devil is their real father.

Lagleyze quotes Dubois as stating that in certain parts of India the natives used to draw and quarter albinos and throw their bodies on manure piles or to ferocious beasts.

Etiology and Pathogenesis

Little is known of the etiology of albinism other than that it is a congenital defect in the mechanism which gives rise to the melanin group of pigments in the body. For many years a battle raged over the question of the etiologic significance of heredity, many authorities denying its influence, but the weight of opinion today regards albinism as a Mendelian recessive characteristic. Mudge, Jablonski, Pardo-Castello and Musser, among others, definitely subscribe to this view. Musser explains the relative rarity of albinism by the fact that the health of albinos usually is poor, and they often die without propagating. Swab records the case of a white man who married a negress; they had a black daughter; when she became 15 years old, her father had incestuous relations with her, and an idiot albino resulted. Wakefield and Dellinger have described a pair of albino identical twins of negro parentage. A view formerly held, that albinism represents an atavistic reversion to a special race of albinos, has been practically abandoned. Consanguinity in the parents seems to predispose somewhat to albinism. Lagleyze studied 27 albinos in 13 families; among these 13 albinos in 5 families had consanguineous parents. The 27 comprised the total number of albinos he had seen among 30,000 patients. In no case did an albino child have an albino parent. In addition to his own cases, Lagleyze studied the data on 48 families in the literature, with 220 children, 104 of whom were albinos. In 10 of these families the parents were stated to be consanguineous without mention of albinotic heredity, in 7 albinism was reported in collateral antecedents, in 5 there was no mention of familial factors.

Garrod suggests three possibilities to explain the pathogenesis of albinism, as follows: (1) a structural peculiarity of the cells which renders them incapable of pigmentation; (2) an absence of the material from which melanin is formed; (3) the lack of a specific enzyme which brings about the formation of melanin.

A number of observations seem to support the last hypothesis at the expense of the first two, among which are the following.

Mudge noted that in albino rats immersion in formalin turned the hairs a vivid yellow. Subsequent immersion in hydrogen peroxide turned them a brownish color. He believes that this proves the presence of a chromogen and indicates the absence of a ferment in albinism that normally converts the chromogen into pigment. He quotes Cuenot as suggesting that the pigmentation of mammalian hair is due to the interaction of a chromogen and a ferment. He also cites the work of Miss Durham, who extracted in water from the skins of young rodents a material which, when incubated with tyrosin to which a small quantity of ferrous sulphate had been added as an activator, threw down a pigment of the same color as that of the hair growing out of that particular portion of skin. Mudge also notes that breeding experiments show that albinos carry some pigment factors. Mudge's findings were confirmed by Sollas. Schultz showed that a piece of albinotic rabbit skin containing growing hair, when kept for from seven to twelve hours under certain conditions of moisture and oxygen at a temperature of from 30° to 36° C., would develop a strong melanin pigment at the hair roots. By a similar method the iris of a newborn albino rabbit became pigmented.

Garrod calls attention to some interesting findings of several investigators as follows: Halliburton, Brodie and Pickering noted that intravenous injections of nucleoproteins in albino animals failed to produce such clotting as in pigmented ones. Mudge found that all albino rabbits were not alike in this respect, but that in general more nucleoprotein must be injected into albino animals to cause death from intravascular clotting than into similar pigmented controls. Pickering also noted that the Norway hare in its winter coat reacts like an albino when injected with nucleoprotein, whereas in summer it reacts like any other pigmented animal. Bickel and Tasawa found that exposure for several weeks to a bright light increased the red cell count in pigmented animals but did not do so to any appreciable degree in albinos.

Symptomatology

Complete albinism presents the following symptoms and physical signs. The skin is milky white and looks thin and delicate. The superficial blood vessels are conspicuous. The hair is fine and almost white, of a very pale silvery flax color. The irides are untinted and appear red, pink or violet according to the intensity of the light by which they are seen, looking red in a very strong light and violet in a very subdued one. There is a red pupil reflex due to the lack of pigmentation within the eyes, which resemble those of a white rabbit. Because of the lack of protective pigment in the eyes, photophobia is marked, and nystagmus is an almost constant finding. The latter usually develops in early infancy, though occasionally it is present at birth. As a rule, it is horizontal, rapid and of wide excursion, though rotary and mixed forms have been described. Lagleyze explains the nystagmus as an effort of the eyes to escape from the irritating light. The nasal side of the eye being more shaded than the temporal, the eyes move back and forth in an effort to relieve the points of momentary maximum irritation.

The extreme photophobia develops a characteristic attitude and facies in which the head is bent forward, the eyes are kept partially closed, there is a constant frown, and in a strong light the patient will nearly always shield his eyes with a hand as with a vizor, unless they are suitably protected. The pressure on the eyeballs from the contracting muscles is considerable, and this soon gives rise to a high degree of refractive error, which may be hyperopic or myopic, and is always complicated by a very marked astigmatism. Chronic blepharitis naturally is the rule. In addition the visual acuity becomes markedly reduced and usually is found to be from $\frac{1}{6}$ to $\frac{1}{10}$ of the normal. This is a true amblyopia which remains after refractive correction. All these phenomena tend to make the albino look abnormally old. Often the optic discs appear about the same color as the rest of the eyegrounds, which are, of course, pale and can be found only by locating the entrance and exit of the retinal vessels. In other cases they may appear a deep red or an ashy gray. Color vision and the visual fields are unaffected. Lagleyze has noted persistence of the pupillary membrane in a few albinos and states that he has not seen it in non-albinos. Concomitant strabismus often occurs in albinism. Shaad noted that albinos adapt their vision to relative darkness less rapidly than normal persons, but their vision became more sensitive in the dark after 10 minutes than that of normal controls and remained so throughout the remainder of a 30 minute test. The name "moon-eyes", sometimes applied to albinos, is based on the fact that they can see better by moonlight than by bright daylight.

Intelligence is unaffected by albinism. All grades of intelligence from idiocy to brilliance have been noted, as in non-albinos.

The skin will not tan in the sun and is very susceptible to sunburn and irritation from other types of ultra-violet radiation. Garrod states that melanotic tumors do not occur in the albino, and that there is no record of an albino with Addison's disease. The hyperpigmented areas usual in pregnancy do not appear in albino women. Hewer reports three cases of multiple epitheliomata in Egyptian albinos which he considers due to the action of the sun's rays on the unpigmented skin.

A number of associated anomalies have been noted in individual albinos, but these probably are to be looked on as coincidental, rather than as bearing any relation to the albinism. The writer has studied a case of albinism in a young woman, a virgin, who had, in addition to a severe dysmenorrhea, a practically complete congenital absence of the muscles of the pelvic floor, the vaginorectal septum being almost as thin as paper.

Albinism may be classified as *complete*, *incomplete* and *partial*. The *complete* form has been discussed. *Incomplete albinism* is a condition in which there is a general deficiency, but not complete absence of the melanin pigments. There are all grades of this, with corresponding degrees of severity of symptoms.

In *partial albinism* there are contrasting albinotic and normal areas throughout the body. If an eye is in an albinotic area, it will be affected, otherwise it will not. Only a portion of an eye may be involved. Hair growing out of albinotic areas is devoid of pigment, that growing out of normal areas has the normal color. A number of instances of red haired albinos have been recorded. Garrod states that the pigment may be present in the eyes alone, in which case the other ocular phenomena of albinism are likely to be absent. Squire reported the case of an albino, whose entire skin and hair system were pigmentless, but whose eyes were dark blue, who had no photophobia, but who did have horizontal nystagmus, so that he had difficulty in reading, though his visual acuity was normal.

A piebald appearance often occurs in partial albinism and probably represents a mosaic inheritance. Pardo-Castello regarded all such cases as probably achromic nevi. Traub, however, has given us a differential criterion, viz., that piebald albinotic areas become hyperemic on friction with ice, whereas achromic nevi do not. Firth has made the interesting observation that individual red hairs from the scalp of a black haired African showed the same characters as the hairs do in red haired albinos.

Diagnosis

Diagnosis of albinism usually is obvious on inspection. Occasionally partial albinism may have to be differentiated from achromic nevi by Traub's method as described above. Vitiligo is distinguished from partial albinism by the fact that it is an acquired condition, whereas partial albinism is congenital.

Prognosis and Treatment

Garrod states that albinos occasionally may acquire pigmentation in childhood or early life. The condition usually is permanent, however. Poor health due to the eyestrain and to various other associated conditions often occurs, so that the life expectancy of an albino probably is less than that of a normal person of the same age.

Treatment is largely a matter for the ophthalmologist, who must be consulted for protection of the eyes from light and for proper refraction. The piebald cases may benefit from dermatologic advice, as certain stains have been devised for use on the pigmentless areas for cosmetic purposes. In such cases the recently introduced "Covermark" also might prove helpful. Strong light should be avoided and special precautions taken against sunburn. Exposure of the body to other forms of potent ultra-violet radiation also is contraindicated.

BIBLIOGRAPHY

FIRTH, D.: Red-headed albinos, Proc. Roy. Soc. Med., 1924, (Clin. Sect.), XVII, 25.

FOLKER, W. H.: Case of a remarkable albino, Lancet, 1879, I, 795.

GARROD, A. E.: Inborn Errors of Metabolism, p. 30, 2nd ed., Henry Frowde and Hodder and Stoughton, Lond., 1923.

GOULD, G. M.: The pernicious influence of albinism upon the eye, Jour. Am. Med. Assoc., 1893, XXI, 685.

GUNN, A. R.: Albinism in man, Brit. Med. Jour., 1907, I, 718.

HEISER, V. G. and VILLAFRANCA, R.: Albinism in Philippine Islands, Philippine Jour. Sci., 1913, VIII, 493.

HEWER, T. F.: Multiple epitheliomata in albino, Brit. Jour. Dermat. and Syph., 1932, XLIV, 469.

JABLONSKI, W.: Ueber Albinismus des Auges im Zusammenhang mit den Vererbungsregeln, Deutsch. med. Wchnschr., 1920, XLVI, 708.

LAGLEYZE: L'œil des albins, Arch. d'Opht., 1907, XXVII, 280, 361, 461.

McLEOD, J. M. H.: Complete albinism in a girl aged 6, with total absence of pigment in the skin, hair, choroid and iris, Proc. Roy. Soc. Med., 1910–11, IV, Dermat. Sect., 7.

MUDGE, G. P.: Problems in Mendelism and some biological considerations: human albinos, Lancet, 1909, I, 857; Jour. Physiol., 1909, XXXVIII, (Proc. Physiol. Soc., March 27, 1909, p. lxvii).

MUSSER, J. H., Jr.: Albinism in the negro, Med. Clin., North America, 1924, VIII, 781.

PARDO–CASTELLO, V.: Congenital partial albinism, Arch. Dermat. and Syph., 1926, XIV, 173.

RILLE: Zwei Bruder mit Albinismus Totalis Congenitus, Münch. med. Wchnschr., 1908, LV, 592.

SCHULTZ, W.: Kältepigmentierung von Albinohaar und -auge im Regensglase. Genetische Physiologie, Pflüger's Arch. f. d. ges. Physiol., 1929, CCXXI, 386.

SHAAD, D. J.: Dark adaptation in albinotic eye, Arch. Ophth., 1933, IX, 179.

SQUIRE, A. J. B.: An atypical albino, Lancet, 1895, I, 282.

STIVEN, H. E. S.: A Sudanese albino, Lancet, 1923, I, 648.

WAKEFIELD, E. G. and DELLINGER, S. C.: Identical albino twins of negro parents, Ann. Int. Med., 1936, IX, 1149.

Sept. 1, 1937

CHAPTER XIII

ADOLESCENCE

By WILLIAM PALMER LUCAS

TABLE OF CONTENTS

INTRODUCTION

THE adolescent period represents the second most rapid period of growth in a child's development. From the anatomical standpoint, this period does not represent as rapid a growth as the period of infancy, but the significance of its anatomical, psychological, and physiological development is greater than at any other period of growth. During this period certain finalities along the lines referred to are definitely established. At the same time the period covered by adolescence is a "fluid" one; the finalities established when adult life is reached have passed through various phases of development. The very character of this period of adolescence, therefore, demands a most careful analysis of the different stages of the development. But more than that, it demands also of the study of medicine a more "fluid" attitude toward this field and a wider knowledge of the social experience through which a child passes during the stage of development. A sympathetic appreciation of the child's world is absolutely necessary if the changing phases of this period are to be intelligently related to the whole field of medicine. The study of the adolescent period is therefore a study of constant changes, and the relation of these changes to each other and to the whole development, is the effort attempted here.

Growth Changes of the Adolescent Period

General Body Growth

The accepted opinions on this subject recognize the so-called time element which must be considered; i.e. the fact that growth, as it takes place at any given period, is a variable. Growth proceeds in curves rather than in straight lines during any period, and the very waves of the curves vary in height and width. Thus during the period of adolescence growth must be considered from the particular part under observation rather than from the general standpoint. Space permits of discussing only the main points of growth during this period. The size of the skull remains practically the same, any slight change being relative to the growth of other parts of the bony structure, such as the increased lengthening of the face by the growth of the jaw bone.

A marked difference takes place in the chest during the adolescent period; the growth takes place laterally and we have increased width in the chest cavities rather than any marked increase in depth. The long bones of the body increase rapidly in growth, and here the growth curves vary at different times during the period, and in the two sexes differences in the time element have been noted. The final attachment of the epiphyses that have not already ossified takes place during this period. The final rounding out of the muscular system is the "normal" muscle limit of this period. This long bone and muscle development of the adolescent period bears an immediate relation to several of the most common characteristics of the so-called "awkward age." When the bones grow more rapidly than the muscles, we often have the "growing pains" of adolescence as the physical result. Also this rapid growth of bone without the muscular development to uphold the bony structure results in poor posture for the child, with far-reaching results of such abnormality.

When the muscles grow faster than the bones, the joints are loose and this often accounts for the ungainly habits of the adolescent child. The clumsiness noted in the child, whose earlier muscular skill had been marked, is often caused by the rapid growth of the large muscles employed in the finer, more detailed use, say of one's hands. Take the emphasis placed upon the piano lessons of the small child. The finer muscles are developed then—if this were not so, they would lose their chance for development during the adolescent period, as that period is mainly devoted to the development of the large fundamental muscles. The end of the adolescent period has, in the main, usually established the final bony structures. Both the shoulder and pelvic girdles in boys and girls develop rapidly during the period. The pelvic development in both male and female is the most clearly defined in the adolescent period, the female pelvis becoming broader horizontally than the male, and parallels in its development the growth of the generative organs. The male pelvis becomes more fixed than the female, as the complete ossification of the female pelvis is deferred to a later period. This is a most important point in the problems of attending maternity.

Finally, within certain broad limits, the appearance and development of metacarpal bones is of value in estimating the different periods of development. This metacarpal development, however, cannot be used as an absolute gauge, either physiologically or chronologically, for any definite age. The rapid increase in height, which includes not only the more rapid development of the extremities but also the slower but gradual lengthening of the trunk, is the essential index of development during the adolescent period. The child should be taught to be proud of his height and not allowed to develop bad posture, which only increases his awkwardness and often leads to permanent deformities, such as scoliosis.

Growth of the Heart

The heart develops rapidly during the period of adolescence. The increase in size and strength is marked, the volume of the heart increasing from 160 to 225 cubic centimeters. This is not only a growth in the size of the contractile fibers but also in the number of fibers. Before puberty, the blood vessels are large and the heart small. With the increase in the size of the heart this relation changes. The more rapid this adjustment between heart and arteries the sooner and more complete is the adolescent development. The general tendency during this period is for the rate of the heart to diminish and the strength of the individual contraction of the heart to increase, but there are many unaccountable variations in the heart rate and the forces of the cardiac impulse. These variations cause at times pronounced palpitation, at other times marked slowing down of the heart rate. This often causes alarm in the child, awakening, so to speak, a consciousness of his heart which he does not understand. These symptoms are very disquieting and often recur without an apparent cause. It is probably more exaggerated on over-exertion, such as muscle or nervous fatigue. This alarm should be sympathetically dealt with, by a simple explanation of this growth to the child, and a carefully planned regimen which avoids the state of over-fatigue of any kind. The disproportion between the general development and the development of the heart, which often accounts for these symptoms, can be demonstrated not only by physical examination but most graphically by radiography.

Growth of the Lungs

The vital capacity increases with the development of the chest. This development, as in the development of the heart, proceeds in curves rather than straight lines, and nothing affects its development more than proper breathing and correct posture. There has been a great deal said about this being the period of marked change in the breathing of the sexes; the boy maintains the more normal and abdominal breathing, the girl develops thoracic breathing. This is not a true sex difference, but is artificial and due to the radical change in dress between the sexes, as has been clearly demonstrated by Mosher ([1]). During the adolescent period, tuberculous affections of early childhood are likely to become active processes. The early infection of the bronchial glands extends to the lungs during this period of the direction of all surplus energy to growth. Hygiene and careful supervision of those who have had gland infection in earlier childhood is most important at this time to prevent this pulmonary extension. Excessive fatigue and acute infections are most important to avoid.

Growth of the Brain

The adolescent period is the most important one in the differentiation of the brain. At this time there are more active cells. The size of the brain and weight of the brain have reached their maximum in the pre-adolescent period, but adolescence marks the intensification of the differentiation of the fibers which represent the higher intellectual powers. The nervous system gives a clear illustration of regular and orderly growth. The higher centers depend on their development upon the growth of the lower centers. This development of the higher centers progresses rapidly during the adolescent period connecting the sensory and motor areas. This growth of association fibers is apparently stimulated by the appearance of our higher intellectual powers. During the adolescent period there is undoubtedly an increased stimulation in new centers. These centers are not limited to sensory or motor aspects, but undoubtedly have to do with the higher centers of volition and will. The inter-reaction of different centers causes development and growth of other centers, so that we have a number of different periods of growth, as it is true that certain fibers become medullated far earlier than others. During the adolescent period new interests and cravings appear and undoubtedly are related to the maturing of certain association centers.

Growth of the Larynx

The larynx grows rapidly at adolescence with quite a marked sex difference, the male growing larger than the female. All the cartilages are enlarged and the thyroid cartilage in the male becomes quite prominent and the glottis nearly doubles in length. This development of the larynx includes the development of the vocal cords, which lengthen and thicken; accounting thus for the change in voice, especially in boys, during this period. A boy's voice commonly breaks at this time and often becomes a full octave lower.

Growth of the Reproductive Organs

The first indication of the growth of these organs is found in the development of secondary sexual characteristics. Hair begins to appear in the pubic regions and the armpits of both boys and girls. In boys, there is a more marked increase in hair on the face, chest, abdomen, as well as all over the body. In girls, there is a marked rounding out of the hips and the development of the breasts. The reproductive organs, themselves, begin to develop in size. The penis and testes of boys show marked change in size as do the uterus and vagina in girls.

Physiological Development and Changes

.The foregoing general discussion of growth leads naturally to the consideration of the effect of growth upon the function of the organs of the body and the resultant physiological changes. At the time of the beginning of the development of the sex organs, we have the first fundamental appearance of the physiological activity of the gonad system or sex glands. This development is one of the most complex processes taking place in the body, because upon it is based the differentiation of the sexes and the power of normal reproduction in both. The development of the gonad system is intimately associated with the normal functioning of other internal glands. Any disturbance in the pituitary glands usually affects the normal development of the sex glands. Changes in the adrenal and thyroid glands also affect the normal functioning of the reproductive glands.

Closely paralleling the development of the internal secretions come the external signs of sex functioning, which at the beginning often cause great mental and nervous suffering. In boys, the appearance of nocturnal seminal emission is not at all regular, recurring at first at infrequent intervals and normally at the height of puberty, not oftener than once in ten days or two weeks. This emission is often accompanied by dreams. The semen is composed of a thick gelatinous secretion containing many active spermatozoa. Menstruation in girls occurs with greater regularity, the normal periodicity being twenty-four days. The duration of the flow varies in normal limit from two to five days. Under conditions of poor hygiene, both physical and mental, the menstrual function is very often disturbed, and this disturbance often produces the common pathological condition of amenorrhea and dysmenorrhea. In a few instances these conditions are undoubtedly due to derangement in the internal gland secretion, but by far the majority are due to improper hygiene.

Menstruation is undoubtedly influenced by the internal secretion of the ovaries. The thymus, the posterior lobe of the pituitary and the thyroid are also supposed to play a part in menstruation. There is undoubtedly a relation between the mammary glands, which become enlarged immediately before the menstrual period. During menstruation the uterus is markedly hyperemic and the flow of blood is the result of this normal condition. This blood contains varying numbers of endothelial cells from the uterus and epithelial cells from the vaginal tract. Changes in the skin occur constantly during this period. In girls the pigmentation is most pronounced in the areola of the nipple. The decided change in the complexion of both boys and girls is marked at this time. The sebaceous glands enlarge and become more easily infected and are responsible for the frequency of acne during adolescence. Blackheads are very common during this period, caused by the growth of the sebaceous glands and the pigmentation. Connected with the skin changes are the presence of characteristic body odors, which are more pronounced in girls during the menstrual period. Perspiration increases in both boys and girls. The activity of the salivary glands increases during this period. The spitting contests of the small boys are familiar to all. During the adolescent period the physiological changes in the organs of sense are on the whole slight. Sight and hearing are not affected. Smell and taste are slightly accentuated. The craving for sweets is a common symptom. The tactile sense may be increased or diminished.

Psychological Development and Changes

Adolescence is the period of great awakening and change both mentally and morally. The child passes from the "gang" stage to the stage of a larger group, society in general. He becomes more conscious of himself as an individual and that consciousness demands his own relation to others as well as to his environment. The desire to count as one and a part of the whole slowly overshadows the former contentment in acting merely in the "gang" spirit. This change cannot be tabulated. It is even more fluid than the physical change. The only wise method is the constant study of each phase as it presents itself. For the first time consciousness of dress appears in both boys and girls. Anything that seems to call attention to oneself is the most sought after, a tie of gay colors, a bizarre ornament worn at an unusual angle, all the many ways in which the individual may be marked by his kind. On the other hand, there may be periods of absolute personal neglect, arising from the same individual awakening and marking a stronger development: "to be in a group yet not of it, is an old standard of moral strength."

The actual mental caliber of boys and girls at this period may be equally baffling. Sometimes it is marked by precociousness in their mental processes. They may show a great power of assimilation in a subject that interests them; again they may be absolutely indifferent to any mental achievement and for the time being have lost interest in anything and everything that has to do with their mental development. These mental states are usually closely associated with their physical development. When their physical development seems to be progressing most rapidly, the mental activity seems to be at a standstill. Often the strength of the child is entirely absorbed by the physical growth. At other times when the physical development progresses slowly the mental activity may develop very rapidly. Again there may be a rapid and even development of both the physical and mental powers, or there may be a slow and even development of both the physical and mental powers and, lastly, that most baffling of all phases, when both the mental and physical developments seem to be marking time. These unevennesses are marked, mentally and emotionally, in various ways.

Sex attraction now manifests itself and often begins with a strong devotion between members of the same sex. Boys have their boy heroes of their own age and older. Girls are more apt to be attracted by older women, especially their teachers. Adolescence is often marked by vivid religious emotions and aspirations, utterly unfounded likes and dislikes, periods of uncontrolled temper, periods of equally unreasonable spells of contrition, periods of great excitement and high spirits, and again periods of deep depression. Taste in food as well as dress suffers from the uneven developments of this period. All these manifestations differ in degree and intensity throughout the whole period of adolescence and there seems to be no consistency in sequence in any two individuals. Therefore the understanding and relative importance of these changes necessitates a careful study of each child. The period is marked by greater variations within the normal than any other period of human development.

In spite of all this ebb and flow, this varied expression of adolescent contrasts and inconsistencies in the relationship between the mental and physical development, certain definite mental finalities are steadily being approached. At the end of adolescence, the power to reason has become stabilized and ready for its mature development. The will power, most unstable during adolescence, if normal in development, becomes more fixed and ready to build upon. The character development during adolescence is but a continuation and molding, so to speak, of processes begun in the very earliest adaptation of a child to its environment. During the adolescent period, the same "fluid" conditions exist in the moral adjustments as in the physical and mental development. We often find that a child during this period of adolescent variation develops weak or vicious traits which, unless properly and sympathetically guided, might become stabilized. If so guided, the child, when adolescence is completed, emerges with the moral finalities that were established long before the adolescent period began. At the same time the child entering the adolescent period with the wrong moral concepts has in the very nature of the period itself, its instability and variation, a new chance to develop the right moral valuation. Such moral development during adolescence is closely related to the development of the mental powers, such as the reason and the will. For reasons such as these, the strongest emphasis must be placed upon the care and guidance of children through this period, as it is the last opportunity for the molding of character. While not as important as the earlier stage, still it is the last opportunity for permanently affecting character formation. Radical changes of character after the completion of adolescence are rare and are usually the result of great or disturbing elements in life, such as religious conversion or exposure to tremendous emotional experiences, great joy, fear or tragedy, as the war has demonstrated.

The Defects of Adolescence

Such a period, marked deeply as it is by constant change, growth and development along physical, mental and psychical lines, is naturally marked by defects of great gravity. These defects naturally fall into two groups—the defects of heredity, and acquired defects. Defects of heredity again fall into the two main groups of those inheriting mental defects and those inheriting moral defects. The mental defects which appear first during adolescence are mainly the moron group. These individuals form a great part of our adolescent juvenile offenders, especially among girls. The increased instability of the period, plus the weak mentality, minus a good environment, leads usually to the breaking of some social law in these cases. In girls, it is more often a sex offense, in which case they are more unmoral than immoral, having been used by normal people who should be the real offenders against the law. As to boys, of the moron group, we find them in the same status, being used by brighter more normal individuals as tools, and the common offenses are larceny, truancy and depredations of various sorts. The moron, it must be remembered, is the individual whose maximum intelligence equals the normal intelligence of twelve years.

During the unstable period of adolescence the moron can be trained into certain habits of life and work that will make him often economically independent. This can be accomplished by vocational training along manual lines under careful supervision. Nor does this mean constant institutional care. By special classes in the public schools, combined with constant careful follow-up work in the homes, many of these individuals can be kept out of trouble and can constructively use the limited abilities they possess. This type of care is possible but it is only possible with community understanding and coöperation between school, family and the follow-up workers. The majority of morons who go wrong during the adolescent period do so from a lack of this coöperative effort and a lack of understanding of a child's limitations. The stress and storm of the adolescent period is much harder on the moron group than upon the normal child because they lack the development of the higher mental traits, reason, will power and judgment, which come to the normal child during that period. The moron's maximum intelligence of twelve years may not be reached until the later years of adolescence, which makes the problem very much more difficult. The adolescent changes have to be met without the stabilizing effect of mental development. On the other hand, many of the moron group do not seem to experience the stress of the adolescent period, but on account of their lack of mental development are just as easily led astray. Many of these children cannot be cared for successfully in communities where general understanding and coöperation are lacking, and as such communities are as yet in the vast majority in the world, the institution becomes a necessity for the care of the moron. The type of institution, however, should be one which embodies all that outside care might, in special instances, accomplish. The old idea of merely shutting such children away from the world has passed forever and the new institution has, as its goal, the final placing of the moron in society again, so stabilized and trained by habit and education fitted to his powers that he can be a self-supporting and self-respecting member of the group. This would always necessitate a certain amount of intelligent supervision, varying with the demands required of the individual and the changing environment. Friendly advice from the modern trained medical social worker should always be available to this group in order that the individual may be able to make his adjustments to new demands without a loss of the training he has had.

Another group which suffers keenly during the adolescent period is that composed of children whose mentality is not below normal but who suffer from lack of moral stamina. These children are much more difficult to detect because their intelligence is normal. They show usually a total lack of the social sense, no perception of right and wrong, and from this group come many of our criminal class and the worst offenders against sex laws. The understanding and management of this group is much more difficult than that of the moron, and the success of training and supervision is markedly less because their intelligence gives them an advantage. If, at early periods, some decided bent or aptitude can be discovered and the training and supervision related to it most carefully and intelligently applied, the chances of success are much greater.

A third group of defectives which appears usually during the adolescent period is that of so-called constitutional psychopaths. These individuals are of varying types, their principal defect being their inability to adapt themselves to the normal environment. Many in this class have what is recognized as a hereditary nervous background (diathesis) which shows itself in the constant impulsive basis from which they act. We find in this group all our cranks, kleptomaniacs, pyromaniacs, agitators, and all the impulsive types that make up our grave social problems. The keen intelligence which often marks these impulsive psychopaths makes them most difficult to treat with the intelligence they demand. During adolescence these types first reveal themselves, and that period should be most carefully studied by students of medicine. In the past there has been little appreciation by the medical profession of the importance of such manifestations during adolescence. But of late, such intensive studies as have been carried on by Healy ([2]) and by the best modern psychopathic hospitals, juvenile clinics and juvenile courts, have brought to the attention of the medical profession a vast amount of material that shows the importance of the understanding of the heredity and environment of these cases.

The fundamental aspect to be stressed in handling these cases is to make every attempt during the plastic period of adolescence to force upon these individuals the realization of their own condition. In this is a surer hope of solution for them. Psychoanalysis, if used at all, should be used not so much in the Freudian sense of establishing all lines of relation of abnormal traits to sexual development, as in the analysis of the individual's own life so that he will understand his own weaknesses and handicaps. In modern social psychology we have a better means of stimulating the child to an appreciation of the development of his instincts and so helping him to gain a more stable control over his defective impulsive bases.

Another group of defectives are those suffering from language and speech defects, which may or may not appear before adolescence, but which do often appear and usually meet medical attention first during this period. Children with these defects are often normal in every other respect. These defects may be permanent or temporary, and the importance of understanding them is in order to be able to classify them, so that the training of these children may proceed along the lines in which they are normal, and in this way to diminish their handicap as much as possible.

Other types are those defective in number work. This often causes a classification of these children as feeble-minded when the defect is limited to this one faculty. Stammering and similar speech defects, which appear during the adolescent period in the nervous or timid child, have a definite neuromuscular and mental or psychological basis. These conditions may be begun through imitation; a sensitive child often acquires an actual speech defect from contact with another suffering from such a defect. Such defects may also be acquired after a definite fright or shock of any kind to the nervous system. Of course, this acquisition of such defects may appear at any age, but before the completion of adolescence they must be handled, if possible, as delay in treatment increases the chance of permanency. The treatment should be carried out by one acquainted with the psychology of childhood as well as the mechanics of voice production and control. Many of these speech and language defects are hereditary, many are acquired, and some have the double basis.

Diseases of Adolescence

This period is marked by the development of definite psychoses, mainly those of mania and melancholia. These states often have an hereditary basis, but are usually brought into evidence by the awakening of the sexual functions. The state of mania is characterized by periods of intense excitement, uncontrolled temper, followed by periods of great fatigue. Sometimes intense jealousy, great selfishness, sharp depression are manifested. The state of melancholia is expressed by constant depression maintained sometimes over long periods. While there are intervals of normality and cheerfulness, depression is the more constant symptom.

The treatment of these states requires as early a recognition as possible and a careful analysis of the causes, either real or imaginary, that have brought on these states. The removal of the causes and the placing of the child in the best possible environment which will prevent a recurrence of the cause, is the best line of treatment to be followed. In the more severe cases institutional care is necessary, but the outcome of these cases is not good because they often become chronic or fall into such bad nutritional condition that they often die of some intercurrent disease. The adjustment of these cases to everyday life is one of the most hopeful fields of modern psychiatry. Careful study of the individual case with the necessary change of environment and the personal follow-up work of a trained psychiatrist and social worker bids fair to be the best solution possible for these cases.

A common mental condition of adolescence is *dementia praecox*. On account of the stress of rapid change of this period, dementia praecox with its gradual decay of mental faculties is very likely to appear in the early and confusional states. At that stage it is often difficult to differentiate the state from an exaggerated adolescent condition of instability which corrects itself. In the most common type of dementia praecox, the hebephrenic type, are found states of increased excitement alternating with foolish laughter and silly speech, an exaggerated impulse to be doing something which is only evidenced by perfectly aimless actions which accomplish nothing. These conditions may persist for a long time without any evident increase in the mental decay, but in general these states terminate in extreme mental weakness followed by the complete destruction of the mind. Other forms of dementia praecox may begin at puberty, such as the catatonic form in which states of depression are followed by alternating periods of stupor and excitement shown by varied motor spasms or retardations. *Paralytic dementia* also has its beginnings frequently at the period of adolescence. All these states when actively manifested are best handled in an institution.

Syphilis is the underlying cause of many of the mental deteriorations during the adolescent period. Hereditary syphilis is sometimes retarded, and without having shown any previous manifestations, either in the physical or mental development of the child, develops very rapidly during puberty. Especially is this true at the time of the development of the sexual functions and manifests itself by rapid mental deterioration or by the development of juvenile tabes. Active treatment with mercury and salvarsan or neosalvarsan begun early may be able to check the condition, but these conditions more often continue to rapid disintegration both mentally and physically. Such cases usually die of some intercurrent infection.

Because of the fundamental change in the brain and central nervous system and marked physiological changes, *epilepsy* reaches its most marked development during adolescence. Instead of the hoped for cessation of symptoms, they are usually exaggerated during this period. When *chorea* appears first at adolescence, it is marked by greater severity and longer periods of duration. The characteristic involuntary movements are usually accompanied by irritability, absent-mindedness and slight mental weakness.

Changes in the composition of the blood during adolescence often take place, especially the anemias which are marked by pallor and great languor. In boys, this usually takes the form of simple secondary anemia, due to the effects of malnutrition or previous infection. During adolescence this secondary anemia may become quite pronounced on account of the increased demands of growth and the disturbances caused by the development of internal glandular secretions on the lymphatic system. In girls these anemias often take the exaggerated form of *chlorosis,* in which there is a definite disturbance of lymph formation. The red cells are not able to carry their normal proportion of hemoglobin so that the characteristic finding of this condition is a very marked reduction in the hemoglobin without a corresponding reduction in the red cells. In severe cases, poikilocytes and normoblasts make their appearance. Connected with these blood findings are marked lassitude and fatigue which chlorotic girls suffer from, and also distinct nervous phenomena such as headache, vertigo, insomnia, and general nervous instability. These conditions are often accompanied by hemic murmurs of the heart and change in the blood pressure. Their treatment requires careful regulation of diet and régime based upon a study of their previous condition, making sure that the cause is neither syphilis nor tuberculosis. Iron in most instances has a very definite effect upon these anemias.

The endocrine glands exert a powerful influence upon adolescent development of both girls and boys, not only on the development of the sex organs and functions but also upon the secondary sexual characteristics. The functional activity of the sex organs depends upon the harmonious action of the endocrine system, upon the efficient and normal action of this system. It is not sufficient to have merely the sex glands develop. The development of the sex glands is so intimately connected with the development of the thyroid and pituitary glands that the two must progress in parallel lines. We know that the thymus gland begins to disappear about the time of puberty. Whether this disappearance of the internal secretion of the thymus causes the beginning of the development of the gonad system with its internal secretion, or whether the appearance at this time of the internal secretion of the gonads causes the disappearance of the thymus gland, is not known. The reaction is probably mutual. Any change in the development of the thyroid or the pituitary, causing an insufficiency of its internal gland secretion, retards the development of the generative organs. A tumor in the pituitary will cause infantilism. Most of the cases seen during adolescence of retarded or abnormal growth are due to a combination of defects in the endocrine system, usually a polyglandular one. The thyroid gland during the adolescent period is very prone to enlarge, especially in girls. Marine ([3]) in his studies, "Thyroid in School Children," found it four times as often in girls as in boys. This increased tendency to thyroidism during adolescence has a definite effect upon the development of generative organs. The period of nervous instability is markedly increased by this tendency. It seems fair to assume that the instability and the varying phases of great fatigue and excitement are caused by the uneven development of the internal glands or the attempt to harmonize their activities. Marine ([3]) has shown that this condition is more prevalent in certain regions, such as that of the Great Lakes. The fact that this condition may be controlled by small doses of iodine offers a simple method of affecting this important period of development when it is complicated by thyroidism.

Disturbance of the suprarenal glands has the opposite effect, that of stimulating the gonad development and in the cases of precocious puberty a tumor of the suprarenals is often found. In other cases, there may be simply an overstimulation from the suprarenals which causes the noted precocity. Each individual case of disturbed adolescence, either delayed or precocious, must receive careful study of the endocrine gland system to determine which glands are at fault. Some very definite effects can be obtained from appropriate glandular treatment, especially in cases where we can determine some definite derangement. Many cases, however, are most baffling, and there is no field in medicine related to the adolescent period that needs more intelligent study than this of the endocrine system.

Growth is not a simple nor a single process but is a multiplex phenomenon, as described by Robertson ([4]) in his discussion of the growth factor found in the anterior lobe of the pituitary. He states that "it would appear legitimate to infer that, at a late stage in the third adolescent growth cycle, the administration of excess of pituitary anterior lobe tissue leads to an acceleration of growth while, at an earlier stage in the development of animals, the administration of anterior lobe tissue leads to retardation of the rate of growth." He concludes that "it is quite conceivable that pre-adolescent hypopituitarism at a certain stage of development might yield effects in some respects analogous to those of late post-adolescent hyperpituitarism." He was able to produce such effects with the extract, tethelin, which he obtained from the anterior lobe, completely changing the growth cycle of adolescence. Clinically we see many cases which during adolescence undoubtedly show some disturbance in the normal development and secretion of the pituitary gland, causing a disturbance in the normal progress of adolescence. Besides the clear-cut cases of hypo- or hyper-pituitarism we probably have many more cases in which there is a dys-pituitarism connected with disturbances in some other gland; most often in my experience this is connected with hypothyroidism.

Treatment of Various Conditions

The treatment of these various conditions demands first of all a careful study of all the changes of the period of adolescence, the anatomical, physiological and psychological developments. The anatomical and physiological disturbances are best handled by the most intelligent consideration of the details of life. The amount of recreation needs careful regulation. Sleep and rest are most important items. Adolescence demands a more nutritive diet than any other period of life. The school studies carried on in this country show that the food and the variety taken by adolescents far exceeds the demands of any other period, amounting to from four to five thousand calories a day for boys. The writer's own experience in studying the "ravitaillement" system in Belgium and the north of France emphasized the great ravages made in this period, due to diminished food. The period of adolescence stood out markedly as one which could not hold its own on the food ration of an adult. This condition is now known to exist over all of war-ravaged Europe and the adolescent period has suffered most from the stern restriction of diet caused by the war. The varied psychological changes, which have almost an infinite number of combinations and aspects, need most sympathetic understanding and firm, skilled handling. As already indicated more than this, the constant interrelation of all these changes must never be lost sight of, as most often the study of the whole gives the key for the particular problem.

Certain Problems of Adolescence

While all the varied changes of adolescence present many problems, conduct, which is the result of the individual's effort to adjust himself to the demands of his environment, during adolescence presents many of the most acute difficulties. The mass of material accumulated by the juvenile courts of the country are crowded with instances of mal-adjustment, of bad conduct which results disastrously for the individual. These cases represent in varying degrees the anatomical, physiological and psychological defects of adolescence. Masturbation, which is one of the most frequent sexual acts indulged in by the adolescent boy and girl, is found much more frequently in these cases of mal-adjustment. Where masturbation is a persistent factor, it is commonly associated with mental or moral defect.

Healy ([2]) has carefully studied these problems of individual conduct and he urges the most intelligent study of the cases accompanied by an honest effort to adequately solve the problem. Ordinarily this solution is left to the judge of the court. In rare instances he has the advice of a trained psychologist. In that case, he may desire to act in the most intelligent manner, but the judge has his limitations. He can do one of three things, place the delinquent child on probation, assign him to an institution, or drop the case. If dropped without any attempt made to change the causes for the delinquency, the case will undoubtedly come up again. Most institutions are overcrowded and not properly equipped for the necessary training, either in trained personnel or the mechanics of handling the cases. Probation officers are comparatively few in number and not particularly well trained. Therefore, the limitations of a judge of a juvenile court are not to be entirely laid at his door.

The education of the community and the training of responsible public opinion to demand adequate laws and adequate budgets for carrying out the laws are absolutely necessary if these problems of conduct during the period of adolescence are to be adequately handled. To gain this community responsibility psychopathic centers for the study of these adolescent problems are essential. At such centers, the best scientific medical and psychological studies can be carried out on these individual problems as they present themselves. More than that, such findings must be interpreted for and to the public in language understood and appreciated in order that the greatest factor in the whole problem of adolescent conduct may be met, the factor of environment.

Environment is after all a lay problem. Only the very few in comparison to the need can have carefully planned and selected environment. The average child passes his adolescence in the average community and that community must be educated in the needs and problems of adolescence. The average community expression toward the adolescent child is either shown by constant repression or complete ignoring of the whole problem. The records of the court prove this beyond any doubt. Case after case of misconduct on the part of both girls and boys record the fact of stern denial on the part of parents to what might have remained more or less normal activity on the child's part, or an absolute lack of interest in or knowledge of a child's activities, which, allowed to seek their own levels during the unstable periods of adolescence, ended in broken laws.

The physician's part is first of all the patient study of the period of adolescence and an appreciation of its effect on the conduct of the individual. But his responsibility does not end here. The education of the person controlling the environment of the individual case must also be undertaken by the physician if the results of his study are to be effective. In this education of the parent, the home, and the community, the physician must have the indispensable service of the medically trained psychological social worker. It is interesting to note that the war has stimulated the formation of a course of training at Smith College for those social workers interested in the psychological and moral problems. But the physician himself must emphasize and help interpret to the community the broader community responsibilities. The kind of recreation offered to the adolescent child of any given community becomes the business of the physician because it is part of his treatment to recommend proper recreation. The dearth of opportunities for proper recreation immediately appals the interested physician. Cheap moving pictures, dealing in so many instances with grotesque and vulgar suggestive humors or intense sex complications, and the unsupervised dance halls make the problem most difficult for the doctor. The adolescent child needs wholesome out-of-door exercise, organized to permit of free self-expression, swimming properly supervised, dancing, dramatics. Often the child of the poor is better off in these respects than the child of moderate circumstances or of the rich. The settlement houses long ago recognized these problems and the club life of settlements has been the attempt to meet them.

The Teaching of Social Hygiene

"The war has forced the issue in sex education." These words of Dr. Mabel Ulrich in her telling pamphlet, "Mothers of America," give the reason for this discussion here ([5]). The past two years of public government propaganda has brought the subject of social hygiene out of the field of private endeavor to that of a distinct public health educational basis. When the Surgeon General's Office ([6]) issues such facts as these, namely, that syphilis and gonorrhea have disabled more men in our army and navy than all other diseases combined, that the draft has proved these diseases to be more frequent among the boys from our own home towns than among those in the regular army, and that in spite of all that was done to prevent contagion, at least 125,000 new cases developed among our drafted boys, the field of social hygiene has become one of the most burning of the public issues. Here we are concerned with two aspects of the question: the relation of preventive medicine to the field and its bearing upon adolescence; and the relation of adolescence to social hygiene. The pre-adolescent period is the time in which the foundation of the education in sex hygiene should be laid. It is then that the questions as to the whys, wheres, and hows of life are asked and upon the frank meeting of these questions depends the future of adolescent attitude. If before ten, the child has met honest, frank answers to his questions, the later sex problems are the more readily approached with frankness and a minimum of sex consciousness.

The importance of the pre-adolescent question as to how life is created, does not lie so much in the information given in the honest answer, but in the frankness and beauty with which the question is discussed, the maintenance of the unconscious curiosity of the child. Sex consciousness, as such, seldom enters into the natural curious inquiry of the child under ten. Sex then is merely accidental, the why is asked about everything which brings new life; babies simply fall naturally into the category of interesting new life that is introduced into the child's immediate environment. It is the same with a new kitten or calf. The truth is wanted and should be given at the period, but it bears no personal relation to the child, while the way in which he is answered makes the more lasting impression. The pre-adolescent period has been left largely to the ignorance or lack of understanding of parents, and the curiosity of other children, which has brought to the adolescent period a false impress. Preventive medicine must begin its work in the pre-adolescent period if it is to have any comprehensive effect on the adolescent period.

It is the business of the physician to stimulate the parents to equip themselves to meet these intimate problems of the children. This can be done largely by intelligent direction on his part to the available literature on the subject, and by giving to the parents his own comprehensive idea of the subject. The child under ten grasps little of the detail of the information given him but the dramatic points, the frank intimacy shared by him and his parents are his best preparation for the sex consciousness of the adolescent period. The adolescent period marks the beginning of his consciousness that these questions that have stirred his curiosity and imagination are personal sex problems and that he must establish his relationship with them. This sex consciousness results often in that impenetrable reserve, often the attitude almost of fear, that causes many of the complex psychoses of adolescence. Information may be given at different times with varying degrees of detail to meet the particular problem facing the individual but the chief problem is to so relate the child to the whole life concept that sex becomes more and more a normal part of a normal whole. The best time to differentiate sex distinction in a child's mind is before he becomes conscious of himself as of a sex. When adolescence comes, the avenue of approach to sex hygiene should be social rather than personal. At no time in life is the need of a background of law more needed or more helpful than during the unstable years of adolescence. One of the most clear and concise expressions of this is set forth in that splendid "Children's Code" prepared by William J. Hutchins ([7]). The theme of the code is patriotism expressed in conduct. The code is given in full because it states in the fewest words the constructive preventive program for the adolescent period:

"Boys and girls who are good Americans try to become strong and useful, that our country may become ever greater and better. Therefore they obey the laws of right living which the best Americans have always obeyed.

"*The Good American Tries to Gain and to Keep Perfect Health.*—The welfare of our country depends upon those who try to be physically fit for their daily work. Therefore: 1. I will keep my clothes, my body, and my mind clean. 2. I will avoid those habits which would harm me, and will make and never break those habits which will help me. 3. I will try to take such food, sleep, and exercise as will keep me in perfect health.

"*The Good American Controls Himself.*—Those who best control themselves can best serve their country. 1. I will control my Tongue, and will not allow it to speak mean, vulgar, or profane words. 2. I will control my Temper, and will not get angry when people or things displease me. 3. I will control my Thoughts, and will not allow a foolish wish to spoil a wise purpose.

"*The Good American is Reliable.*—Our country grows great and good as her citizens are able more fully to trust each other. Therefore: 1. I will be honest, in word and in act. I will not lie, sneak, or pretend, nor will I keep the truth from those who have a right to it. 2. I will not do wrong in the hope of not being found out. I cannot hide the truth from myself and cannot often hide it from others. 3. I will not take without permission what does not belong to me. 4. I will do promptly what I have promised to do. If I have made a foolish promise, I will at once confess my mistake, and I will try to make good any harm which my mistake may have caused. I will so speak and act that people will find it easier to trust each other.

"*The Good American Plays Fair.*—Clean play increases and trains one's strength, and helps one to be more useful to one's country. Therefore: 1. I will not cheat, nor will I play for keeps or for money. If I should not play fair, the loser would lose the fun of the game, and the winner would lose his self-respect, and the game itself would become a mean and often cruel business. 2. I will treat my opponent with politeness. 3. If I play in a group game, I will play, not for my own glory, but for the success of my team and the fun of the game. 4. I will be a good loser or a generous winner.

"*The Good American Does His Duty.*—The shirker or the willing idler lives upon the labor of others, burdens others with the work which he ought to do himself. He harms his fellow citizens, and so harms his country. 1. I will try to find out what my duty is, WHAT I OUGHT TO DO, and my duty I will do, whether it is easy or hard. What I ought to do I can do.

"*The Good American Tries to Do the Right Thing in the Right Way.*—The welfare of our country depends upon those who have learned to do in the right way the things that ought to be done. Therefore: 1. I will get the best possible education, and learn all that I can from those who have learned to do the right thing in the right way. 2. I will take an interest in my work, and will not be satisfied with slip-shod and merely passable work. A wheel or a rail or a nail carelessly made may cause the death of hundreds. 3. I will try to do the right thing in the right way, even when no one else sees or praises me. But when I have done my best, I will not envy those who have done better, or have received larger reward. Envy spoils the work and the worker.

"*The Good American Works in Friendly Coöperation with His Fellow-workers.*—One man alone could not build a city or a great railroad. One man alone would find it hard to build a house or a bridge. That I may have bread, men have sowed and reaped, men have made plows and threshers, men have built mills and mined coal, men have made stoves and kept stores. As we learn better how to work together the welfare of our country is advanced. 1. In whatever work I do with others, I will do my part and will help others do their part. 2. I will keep in order the things which I use in my work. When things are out of place, they are often in the way, and sometimes they are hard to find. Disorder means confusion, and the waste of time and patience. 3. In all my work with others, I will be cheerful. Cheerlessness depresses all the workers and injures all the work. 4. When I have received money for my work, I will be neither a miser nor a spendthrift. I will save or spend as one of the friendly workers of America.

"*The Good American is Kind.*—In America those who are of different races, colors, and conditions must live together. We are of many different sorts, but we are one great people. Every unkindness hurts the common life, every kindness helps the common life. Therefore: 1. I will be kind in all my Thoughts. I will bear no spites or grudges. I will not think myself above any other girl or boy just because I am of different race or color or condition. I will never despise anybody. 2. I will be kind in all my Speech. I will not gossip nor will I speak unkindly of anyone. Words may wound or heal. 3. I will be kind in all my Acts. I will not selfishly insist on having my own way. I will always be polite. Rude people are not good Americans. I will not trouble unnecessarily those who do work for me. I will do my best to prevent cruelty, and will give my best help to those who need it most.

"*The Good American is Loyal.*—If our America is to become ever greater and better, her citizens must be loyal, devotedly faithful, in every relation of life. 1. I will be loyal to my family. In loyalty I will gladly obey my parents or those who are in their place. I will do my best to help each member of my family to strength and usefulness. 2. I will be loyal to my school. In loyalty I will obey and help other pupils to obey those rules which further the good of all. 3. I will be loyal to my town, my state, and my country. In loyalty I will respect and help others to respect their laws and their courts of justice. 4. I will be loyal to humanity. In loyalty I will do my best to help the friendly relations of our country with every other country, and to give to everyone in every land the best possible chance.

"If I try simply to be loyal to my family, I may be disloyal to my school. If I try simply to be loyal to my school, I may be disloyal to my town, my state, and my country. If I try simply to be loyal to my town, state, and country, I may be disloyal to humanity. I will try above all things else to be loyal to humanity; then I shall surely be loyal to my country, my state, and my town, to my school, and to my family."

Thus are given the social objectives by which the youth hitches his sex consciousness to the stars!

At the same time sex consciousness has its very definite physical aspects and developments and these must be explained and understood. But all this is more possible when the child's relation to the larger physical and social life has been firmly developed in him. Adolescence is not a pleasant period for a child—change and upheaval seldom are. But the awakening of the sex life is for the great purpose of reproduction and even though the adolescent child may have no personal interest as yet in that great purpose, he may be appealed to to play the game fairly in order that he may do his part when the time comes. The period of adolescence always necessitates a restatement of the facts of life and then they are related to the new sex development; physical rightness is the aspect to be most thoroughly emphasized because of its wider social responsibility.

The old method of fear and penalties for breaking rules of health is not to be employed during the adolescent period, particularly because of the bad psychical effects. The constructive side is always to be emphasized. In the mass of literature on this subject certain publications stand out with refreshing strength and wisdom along these lines. The Armstrongs' (8) pamphlets for boys and girls from twelve to sixteen years: "Sex in Life" and "Sex in Life, the Development of the Mind and Will," are of the best, and a vigorous contribution to preventive medicine. Doctor Ulrich's (9) booklets are a happy combination of the physical problems of adolescence and their immediate bearing upon the purpose of life and its responsibilities. Sex hygiene is social hygiene, and in the teaching of it there must be constant recognition of the constant relation of the individual to the social group. The petulant remark of a nervous girl during her adolescence, "I don't care what organs I have—I want to know why I feel as I do," is natural and characteristic of the period. The most carefully selected and frank information along physical lines leaves the feelings untouched, and feelings are but the golden links between the physical facts of life and the social purpose.

Kirkpatrick states in that illuminating book, "The Individual in the Making," "never does one feel so vividly that he can be anything or do anything that he desires. This assurance should and often does lead to immediate direction of effort toward ends that are desired (10)." Thus the teaching of social hygiene becomes a great incentive in the field of preventive medicine to a more clear-cut development of the many physical, anatomical and psychological changes of the adolescent. The period gains in the strength of its "finalities" by the careful, intelligent relation of all its variableness to the great social purposes of life.

BIBLIOGRAPHY

Direct Text References

1. MOSHER, CLELIA DUEL: Health and the Woman Movement. Nat. Board Y. W. C. A., 1916, 11.
2. HEALY, WILLIAM: The Individual Delinquent. Little, Brown & Co., 1915.
3. MARINE, DAVID, and KIMBALL, O. P.: Jour. Lab. and Clin. Med., 1917, III, 40.
4. ROBERTSON, T. BRAILSFORD: Endocrinology, 1917, I, 30.
5. ULRICH, MABEL S.: Mothers of America. Minn. State Board of Health, Division of Venereal Diseases, 1918, 5.
6. ULRICH, MABEL S.: Mothers of America. Minn. State Board of Health, Division of Venereal Diseases, 1918, 3.
7. HUTCHINS, WILLIAM J.: The Children's Code of Morals. University Society, New York City.

8. ARMSTRONG, DONALD B., and EUNICE B.: Sex in Life, Soc. Hyg., 1916, II, 331; Sex in Life, Development of Mind and Will, Pamphlet No. 2, ibid., 549.
9. ULRICH, MABEL S.: Uncle Sam Needs Leaders: The Girl's Part. Minn. State Board of Health, 1918.
10. KIRKPATRICK, E. A.: The Individual in the Making. Houghton, Mifflin Co., 1911, 249.

General Chapter References

BEEKMAN, F.: Arch. of Pediat., 1915, XXXII, 4.
BELL, W. BLAIR: The Sex Complex. Balliere, Tendall & Cox, London, 1916.
BENEDICT, FRANCIS G.: Boston Med. and Surg. Jour., 1919, CLXXXI, 107.
BIEDL, ARTHUR: The Internal Secretory Organs. Wood, New York, 1913.
BRIDGMAN, OLGA L.: Boston Med. and Surg. Jour., 1918, CLXXIX, 505.
CANNON, W. B.: Endocrinology, 1917, I, 50.
ELLIS, HAVELOCK: Studies in the Psychology of Sex. Davis, Philadelphia, 1910.
ENGELMANN, G. J.: Jour. Am. Med. Assoc., 1901, XXXVI, 1,650.
GEPHART, F. C.: Boston Med. and Surg. Jour., 1917, CLXVI, 107.
GODIN, PAUL: Comptes Méd. des Séances de l'Acad. des Sciences, 1911, CLIII, 967; 1912, CLV, 66.
GULICK, LUTHER HALSEY, and AYRES, LEONARD P.: Medical Inspection of Schools, N. Y. Charities Pub. Com., 1910.
GARRIGUES, HENRY J.: A Text Book of the Diseases of Women, 3d ed., Saunders, Philadelphia, 1910.
GUYER, MICHAEL F.: Being Well Born. Bobbs, Merrill, 1916.
HALL, G. STANLEY: Adolescence, I and II. Appleton, New York, 1916.
HALL, W. S.: Am. Acad. of Med., Bull., 1914, XV, 86.
LATIMER, CAROLINE WORMLEY: Girl and Woman, 1909.
LOMBROSO, CESARE: Revue de Psych., 1901.
McDOUGAL, WILLIAM: Social Psychology. John W. Lucas & Co., 1916.
MORRO: "Le Puberte."
OSBORNE, T. B., and MENDEL, LAFAYETTE B.: Jour. Biol. Chem., 1914, XVIII, 95; Am. Jour. Phys., 1916, XL, 16.
PIERSOL, GEORGE A.: Human Anatomy, 5th ed. Lippincott, Philadelphia, 1907.
PUFFER, J. ADAMS: The Boy and His Gang.
ROBERTSON, T. BRAILSFORD: Am. Jour. Phys., 1915, XXXVII, 74; Am. Jour. Phys., 1916, XLI, 547.
ROTCH, THOMAS MORGAN: Living Anatomy and Pathology by the Roentgen Method. Lippincott, 1910.
SEITZ, PROF. C.: Diseases of Puberty, 111-130, Pfaundler and Schlossmann. Lippincott, 1908.
STARR, LOUIS: The Adolescent Period. Blakeston, Philadelphia, 1915.
TALBOT, FRITZ B.: Am. Jour. Dis. of Ch., 1919, XVIII, 229.
TYLER, JOHN MASON: Growth and Education. Houghton, Mifflin Co., Boston, 1907.
VINCENT, SWALE: Internal Secretions and the Ductless Glands. London, 1912.

CHAPTER XIV

AVIATION MEDICINE

By LOUIS HOPEWELL BAUER

TABLE OF CONTENTS

INTRODUCTION

Aviation is a comparatively new subject which had its origin in the rapid development of aeronautics which took place during the first World War. Except for the effects of high altitude, as observed in mountain expeditions and certain researches on the vestibular mechanism, nothing was known pertaining to the physiology of flight. Man was not designed by nature to fly and hence, what its effect on him might be, had hardly been considered.

In the early days of flying, at the time of the Wright brothers' epochal accomplishment and for some time thereafter, flying was hardly even a science. A man was taught what he could be taught on the ground, and then he tried to apply it in the air. If he were lucky, he flew. If he were unlucky, he was killed or severely injured. The one physical attribute considered necessary was "nerve", and there is no doubt that it took plenty of that.

Development in aeronautics was desultory until the first World War broke out, and then the possibilities of flying from a military standpoint were so impressed on the Allies and the Central Powers that a tremendous advance was made from the mechanical standpoint. The physical factor still was not considered especially important. Only the ordinary physical examinations were required for duty in aviation services. Soon, however, it became apparent that there were many accidents from a physical cause. Pilots were wearing out too fast, and there were too many deaths attributable to physical causes. Research work, stimulated by the necessity of man-power conservation, indicated that certain factors of a physical nature, not important in ground fighting, were paramount in the air.

Gradually, therefore, special examinations developed which became more or less similar in all countries. By the time the United States entered the war much experience in the subject had been gained by the Allies of benefit to our own country. As would be expected, many mistakes were made; stress was laid where it should not have been in some instances, and other points which should have been stressed were overlooked.

Following the war civil aeronautics began to develop in Europe, although it was not until 1927 that any progress was made in this country. It was found that civil flying is somewhat different in its demands from military flying and consequently, the regulations had to be modified. With the development of transport planes with their complicated instrument panels and safety devices, with the increasing altitude of flight including flights into the stratosphere and with the steadily increasing speed of planes, the medical aspects of flying became increasingly important. Finally, with the development of high altitude bombing and dive-bombing, the resulting onset of aero embolism and emphysema and the damaging effects of marked centrifugal force, new problems have had to be conquered.

Definitions. — *Aviation Medicine.* — Out of a mass of experience, research and statistics a subject known now as aviation medicine has developed as a distinct specialty. This specialty is really a branch of preventive medicine, as its sole basis is the prevention of aircraft accidents from the human standpoint. It has drawn to itself portions of other specialties, namely, physiology, internal medicine, ophthalmology, otology, neuropsychiatry and psychology. It is a correlation of certain parts of these specialties as they relate to flying. The specialist in aviation medicine is known as the flight surgeon.

The Flight Surgeon. — The flight surgeon is a physician trained in aviation medicine. He is familiar with the branches of medicine concerned with aeronautics and their application thereto. He is skilled in making the various examinations required. He is sufficiently familiar with flying and its attendant strains and stresses to be a useful medical advisor to pilots and operators. He is familiar with the effects of oxygen want and lowered barometric pressure; he knows the effects of increased gravity drags on the human body, and he knows how by applying his special knowledge he can prevent accidents from a physical standpoint by careful selection and careful supervision of flying personnel.

The flight surgeon is preferably a fairly young man, as most flyers are young, and they are more apt to make a confidant of one not too old. His personality must be one to inspire confidence and respect.

He should fly under all conditions and with all types of pilots. The flight surgeon, who remains on the ground, gets scant consideration from the flying personnel. He must experience the conditions the flyer meets almost daily in order to appreciate them and be competent to advise regarding their effect. He must have a thorough grounding in physiology of respiration and circulation, in psychiatry and psychology, in internal medicine, and he must know sufficient ophthalmology to make the special examinations required and interpret their results.

Varieties of Flying

Flying is divided into heavier-than-air and lighter-than-air. Heavier-than-air flying is divided into military, civilian and glider, which may be either military or civilian, and civilian flying into airline, commercial and sport flying.

The requirements vary according to the type of flying to be done.

Military. — Military flying is divided into fighting, formerly known as pursuit, air support and bombing. There are three types of bombers, light, medium and heavy.

Pursuit. — Acrobatic flying, which we sometimes think of as stunt flying, is absolutely essential for a military pilot. For the combat pilot it is life-saving. The pursuit or fighter plane is fast and easily maneuverable. It is a single seater. The pilot's decisions must be automatic. He must always be one jump ahead of his opponent. His vision must be perfect. He must be able to identify other aircraft in the air often by silhouette alone. His depth perception must be perfect, as he flies in formation with only a few feet between wing tips. His reaction time must be immediate, and his coolness in danger is absolutely essential. The fighter pilot must not only be a flyer but a gunner.

Air Support. — This includes military flying not covered by the fighters and bombers. It includes support of the ground troops with attack by machine guns and small bombs.

Bombardment. — This has become more complicated during the present war. The heavy bombers are 4 motored ships and virtually flying fortresses with a crew of several men, including pilot, co-pilot, navigator, radioman, gunners and bombardiers. They fly at high altitudes and for long distances. Then there are the medium bombers, which are faster but have a shorter range and are small. They are used for either horizontal or dive-bombing. In dive-bombing the planes swoop down from a high altitude, drop their bombs and zoom up again. These pilots are subject to change of direction at speeds up to 500 miles an hour. Light bombers fly at low altitudes and attack troops.

Naval. — Naval pilots. besides the above, have to learn to land on the deck of a carrier which calls for coolness and excellent depth perception. Landing on the water calls for more accurate depth perception than landing on land.

As a whole military flying is a young man's game, fighter and dive bombing flying calling for the greatest skill, quickest reaction time, greatest daring and coolness. Long and moderate distance high altitude bombing probably are a close second.

Civil Flying. — Civil flying in the United States is divided into three classes, (1) air-line, (2) commercial and commercial lighter-than-air and (3) private, student and private or student lighter-than-air and free balloon.

The air-line pilot flies commercial transport planes, day and night, over scheduled air routes. He is responsible for passengers, mail, freight and property. He must be an accomplished pilot, navigator, radioman and blind flyer.

The commercial pilot, either heavier or lighter-than-air, carries passengers and often is an instructor. He may be a co-pilot on an air-line.

The private pilot may fly for his own amusement or recreation but may not engage in any phase of commercial flying.

The student, of course, is the novice learning to fly. He must take his instruction from a licensed commercial pilot and in a licensed plane.

The air line or commercial pilot does not, in fact, he is forbidden to, indulge in acrobatics while flying commercially. He flies over known territory adequately equipped with landing fields and beacons and the air line pilot, in addition, flies on a radio beam. He may strike bad weather, but an efficient meteorological service keeps him in touch with weather conditions. His responsibility is heavy, however, as he has the lives of passengers in his hands. Often his flying is done at night. While commercial flying does not call for quite the same qualifications as certain phases of military flying, nevertheless it does call for physical soundness and technical proficiency.

The commercial pilot is a potential transport pilot, and therefore, the same applies to him.

The private pilot may reasonably have a lower physical standard than the transport grade. He, however, must meet a standard that insures his not being a menace to other flyers and the general public.

Blind flying has become essential for air line pilots in order to insure safety in unexpected or expected poor weather conditions or above the clouds. Transport flying is fatiguing and calls for endurance and sober judgment as well as constant alertness and keenness.

Taken as a whole, air-line flying and military flying are equally difficult and call for the highest type of physical and mental makeup.

Lighter-than-air. — Lighter-than-air flying pertains to airships, dirigibles and blimps, and to balloons. The general physical requirements need not be so high, in that visual defects may be corrected with glasses. Minor structural defects may be passed also.

Glider Pilots. — Glider pilots fly motorless planes. Originally this was a sport only. Now, however, it has become a military function also, as often great fleets of gliders are used to transport troops. The physical qualifications of glider pilots have not been definitely set, but they should be at least those of private pilots.

Physical Requirements of Flying

At the present time we may group the physical standards of aeronautics into two distinct classes. First, the standard for the military pilot and the commercial pilot and second, the standard for the private or sport pilot.

The detailed requirements may be obtained in the regulations of the various countries. They vary somewhat but more in methods of examination than in actual standards. In this chapter we shall discuss requirements in general rather than in detail.

The Eye

Central Vision. — It is recognized both by the physicians concerned and by successful pilots that good vision is a prime necessity. Not only is it of importance to the military pilot, who has fighting, bombing or reconnaissance to carry out, but it is important to any flyer. Traffic in the air is rather congested at many airports, and the obstructions around many airports are not always easily seen. Planes in the air must be detected. When two ships are traveling at a rate of well over 300 miles per hour, they cannot be seen by each other too promptly. By good vision is meant normal vision without correction. Corrected vision, while permitted in the private pilot, is a poor substitute for good, uncorrected vision. Corrections worn in goggles are very unsatisfactory, as they correct only straight ahead vision, and when misted or fogged, necessitating their removal, the pilot is rendered helpless. Furthermore, the wearing of corrected goggles restricts the peripheral field of vision. With the development of cabin planes there is less objection to moderate corrections being worn as glasses.

Practically all countries require for military and air line pilots normal or 20/20 vision in each eye uncorrected. Some countries, notably France, Holland and Hungary, permit one eye to be 25 per cent. less than normal, if the other eye be normal. Germany accepts 80 per cent. of the normal in both eyes. For private pilots the standard varies, but the majority require at least two-thirds normal vision or better with correction.

During the present war standards of visual acuity in several countries have become gradually lowered owing to the shortage of man power with normal vision. Neither the United States Army nor Navy, however, has yet lowered its visual standards.

Peripheral Vision. — Peripheral vision is important, for the flyer must see on all sides of him at once, particularly in landing, taking off, in formation flying and above all, when on a military mission. Peripheral vision is also of importance in night flying, as defects of the color fields are sometimes associated with night blindness.

Visual fields are tested by means of a perimeter or campimeter in the great majority of countries. The notable exception is Great Britain, which relies on the confrontation test. Berens[6] believes that all military and passenger-carrying pilots should be examined by the perimeter on an eight point field.

Central color vision is almost universally recognized as important for the flyer. He needs to detect colored lights on the airdrome, navigating lights on other ships, colored signal panels and signal lights and what is

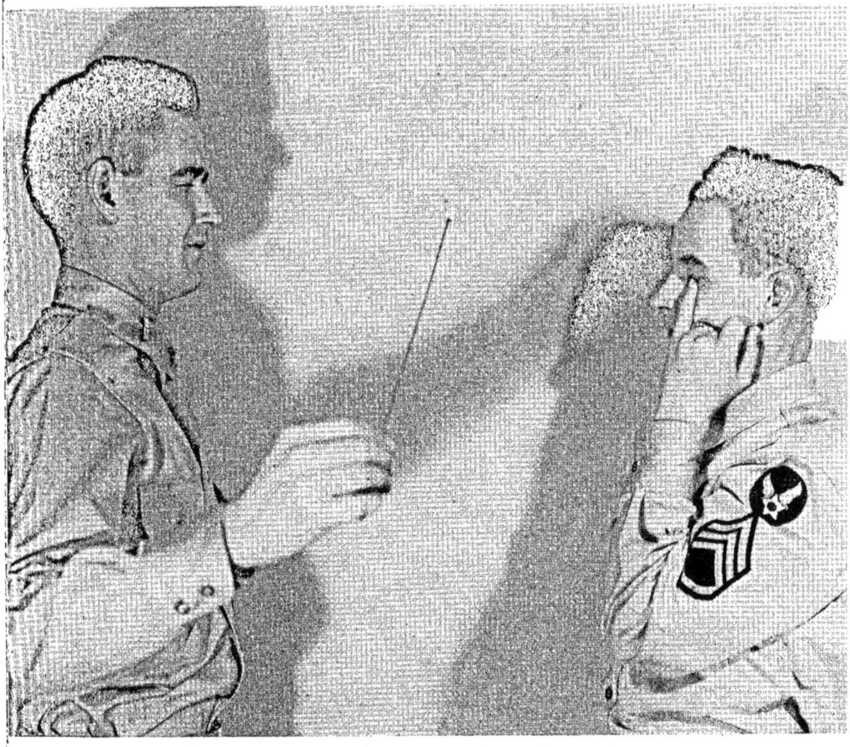

FIG. 1. Confrontation test for gross peripheral visual field determination. (Courtesy, The School of Aviation Medicine, Randolph Field, Texas.)

more important, to determine from the color the character of the terrain over which he is flying in case of an emergency landing. As one ascends, the perspective of the third dimension gradually fades, and one depends more and more on color vision to identify the characteristics of the terrain.

The Ishihara and Stillings' plates, which are used by many countries, are delicate color tests. Many cases of partial color blindness are detected by them that are not revealed by a simple test such as the Holmgren or Jennings. It is questionable whether such perfect color vision is essential in flying. The Department of Commerce does not require anything more than correct identification of individual colors.

A study of partial red-green color blind cases by Cooper[9] revealed that only 14 per cent. of partially color blind students were able to obtain licenses as against 30 per cent. of the normal. Wright[36] states: "those of you, who have flown along the air lanes at night in thick weather and tried to distinguish the red flashing intervals between the white beacon lights from those which flash green, know how difficult a matter it is at best. The red backed beacons denote the course of the flight, and the green backed beacons indicate emergency landing fields. Any serious defect in color vision would certainly make it difficult for a pilot to distinguish the two in rainy or foggy weather. The wind tees, which indicate the direction of the wind at air fields, often are lighted at night by green or red neon tubes, which are not brilliant shades of the color they are supposed to represent, and show shades, which are difficult for color blind persons to distinguish from other nearby lights. In the daytime, if a forced landing is to be made, an instantaneous decision must be arrived at as to which field is to be used for the attempt at landing. Inasmuch as the length of the grass, the presence of holes or irregularities of the ground are only discernible from above by the different shades of green in a grass field, and because the undertone of brown in a marsh may look similar to the overtone of green to a color blind pilot, who is above this type of ground, we believe that the element of danger is considerably increased by allowing color blind pilots to fly passengers."

Light Perception. — Light perception is now considered by more and more countries. Berens[6] states that night flying and flying at dusk necessitates normal light perception. Onfray[26] believes that the visual acuity at night should be equal, at least, to $\frac{5}{100}$ for an illumination of 0.0015 lux after 20 minutes of adaptation. Flynn[12] recently has described a clinical test for dark adaptation which he feels every pilot should be required to pass. It consumes but five minutes. It is important also in bringing out avitaminosis. Of 32 pilots, who were demonstrated to have a deficiency in dark adaptation, 22 were successfully treated with 10,000 units of vitamin A three times a day for fourteen days. Three weeks after the treatment all were retested and found to be well within normal limits. In 500 cases tested 6.4 per cent. were found to be deficient in vitamin A.

Ocular Muscle Balance. — Ocular muscle balance is tested in the United States rather more carefully in the military services than in

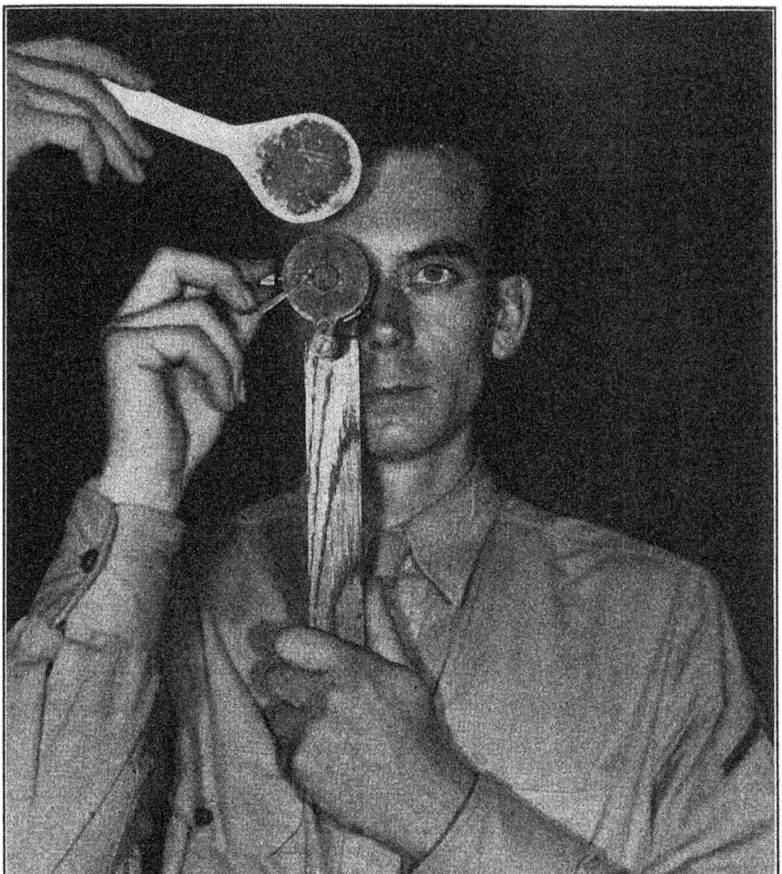

FIG. 2. Determination of heterophoria. (Courtesy, The School of Aviation Medicine, Randolph Field, Texas.)

commercial flying. It is also tested in certain other countries but not with the same detail. Berens[6] states that latent heterophoria often becomes manifest or results in diplopia under flying conditions. It certainly is a fact that fatigue and high altitude affect ocular muscle balance. Flying certainly is fatiguing. Heterophoria is a suppressed condition. It causes fatigue and results in inattention and eventually carelessness. Poor muscle balance is also a factor in faulty judgment of distance as will be seen later.

Limits of 1 diopter of hyperphoria and a minimum of 7 diopters of convergence and 3 diopters of divergence are accepted for civilian flyers in this country; also there must be no diplopia develop with the head in

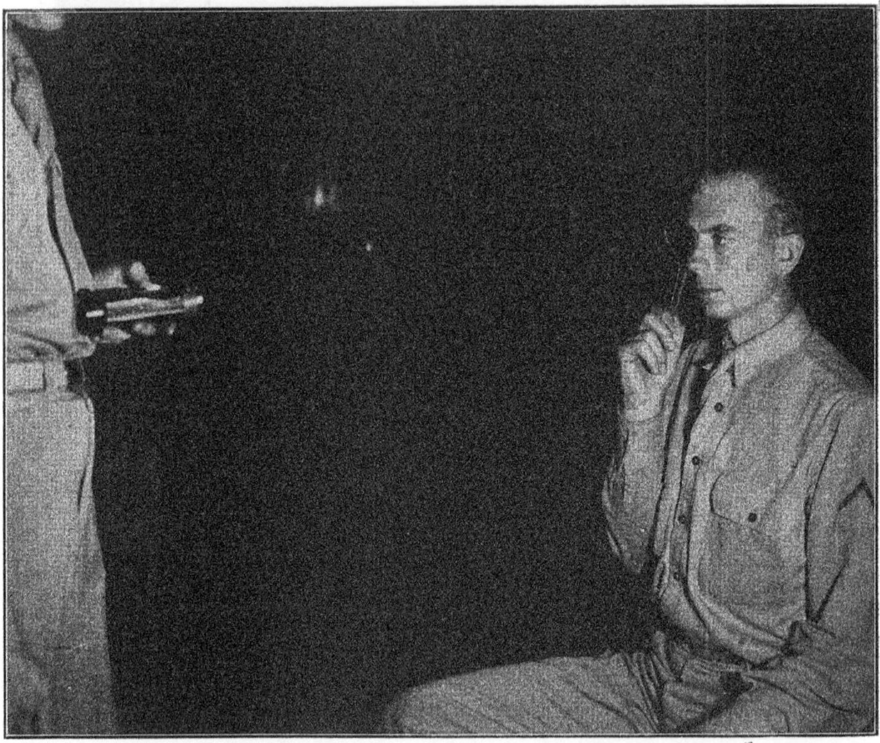

FIG. 3. Red lens test for determination of diplopia. (Courtesy, The School of Aviation Medicine, Randolph Field, Texas.)

any position except extreme angles on gazing at a light 20 feet distant with a red glass in front of one eye. The military services also test esophoria and exophoria at 20 feet and 33 inches, and the angle of convergence also is measured. The British use the red-green test and the Bishop-Harman apparatus. Berens[6] believes the near point of convergence is important, and that any near point over 80 mm. should be disqualifying.

Accommodation. — Accommodation is not universally tested, but the United States requires a certain amount of accommodation. The Army and the Department of Commerce require a minimum of 2 diopters. The Navy requires normal accommodation for age. The flyer must rapidly

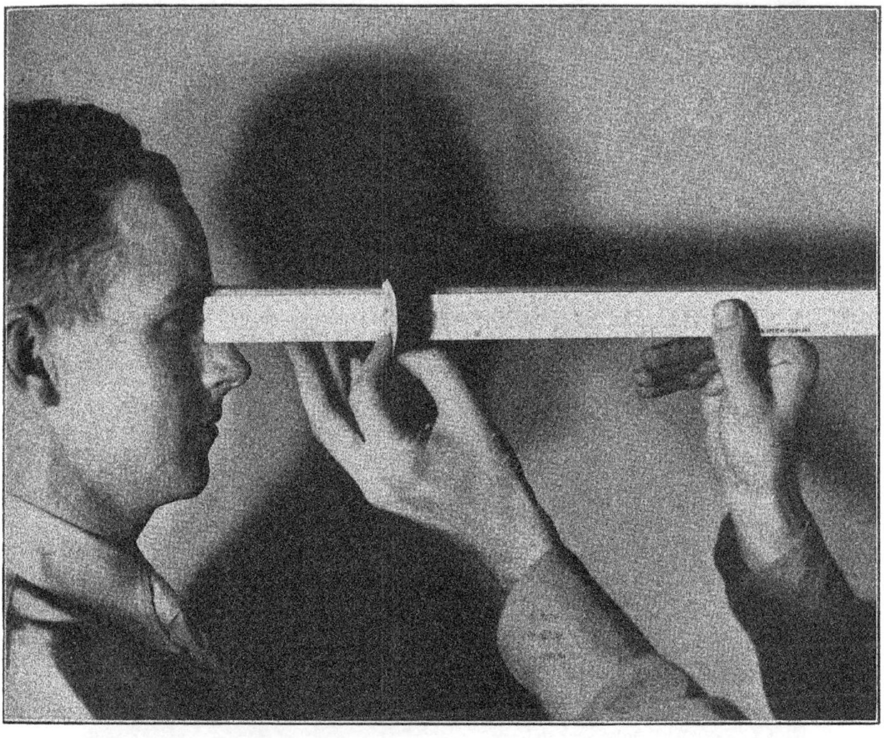

FIG. 4. Determination of the near point of accommodation. (Courtesy, The School of Aviation Medicine, Randolph Field, Texas.)

change his accommodation from that required for reading his maps and instrument board to the relaxation necessary for observing distant objects.

Depth Perception. — Judgment of distance is a highly important factor. The flyer must judge distance, when taking off or landing, from the ground, trees, buildings, telephone poles, wires, other planes, etc. In formation flying the wing tips are but a few feet apart, and a miscalculation of distance may prove fatal.

FIG. 5. The Howard depth perception apparatus in operation. The candidate is seated 20 feet away from the apparatus and looks at the rods through the window in the front. The rods are widely separated, and he endeavors to bring them parallel. At least three trials are given, and the average discrepancy must not be more than 30 mm. The apparatus is 40″ long and 12″ wide. The front and rear ends are 12″ square. The window in the front end is 5″ by $7\frac{1}{2}$″. The rods are $10\frac{3}{4}$″ high and $\frac{5}{8}$″ in diameter. One rod is fixed, and the other moves forward or backward in a slide groove. The entire apparatus is painted black except the front face of the rear screen, which is painted white. (Courtesy, The School of Aviation Medicine, Randolph Field, Texas.)

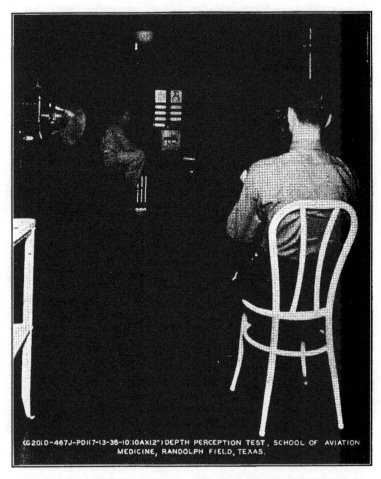

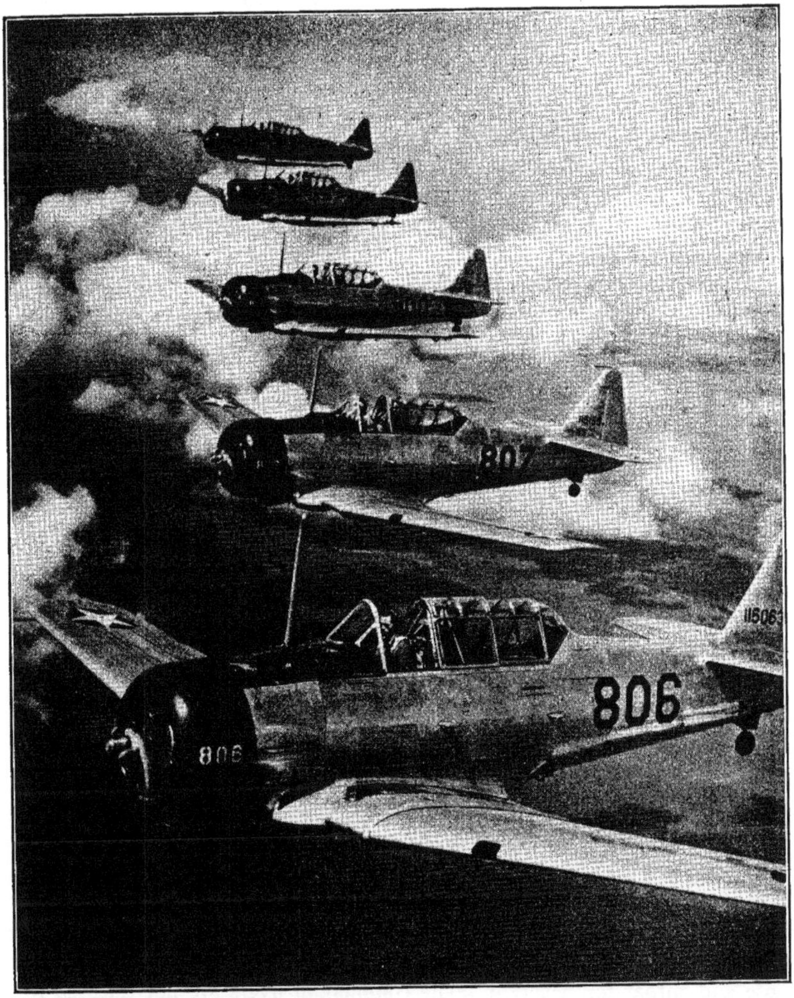

FIG. 6. Formation flying. This calls for excellent depth perception. (Courtesy, Photo Section, U. S. Army Air Forces.)

No special tests of depth perception or judgment of distance are required by many countries as they depend entirely on visual acuity and normal muscle balance. Some countries require a test of stereoscopic vision with a stereoscope. The United States uses the Howard depth perception apparatus[16] requiring a depth perception of not more than 30 mm. at 20 feet on the average of several trials.

Stereoscopic vision requires two eyes, and hence monocular individuals and those who have markedly different vision in the two eyes usually have poor depth perception. Poor ocular muscle balance also affects depth perception adversely. Clements of the Royal Air Force found that many students making poor landings were doing this because of defective ocular muscle balance and on having this defect corrected 87 per cent. of them made satisfactory landings.

There are a few one-eyed pilots who can judge distance fairly well and are good flyers. There is no question but these men acquire a method of judging distance which the average two-eyed man does not use. Jarman[17] believes this to be by means of moving the head from side to side. Having lost the function of binocular parallax, he uses one eye twice in an endeavor to make up for this loss of normal function. Only old, experienced pilots, however, should be considered for waiver of such a serious defect.

The time factor usually is not considered in this test, but it undoubtedly is an important factor, as the individual who judges distance quickly as well as accurately, is safer than one who judges it slowly, although perhaps as accurately.

Ocular Disease. — The eyes are inspected and the fundi examined for ocular disease and abnormalities and diseased conditions which, revealed, serve as a cause for rejection.

The Ear, Nose and Throat

The ear, nose and throat are surveyed for defects and disease. It has been demonstrated that under exposure to cold and extremes of weather and as a result of fatigue in flying diseased tonsils, sinuses and low grade ear infections are apt to light up into acute infections. Such should, therefore, be eliminated at the start.

Requirements are much more rigid in the military services than in civilian flying. The military services require a practically perfect ear, nose and throat for selection. The commercial flyers are not rejected for minor abnormalities, and in the private pilot gross defects sometimes are passed, such as perforated ear drums, for example. Middle ear conditions usually are accompanied by blocked or partially blocked Eustachian tubes, and on sudden changes of altitude the ear drum may be ruptured, or at least its sudden retraction may cause excruciating pain.

Hearing. — So far as hearing is concerned, up until recently it was not considered very important. It is well-known that the majority of old flyers, old in the sense of experience, have diminished hearing. This is due to the constant roar of the motor or motors. Protection is advised, but flyers for some reason are loath to wear it. The majority of pilots flying open ships wear large sized powder puffs sewn into the ear flaps of the helmets, but pilots of closed ships rarely wear any protection. In closed ships the noise is not nearly so severe, but even there it is sufficient to damage hearing.

Furthermore, the increased use of radio has made the use of any protection difficult. The pilot likes to keep his radio tuned in as low as possible. Wright[36] reported that a radio head piece with cup-shaped ear phones with sponge rubber inner surfaces was being worked out, and it is hoped that it or some other device will prove satisfactory.

The increased use of radio necessitates a certain amount of hearing and it is causing many of the older pilots some worry because they feel they are losing their hearing. It is a fact, however, that the pilots, who are somewhat deaf to ordinary tones, can still hear radio signals, the tones required by the radio not being those to which they are deaf. Good hearing then should be required in all pilots who are starting in with the idea of becoming commercial or military pilots. McFarland and associates[23] reported that with increasing age there was a gradual decrease in acuity of hearing the higher frequencies. He found this decrease was the same in non-flyers.

Equilibrium

This has been a much discussed point. During World War I two-thirds of the articles written by Americans were on the vestibular mechanism of the internal ear. The Barany tests were stressed and made much of. The French and Italians used them largely also. The British never did have any use for them. The Barany tests are now largely in the discard so far as flying is concerned. In this country they are used only by the Navy. The Army formerly used the British self-balancing test but has since discarded it. The Army now has no specific test of equilibrium as such. The Barany chair may be used as an emotional stimulus in cases of suspected neurocirculatory asthenia and doubtful nervous stability.

The Department of Commerce uses the self-balancing test alone. It consists in demonstrating the ability to stand on one foot with the other leg flexed at the knee, with the eyes closed, for 15 seconds. Three trials

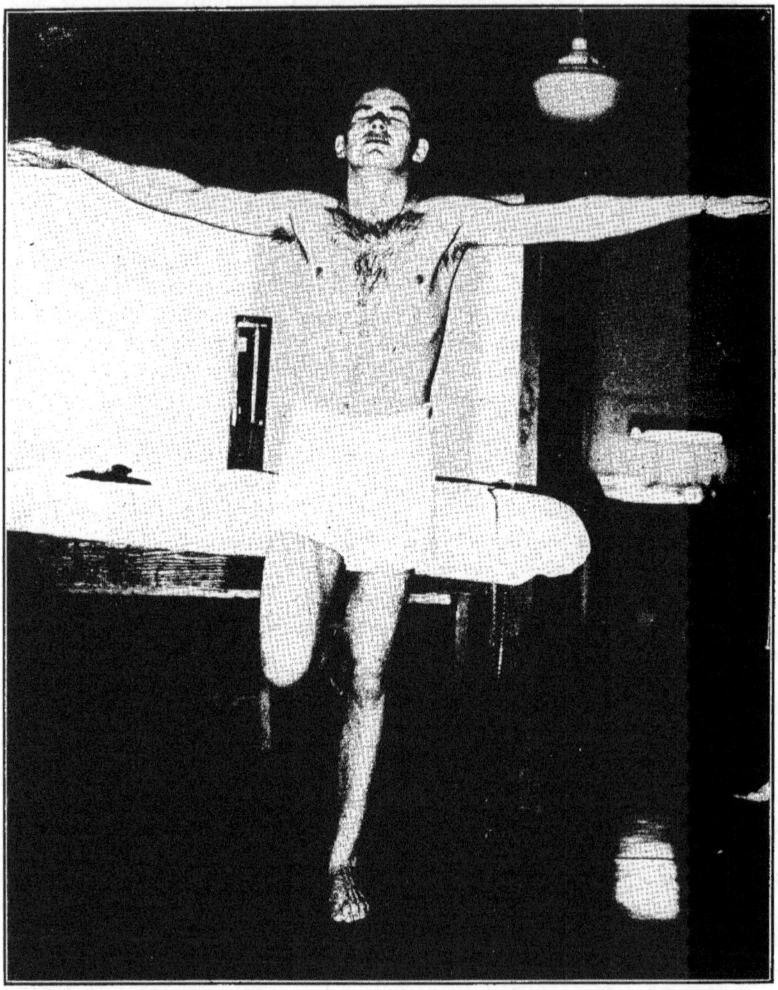

FIG. 7. The self-balancing test for equilibrium. (Courtesy, The School of Aviation Medicine, Randolph Field, Texas.)

are given. It is then repeated on the other foot. It is satisfactory for all practical purposes and does away with cumbersome apparatus that, at best, was not wholly satisfactory.

Equilibrium depends on the sensations received from our whole proprioceptive mechanism. Its various parts cannot be considered too individually. Vision is undoubtedly the most important factor in the flyer. The tactile sense is largely non-functioning in a flyer, but the internal ear, visceral sensations and sensations received from the bones, joints and muscles should be considered collectively.

Equilibrium has received a new importance with the advent of blind flying, of which more will be said later.

The General Physical Requirements

The general physical requirements are the requirements of any thorough physical selection. Sound heart, lungs, kidneys, a normal endocrine system, freedom from structural defects and disturbances of cardiovascular function and a good medical history are required and are essential. The examination consists of a thorough physical examination.

Stature. — Stature is not so important as it used to be, but a very small or a very large man is not ideal because of the resultant mechanical difficulty in reaching or operating the controls. Men of average stature are preferred for fighter pilots rather than very tall men.

Age. — Age is a disputed factor, but flying is still for the younger generation. After 35 to 40 a conservatism and slowness of reaction develop that prevent one from becoming a high class flyer, if he does not learn until that age. Those, who learned young and are now between 40 and 50 years of age, are in a different class. They have passed the most difficult stage of their careers, namely training and early experience. They seem to continue to do well. Fighter and dive-bomber pilots definitely are preferred of the younger age, below 28 years. The international regulations impose an age limit of 19 to 45 for transport license.

Structural Factors. — Complete use of the four limbs is an international requirement. Loss of 2 or 3 fingers, slight limitations of motion of the ankle, wrist or knee may be permitted, but complete mobility of shoulder, elbow and hip are essential and only minor limitations of the excepted joints permitted. The manipulation of the controls, brakes and stabilizer require this much as a safety factor. There are a few pilots flying who have had one leg amputated below the knee, but they all learned to fly before the amputation and are in a special class, therefore. Hernias in the case of transport or military pilots should disqualify until they are repaired. Flying often is strenuous, and strangulation a danger.

General. — The military, of course, require freedom from organic disease of the heart, lungs, kidneys, endocrine glands and digestive system. That pilots, who are to carry passengers, should likewise be physically sound goes without saying. There are a few exceptions. An old arrested tuberculosis without symptoms may be passed for commercial flying. Acute infections need be causes for rejection only temporarily unless they leave manifestly disqualifying defects.

Cardiovascular System. — The cardiovascular system should not only be free from organic disease, but there should be no evidence of neurocirculatory asthenia. The nervous mechanism is under a severe strain in flying anyway, and the "weak sister" drops by the wayside. More will be said of this under the nervous system.

Fatigue, altitude and stress all impose strain on the cardiovascular mechanism, and hence it must be normal to start with. Many applicants come in for their first examination in a state of apprehension. High pulses and blood pressures are encountered frequently. The examiner must eliminate organic cardiovascular disease, thyroid disease and neurocirculatory asthenia. Reassurance and obtaining the confidence of the applicant often will result in the pulse and blood pressure returning to reasonable limits. The response of the pulse to exercise and the length of time it takes it to return to its pre-exercise rate are often more important than the rate itself. Any pulse that gives an exaggerated response to exercise and is slow in returning should be a cause for rejection, even if no organic disease is demonstrable. Such an applicant probably is in the class of the nervously unstable and will make poor flying material. Those applicants, who show hypertension on several examinations but who have no history of hypertension when not under stress, rarely make good pilots. Many are potential cases of essential hypertension, and most of them are somewhat emotionally unstable.

Urine Examination. — Nephrosis, nephritis and diabetes are, of course, disqualifying because of the serious constitutional effects. A urine examination is manifestly a requirement.

Digestive System. — The digestive system seems to be particularly important in flyers. They have irregular hours and irregular meals with food of all kinds and at all sorts of places; their bowels may of necessity be irregular because of their flying schedules, and disturbances of the gastrointestinal tract are common. Hence, the history of any symptoms suggesting ulcer, gall bladder disturbance, colitis, etc. must be gone into with considerable care, and all cases that seem to have a definite gastrointestinal condition should be rejected.

Syphilis. — Syphilis is, of course, disqualifying. A Wassermann reaction is not required for a commercial license unless a history or suspicious signs are unearthed. It would be best if a Wassermann test was required on all prospective commercial pilots. The military do require it, of course, as a prerequisite to commission.

The Nervous System

The nervous system was passed over superficially in the early days of flying. Other than examination by means of a few neurological tests, such as pupillary reactions, station, knee jerks, etc., nothing was done.

It soon became apparent that the nervous system was subject to great wear and tear in flying, and one of the commonest causes for removal from flying status was nervous instability. Consequently, the development of a searching neuropsychic examination took place. It has reached its highest peak in this country in the Army examination. The Navy and Department of Commerce also require searching examinations.

For practical purposes the following points are all that it is necessary to cover.

Neurological Examination. — (1) Pupillary abnormalities, the cause of which must, if possible, be elicited and syphilitic conditions suspected.

(2) Knee jerks, with the usual interpretation of findings.

(3) Station; both a Romberg and modified Romberg are done which must be satisfactory.

(4) Gait; walking backward, forward and in a circle with eyes open and closed.

(5) Tics, the presence of which leads one to suspect an unstable nervous system.

(6) Tremors of hands, eyelids and tongue; if abnormal, neurological conditions, hyperthyroidism and neurocirculatory asthenia must be considered.

(7) Other motor abnormalities, such as residual from infantile paralysis.

(8) Psychomotor tension, the ability to relax voluntarily. If unable to relax, the applicant usually is emotionally unstable and will not learn to fly readily.

(9) Peripheral circulatory flushing, mottling, acrocyanosis, sweating, cold extremities, the presence of which suggest neurocirculatory asthenia or a more serious nervous system derangement.

Psychic Examination. — This part of the examination, as Longacre[19] so aptly states, "should begin when the candidate first comes into view and ends only when he has passed from sight and hearing".

The psychic examination specifically includes a search for a family history of epilepsy, hyperthyroidism, psychosis and psychoneurosis. The family history of any may indicate a transmitted nervous instability. Past personal history should be searching and covers not only the history of severe illnesses and injuries, but a complete personality study is made. This covers childhood environment and reaction to discipline, educational history and progress, athletic life, social trends, somatic demands, self-expression, psychomotor activity, self-criticism, temperament, philosophy of life.

Longacre[19] has stated that the purpose of this personality study is to study the condition of the candidate's nervous system. An effort is made to determine whether or not there are deviations from the normal, and if so, whether or not these deviations are sufficient to disqualify him from flying, to study the candidate's temperament, intelligence and volition and again to determine deviations from normal for the same reason, to study the manner of the candidate's reaction to his environment and to unearth latent tendencies which, under the stress of flying, might become accentuated in such a manner as to render him inefficient, and to determine the personality trends, resistances and potentialities.

During this personality study, we may find the following favorable factors: (a) Temperament. — Cheerful, stable, self-reliant, aggressive, modest, frank, fond of people, satisfied, punctilious, serious, good coöperation in work and in examination, good sportsmanship, moderate tension, enthusiastic, adaptable; (b) Intelligence. — Precise, penetrating, sharp, alert, resourceful; (c) Volition. — Energetic, quick, deliberate, or moderately impulsive, controlled, good tenacity of purpose.

We may also find the following unfavorable factors: (a) Temperament. — Depressed, unstable, submissive, pacific, vain, withholding, secretive, loquacious, likes to be alone, hypercritical of conditions, careless, frivolous, poor coöperation, irritable, poor sportsmanship (under adverse circumstances, querulous and complaining), exceedingly high tension, lost enthusiasm; (b) Intelligence. — Vague, superficial, dull, hesitant, without initiative, untrained; (c) Volition. — Sluggish, slow, recklessly impulsive, restless, poor tenacity of purpose.

No one, of course, will exhibit all favorable or all unfavorable factors, but the preponderance one way or the other will determine whether or not he will make a satisfactory flyer. The importance of this part of the examination will be realized when a study is made of the reasons given by instructors why men fail to learn to fly. Longacre[20] made such a study of the failures at the Army primary flying school. He found the following reasons for failure as stated by the instructors: slow, mentally and physically; unable to analyze and correct errors; inconsistent, erratic from day to day; poor on simple manœuvres and lost in acrobatics; unable to absorb or retain instructions; poor in speed, distance, coördination, altitudes and balance; no feel of ship; does not realize his mistakes or when he is right and when he is wrong; unable to sense slips, skids, stalls, etc.; easily confused; lacks initiative and aggressiveness; learns nothing for himself; fusses with controls; inattentive to instruments, traffic, obstacles, wind directions; jerky and rough on controls; kicks or rides the rudder; mechanical flyer, and in connection with that one instructor very aptly completes the picture by saying "no instinctive performance, all mechanical"; unable to coördinate controls; headwork poor; judgment poor; tense, apprehensive, nervous and excitable; danger in power-off; poor headwork on forced landing; excitable and blows up on slightest provocation; had difficulty because left-handed; repeats his mistakes over and over again; forgets instruction over night, over the week-end, over the Christmas holidays and so on; perhaps too much diversified interest; inattentive to details; reaches his saturation point and fails to progress; concentrates on flying the plane to the exclusion of everything else, i.e., he excludes every factor in the environment, he is oblivious to the traffic, the wind directions, lights and everything of that sort; lets plane fly; never seems to control it; hopelessly unable to fly; entirely out of his element; too easily confused; unable to execute manœuvres requiring finer timing and coördination; unable to decide promptly and act decisively; unable to relax. He states that, of 687 failures, 404 were reported as incurably tense and apprehensive.

Carlson[8] reported that instructors "washed out" students frequently with the following remarks; slow learner, poor comprehension, poor retention, poor headwork, slow progress, unable to understand, forgets instructions.

Longacre[19] further states the following traits are indices of such future poor performance and in a careful examination could be unearthed; "indecisiveness, inattentiveness, uncertainty, indefiniteness, evasiveness, hesitancy, timidity, overdeveloped self-preservative instinct, vagueness, superficiality, recklessness, clumsiness, awkwardness, slow comprehension, delayed or slow motor response, sluggishness, poor retention, lack of initiative and aggressiveness, self-depreciation, tenseness, inability to relax, being oversensitive, being unduly introspective, being handicapped by an inability to respond correctly to diversified stimuli, i.e., to instruments, ships, etc. and environments simultaneously."

We must, therefore, endeavor to forecast the candidate's probable reaction to this new experience of flying. Again to quote Longacre[19] "the examination must reveal latent tendencies which under the stress of flying might become so accentuated as to make him, the pilot, inefficient and lead to nervous and mental breakdown; or on the other hand, make clear such stability of organization as will be proof against stresses admittedly exceptional and foreign to average experience. It is not conceded that nature has at last achieved her highest objective and in the flyer produced a superman. It is, however, required that he be equal to the requirements of any situation, usual or unusual and with respect to the unusual, be capable of the instantaneous and correct response demanded by the emergency."

Vasomotor Instability. — Examination for this condition is conducted as part of the cardiovascular examination and as part of the neuropsychic examination. The Army[11] states that, if persistently present in marked degree, it is disqualifying for pilot training. The following manifestations are listed; (1) rapid pulse, (2) labile pulse, (3) labile low blood pressure, (4) low Schneider index, (5) cyanotic extremities, (6) cold clammy extremities, (7) mottling of extremities, (8) profuse axillary perspiration, (9) palmar and plantar perspiration, (10) tremors of extended hands, (11) tremors of closed eyelids, (12) tremulousness of muscles of face and lips, (13) tremulousness of speech.

In each case the flight surgeon is cautioned to evaluate any of the signs of vasomotor instability with all the other findings in the complete examination to determine the individual's ability to withstand the signs of military aviation.

Reaction Time and Flying Aptitude

Reaction time has always been considered an important factor in flying, and various attempts have been made to devise a satisfactory apparatus. During World War I simple reaction times were tested, but they have been discarded nearly universally as being worthless. It was found that the promptness with which an individual might tap a telegraph key in response to a stimulus of a light, a bell or an electrode on the hand was no indication of how he might respond with a complicated arm and leg movement under the proper stimulus in the air.

The Ruggles orientator was devised in this country and was used considerably. It consisted of the cockpit of an airplane suspended in three concentric rings controlled by motors and governed either from the cockpit or the ground. The candidate could be placed in every conceivable position with relation to the horizon and put through any rotary motion. The disadvantage of the apparatus was that the results of training in it were purely a matter of personal opinion of the operator. There was no graphic record, and it has been discarded.

The Reid reaction apparatus is an improvement in that it has a graphic record of the candidate's performance. It consists of the cockpit of a plane fitted with seat, stick and rudder bar. On the instrument

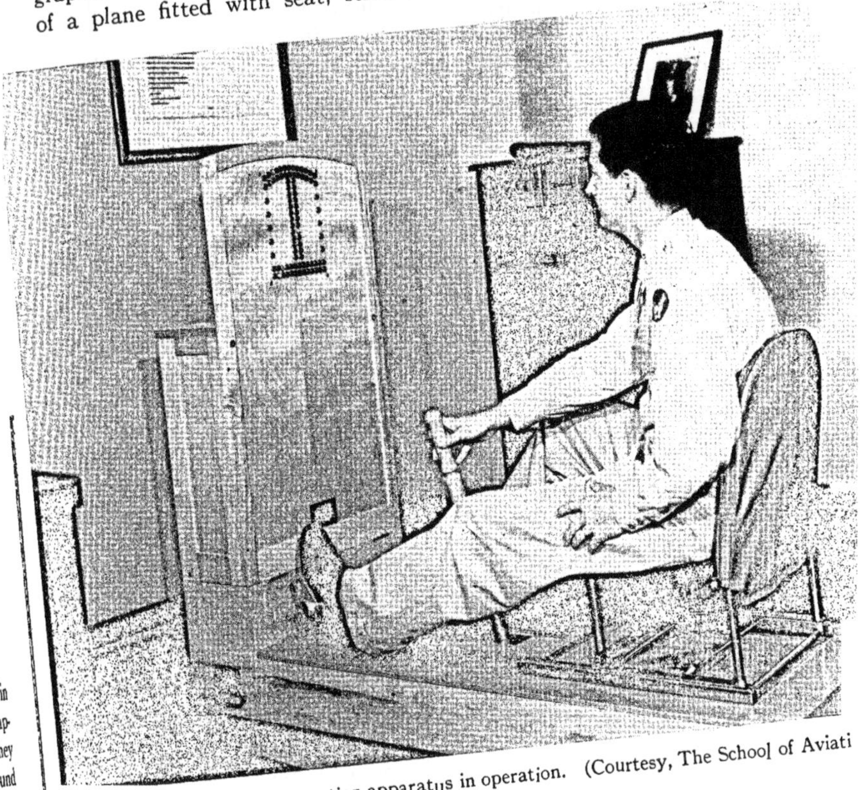

FIG. 8. The serial reaction apparatus in operation. (Courtesy, The School of Aviati Medicine, Randolph Field, Texas.)

board are two rows of lights, one for the stick and one for the rudd When in an extreme position all the lights are lighted. They gradua go out as the controls approach neutral. Whenever the controls are neutral, a recording pen continues writing until the neutral point reached and maintained. A chronometer measures the length of tim fractions of a second that the controls are off neutral.

The test, after a practice period, consists in having the controls placed in an extreme position. The chronograph starts, the pen writes, and the length of time it takes to neutralize the controls is recorded graphically. Ten tests of rudder, 10 of stick and 20 of combined stick and rudder are so made. Then, while one test is being made, a klaxon horn back of the candidate is blown suddenly, and the effect of the emotional disturbance in prolonging reaction time is noted and also in succeeding tests the length of time it takes to come back to his average performance before the horn was blown.

The average reaction time is figured and the candidate rated accordingly. The British claim remarkable results with it. They state that there is an 80 to 90 per cent. correlation between the results of the test and the actual flying record in the schools of instruction.

The slower the reaction time, the poorer the flyer, as a rule, and anyone whose reaction time is below 4 seconds is not considered worth training, and those who cannot do better than 3.5 seconds probably will make only mediocre pilots at best.

A serial reaction apparatus was devised in 1934 by Mashburn and Constable and reported by Mashburn as an automatic apparatus designed to present a continuous series of stimuli[21]. The responses to the signals are made by a coördinated movement of a series of controls operated by the hands and feet. The correct response to a set of signals automatically sets up the succeeding signals until the whole series is completed. A reactor's score is the total time required to run through the complete series.

This test still is being used at certain reception centers in the Army in conjunction with five other psychomotor tests in an effort to find a group of tests which will have a high correlation rate with the successful completion of flying training.

For commercial flying no such complicated tests and no expensive apparatus as those just described can be used. We must depend on the neuropsychic examination, already outlined. With careful examinations and with particular lookout for the factors, enumerated by Longacre as indicating poor aptitude, we can arrive at fairly satisfactory results.

The Army has adopted an adaptability rating for military aeronautics aptitude[35]. This is based on an even more detailed personality study than the one outlined under the nervous system. The following factors are studied and a maximum rate for each factor is reckoned as follows on the next page:

Family history	05
Environment	05
Morphology	10
Intelligence	60
Achievement	20
Psychomotor activity	20
Emotionality	35
Somatic demands	25
Sociality	15
Philosophy of life	05
Total	200

160 points are required to qualify. An unsatisfactory adaptability rating must be supported by at least one of the following 18 reasons: (1) history of multiple, 2 or more, instances of mental disturbances in the immediate family (father, mother and siblings); (2) intelligence is considered below the required standard because of (a) many failures in the grades and high school requiring extra months or years to complete high school, (b) inability to accomplish two years of college work because of many academic failures, (c) complete lack of accomplishment to date and failure to take advantage of opportunities (school and work), (d) specific instances of applicant's behavior indicating questionable intelligence. Record must be made of evidence demonstrating poor judgment, poor comprehension, poor memory, poor attention, poor learning or other faulty intellectual operations. These must be so obvious that they outweigh any educational attainments; (3) a history of somnambulism; (4) a history of stammering or presence of a tic; (5) a history of migraine or migraine type of headache; (6) a history of amnesia, (psychogenic); (7) a history of skull fracture or severe concussion with persistent symptoms, any period of unconsciousness of 2 hours or longer; (8) a history of epilepsy or convulsions; (9) a history of fainting due to inadequate cause subsequent to age 12, the only adequate causes being (a) pain following a severe injury, (b) during convalescence from an acute illness, (c) moderate to severe loss of blood; (10) persistent insomnia (anxiety); (11) obsessions or phobias which motivate conduct; (12) instability manifest by combinations of the following, one or even two not necessarily disqualifying; (a) convulsions in minor illness, (b) prolonged enuresis; if to present time, it alone is disqualifying, (c) frequent headaches, (d) multiple histories of momentary unconsciousness in minor injuries, (e) pavor nocturnus (anxiety), (f) mild insomnia (anxiety), (g) nail biting, (h) mannerisms, (i) excessive tobacco, (j) a

low Schneider index, (k) tenseness; (13) excessive alcohol or criminal history; (14) any major psychosis; (15) any minor psychosis (psychoneurosis); (16) any constitutional psychopathic state; (17) the following personality trends, if present to a considerable degree, seclusive, overactive, depressive, suspicious, egotistical, irritable, sexually abnormal and criminalistic; (18) any neurological disqualification.

Periodicity of Examinations

All countries require some sort of physical examinations for their military air forces, and most countries require stringent examinations as already described for both military and civilian pilots. The United States and many other countries require a satisfactory physical examination for flying before an individual may solo in licensed aircraft. It is a universal practice to require re-examinations of licensed pilots at stated intervals. All civil pilots are examined once a year. Air-line pilots are examined at least twice a year. All pilots must be re-examined following an accident before resuming flying. The United States requires its military pilots to be re-examined twice a year. The mid-year examination is only a check of the more important points. The annual examination is complete. Following accidents or serious illness, an examination is required also before resuming flying. Air-line pilots in the United States are examined at least twice annually and other pilots annually.

Physical Defect and Flying Ability

Much has been said already about the necessity of a normal physical makeup for flying and how the examinations for selection of the flyer have grown more stringent. It may be well at this point to consider what happens to the flyer who is not physically sound, particularly in his training period.

Bauer and Cooper[9] studied the records of 9,000 students without previous experience and the records of about 2,000 accidents in trained flyers. Later Cooper[10] carried it further to cover about 30,000 students and over 4,000 accidents.

In the first study the records of all student pilots licensed by the U. S. Department of Commerce, who had had a year or more since the issuance of their student permits in which to obtain a higher grade of license, were studied. No student was included who had had previous experience in flying. The students were classified according to their physical condition. The study showed that of those with no defects, 35.4 per cent.

obtained a private license or better in a year; those with minor defects, 30.3 per cent. advanced; those with major defects, 18.5 per cent. advanced and of those with disqualifying defects, only 12.5 per cent. advanced. In other words, as the defect increased in magnitude, the less chance the individual had of learning to fly.

Cooper's[10] study of 30,000 students showed similar but more marked discrepancies between the groups. In this study the normal group showed a progress rate of 30.5 per cent.; the minor defect group, 17 per cent.; the major defect group, 14.7 per cent. and the disqualified group, 4.1 per cent. He found also as to the group with disqualifying defects that, all told, 286 permits had been issued to students with disqualifying defects, and of these 286 only 6 at the time of the study held a license of any sort. In other words, if regulations did not stop their flying, nature did.

Cooper[10] went a step further in this latter study and broke down the large groups into classes of defects. As would be expected, he found that some defects were more serious than others. For example, in the group of so-called minor defects he found that mild structural defects and minor defects of hearing showed a progress rate of 21.5 per cent. as against 17 per cent. for the group as a whole and 30.5 per cent. for the normals. Moderate defects of color vision showed a progress rate of only 14 per cent., thus bearing out Wright's contention already mentioned. Those with high pulses and blood pressures had a progress rate of only 8 per cent. This is in line with Longacre's findings that nervousness and apprehension are common causes of failure in learning to fly. In the group of major defects defective vision showed a progress rate of 21.5 per cent. as against 14.7 per cent. for the group as a whole and 30.5 per cent. for the normals; general physical defects, a rate of 5.8 per cent.; ocular muscle imbalance, a rate of 4.1 per cent.; inferior neuropsychic makeup a rate of 3.5 per cent., again emphasizing the importance of a sound nervous system; while structural defects and defective equilibrium showed a rate of 0.

All this proves rather conclusively that physical condition and the ability to learn to fly are closely related. The greater the physical defect, the poorer the chance of becoming a flyer.

The study of accidents by Bauer and Cooper[9] showed that in 1928 the accident rate in normal pilots was 13.6 per cent.; in pilots with some physical defect, the rate was 18.2 per cent. In 1929 the rate for the normal group was 12.3 per cent. and for the defective group 18.2 per cent. Figured in another way, in 1928 the percentage of normal pilots who had accidents was 10.5 per cent. and the percentage of defective pilots who had accidents was 18.5 per cent. In 1929 the figures were 10.6 for the normal and 15.6 for the defective. The normal pilots showed a fatality rate in accidents of 1.55 per cent. and the defectives a rate of 2.36 per cent.

Cooper[10] studied 4,227 accidents and considered the transport, the limited commercial and the private pilots separately. He found the private pilots, who had physical defects, had accidents 33⅓ per cent. more often than the normal, and the fatal accidents were 66⅔ per cent. more numerous among the defective than among the normal. In the limited commercial grade the figures were the same as for the private pilots for accidents, and the fatal accidents were 50 per cent. greater among the defectives than among the normal.

In the transport grade the accident rate in the physically defective group was 50 per cent. greater, and the fatal accidents were the same in both groups. Cooper explains the latter fact by stating that transport pilots in view of their greater experience are more apt to get out of serious situations with less damage.

The work by Bauer and Cooper has been criticized as not being borne out by facts. However, Herbolsheimer[15] has just made a study of 300 unselected aviation accidents and found that the accident rate in pilots with physical impairments was one-third greater than the ratio of physically defective pilots certificated. This study was on reported civil air accidents in 1941.

As a check the last 100 accidents reported up to August 1942 were analyzed, and the figures were in close agreement with the 1941 figures. From the results of the study Herbolsheimer states: "It appears safe to conclude that pilots with physical impairments can reasonably be expected to be involved in aviation accidents more frequently than persons with no impairments".

These figures are not radically different from those of Cooper, who found the rate of accidents in various types of pilots was from 33 to 50 per cent. greater in the group with physical impairments.

It has been alleged that flying experience is a greater deterrent of accidents than physical condition. No one denies that the experienced pilot is less prone to accidents, but it must be remembered that aviation accidents are apt to be fatal, and hence, as Herbolsheimer states, "there are few 'repeaters'", so that those prone to accidents are eliminated. Furthermore, in any study of experienced pilots the type of flying done, type of aircraft flown, whether local hops or cross country, blind flying, weather conditions, etc., must be known, as they all affect the pilot's "accident exposure".

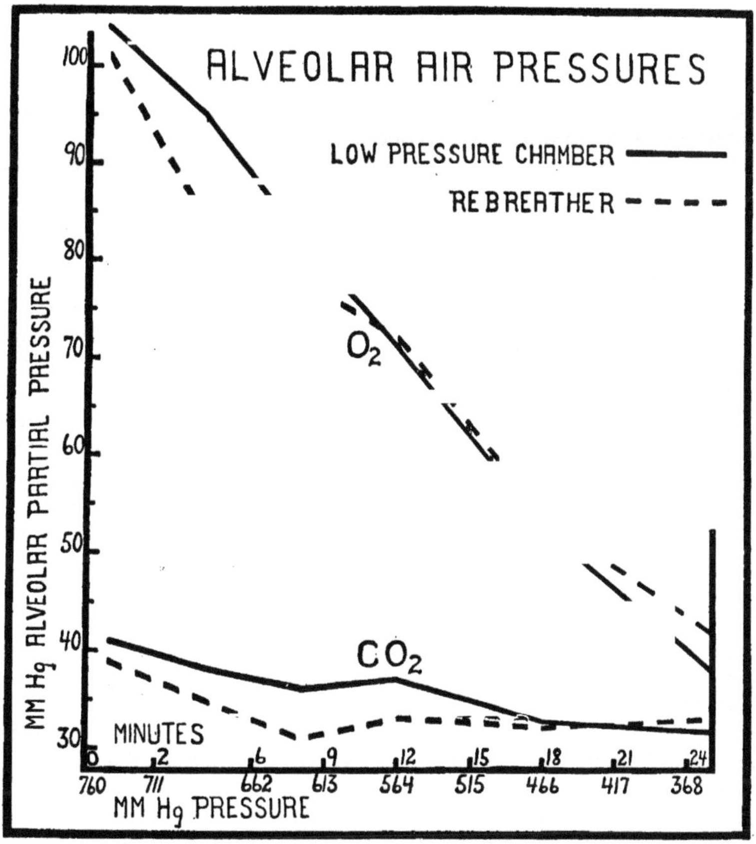

FIG. 9. Alveolar air pressures. (From Bauer, Aviation Medicine, courtesy, Williams and Wilkins Co.)

THE EFFECTS OF HIGH ALTITUDE

Military flying is being done at increasingly high altitudes, 30,000 to 40,000 feet. In commercial flying, except when flying over mountainous country, 8,000 feet is about the limit except in the so-called "stratosphere planes". In crossing the Rocky Mountains altitudes of 10,000 to 14,000 feet may be reached. Stratosphere planes are now in use on some of the air-lines. They are really substratosphere planes and not stratosphere. They fly at about 20,000 feet. They have a hermetically sealed cabin in which the atmosphere is kept at a level which does not require supplementary oxygen. Recently much has been heard about building planes that can fly in the stratosphere, above 50,000 feet, in order to take advantage of the wind direction and speed at that height.

In this connection it must be borne in mind that the average unacclimatized person becomes unconscious without oxygen at about 25,000 feet. With oxygen he may go considerably higher. What the exact limit is varies probably with the individual, his physical condition and weather conditions. However, it is somewhere near 47,000 feet. At this level, or near it, the pressure of oxygen, even when the individual is breathing pure oxygen from a supplementary supply, is too low to sustain life, and the individual dies.

The early effects of oxygen want are evidenced by an increased volume of respiration per minute. The pulse accelerates, possibly in an effort at compensation, but probably chiefly as a sign of distress. The blood pressure may remain level until just before unconsciousness, when there may be a gradual rise of the systolic pressure and a gradual fall of the diastolic. In some cases either the systolic or diastolic pressure may fall suddenly, causing circulatory failure with fainting.

The effects of oxygen want on the brain are evidenced first by a feeling of exhilaration. Then there is a loss of attention, particularly a restriction of the field of attention, and an inability to coördinate the finer muscular movements. This may be seen experimentally in the handwriting of an individual. Finally, judgment is lost. Vision and hearing do not diminish until just before unconsciousness. The effects develop insidiously, and frequently they are compared to the effects of alcohol. Unconsciousness may ensue without the individual being at all aware of anything wrong.

As one ascends into higher altitudes, the barometric pressure gradually falls, and the oxygen percentage remains constant. The oxygen pressure in the atmosphere is determined by the formula:

$$\text{Oxygen percentage} \times \text{barometric pressure.}$$

For example, at sea level, the oxygen pressure is 760 mm. $\times$ 0.21 = 159+ mm. Hg.

Alveolar oxygen pressure determines the amount of oxygen absorbed into the blood. Alveolar oxygen pressure is determined by deducting the pressure of water vapor accumulated in inspired air (47 mm. at any level) and multiplying the remainder by the oxygen percentage. The oxygen percentage in the alveoli, however, is not 0.21 but approximately 0.145 per cent. as it has become diluted by the time it reaches the alveoli. Hence at sea level the alveolar oxygen pressure is

$$760 - 47 = 713 \times .145 = 103+ \text{ mm.}$$

As one ascends, the alveolar oxygen pressure falls. If one adds supplementary oxygen to the inspired air, he increases the oxygen percentage and can, therefore, increase the alveolar oxygen pressure. This, as will be seen, is true only up to a certain point.

The pressure of oxygen is what man depends upon for life. At 47,000 feet the barometric pressure is 100 mm. of mercury and 47 mm. of water vapor accumulates in inspired air before it reaches the alveoli of the lungs. This must be deducted from the atmospheric pressure. This leaves us 53 mm. of available atmospheric pressure in the alveoli. From this must also be deducted the carbon dioxide pressure. There is no known method of breathing supplementary oxygen that prevents dilution by outside air, and hence this less than 53 mm. of possible O_2 pressure is reduced still further. Forty mm. of pressure in the alveoli is about the minimum at which man can exist for more than a few minutes. Even then, the blood is somewhat venous and the individual suffering from extreme oxygen want. In addition the carbon dioxide pressure has fallen, due to the increased ventilation of the lungs, and this fall in carbon dioxide pressure decreases the dissociation of oxygen from the hemoglobin in the tissues. Hence, somewhere about 47,000 feet is the absolute limit for man even when breathing pure oxygen.

From 10,000 feet to about 34,000 feet the use of supplementary oxygen in gradually increasing percentages will restore the aviator to sea-level conditions. At 33,000 feet he needs 100 per cent. oxygen. From then on up even with 100 per cent. he again suffers from increasing oxygen want, due to the diminished partial pressure of oxygen available. It has been estimated that a man at a little over 40,000 feet breathing pure oxygen is in the same condition as a man at 18,000 feet without oxygen, and somewhere around 47,000 feet he will die even though breathing 100 per cent. oxygen.

The flights in a balloon to the stratosphere by Piccard were accomplished by the observers being sealed in a metal ball in which the atmospheric pressure was kept up to a point compatible with life. In flights of airplanes to this level the cabin was sealed hermetically and the pressure within the cabin artificially kept at a level compatible with life as well as a means provided for elimination of carbon dioxide, as an excess of the latter is as bad as too little. In pressure cabins the atmosphere is kept at a level of 8,000 feet. At altitudes of 40,000 or more feet, if a leak ensues, not only will acute oxygen want develop, but unconsciousness will ensue rapidly and air "bends" are apt to occur.

On repeated flights to high altitudes above 10,000 feet oxygen should be used. On any flight above 12,000 feet it should be used. No flyer can perform his mission safely and efficiently at high altitudes without oxygen. Barach states that impairment of reason, memory and judgment takes place at altitudes as low as 12,000 feet[4].

Gaseous oxygen is the type commonly used. It is fed to the pilot through a face mask of the B.L.B. or similar type[7].

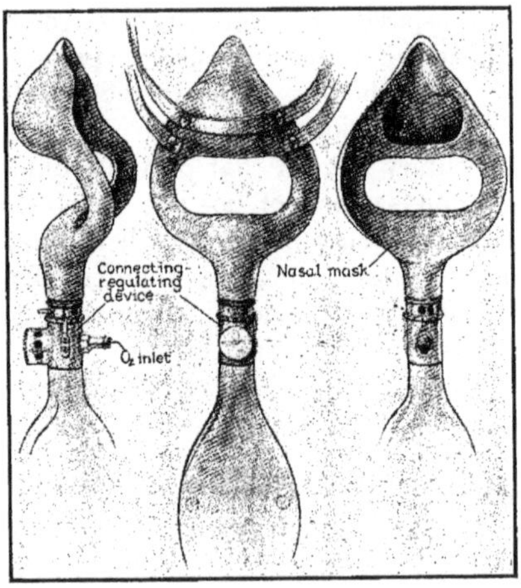

FIG. 10. The Boothby-Lovelace-Bulbullian (B.L.B.) nasal oxygen mask. (Courtesy Walter M. Boothby and the Bruce Publishing Company.)

AERO EMBOLISM AND EMPHYSEMA

At levels above 25,000 feet we encounter not only the effects of oxygen want but the effects of greatly lowered barometric pressure. With rapid ascents through these high altitudes nitrogen is given off in gaseous form into the blood and tissues. If the gaseous bubbles are in the blood, they may form air emboli. If they penetrate the tissues emphysema results. The condition is the same as what has long been known as caisson disease or the "bends". The condition may be sufficient to cause discomfort, actual distress or even total disability. It occurs frequently at levels between 30,000 and 40,000 feet. Paralysis may result from air embolism to the spinal cord.

Behnke[5] states that "bends" will develop between 25,000 and 28,000 feet without preoxygenation. By this is meant breathing 100 per cent. oxygen prior to the take-off. He found that with 45 minutes of preoxygenation bends did not develop until 30,000 feet were reached; with 90 minutes, not until 34,000 feet; with three hours, not until 37,000 feet and with five hours, not until 40,0000 feet. He found also that using a mixture of oxygen and helium instead of pure oxygen shortened the time necessary to accomplish the same end. For example 90 minutes of breathing the oxygen-helium mixture was equivalent to 5 hours of pure oxygen. Behnke found also that the younger group of pilots was far less susceptible to aero embolism than the older group. He recommends preflight tests for selection of those to do high altitude flying.

Effects of High Speed

High speed in flying is becoming more and more common. Passenger airplanes now frequently travel at 200 or more miles per hour. Such a speed, however, is not particularly dangerous. The speed planes, however, flying 300 or more miles per hour are a different matter. Dive-bombing in which the plane attains 500 miles per hour before the pull-out is serious.

Straight ahead speeds are far less dangerous than speed on turns, because the acceleration is gradual, and there is no change of direction. In turning, however, there is danger of unconsciousness. Even turning sharply at 200 miles an hour may cause everything to become blotted out for the flyer. This usually is transitory, and the flyer promptly recovers. Sometimes the "blotting out" persists for several seconds. One flyer, who pulled his ship up in a test at 190 miles an hour, states that everything remained black for 45 seconds. One Army officer did not fully recover his vision for several hours. Garsaux[14] in experiments on dogs rotated the animals on a wheel at speeds varying from four to six turns per second. Some of the dogs showed actual brain damage due to the pressure of the brain against the skull. Autopsies showed an anemia of the brain and an engorgement of the vessels of the abdominal area.

In dive-bombing the pull of centrifugal force on change of direction at about 500 miles per hour amounts to 5 or more G's. 1 G is equal to the pull of gravity, namely, the pull to which we are accustomed and which keeps us from falling off the earth. When this pull is increased, we feel the effects. At a pull of 5 G's muscular power is overcome, and breathing becomes almost impossible. The blood is drained away from the upper part of the body, and unconsciousness ensues. There may be, according to some, a factor of vasomotor relaxation in addition to the pull of centrifugal force.

The exact point of unconsciousness depends somewhat on individual tolerance, but it occurs between 6 to 8 G's. There is a fall in blood pressure in the upper half of the body and an increase in the lower half as would be expected. Fulton[13] states that at 7 G's a man weighing 180 lbs. would weigh 1,260 lbs., the weight of the hydrostatic column of blood on the arterial side would be more than the heart could cope with, and the venous blood would fail to return from below the cardiac level.

All these remarks pertain to positive acceleration, which is the common condition met in flying. Negative accelerations are met in certain acrobatic manœuvres. Here we find the reverse, the blood being drawn to the upper part of the body with resulting seeing "red" instead of "black", with cerebral congestion, conjunctival and even cerebral hemorrhages being a possibility. Armstrong[2] states that at $4\frac{1}{2}$ G, the highest negative acceleration studied in man, there is mental confusion, persisting for several hours, accompanied by severe throbbing headache. The face is congested, petechial hemorrhages result in the skin and conjunctivæ, and subcutaneous ecchymoses may remain for hours or days.

Prevention of the effects of positive accelerations may be obtained in part by (1) the pilot wearing an inflatable abdominal belt exerting sufficient pressure to prevent pulling of the blood to the lower half of the body, (2) placing the pilot in a crouching posture, so as to bring the pull of centrifugal force more transversely rather than from head to feet and (3) by having him yell at the top of his lungs, thereby fixing his diaphragm and causing some cerebral congestion.

Effects of Cold and Wind

Considerable work has been done recently on the effects of cold in flying. We know that during the first mile of ascent the temperature falls 1° F. in every 540 feet of ascent. From 14,000 to 16,000 feet there is a fall of 1° F. in every 360 feet of ascent. From 23,000 to 29,000 feet there is a fall of 1° F. in every 188 feet of ascent. Above 35,000 feet is the zone of constant temperature, −67° F. below zero.

Schneider[18] states that in flight cold increases by stages. First there is a sensation of chilling, a development of goose-pimples and pallor; if there is not sufficient protection, the chilling accentuates, there is a development of painful sensations, the extremities become stiff followed by

numbness and a tendency to sleep. The fall in temperature stimulates metabolism, and, therefore, the demand for oxygen is increased, a fact worthy of note, at high altitudes, where extremes of cold and low oxygen tension are encountered. Heavy clothing is inadequate at very low temperatures, and it further restricts free movement. Armstrong[2] states that at $-40°$ F., there is a loss of morale, distraction, acute physical suffering, muscular sluggishness and incoördination with finally a tendency to stupor.

The effects of wind in flying, according to Aggazzotti[1] and Galeotti, are such as to cause irregularity and acceleration of respiration and a diminution in alveolar carbon dioxide. Strong winds may interfere with the entrance of air to the lungs, hinder movements of the thorax and decrease lung ventilation. Metabolism will be increased by the effect of wind in flying, and this increases the demand for oxygen.

With the use of cabin ships the effects of wind are less important than in open ships so far as the effect on the pilot is concerned. Pinson and Benson[28] state that the final solution to the problem of maintaining body heat under the varied and extreme conditions encountered in flight is dependent to a great extent on future developments in airplane design. In pressure cabin planes heating of the cabin with a provision for defrosting the windows may be the answer. At present they recommend using the best features of the electrically heated suit with the use of insulative clothing of maximum bulkiness commensurate with normal personal comfort and efficiency.

Blind Flying

This comes rather under the head of flying training than under aviation medicine. Nevertheless, the difficulties of blind flying are physiological, and so a few words must be said on this subject. By blind flying is meant flying without a horizon for guidance. This occurs in fogs, thick weather and above the clouds. We have seen that equilibrium depends on several factors and one of these, the most important in the pilot, is vision. Vision is of no use in blind flying. Our other senses are unreliable, and hence the flyer must depend on instruments to determine his position in space. This sounds simple but is not, because one's physical sensations are overpowering unless he has been specially trained.

That vertigo results from spinning and turning is well known. That this vertigo is not only confusing but causes false sensations of direction is not so well understood. However, that such is the case can be easily demonstrated by a Barany or other turning-chair.

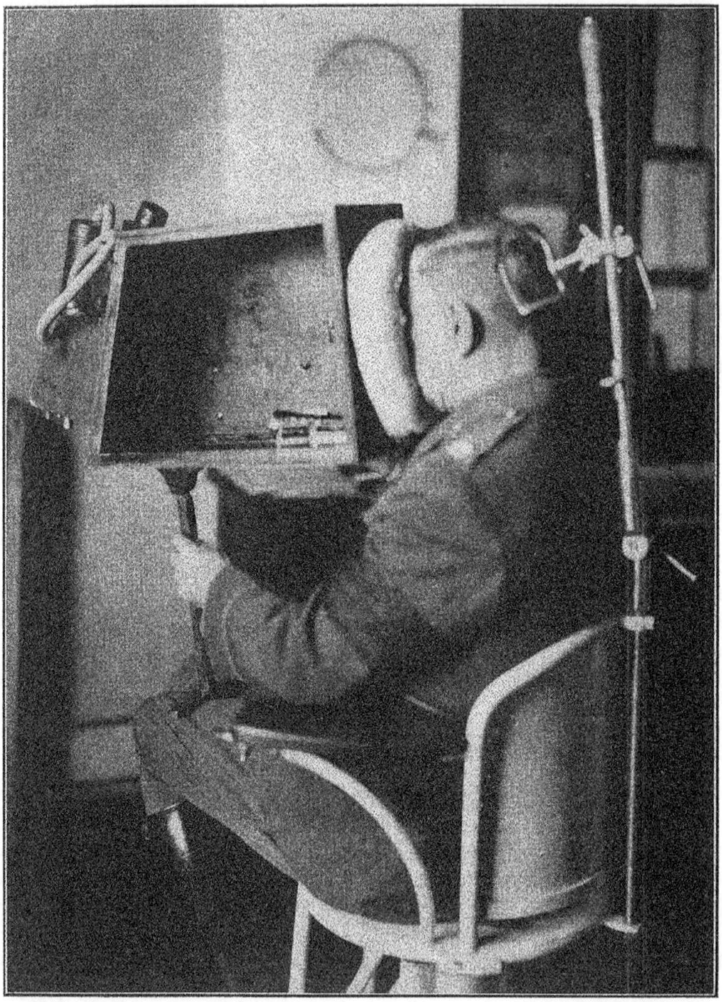

FIG. 11. Apparatus for demonstrating to a pilot the falsity of his sensations after turning. The side of the camera has been removed to show the interior. The scheme was first suggested by Colonel D. A. Myers, U. S. Army (Ret.). Apparatus perfected by Colonel W. C. Ocker, U. S. Army.

For example, if the applicant is turned to the right with his eyes closed say 10 times in 20 seconds, he at first has a sensation of turning to the left, then a sensation of turning to the right, and if the turning rate then is slowed or stopped altogether, he has the sensation of turning to the left. If he opens his eyes, the falsity of his sensations is apparent at once.

The cause of these sensations is due to stimulations of the end organs of the vestibular branch of the eighth nerve in the semicircular canals. The exact physiological phenomenon has been a source of great dispute among otologists, but it is pretty generally agreed now that the cause is a change of tension in the fluid in these canals. For our purposes, however, the exact cause is not important; the fact that such sensations occur is the factor to be considered.

The practical application of this to flying is the following: If a pilot flying in a fog gets into a spin and then comes out of it, he has the sensation of spinning in the opposite direction. If he depends on this sensation, he will correct for the supposed spin and this "correction" at once puts him into another spin. This may keep up in a vicious circle until he crashes. His only hope is to disregard his sensations and fly by instruments.

Many flyers have, in the past, complained after blind flights, from which fortunately they returned, that their instruments were wrong and were disconcerting. Without some such demonstration as has been outlined above it would be impossible to convince these flyers that their instruments were right and that they or their sensations actually were wrong.

To follow one's instruments is difficult without special training, because these erroneous sensations one receives are overpowering until he has been trained to disregard them. In this connection it is interesting to note that Ocker[25] found trained flyers were unable to fly a course by instruments without re-education, even though they realize its necessity. They had been flying too long "by feel" to be able suddenly to disregard their sensations. On the other hand, they found that an untrained or rather a very slightly trained flyer could do fairly well because he had nothing to unlearn.

Military pilots are now trained in blind flying, and all air line transport companies also train their flyers in it. The instruments used include not only an altitude indicator, an air speed indicator, tachometer, turn and bank indicator, a gyro compass as well as a magnetic compass but an instrument giving an artificial horizon, such as the flight integrator of Ocker and Crane[25] or a gyro horizon.

Care of the Flyer

Selection of the flyer is only part of the problem, important though it is. Once selected, the pilot must be maintained in at least as good condition as he was at the time of his selection. This requires frequent observation. In the Army and Navy flyers are all under the constant supervision of a trained flight surgeon. Both services require the flyer to check out daily through the flight surgeon before flying. This is the ideal arrangement. The flight surgeon becomes thoroughly acquainted with his flyers and knows their habits and weaknesses. He knows which flyer needs more supervision, which takes good care of himself. Aside from the required semi annual examinations frequent checks of certain physical points are made as developments warrant. In the service, whenever a student flyer begins to fall off in his flying, makes poor landings or what not, he is sent to the flight surgeon for an overhaul.

Fatigue. — Flying is fatiguing, and too much of it results in "staleness" or neurocirculatory asthenia. Not only too much flying will bring on this condition, but too little exercise, too little recreation or too much dissipation likewise will do it.

Schneider[30, 31] has defined fatigue as "a progressive flagging of efficiency together with a subject sensation of the loss of control of the muscles". Physiological activity becomes lowered and the ability to work is diminished. When a person engages in normal activity, it is a natural result that fatigue ensues. However, this fatigue should be relieved completely by a night's sleep. When it is not relieved and the activity responsible for it continued, there will be an accumulative fatigue which eventually burns up the reserve, and we have "staleness" resulting.

Staleness. — Schneider[31] has defined the various types of "staleness" as follows: (1) Cardiorespiratory. — Pulse increase in rate, poor in volume and low in tension. There is distress on slight exertion accompanied by an inordinate rise in pulse rate and prolonged time of return of the pulse after exercise; breathing shallow and rapid; extremities poor in color, cyanotic and cold. (2) Nervous type. — Poor muscular control of balancing movements; fine tremors of the hands, eyelids and tongue; apprehensive starts with sudden sensory experiences; disturbed sleep; loss of sleep; nightmare. (3) Muscular type. — Tenderness of the muscles with loss of tone, flabbiness, loss in power which may be marked or slight. These symptoms may be confused with rheumatism. (4) Staleness may be brought about also by disorders of digestion characterized by removal of normal inhibitions, i.e., reponse to sensory stimuli by excess of motion, hypersensitiveness, annoyance by bright light, little noises, etc., restlessness.

Bainbridge[3] considers "staleness" as nothing more or less than "effort syndrome". It results from severe exertion or in the course of training, and the circulatory and respiratory changes which occur normally are increased. He further believes that the contractile power of the heart is diminished and that oxygen want plays a part in functioning of the muscles and nervous system. The changes in pulse, respiration and blood pressure result from an insufficient supply of oxygen.

Effort syndrome or neurocirculatory asthenia was described first by Lewis[18]. He describes four groups of cases. These are (1) constitutional or hereditary group, (2) a group due to exposure and mental or physical strain, (3) convalescent group, (4) toxic group.

The symptoms are, in the order of importance, breathlessness brought on by exertion, the rate of breathing being markedly increased by exercise; pain, usually this is exaggerated by exercise; exhaustion, even mild cases show fatigue on moderate exertion, and palpitation is common; giddiness is more or less constant and is associated with change of posture and effort; fainting may occur; other symptoms are headache, lassitude, irritability, sleeplessness, inability to fix attention, coldness of the hands and feet, sweating, particularly of the hands, feet and axillæ.

The physical signs are increased heart rate and particularly an exaggerated response of the heart to exercise with a slow return of the pulse after exercise. There are exaggerated responses of the blood pressure, although frequently we find that upon change of posture the blood pressure falls rather than rises. The apex beat may be diffuse and the heart sounds accentuated. Functional systolic murmurs may be present. There is an exaggeration of the deep reflexes and coarse tremor of the hands and tongue. The symptoms of an individual case may be anything from breathlessness up to a definite picture presenting the above symptoms. The stale flyer presents much the same picture. The flight surgeon should be continually on the watch for the development of this condition. It must be caught in its incipiency, for if it is allowed to develop, not only may a serious accident occur, but recovery becomes prolonged and uncertain. Staleness may be prevented by maintaining a condition of physical fitness. Exercise and proper rest are the essential factors in this program.

Bainbridge[3] states that training develops the skeletal muscles and also the heart. A person in training shows a slower pulse, lower blood pressure and a lessened minute volume of the heart. The heart output is greater per beat, and the oxygen carrying power of the blood has a greater coefficient of utilization. Movements are better coördinated, and there is a better economy of effort.

The development of staleness results in a dislike of flying and a loss of flying efficiency. Poor landings, the loss of the "feel of the ship", neglect of details such as attention to instruments, position of stabilizer, neglect of altitude adjustment and incorrect computations of gas expenditures may result. Poor judgment becomes common, and the flyer does not make prompt decisions.

Staleness is insidious in its development, and frequent medical supervision is important. In civilian flying constant medical supervision is not practicable. Its importance, however, is considered so great that several air lines in the United States employ flight surgeons to check the physical condition of their pilots monthly.

Wright[36] feels that a pre-employment examination is essential in order that the pilots can be certified for their positions, not only in regard to their present state of health and efficiency but to prognosticate their adaptability to conditions, their reliability and stamina. He feels that the Schneider index is an excellent method of keeping track of the flyer's physical efficiency. This test was devised by Schneider[30] primarily for use in following the physical condition of aviators. It will be described later in the chapter.

Miller and Ginsberg[24] studied metabolic and serological changes in flight fatigue in a group of pilots. They found hypotension was common after flight and wondered whether or not this was an evidence of fatigue. They made determinations of basal metabolic rate, blood sugar, creatinine and non-protein nitrogen before and after flight in a group of 15 pilots. They also took Schneider tests and flarimeter tests on the same group. A brief summary of the work follows: "Fifteen veteran pilots have been studied. Forty-six and six-tenths per cent. of these pilots show a lower basal metabolic rate after flying in comparison to the basal metabolic rate found after resting. Blood sugar values were low. Identical values were almost always found for blood sugar after flying and after rest. Creatinine determinations show no change. Non-protein nitrogen determinations show that forty-six and six-tenths per cent. give higher values after rest, but this group is not related to the group showing higher basal metabolic rates after flying. The Schneider index permits us to conclude that a pilot has a more efficient neurocirculatory mechanism after rest." They suggested that the hypotension may be a sign of physical fatigue caused by drain or exhaustion of the adrenals. Flying causes fear in the novice, and this gradually becomes more or less repressed into the unconscious. Fatigue is induced more quickly by flying in bad weather or over unfavorable territory. This, they feel, forms the basis of emotional stress. They state: "Our findings lead us to believe that there is possibly a drain on the suprarenals during flying, whether it is physical or mental. It might then follow that an exhausted suprarenal gland may affect the sympathetic nervous system in such a way as to reduce its tonicity. Further, this drain or exhaustion of the adrenals is probably the cause of fatigue with its associated hypotension. Our opinion is that, due to prolonged emotional stress, the sympathetic nervous system stimulates adrenalin secretion, which causes a decrease in the liver and muscle glycogen. Exhaustion of the liver glycogen calls forth the manufacture of carbohydrate from protein and possibly fat, resulting in the tearing down of tissues. This anabolism produces an increase in the acids, and these acids in turn stimulate the respiratory centers to cause increased pulmonary ventilation. This is necessary to keep pace with the demand for oxygen. Our blood sugar findings are low. This denotes increased sugar consumption, and as the energy is needed, the demand becomes greater on the adrenals until we have a depletion and adrenalemia with resulting fatigue and hypotension."

Padden[27] reports that irregular hours and excessive flying affect ocular muscle balance early. He lays great stress on goggles and states that many difficulties are encountered due to optically imperfect lenses in the goggles. He recommends frequent checking of goggles to protect the eyes of the flyer.

Flyers are particularly prone to develop gastrointestinal upsets, probably due partly to emotional stress and partly to the irregular hours and irregular meals. One transport operator had 16 per cent. of his pilot personnel develop acute appendicitis in 13 months. All these cases were operated on, and in all instances the attack came on from within 5 minutes to 2 hours of takeoff and in one pilot while flying his run. Gastric ulcer is not infrequent and probably due to the same causes.

Diseases of the upper respiratory passages due to exposure to cold and fatigue, middle ear troubles, particularly in altitude flights, are common.

All these factors show the need for medical supervision. One flight surgeon reported that the effect of irregular schedules, meals, sleep and recreation showed by frequent minor accidents, poor morale among pilots, staleness and a marked decrease in general physical fitness. Flying then causes fatigue, and this may cause various physical ailments and eventually may develop into staleness; a falling off in flying ability occurs, and nervous instability results.

The flight surgeon must detect such conditions early and take the necessary measures to prevent a state developing that will necessitate complete removal from flying status, or that will result in accidents. Careful selection, regular exercise, avoidance of too much flying, adequate rest and recreation will prevent staleness. Laboratory examinations should play a part in the supervision of pilots as pointed out by Tillisch and Lovelace[33]. They found 73 of 103 pilots had defects, which did or could affect their health. Many of these defects would have gone unrecognized in an ordinary physical examination.

The Army Flight Surgeon's Handbook[11] recommends that the limitation of flying hours, as given later under "Flying time," should be adhered to. The Army also feels that on completion of a mission crews should be taken 3 to 5 miles away from the airdrome for rest and sleep. Attention is called to the fact that mild degrees of anoxia increase fatigue. Strict oxygen discipline should be insisted upon. New personnel joining operational units should be watched carefully, as inadequacies are apt to crop up early. It is advised that flying stress, once developed, should be treated only in a hospital. They consider flying stress is "infectious".

McFarland[22] in an excellent treatise on fatigue in aircraft pilots shows that a pilot whose muscular activity in flight is limited could hardly exhaust the energy reserves sufficiently to explain the fatigue and exhaustion often observed in airmen. He ascribes the acute and chronic pilot fatigue and exhaustion to psychological factors such as emotional stress regardless of whether it is related to adverse flying conditions, fear of accident, economic and social insecurity and unhappy marital adjustments. He also considers lack of exercise, reduced oxygen tension in high altitude flights, poor selection of food and excessive use of tobacco and alcohol as contributing factors to fatigue. Other variable contributing factors are noise, vibration, poor illumination, glare, static from the radio and poor regulation of ventilation and temperature.

Physical fitness is more important in flying than in any other occupation. The necessity of constant medical supervision, or as near constant as practicable, cannot be too strongly emphasized.

The technique of the Schneider test already mentioned is described below:

DIRECTIONS FOR PROCEDURE IN THE CIRCULATORY EFFICIENCY TEST (SCHNEIDER INDEX)[30]

Preliminary: Subject reclines for five minutes.

1. Heart rate is counted for 20 seconds. When two consecutive 20 second counts are the same, this is multiplied by 3 and recorded.
2. The systolic pressure is taken by auscultation and recorded. Take two or three readings to be certain.

3. The subject then rises and stands for two minutes to allow the pulse to assume a uniform rate. When two consecutive 15 second counts are the same, multiply by 4 and record. This is the normal standing rate.
4. Standing pulse minus the reclining pulse gives the increase on standing.
5. The systolic pressure is taken as before and recorded.
6. Timed by a stopwatch, the subject steps upon a chair 18½ inches high five times in 15 seconds. To make this uniform the subject stands with one foot on the chair at the count one. This foot remains on the chair and is not brought to the floor again until count five. At each count he brings the other foot on the chair, and at the count "down" replaces it on the floor. This should be timed accurately so that at the 15 second mark on the stopwatch both feet are on the floor.
7. Start counting the pulse immediately at the 15 second mark on the stopwatch and count for 15 seconds. Multiply by 4 and record.
8. Continue to take pulse in 15 seconds counts until the rate has returned to normal standing rate. Note the number of seconds it takes for this return and record. In computing this return count from the end of the 15 seconds of exercise to the beginning of the first normal 15 seconds pulse count. If the pulse has not returned to normal at the end of 2 minutes, record the number of beats above normal and discontinue counting.
9. Check up points and enter final rating.
10. Enter history of case, including amount of sleep, amount of smoking, kind of work (outdoor or indoor, active or sedentary, etc.), time since last meal, any personal worries or any pathological condition which might affect the condition of the subject. The test should not be made within 2 hours after a meal, and the habits of the individual must be taken into consideration.

Roughly, an index of 14 to 18 is excellent; 10 to 13 very good; 7 to 9 borderline; below 7 unsatisfactory.

Scott[32] by means of systematic exercise over a period of one month improved the average index of a group of flyers. The results before the exercise was started were 20 per cent. 14 or above; 60 per cent. 8 to 13; and 20 per cent. 7 or less. At the end of the month the results were 80 per cent. 14 or above; 10 per cent. 8 to 13 and 10 per cent. 7 or less.

As a gauge of condition in athletes, flyers and those subjected to constant mental strain, whose condition may be checked from time to time, it is probably the most satisfactory test yet devised.

Flying Time for Pilots

This is a much mooted question, but as flying is fatiguing and apt to induce staleness if overindulged in, a limit in the amount of flying a man should do must be set in the interest of safety and efficiency. The Army considers 100 hours per month as the limit, and its pilots are under constant medical supervision. Taken as a whole, peace time flying in the Army with its associated military duties may be compared with transport flying from the physical standpoint.

TABLE OF POINTS FOR GRADING CARDIOVASCULAR CHANGES IN THE SCHNEIDER INDEX

A. Reclining pulse rate		*B.* Pulse rate increases on standing				
Rate	Points	0–10 beats, points	11–18 beats, points	19–26 beats, points	27–34 beats, points	35–42 beats, points
50–60	3	3	3	2	1	0
61–70	3	3	2	1	0	–1
71–80	2	3	2	0	–1	–2
81–90	1	2	1	–1	–2	–3
91–100	0	1	0	–2	–3	–3
101–110	–1	0	–1	–3	–3	–3

C. Standing pulse rate		*D.* Pulse rate increase immediately after exercise				
Rate	Points	0–10 beats, points	11–20 beats, points	21–30 beats, points	31–40 beats, points	41–50 beats, points
60–70	3	3	3	2	1	0
71–80	3	3	2	1	0	0
81–90	2	3	2	1	0	–1
91–100	1	2	1	0	–1	–2
101–110	1	1	0	–1	–2	–3
111–120	0	1	–1	–2	–3	–3
121–130	0	0	–2	–3	–3	–3
131–140	1	0	–3	–3	–3	–3

E. Return of pulse rate to standing normal after exercise	
Seconds	Points
0–30	3
31–60	2
61–90	1
91–120	0
After 120: 2–10 beats above normal	–1
After 120: 11–30 beats above normal	–2

F. Systolic pressure, standing, compared with reclining	
Change in millimeters	Points
Rise or 8 or more	3
Rise of 2–7	2
No rise	1
Fall of 2–5	0
Fall of 6 or more	–1

The test must be performed accurately and painstakingly. Also one index is not of much value. Several should be had in order to afford a basis for comparison.

Air-line flying may be divided into day and night flying. To deal first with the former, it is believed that the air-line regulations, which in peace time limit the total flying of any pilot to 85 hours per month, is reasonable. Poor terrain, heavy passenger loads, poor average weather conditions and lack of a co-pilot should reduce the maximum. Good terrain, the presence of a co-pilot and good average weather conditions may increase it somewhat, perhaps to 100 hours. Or in the case of repeated short flights under good conditions, perhaps slightly more.

As to night flying, this is admittedly more hazardous and more of a strain. With the same factors acting in modification, a limit of 60 to 75 hours per month is desirable.

In advancing any limits, however, it should be assumed that the pilot obtains sufficient sleep each day under restful conditions to give the necessary recuperation from exhaustion and place him in condition to resume flying.

The commercial pilot should have one or more days a week off from flying. Under good flying conditions one day may be sufficient, but under more trying conditions every third or fourth day should be taken off. In addition, the pilot should have from three to four weeks a year off. Whether one vacation of four weeks is better than two vacations of two weeks each is, perhaps, still open to argument, but that it should not be subdivided more than that is generally agreed by medical men.

Because of the war limitation of flying hours has been removed, and already many pilots have complained of marked fatigue, inadequate rest periods, and the excellent record for safety made during the past several years by the air lines of the United States will be in grave danger.

In military operations it is important to space operations for the pilot as evenly as possible. Ninety to 110 operational hours in six weeks has been recommended for fighter pilots and 120 to 139 hours of operational flying for bombers in three months. Leaves should be given then followed by a period of flying not involving operations before return to operational duty.

The Army feels that 7 days is as long a leave as should be given but that this should be given at stated intervals. One-half a day off should be given every 3 or 4 days; 48 hours every 2 weeks and 7 days at the end of the operational limit.

Air Sickness

Sea-sickness has been known ever since man took to the sea, and air-sickness became fairly common after flying became prevalent. The cause of air-sickness is the same as the cause of sea-sickness, namely unaccustomed motion with overstimulation of the vestibular mechanism. We have other similar forms of sickness, namely train sickness, swing sickness, etc., all of which are due to the same cause.

The airplane moving through a rather unstable medium is similar to a ship plowing through pitching seas. The air is smooth on some days and rough on others. On windy or gusty days the air is rough. Likewise on days, on which there has been a sudden drop in temperature, the air is rough and bumpy, due to the fact that the air is not uniformly cooled, and we meet warm and cold currents of air alternately. The air usually is bumpy over mountains and in crossing bodies of water from the land. This unaccustomed motion stimulating our motion sensing apparatus causes a certain amount of vertigo and nausea.

Some people are more prone to air-sickness than others, just as is the case with sea-sickness. The nervous, high strung type of individual is more apt to be air-sick than the phlegmatic type. Fear often acts as an exciting cause for air-sickness. There is, therefore, a psychological factor in air-sickness aside from the physical factor. The person, who is car-sick or sea-sick, probably will be air-sick also.

There are certain measures to be carried out as a prophylactic. The passenger, for pilots are rarely air-sick, should avoid eating rich or heavy food before flying. He should be instructed to swallow frequently as this keeps his Eustachian tubes open and prevents pain developing from retracted ear drums on sudden change of altitude. Chewing gum facilitates keeping the Eustachian tubes open. The passenger also should have his attention diverted as much as possible. If he can be encouraged to follow a map, it takes his mind off himself and prevents fear. If he actually becomes sick, he should be made to go to the wash-room to avoid upsetting other passengers. An alkaline effervescent drink is recommended by Wright[36] as a cure for nausea in the air. If food is taken, toast, plain crackers or an apple are less upsetting to an air-sick passenger than heavy food or liquid except for an alkaline drink.

Both Padden[27] and Wright[36] recommend a grain or two of amytal for a nauseated passenger. Wright states such a passenger often will drop off to sleep and awake feeling refreshed enough to enjoy the remainder of the trip.

Just as the person used to the sea is less apt to be sea-sick than one who rarely sails, so the one who flies frequently is less apt to be air-sick. Pilots rarely are air-sick, partly because they are so used to flying and partly because they are busy and have no time to think about themselves.

The frequency of air-sickness is disputed. Some authorities claim it occurs in 5 per cent. of passengers, but this probably is too high. A great deal, of course, depends on flying conditions. On a smooth day only rarely is a person air-sick, while on a rough day more are sick. Tuttle[34] found in a survey of the United Air Line flights that the rate of air-sickness was only 3 per 100. He classified all discomfort in air-line planes as follows:

Air-sickness	0.33%
Nervousness	0.09%
Oxygen want	0.08%
Ear trouble	0.05%
All others	0.05%
Total	0.60%

Conclusion

Aviation Medicine, therefore, has an important field. By means of it the public is assured of safety in flying so far as the physical side is concerned. It includes a broad knowledge of medicine and psychology and a personality in the flight surgeon that inspires confidence and respect.

BIBLIOGRAPHY

1. AGGAZZOTTI, A.: Influenza del vento sulla funzione respiratoria e nil polso, Gior. di Med. Mil., 1919, LXVII, 107.
2. ARMSTRONG, H. G.: The Principles and Practice of Aviation Medicine, Williams and Wilkins Co., Baltimore, 1939.
3. BAINBRIDGE, F. A.: The Physiology of Muscular Exercise, Longmans Green, New York and London, 1919.
4. BARACH, A. L.: Principles of aviation medicine, War Medicine: a symposium, Philosophical Library, N. Y., CCCXXXVI, 1942.
5. BEHNKE, A. R., Jr.: Investigations concerned with problems of high altitude flying and deep diving; application of certain findings pertaining to physical fitness to the general military service, Mil. Surg., 1942, XC, 9.
6. BERENS, CONRAD: Present ophthalmologic standards for commercial aviation in the United States, Jour. Aviation Med., 1932, CXI, 55.
7. BOOTHBY, W. M. and LOVELACE, W. R., II: Oxygen in aviation, Jour. Aviat. Med., 1938, IX, 172.
8. CARLSON, W. A.: Psychology and aviation, Jour. Aviat. Med., 1939, X, 216.
9. COOPER, H. J.: The relation between physical deficiency and decreased performance, Jour. Aviation Med., 1930, I, 5.

10. COOPER, H. J.: Further studies on the effect of physical defects and flying ability, Jour. Aviat. Med., 1931, II, 162.
11. Flight Surgeon's Handbook, The School of Aviation Medicine, Randolph Field, Texas, 1942.
12. FLYNN, V. P.: Clinical test for dark adaptation, Jour. Aviat. Med., 1942, XIII, 216.
13. FULTON, JOHN F.: Physiology and high altitude flying; with particular reference to air embolism and the effects of acceleration, War Medicine: a symposium, Philosophical Library, N. Y., CCCXXXVI 1942.
14. GARSAUX, P.: Results of the experiments on the 12th and 17th of July, 1918 from the action of centrifugal force on dogs (translation), Experimental service, technical section, military aeronautics, Office of Minister of War, Paris, 1918.
15. HERBOLSHEIMER, A. J.: A study of 300 non-selected aviation accidents, Jour. Aviat. Med., 1942, XIII, 256.
16. HOWARD, H. J.: A test for the judgment of distance, Am. Jour. Ophth., 1919, 3 s., II, 656.
17. JARMAN, B. L.: Monocular vision and other peculiar phases of flying as regards depth perception, Jour. Aviat. Med., 1932, III, 194.
18. LEWIS, T.: The Soldier's Heart and the Effort Syndrome, P. B. Hoeber, N. Y., 1920.
19. LONGACRE, R. F.: Personality study, Jour. Aviat. Med., 1930, I, 33.
20. LONGACRE, R. F.: Department of Commerce conference, Jour. Aviat. Med., 1931, II, 361.
21. MASHBURN, N. C.: Mashburn automatic serial reaction apparatus for detecting flying aptitude, Jour. Aviat. Med., 1934, V, 155.
22. McFARLAND, ROSS A.: Fatigue in aircraft pilots, War Medicine, Philosophical Library, N.Y., CCCXXXVI, 1942.
23. McFARLAND, ROSS A., GRAYBIEL, A., LILJENCRANTZ, E. and TUTTLE, A. D.: An analysis of the physiological and psychological characteristics of two hundred civil air-line pilots, Jour. Aviat. Med., 1939, X, 206.
24. MILLER, W. H. and GINSBERG, A. M.: Metabolic and serologic changes in flight fatigue; preliminary report, Jour. Aviat. Med., 1931, II, 155.
25. OCKER, W. C. and CRANE, C. J.: Blind Flight, in Theory and Practice, Naylor Printing Co., San Antonio, Tex., 1932.
26. ONFRAY, R.: Aviateurs, XIII, Concilium Ophthalmologicum, Hollandia, N. V. Boeken Steendrukkerij, Edward Ljdo, Leiden, 1929.
27. PADDEN, E. H.: Observations of monthly examinations on flying personnel, Jour. Aviat. Med., 1930, I, 154.
28. PINSON, E. A. and BENSON, O. O., JR.: Problems inherent in the protection of flying personnel against temperature extremes encountered in flight, Jour. Aviat. Med., 1942, XIII, 43.
29. SCHNEIDER, EDW. C.: The human machine in aviation, Yale Review, March 1922, New Haven.

30. SCHNEIDER, EDW. C.: Further observations on a cardiovascular physical fitness test, Mil. Surg., 1923, LIII, 401.
31. SCHNEIDER, EDW. C.: Unpublished lecture notes on aviation physiology, The School of Aviation Medicine, U. S. Army, 1924.
32. SCOTT, VERNER T.: Daily exercise a factor in preventive medicine, Mil. Surg., 1922, I, 648.
33. TILLISCH, J. H. and LOVELACE, W. R., II: The physical maintenance of transport pilots, Jour. Aviat. Med., 1942, XIII, 121.
34. TUTTLE, A. D.: Safety and comfort aloft, Jour. Aviat. Med., 1939, X, 72.
35. U. S. Army: Outline of Adaptability Rating for Military Aeronautics, to be published.
36. WRIGHT, HERBERT B.: Medical supervision of air lines, Jour. Aviat. Med., 1932, III, 182.

General References

ARMSTRONG, H. G.: The Principles and Practice of Aviation Medicine, Williams and Wilkins Co., Baltimore, 1939.
BAUER, L. H.: Aviation Medicine, Williams and Wilkins Co., Baltimore, 1926.
Handbook for Medical Examiners, Dept. of Commerce, Civil Aeronautics Administration, 2d edition, Washington, 1942.

March 1, 1943.

Pages 594 to 618 will be supplied at a later date by another article.

CHAPTER XV .

THE RATIONALE OF CLINICAL DIAGNOSIS

(*Medical Logic*)

By LEWELLYS F. BARKER

TABLE OF CONTENTS

IN making a diagnostic survey, we recognize the existence, or absence, of " disease " in a person through determining the presence, or absence, of certain symptoms or signs, drawing inferences from our findings, reasoning out the implications of these inferences, testing them for their validity, and finally arriving at the concluding belief that " disease " has been identified, or that the person is " healthy." It is, mainly, the logical basis and the technique of the process that will be discussed in the present article.

DEVELOPMENT OF CLINICAL DIAGNOSIS

During the long period in which human beings have lived, enjoyed, and suffered, there has gradually grown up a body of opinions and beliefs regarding health and disease. At all times, animals and human beings have been subject to accidents and diseases that entail suffering or disability. A human being who suffers pain or who is conscious of disability desires, and seeks, relief. Other human beings who see him suffer have their interest and sympathy aroused and desire to help him or to find someone who can help him. Even among the primitive healers, who called upon the gods to cure, or made use of magic arts and enchantments, there must have been a recognition of different kinds of suffering and of the need of a corresponding variety of remedial measures. Among these healers, too, there doubtless early arose, as incentive to discrimination, in addition to the desire to help and the desire for knowledge, the desire to be successful for the sake of livelihood, power, prestige, and other personal rewards. In the effort to satisfy these desires, partly private, partly social, the art of diagnosis had its crude, empirical beginnings. Listening to the complaints of those who suffered, watching their behavior, comparing the observations made on a given case with those made on others earlier in their experience, primitive healers gradually acquired experience and handed down their observations, opinions, beliefs, and customs to their successors (medical tradition).

The striking character of certain illnesses and accidents unquestionably helped to determine the order of development of medical observation and opinion. Wounds, hemorrhages, fractures, and dislocations, large tumors, phlegmons, convulsions, paralyses, chills, fevers, anasarca, deliria, violent pains, blindness, deafness, jaundice, persistent vomiting, madness, melancholy, and other gross manifestations doubtless earliest attracted attention; an acquaintance with these that permitted him to recognize them when he met them constituted the diagnostic knowledge of the ancient practitioner. It is easy, then, to understand why, in earlier times, external medicine should have developed before internal medicine, and why the observation of the natural course of disease should have yielded important facts that bore upon prognosis long before a therapy that could lay any claim to rationality could be applied.

The study of the natural course of disease and of prognosis was doubtless an inspiration to further diagnostic discrimination and resulted in the general growth of diagnostic knowledge. The course and the outcome were so different in different cases of hemorrhage, of fever, and of paralysis, for example, that curiosity must early have been stimulated to seek explanations by attempting an analysis of the different kinds of hemorrhage, of fever, and of paralysis. The primitive descriptions of disease were, perforce, vague and indefinite. The class names that were first used in diagnosis were names of what we now call symptoms and signs. The groupings that the earlier diagnosticians made use of were probably the best that could be selected for the purposes of their time; but we can be sure that then, as now, there were only a few who recognized that groupings are conceptual, and that they must be changed when the purposes for which they are wanted change. The rank and file are, at all times, prone to accept classes and class-names as given facts that need no further investigation. The value of a class-name is to assemble (for convenience in making general statements) individuals that have points of resemblance or "common attributes" despite the fact that they also differ from one another; the class-name stands for "unity in spite of difference." When, for example, diagnosticians assembled a group of cases under the class-name "paralysis," they sometimes forgot that the differences between one member of the class and other members of that class might, for certain purposes, be more important than the resemblances. Thus, a gumma pressing on the thoracic portion of the spinal cord causes paralysis; a metastatic carcinoma in the same region causes paralysis. For the purposes of description, the class-name "paralysis" has its value for both instances; for purposes of prognosis and therapy, other class-names (syphilis and cancer) are more important. In other words, in assigning an individual to a class, the value of the assignation depends upon the aim or purpose we have in view. We have gradually to find out the "degrees of generality" that exist, for one class possesses higher generality than another if it includes not only that other but also more. The older logicians recognized these scales of generality, and arranged tables of higher classes (general) and lower classes (special) in order—the so-called "tree" of division or classification (e.g. Porphyry's tree). And advance in diagnosis has resulted from discovering specific differences (differentiae) between members of general classes made for certain purposes, and discovering features that make assignation to other classes that we create for other purposes more important. By examining closely the members of a class for portions that for some clearly-seen purpose differ essentially from one another, diagnostic thought moves ever towards clearer definition. This movement from vagueness towards definiteness is on the one hand the effect, on the other the cause, of each advance in the growth of diagnostic knowledge.

Now, it is this movement of diagnostic thought, impelled by the desire for more effective treatment based upon more accurate and ever more definite knowledge, that accounts for the growth of the medical sciences as a whole and for the subdivision of diagnosis itself into three parts (pure science, applied science, and art). In order that diagnosis may become something more than merely regional and external, a knowledge of the interior of the body and its development, a knowledge of the mind and its development, and a knowledge of the environment of the body and mind, including a knowledge of the modes of interpenetration of associated minds, become important. Anatomy, physiology, pathology, and psychology are the sons and daughters of diagnosis, children that, in turn, contribute lavishly to the parental larder. Diagnosis gradually became internal as well as external; organal, histological, cytological, and chemical as well as regional; functional and dynamic as well as structural and static; psychic as well as somatic; social and situational as well as personal; etiological and pathogenetic as well as symptomatic and descriptive. Diagnosis has become partly a pure science based upon data derived from a large number of subsidiary sciences; partly an applied science in which the utilities of the truths of the pure science are perceived and the necessary adjustments for realizing them are made; and partly an art in the exercise of which practitioners employ more or less skillfully the inventions that the applied science affords.

The Position and the Relationships of the Science of Clinical Diagnosis

The meaning of diagnosis has, during the centuries, become gradually enlarged. The term "diagnosis" came to us through Latin from the Greek *dia-*, through, or thorough, and *gignōskō*, recognize. As applied to-day it is, of course, attached to a far more complex subject than could have been anticipated by those who first used the name. Through the development referred to above, a development that is going on in our time more rapidly than ever before, a pure science, an applied science, and an art of diagnosis may be said to have come into existence, for we now possess (1) laws and principles that hold in diagnosis ("pure," or "theoretical," diagnostic science), (2) perceptions of the possibilities of utility and inventions through which the principles are applied ("practical," or "applied," diagnostic science), and (3) skill and experience in employing these inventions in practice (diagnostic art).

The "pure" science of medical diagnosis treats of the phenomena and laws of disease, explains the processes by which pathological phenomena occur, tracing each phenomenon back through a series of antecedent conditions, and inquires into the anatomical, physiological, biological, chemical, physical, psychological, and social causes of disease-states. This "pure" science of diagnosis, like every other "pure" science, is interested in facts and their regular occurrence. It reasons about the facts and discovers "truth," but it rests upon faith, namely, "faith that causation is universal," faith that "all effects have causes and all causes have effects," and faith that "beneficial results will follow the discovery of truth."

The progress of any science is irregular and more or less paroxysmal, but the general methods used for making progress are the same for all the sciences. Progress in the science of diagnosis results from the work of a huge army of clinical and laboratory investigators, each of whom has his individual peculiarities, has had his own special training, and lives and works in his own particular environment. It is not strange, therefore, that even men who are trying to solve the same problem should approach it in different ways, should use different methods, and should attain to somewhat different results. Still the general method employed by all serious scientific research workers is the same. A problem is set; a special technique suited to the particular purposes of the investigator is constructed; observations and experiments are made; the results are recorded. If these results prove to be important, they, and the methods by which they have been obtained, are published. Other workers, noticing the publication, try to verify or to disprove the results, using other similar materials but working by somewhat different methods in a different environment with a background of a different natural endowment and a different past experience. They criticize and are led through their criticisms to make further observations and experiments. All of the earlier results may be disproved or all of them may be verified; more often, some of the earlier results stand the crucial test and come to be admitted as truths by everybody, whereas others of the results fail to stand the test and are rejected. Gradually, the tested and accepted results in connection with special problems in a number of circumscribed fields make a considerable mass and attract the attention of some worker with a synthesizing mind who coördinates the new results in comprehensive papers. Later, the results thus coördinated get into textbooks and the knowledge is made widely accessible; the achievements of the relatively few workers in each circumscribed field can thus be appropriated by the many who are distributed over the whole area of medical research and medical practice. Thus, though advances in diagnosis may have been made by fits and starts, the forward strides have been due to the application of the method of science.

The science of medical diagnosis, or science of the thorough recognition of disease, is, like every other true science, a domain in which phenomena occur in regular order as the effects of natural or efficient causes, such that a knowledge of the causes renders it possible to predict the effects. In the last analysis, the causes are natural "forces"; they obey the Newtonian laws of motion. The word "law" in science implies "uniformity of movement." In the sciences of mechanics, astronomy, and physics, the phenomena can be, in large measure, reduced to exact measurement and in them the "theory of units" (mass, space, time) is easily applicable. In the more complex sciences, the phenomena cannot yet be reduced to exact measurement, except to a limited extent. We *believe,* however, that exact laws do prevail in medical science as well as in all natural domains, though our knowledge of these laws is as yet exceedingly imperfect. It is "faith in the order of the universe," belief that laws are uniform and invariable in the fields of life, mind, and society (as well as in other cosmic fields) that makes the sciences of biology, psychology, sociology, and medicine possible. Social, psychic, and biotic phenomena are exceedingly complex, but study of them by exact methods reveals the existence of uniformities among them. They occur in order. They are subject to law just as rigorously as are the phenomena of chemistry and physics. To discover the laws that health-phenomena and disease-phenomena obey, we must use the method of science, the method that has revealed to the physicist the laws to which heat, light, electricity, and magnetism conform. The diagnostician must know in order that he may accurately predict and successfully control.

A word may be said as to the place of diagnosis and of the other medical sciences in the classifications of all the general and special sciences that have been attempted. The fundamental sciences, as they have been arranged serially (and more or less genetically), are astronomy, physics, chemistry, biology, psychology, and sociology. As complexity increases in the series, the degree to which the phenomena can be exactly determined, what Comte called the "positivity," decreases. Comte made each of these coördinate fundamental sciences stand at the head of a hierarchy of sciences that can be arranged in a logical, or synoptical, order. It is obvious that, if we adopted such a classification, the natural place for the sciences of medicine would, like those of technology, be within the hierarchy of which sociology is the head.* Properly to understand the complex and less exact clinical science of diagnosis, a comprehensive grasp (but not necessarily a mastery of the details) of all the simpler and more exact sciences (physiological, biological, chemical, etc.) below it is necessary. Classifications of the sciences, imperfect as they are, do help us to understand the manifold relations of our own science and give useful pedagogic hints for the most suitable arrangement of curricula.

To understand just what diagnosis is, and what it is not, it is necessary to determine its boundaries, to differentiate it clearly from other

* No classification of the sciences as a whole can be regarded as entirely satisfactory. A very good attempt at a more elaborate classification than the simple one given by Comte is that of Karl Pearson. See his "Grammar of Science," 2 d ed., 1900.

sciences, and especially, perhaps, from those to which it is most closely related. "The view or theory of the relations of the subject to other subjects and to the known world in general, as distinguished from the view or theory of it as isolated or in itself," has been given as a definition of the "philosophy" of a subject as distinguished from its "science." Though the distinction drawn between science and philosophy is now less sharp than that formerly drawn, there is something to be gained by considering separately the philosophy of a science in the sense mentioned above, namely, its relationships, and the definite delimitation of its field.

Relations of Diagnosis and Physics

Of all the natural sciences to which clinical diagnosis is related, none is more fundamental than the science of *physics*. Under physics are grouped the subjects (excluding chemistry and biology) that treat of the properties of matter and energy and of the action of the different forms of energy on matter. The conceptions of matter and energy, of mass and motion, and of space and time, dealt with by physics, lie at the basis of the scientific analysis of all natural phenomena, including those that we deal with in diagnosis.

The laws of dynamics, which deal with the action of force on bodies whether at rest or in motion, hold for the processes that go on within the human body, which the diagnostician studies. The prospective student of diagnosis, who in his early education gains some acquaintance with theoretical mechanics, not only acquires conceptions that aid him in the understanding of the problems of the pre-clinical and clinical medical sciences but also, through dealing with these ideal representations, secures a training in abstract thought that should be helpful to him in the whole of his subsequent career. The methods and principles of applied mechanics, the subject that deals with the theory of structures and with the theory of machines, are likely, as the medical sciences grow, to be ever more applicable to the solution of problems connected with the structures and mechanisms of the human machine.

That the study of the physics of heat, light, sound, electricity, and magnetism stand in intimate relation to the study of the functions of the human body in both normal and abnormal conditions, goes without saying. The diagnostician could not view intelligently the phenomena of fever and of metabolism if he were unacquainted with the effects produced by heat on material bodies, with the laws of transference of heat and with the laws that govern transformation of heat into other kinds of energy. Thermometry and calorimetry are simple and direct applications of physics to clinical diagnosis. And how unsatisfactory would be the work of the general as well as of the ophthalmic diagnostician who had not studied the physics of light, the laws of its rectilinear propagation, of its reflection and of its refraction, and the relations of light to the phenomena of vision and of color perception! In the construction of instruments of precision for diagnostic work, applied optics has made a very great contribution. To recall this fact vividly to mind, I need refer only to the microscope, the polariscope, the photographic camera, the ophthalmoscope, the speculum, the cystoscope, the bronchoscope, the sigmoidoscope, and the refractometer, and the uses to which they have been put in clinical diagnosis. The manifold applications of mirrors and lenses of different sorts in clinical diagnosis nowadays are contributions of optics that command the gratitude of every worker in the field of clinical diagnosis. Almost as important, too, are the applications of the physics of sound to the work of clinical inquiry. The art of auscultation in physical diagnosis can be practiced only inefficiently by one who is ignorant of the physical phenomena that correspond to the loudness, the pitch, and the quality of sounds. Instruments of precision like the stethoscope, the microphone, the phonocardiograph, the tuning fork, the continuous tone series, and the noise apparatus are direct contributions of applied phonetics to clinical diagnosis. It is astonishing, too, how various the applications of electrical science to diagnostic technic have been. In recent years, these have grown very rapidly. The testing of the functions of muscles and nerves by the faradic current and by the galvanic current were early methods of employing electrical science in the service of medical diagnosis. The uses of electricity for the illumination, when instruments of inspection are employed on clinical examination, have been more recently recognized and these modes of applying electricity in medical practice have become ever more important and helpful to the diagnostician and therapeutist. Furthermore, the applications of electricity in roentgenological work are now manifold and by no means simple, as every expert X-ray worker sooner or later learns. A general knowledge of heat, light, sound, electricity, and magnetism is, therefore, obviously essential for good work in medical diagnosis.

One of the most important influences of the study of physics on the science of diagnosis is the understanding that the former subject gives of the different forms of energy, and of the law of conservation of energy during transformation, as they concern the human body. When we recall that stimuli are, in the last analysis, physical agencies, namely forms of energy that excite or depress the several functions of the living body, we realize how important a rôle applied physics must ultimately play in physiology and, accordingly, in diagnosis. The studies of directive stimulation in lower forms of life (phototaxis, chemotaxis, thermotaxis, galvanotaxis, etc.) show us clearly certain of the directions that research must take if we are, later on, to understand more clearly than we do now the activities of the cellular constituents of the human body in health and in disease.

As diagnostic work grows gradually more precise, it makes ever greater use of certain standards of measurement that we owe to the physicists. Quantitative work in physics has been greatly facilitated by the selection for each measurable magnitude of a physical unit, or standard of reference; with the aid of these units, other similar quantities can, by comparison, be numerically defined. Fortunately, since physicists have become convinced that one form of physical energy is convertible into another and that the change takes place according to definite laws, it has been possible to coördinate these several physical units. The most fundamental units are those of length, mass, and time—the centimeter, the gram, and the second (hence the name CGS-system of units). All other physical units of measurement take account of these fundamental notions of length, mass, and time. In mechanics the unit of force is the dyne, the unit of work is the erg, the unit of power is the watt, the unit of energy is the joule. In the physics of heat the unit of heat is the calorie. In electricity the unit of resistance is the ohm, the unit of current is the ampère, the unit of electromotive force the volt, etc. These units are coming ever more into use in clinical diagnostic work. Their general adoption in scientific work is a forcible example of the fundamental relation in which physics stands to all the more complex sciences of nature.

The physical sciences, then, including, as they do, dynamics, mechanics, the physics of heat, light, sound, electricity, and magnetism, energetics, and the setting up of units to be used as standards of measurement, are seen to be essential as a part of the basis upon which a science of diagnosis can be built. Medical educators have been wise, therefore, in making knowledge of the theory and some skill in the use of the practical-technical methods of physics a prerequisite to the study of medicine and of diagnosis.

Relations of Diagnosis and Chemistry

The science of *chemistry* stands in almost as fundamental a relationship to the science of diagnosis as does the science of physics. Chemistry has to do with the study of the composition of substances and of the changes in composition that substances undergo, whereas physics, which we have just considered, studies rather the properties of substances. In physical chemistry, in process of development, we see a new science that attempts to correlate the physical properties of substances with their chemical composition. Our knowledge of the composition of the substances in the cells and in the fluids of the human body has already become very important for the student of the science of diagnosis. Indeed, it could scarcely be otherwise since the fact of the life of the human body is metabolism. The living substance is, on the one hand, ever undergoing decomposition (dissimilation or catabolism), and, on the other, is ever undergoing reconstruction (assimilation or anabolism). With the exact composition of the most complex types of chemical substances existing in the body—the hypothetical biogens—we are as yet unfamiliar, but of the importance in their composition of the long chains of amino-acids known as proteins we have now become convinced. Physiologists and physiological chemists have already gone far toward demonstrating to us how the foods taken into the body are changed in order that suitable building-stones may be available for the construction of the complex biogen-molecules of protoplasm, and they are also revealing to us the various stages in the degradation processes through which these biogens form secretions and excretions as end-products of the body metabolism. The fascinating studies that deal with the morphological changes, with the chemical changes, and with the energy changes that accompany the body metabolism were growing yearly more numerous before the outbreak of the great war; they will doubtless be resumed with even greater vigor now that the war is over and the nations can again settle down to the leisurely and undisturbed cultivation of medical science. The principles and the practical-technical methods of chemistry are now a part of the stock-in-trade of the well-equipped student of diagnosis.

If, then, the modern diagnostician needs to be tolerably familiar with the principles and the methods of chemical science, his preparatory studies should include inorganic chemistry, organic chemistry, analytical chemistry, and physical chemistry. The medical diagnosis of to-day makes extensive use of the principles, of the terminology, and of the machinery, of all these subdivisions of chemistry. The work of diagnosis in the clinical laboratory demands considerable practical acquaintance with the apparatus and the technique of chemical manipulations. In the clinical investigation of metabolism, especially, a knowledge of chemistry and an acquaintance with chemical methods is essential. I need refer only to the chemistry of the proteins and of their derivatives, and its applications to metabolism in the renal diseases and in the amino-acid diatheses; to the chemistry of the carbohydrates and its applications to metabolism in diabetes mellitus and allied disturbances; to the chemistry of the fats and its relations to obesity on the one hand, and to acidosis on the other; to the chemistry of the mineral substances in the body and its relations to the metabolism in rickets, in osteomalacia, and in tetany; to the chemistry of the nucleins, purins, and pyrimidins and its relations to the metabolism in gout; and, finally, to the as yet little known chemistry of the vitamins and its relations to the metabolism in beri-beri and in other diseases in which there is believed to be vitamin deficiency. If I were to-day a student in my teens, looking forward to the study of diagnosis and therapy, and could realize at that age as I do now the fundamental importance of physical and chemical science for the future of the biological and medical sciences, I should make a great effort to become firmly grounded in the different branches of physics and chemistry, securing also sufficient training in mathematics to permit of their higher study. Young students of to-day who will avail themselves of this hint before going on to the study of the biological and medical sciences will, I feel sure, be richly rewarded when they become the diagnosticians and therapeutists of twenty years from now. The time and energy expended in the acquisition of sound and thorough physical and chemical experience as a preliminary to medical study could scarcely be better employed.

Relations of Diagnosis and Biology

The relationship of the science of diagnosis to the science of *biology* is obvious and yet there should be no confusion or overlapping as regards their respective fields. As abstract sciences, biology deals with the laws of life, diagnosis with the laws of the recognition of health and of disease in living organisms. Each science is important for the other though each differs from the other. From biology we learn that the tendency of evolution is to " transfer the maximum amount of inorganic matter to the organized state " as a part of the general process of storing cosmical energy. The most complex chemical combination known is protoplasm, the " physical basis of life." In biotic organization, the unit is the cell, a very complex structure when compared with the relatively simple constitution of protoplasm. Biology treats of unicellular and multicellular organisms, of their structures and functions, of their origin, growth, and destiny. It reveals the advantages of living beings as organized mechanisms for the storage and expenditure of energy. It studies reactions between organisms and their environment and shows how capacity for suitable adjustment makes for success and survival, and how inability adequately to adjust leads to failure and extinction. It explains the origin of anatomical structures and the relations of structures to functions. It discovers that at certain stages of biotic organization feeling becomes important for the preservation of life, that pleasure and pain are conditional to the existence of plastic organisms, and that, out of sentiency, mind develops. Knowing, feeling, and striving become ever more important factors in the living of higher organisms. Some kinds of structure, some varieties of function, and some modes of feeling, striving, and knowing are advantageous to organisms and make for their survival; others are disadvantageous and lead to disease or death of individuals and of species. Evolution, heredity, variation, adaptation, and selection, as studied by the biologist, are all important as building-stones in the foundation of a science of diagnosis.

The relation of diagnosis to one of the special biological sciences, *anthropology,* may be considered from two points of view. The student of diagnosis looks upon the science of anthropology as a part of the foundation for the science of diagnosis, whereas the anthropologist will look upon that part of diagnosis that deals with the recognition of health and of disease in man as belonging to the science of man. Undoubtedly, the two sciences overlap and the facts and phenomena of each are important for the other science. Anthropology as a descriptive science is really a branch of zoölogy. A knowledge of the peculiarly human characteristics, which anthropology supplies, is too often disregarded by students of the science of diagnosis who transfer, without criticism, conclusions drawn from observations upon experimental animals directly to the human sphere. Of the different departments of anthropology, it is somatology (dealing with man's physical constitution) and technology (dealing with man's products, material and institutional) that are most important for the student of diagnosis. Among the institutions man has produced are languages, customs, governments, religions, industries, art, and literature. How inadequate would be the work of the student of diagnosis who lacked familiarity with these achievements of man! Both the "natural history of man" and the "history of culture" supply data that are essential for the construction of a science of diagnosis.

The biological sciences deal, then, with living organisms, and patients who consult physicians are living organisms that conform to biological laws. All the special biological sciences, including (1) Morphology, which deals with the statical aspects of the organic world, or with the structure of living organisms, (2) Physiology, which deals with the dynamical aspects of the same world, or with the properties, processes, and functions of living organisms, (3) Distribution, which deals with the number of organisms of different kinds in different parts of the world, and (4) Evolution, or Etiology, which deals with the natural history of the cosmos, in as far as it concerns organic beings, can contribute to the science of diagnosis. That training in the principles and methods of the biological sciences should, like similar training in the sciences of physics and chemistry, be now regarded as an essential prerequisite to the study of medicine and diagnosis seems, therefore, a reasonable opinion for the medical educator to hold.

Relations of Diagnosis and Psychology

Turning to another subject, it is surprising how little attention has been paid by those who frame pre-medical curricula to the importance of the relations of the science of *psychology* to the science of diagnosis.

Psychology, as the science of mind, embraces not only the phenomena of "intellect" but also those of the "affections" and those of the "will." Students of human psychology study the knowing, the feeling, and the striving of man. Biology has shown us that feelings of pleasure induce lower animals to look for food and to eat it and to perform the acts that reproduce their kind, whereas feelings of pain lead them to make efforts to escape from enemies and from other dangers. Among higher animals, the knowing element became ever more helpful to the feeling and the striving elements of mind in attaining the purposes of the organism. Man is the most highly favored of all living creatures in this respect and by virtue of his intellect has not only obtained dominion over other forms of life, but has also become the conqueror of the physical forces of nature. Feeling is dynamic; intellect is directive; the will is an activity of purposive behavior that is determined by feeling and intellect.

In the animal series, the intellect seems to have developed, at first, as a means of increasing agreeable feeling, of overcoming obstacles to the satisfaction of desires. The "knowing" element gradually became a most important servant of the "feeling" and "striving" elements of the mind. The human pleasures include the realization of certain objective ends—the nutritive, the reproductive, the esthetic, the emotional, the moral, and the intellectual. The desire for self-realization and to obtain pleasure ("lower" or "higher") is the motive to effort. The intellect is to be looked upon as a directive agent to guide the organism in the achievement of its purposes, that is, in the satisfaction of its desires, and in the fulfilling of all its capacities. It manifests itself in foresight, cunning, shrewdness, sagacity, wisdom, tact, ingenuity, inventiveness, art, science, and philosophy.

The psychologist observes and studies his own consciousness and the behavior of men and of animals, and builds up his science upon the basis of the facts thus accumulated. He desires to understand and to explain his own behavior and that of other men and of animals. Knowledge of consciousness and of behavior will, he believes, yield the power to guide and control behavior. He defines behavior as the manner in which an organism possessing mind conducts itself in the active pursuit of its own welfare and in the effort to reach its own ends or to effect its own purposes. By studying himself and observing the phenomena of his own consciousness and his own behavior (as he, himself, thinks and feels and strives), he deepens his understanding of the behavior of all living things and draws conclusions regarding the consciousness he believes they must possess when they exhibit behavior. By systematic studies of this sort the laws of mind are established.

In analyzing and describing the stream of his own consciousness, the psychologist meets with very great difficulties and the overcoming of these constitutes an important part of his problem. He designates the knowing aspect of mind as "cognitive," the feeling aspect as "affective," and the striving as "conative." He seeks to explain both what goes on in consciousness (and the accompanying behavior) on the basis of the "constitution" or the "structure" of the mind, as it develops during the life of the organism, a development that is determined partly by heredity and partly by environmental influences that favor or prevent the realization of the various hereditary possibilities. He conceives of the mind as constituted of a large number of "mental dispositions," which form organized systems. The totality of cognitive dispositions he speaks of as the "knowledge" possessed by the mind; the totality of affective and conative dispositions he refers to as the "character" of the individual. Acquaintance with the knowledge and character of a person gives the clue to his conduct in a given situation. Despite the difficulties of analysis and description, psychologists are gradually arriving at conceptions that are helpful both for theory and practice.

Now, the science of diagnosis is very largely dependent upon observation of the behavior of patients and necessitates inquiry into their mental states in their cognitive, affective, and conative aspects. Most physicians, whether or not they have had any academic training in psychology, acquire a certain power of estimating intellectual capacity and of recognizing types of character. For the higher reaches of diagnosis, however, a much fuller acquaintance with the laws of mind and the phenomena of human behavior than can be obtained without special training in psychology is requisite. Diagnostic science and the art of diagnosis are now being rapidly promoted by men who have been thoroughly trained in psychology as a whole or in one or more of its branches. A larger acquaintance with the psychology of the normal human adult, with the psychology of animals, with the psychology of children, with the individual psychology that deals with the peculiarities of individual minds, with abnormal psychology, and with the social psychology that studies the folk-mind, the crowd-mind, and the group-mind, and their influences upon individual minds through the processes of suggestion, sympathy, imitation, and interpenetration, will doubtless, before long, be regarded as an essential part of the equipment of the earnest student of diagnosis.

Relations of Diagnosis and Sociology

We come next to the kinship of diagnosis and sociology. It is not easy sharply to separate sociology from psychology; social psychology is a link that joins these two sciences. In studying psychology, nowadays, the prospective student of diagnosis learns, as has just been said, of the importance of the crowd-mind or "mass-mind" exhibited by large masses, and of the group-mind that is manifested by smaller associations in every highly organized human society. He studies the principles of collective thinking, collective feeling, and collective acting, and he makes an effort to observe the influence of the social *milieu* upon the development of the individual mind. But the science of *sociology* itself is also closely related to the science of diagnosis, and a fairly comprehensive grasp of its methods and principles should be acquired by those who expect to study, and to practice, diagnosis. Diagnosis has to deal with the recognition of "disease" in individuals, but these individuals are members of social groups. To understand an individual thoroughly one must know much about the social groups to which he belongs and their origin by ascent or descent. A knowledge of sociology should therefore be helpful to the student and practitioner of diagnosis.

Sociology, the science of society, studies the structure, functions, and genesis of the social body, just as anatomy, physiology, embryology, and psychology study the individual organism. It discovers what it is in man's nature that induces him to associate himself with others; what the effects of association are upon his interests, his feelings, his emotions, his desires, and his acts; what purposes association and coöperation subserve and what means are adopted for favoring them; what relations become established among men as a result of different kinds of aggregation and coöperation; and what influence these relations exert upon the thought, the feelings, and the behavior of man. Sociologists like J. S. Mill, A. Comte, and Lester Ward have traced the broad outlines of the science and a host of workers are filling in the details. The data of sociology are drawn from a large number of special social sciences (ethnography, ethnology, technology, archeology, demography, history, economics, jurisprudence, politics, and ethics); these data form the basis of the reasoning and the generalizations of the more general science. The forces studied by the sociologist are psychic; they consist of human motives, the unsatisfied appetites and desires of men. These forces are preservative, reproductive, esthetic, moral, and intellectual—in other words, the "forces of individual preservation," the "forces of race continuance," and the "forces of race elevation." Feeling is the dynamic agent in society and intellect is the directing agent. Resulting from the collision of social forces, states of approximate equilibrium occur among them, and social structures (including the family, the clan, the tribe, the state, the church, and other voluntary associations) and social institutions (including marriage, customs, language, codes, religions, arts, literatures, and sciences) arise. These structures and institutions, while relatively stable, are constantly undergoing change; though there is at every time a social order, there is at all times some social progress, and this progress is described by the sociologist as partly the result of an unconscious evolution (social genesis), partly the result (and increasingly so now) of the conscious application of the intellect as a guide to human desires in avoiding obstacles to their satisfaction (individual and collective telesis). Knowledge of these social structures and functions and of their evolution, therefore, constitutes the science of sociology. None of the better diagnosticians of our time is likely to underestimate the importance for his own science of a knowledge of society, of social structures, of social institutions, or of social functions. For the physician is constantly called upon, nowadays, to recognize in his patients states in which there is maladjustment of the individual to his environment, states in which the reciprocal relations of the individual and of the social groups to which he belongs are unsatisfactory, states that cannot be properly understood or adequately modified by a therapeutic regimen when the individual is studied alone without concomitant consideration of the group, or groups, of socii to which he belongs. The prospective diagnostician should, therefore, receive sufficient training in the science of sociology and should familiarize himself with the laws of association and with the subtle psychic processes of interpenetration that characterize the activities of concrete groups.

Relations of Diagnosis to the Preclinical Medical Sciences

Though some acquaintance with the sciences of physics, chemistry, biology, anthropology, psychology, and sociology, including ethics and politics, is, as has been emphasized above, highly desirable as preparatory experience for the student of the science, and for the practitioner of the art, of diagnosis, a still more comprehensive training is necessary in certain distinctively medical sciences, namely, in a group of sciences intermediate between the fundamental sciences above referred to and the clinical sciences of diagnosis and therapy. This intermediate group of sciences, training in which is indispensable for the prospective clinician, is usually taught in the first two years of the course in the medical school; these sciences we may include under the general name of *preclinical medical sciences.* This group includes several sub-groups: (1) an anatomical sub-group (gross human anatomy, microscopic anatomy, histology, cytology, and embryology); (2) a physiological sub-group (general and special physiology, physiological chemistry, and pharmacology); and (3) a pathological sub-group (general pathology, special pathological anatomy, and histology, bacteriology, parasitology, immunology, psychopathology, and social pathology). These preclinical sciences were largely developed in the first place by diagnosticians (as postclinical sciences), because their development was necessary for the growth of diagnosis and therapy, but as knowledge has grown and technique has become ever more complex, they have come to be cultivated as sciences for their own sake by men who devote their whole time and energies to the single provinces; and they are now taught, and should be taught (as far as developed), as prerequisite to work in diagnosis. The facts and principles of these preclinical sciences supply data that are necessary as a basis for the science of diagnosis. It is essential that the scientific diagnostician shall himself have had a general training in the methods and principles of each of these preclinical medical sciences and that he shall have acquired such a comprehensive grasp of them as will permit him, first, to keep pace with their progress during his lifetime, and, secondly, to make applications of them in any direction that will be helpful to his own science and art.

It must be emphasized, however, that the problems of the preclinical medical sciences, though closely related to the problems of the science of diagnosis, are by no means identical with them. There is much overlapping, but it is desirable that the purposes of each of the sciences should be kept clearly in view by those who represent it. The anatomist should work at the problems of his science for their own sake, for the sake of discovering facts and truths regarding the form and genesis of the structures in organisms, and especially in the human organism, without special reference to their applicability in the science of diagnosis. It is the business of the investigator in the science of diagnosis to make the application of the facts and truths of the anatomical sciences and their methods to the solution of diagnostic problems. The same is true as regards the physiological sub-group of the preclinical medical sciences. It holds even for the pathological sub-group, which many would look upon as an integral part of the science of diagnosis; but the aims, purposes, and methods of the representatives of the special sciences of pathological anatomy, pathological physiology, and bacteriology are, and should be, somewhat different from the aims, purposes, and methods of the representatives of clinical diagnosis. Closely related as the clinical and preclinical medical sciences are, they are still separate and distinct, and much is gained for both groups by the maintenance of this separation and distinction.

Each science will help its kindred sciences most by defining strictly the limits of its province, and cultivating industriously, intensively, and conscientiously its own fields within that province. The clinician must not expect the anatomist, the physiologist, and the pathologist to leave their own special tasks to solve his diagnostic problems for him, nor should the worker in clinical diagnosis be expected by his preclinical colleagues to neglect the crops on his own acreage by yielding to the temptation to till promising neighboring fields. When special needs are felt and lead to a division of work, dormant capacities are aroused and new powers are called into being. The differentiation of purposes and of labor is one of the most powerful influences for increasing the range of intellectual activities and for stimulating their development.

In diagnosis itself, the field is so large that no single person can expect to work equally well in all parts of it. A division of labor in diagnosis, partly methodological and partly regional and systematic, has proved profitable, as in science at large. As evidences of this division we find diagnostic workers distributing themselves more or less (1) according to the methods they employ (applied physics, applied chemistry, applied biology, applied psychology, applied sociology, applied physiology, applied pathology, etc.) and (2) according to the systems and regions they especially study (angiology, neurology, psychiatry, gastroenterology, dermatology, laryngology, ophthalmology, orthopedics, gynecology, etc.). Diagnosis by coöperative groups, with an integrator who, after collection of data and consultations with collaborators, synthesizes the total findings of the group and composes the clinical picture with balanced ordination of its parts, is the highest expression by the diagnostic art of to-day of the unity obtainable despite this differentiation, and of the profit derivable from specialization.

The Pure Science of Clinical Diagnosis

Though the pure science, the applied science, and the art of diagnosis are most often treated together, it is helpful, for purposes of analysis, to make the division and to understand how the three differ one from another.

By the *pure science of diagnosis,* we mean the part of the subject that deals with the general laws and principles of diagnosis, that is, with the laws and principles that govern the recognition of health and of disease. The laws of diagnosis are generalizations that epitomize in brief formulae uniformities of coexistence and of sequence among the phenomena of health and of disease. The causes of these uniformities are natural forces operating under like conditions. The forces concerned are physical, chemical, biotic, psychic, and social, and the pure science of diagnosis is gradually moving toward the recognition of the workings of these forces as manifested in the phenomena of health and of disease. In the construction of this pure science of diagnosis, the data are derived from all the sciences already referred to as fundamental for diagnosis, as well as from all the special diagnostic sciences. The storehouse of knowledge and of truths discovered in the science of diagnosis is already a very large one. Facts have been classified and are ever being more successfully reclassified as the laws underlying them and the causes of the uniformities are being ever better recognized. Subjective symptoms and physical signs are grouped together as symptom-complexes (or syndromes), and these are uniformities of coexistence and of sequence that betoken underlying causes acting under like conditions; and these causes and these conditions are slowly being determined by the host of investigators who are ever eagerly striving to discover them. Through observation, experimentation, and reflective thinking, knowledge concerning the symptoms of disease, disease-complexes, the sites of disease, the structural and functional alterations in disease and their genesis, the forces concerned, and the conditions under which they act, is being organized as a science of diagnosis with some well-established principles. The diagnosis of disease now includes (1) a recognition of disturbed function in disease (pathological-physiological diagnosis), (2) a recognition of the site and nature of the structural changes in disease (pathological-anatomical diagnosis), (3) a recognition of the causes of disease (etiological diagnosis), and (4) a recognition of the relation of causes to the sequence of conditions in the disease (pathogenetic diagnosis). The data accumulated by workers in all the medical sciences are gradually being summarized, arranged, and classified by workers in the science of diagnosis, so that the laws and principles underlying them are slowly becoming evident.

The Applied Science of Diagnosis

Pure science, applied science, and art, progress contemporaneously. Each plays into the hands of the other two; there are ever reciprocal contributions to healthy growth.

The applied science of diagnosis has the task of finding out how the laws and principles of the pure science of diagnosis can best be applied in the practical work of recognizing health or disease in persons who present themselves for examination. This applied science of diagnosis perceives the utilities of the truths of "pure" science and sets about devising the means of adjustment that are necessary to actualize them. It invents methods, tools, contrivances, and systems of procedure, in other words, the "machinery of diagnosis." It calls to the service of diagnosis, from the other sciences, any fact, truth, principle, or invention that it can make use of, directly or indirectly, as an aid. It becomes familiar with the methods and instruments of mathematics, chemistry, biology, psychology, physics, anatomy, physiology, pathology, bacteriology and immunology, modifying them where necessary to meet its own needs. It extends the simpler methods of observation of patients by utilizing instruments of precision or special methods that enormously multiply and refine the possibilities of sense-impressions. Thus the sense of sight is extended by photography, and by the use of the microscope, the spectroscope, the ophthalmoscope, the bronchoscope, the cystoscope, the roentgenoscope and a hundred other devices. The senses of smell and of taste are chemical senses that, unaided, carry us only a short way in collecting chemical data as compared with the fact-accumulation regarding chemical conditions in the blood, secretions, excretions and effusions made possible by the clinical chemists' adaptations of methods devised by workers in physiological and pathological chemistry. The sense of hearing is extended by the stethoscope, the microphone and the phono-cardiograph. The temperature-sense is supplemented by the clinical thermometer. The sense of touch and pressure is subtly refined, or replaced, by various ingenious devices such as the sphygmograph, the tonometer, the balance, the dynamometer and the string galvanometer. The time-honored methods of inspection, palpation, percussion, auscultation and mensuration have gradually become expanded into an observational and experimental technique that is subtle and complex, but which makes for ever greater objectivity and precision. Thus by devising practical technical methods that can be easily made use of in examining patients, the applied science of diagnosis is ever better able to turn to account the truths and principles that students of the pure science of diagnosis have established.

Workers in the applied science of diagnosis are also making many efforts better to organize the mode of conducting clinical examinations and more logically to arrange the several steps that necessarily must be taken to arrive at satisfactory diagnostic conclusions. That the procedure of collecting the data upon which a diagnosis is based and of making clinical records of the course of disease-processes has been systematized in the interests of thoroughness, completeness and accuracy, can easily be seen by comparing the contents of the clinical histories kept to-day (anamnesis, status praesens, catamnesis, epicrisis) with those that have come down to us from the diagnosticians of earlier generations. Moreover, the methods of applying reflective thought to the consideration of the phenomena observed for the purpose of recognizing syndromes, lesions, causes and prospects are being brought into accord with the general method of science and with the newer logic. The purpose of a diagnostic study decides what methods shall be applied and how. In every case there must first be a recognition of the existence of a diagnostic problem; observations and experiments are then made to locate, and more accurately to define, that problem; the phenomena observed are arranged and brooded over until suggestions of possible explanation, or recognition of meaning, occur to the mind; the implications of each interpretative suggestion are reasoned out; a comparison is made between each suggestion, with all its implications, and the facts, as already collected, or as extended by further observation and experiment; and finally, a decision is reached that there is sufficient reason for the acceptance of one or another of the diagnostic inferences through corroboration, and for the rejection of other suggestions that are proved invalid through failure of corroboration. If no suggestion that has been entertained can be found to be valid, no diagnosis is made; the mind is still kept open and judgment is kept suspended until the process has been gone through with again. An attempt to accumulate more facts has then to be made, the occurrence of further diagnostic suggestions is thus favored, and these in turn are reasoned out as to their bearings and tested for their validity. In this way the best diagnoses of which the examiner is capable, in the existing state of his knowledge, ability and opportunities, are reached. The representatives of the applied science of diagnosis, through devising new and better methods of examination, through arranging for their more orderly employment, and through conforming to the usages of a sound logic, occupy therefore an important position mediating between that of the pure science of diagnosis and that of the diagnostic art.

The Art of Clinical Diagnosis

By the exercise of *the art of diagnosis* is meant the skillful carrying out of the plans and methods of the applied science of diagnosis (based upon the laws and principles of the pure science) in solving actual problems of recognizing health and disease in persons who present themselves for examination.

Expertness in performance and capacity to make and deliver a valuable product characterize the diagnostic artist, whether he is active in special domains only or whether he attempts to make a more general diagnostic survey. Many physicians have acquired an extensive knowledge of the classifications of disease, of pathological anatomy and physiology, and of etiology, have become familiar with descriptions of the practical-technical methods in use, and have observed skillful practitioners of the art of diagnosis at work, but have never arrived at expertness and facility, themselves, in the actual performance of diagnostic tasks. There are other physicians who, though they may have attained to real skill in the execution of certain diagnostic procedures, have never become good general diagnosticians owing to lack of a comprehensive grasp of the fundamental laws and principles of diagnosis or owing to insufficient acquaintance with the practical-technical methods of diagnostic work other than a few in which they have acquired accuracy and facility. Mere exactness in outlining an area of dulness by percussion, mere faultless objectivity in description of the sounds audible over the heart and lungs, or mere precision in the conduct of a roentgenoscopic examination of the cardiovascular stripe, in the recording of a sphygmogram, or in the quantitative estimation of blood sugar, valuable though any or all of these procedures may be in collecting data to be used in the reasoning process that precedes the arrival at a legitimate diagnostic conclusion, can be exhibited by men who dare lay no claim to mastery of the general art of diagnosis. As a matter of fact, a laboratory *Diener* may learn to carry out the technique of the Wassermann reaction, or of the differential count of the white corpuscles of the blood, just as accurately, and perhaps more speedily, than the physician who employs him and who has instructed him, but no one would think of regarding such a laboratory helper as proficient in the general art of medical diagnosis. Owing to the lower dignity of his employment, he must be regarded as an artisan rather than as an artist. An adept in an art of medical diagnosis that is not merely local or special in its aims must have acquired at least some skill in the collection of data in all the domains pertinent to general medical diagnosis and must possess that wide understanding of the truths and principles of diagnostic science and that ability in applying them that will permit him, on reflective thinking about the phenomena observed by himself or by those who are associated with him, to arrive at a diagnostic conclusion or belief that is warranted. Ability to do diagnostic work quickly, accurately, and effectively and capacity to produce diagnostic results that are adequate to the purpose in view are, then, the marks of an operator who is skilled in the art of diagnosis.

The attainment of real skill in the general diagnostic art is no easy matter. It presupposes in addition to good natural endowment, a thorough general, and special education for the developing artist. At the basis of our present-day conception of the training of medical students lies the recognition of (1) the desirability of a collegiate education preliminary to the study of medicine, (2) the need of a thorough instruction in the preclinical sciences and in the organized body of knowledge that we call the pure science of medical diagnosis, and (3) of the importance of a closely-supervised systematic education in the practical-technical methods of accumulating facts pertinent to diagnosis and in the logical way of making use of these facts (by grouping them, by drawing inferences from them, by testing these inferences carefully for their validity and by finally reaching legitimate diagnostic conclusions). The requirements for admission to the better medical schools of our time are such that the students entering the schools have had ample opportunities for becoming habituated to the method of science and for acquiring a good general knowledge of nature and of man as an individual and as a member of social groups. The students have all had instruction in mathematics, physics, chemistry and biology, and many of them have studied also psychology, logic and sociology. In addition to a training in the use of their native language, they have acquired a reading knowledge of one or more modern foreign languages, have learned the technique of using libraries, and have discovered the value of consulting sources through bibliographies. The prospective medical students with such a preliminary training can scarcely have avoided becoming acquainted with the general methods and tools of scientific inquiry. They have learned how problems are set and solved. They have been taught the necessity of taking pains in collecting facts by the accurate and detailed observation of phenomena and have come to appreciate the special value of experimentation in which observations are made under rigidly controlled conditions. Under the guidance of good teachers they have begun to acquire the habit of reflective thinking in dealing with their perplexities. They have become unwilling to jump to conclusions and have learned to insist, when confronted with a difficulty, on temporarily suspending judgment and on collecting information that will more rigidly define and locate that difficulty; and when suggestions of possible solution of a problem have occurred to them on brooding over their facts, they have been taught to reason out the bearings of these suggestions, to compare them and their full implications with the actual facts before them, and thus to test the tentative ideas of solution for their validity; they have learned the importance, when necessary, of making more observations and experiments that will either corroborate or refute. In other words, they have had the opportunity to practice deliberative thinking before undertaking their medical studies proper. On entering the medical school they spend a couple of years in work in the simpler preclinical medical sciences before engaging in the much more complex work of the clinical sciences of diagnosis and therapy. In the laboratories of anatomy, of physiology, of physiological chemistry, of pharmacology, of pathology and of bacteriology they continue their training in the applications of the method of science to the study of the phenomena dealt with by these special sciences, and they should come out of these laboratories with that background of knowledge and that familiarity with methods that is indispensable for any proper study of the science, and any skillful practice of the art, of medical diagnosis. In the clinical departments of the medical school the students then enter courses of instruction in the laws and principles of diagnosis and therapy, begin their education in the technical methods of these sciences and, under the closest supervision, make a start in the practice of the corresponding arts. Not only must the methods be learned (the applied sciences of diagnosis and therapy), but skill in carrying them out (the arts of diagnosis and therapy) must be acquired, in order that the students may acquire confidence in the reports that their sense-organs (thus refined) yield and in the warranty for the diagnostic conclusions that can be reached and the therapeutic regimens that can legitimately be outlined by the application of reflective thought to these reports. This training in the clinical departments includes instruction in history-taking, in general physical diagnosis, in clinical laboratory work, in X-ray work, and in the technique of a whole series of special and instrumental methods of examination. The students learn the clinical application of bacteriological and immunological methods to be used in the diagnosis of the infectious diseases; they are taught how to examine the respiratory apparatus, the circulatory apparatus, the blood, the digestive system, the urogenital system, the locomotor system, and the nervous system and its functions; and they also receive instruction in the methods of clinically investigating the processes of metabolism and the functions of the endocrine apparatus. After this more or less thorough drill in the use of the methods of collecting facts regarding each special domain, they begin, as clinical clerks working in hospital wards and dispensaries, to take up the complete diagnostic study of single unknown cases. In close association with, and under the strict control of, experienced diagnosticians, they record anamneses, make physical and psychical examinations, resort to laboratory tests and X-ray tests, are present at and observe closely the examinations made by experts in special domains, summarize and rearrange the total findings, entertain tentative ideas of diagnosis based upon these, consider all the implications of such suggestions, and try to arrive finally at diagnostic ideas that can be corroborated. Though the students are encouraged to work independently as far as possible, they have also the great advantage that the facts they collect and their reasoning about the facts are subjected to frequent review and criticism by the resident hospital assistants and by the older and more experienced visiting physicians. Only after this long training in college, medical school, and hospital is the student fitted to undertake the perfecting of his skill in the art of diagnosis, and long experience in practice may still be required to make him truly expert.

The Actual Process of Clinical Diagnosis

If diagnostic results commensurate with the medical knowledge of the time are to be reached when an internist is asked by a patient to make a diagnostic study, the procedure that he must adopt will be somewhat prolonged and complex and may be divided into several different stages: (1) the recognition of a problem to be solved, and the feeling of a diagnostic difficulty; (2) the accumulation of data that help to locate, and to define the diagnostic problem; (3) the consideration of the data (accumulated, summarized, and arranged) that suggestions of possible solution of the diagnostic problem may occur to the mind; (4) the elaboration by reasoning of the detailed bearings of the several suggestions of solution; and (5) the careful testing of the suggestions thus minutely worked out as to their bearings by comparison with the facts accumulated, supplemented when necessary by other facts obtained by further observations and experiments, this careful testing leading to disbelief in the unverifiable suggestions and finally to belief in the suggestions that are found to be valid; in other words, the arrival at diagnostic conclusions. Each of these five stages is a necessary part of any diagnostic study that aims at accuracy and completeness.

The course pursued by a worker in clinical diagnosis, then, is similar to that followed by everyone who engages in reflective or deliberative thinking in order to solve his problems. Thus the same five stages must be passed through by a business man of the higher type when he is confronted by a new and problematic industrial adventure. The same stopping-places occur in the path of an engineer who is given the task of constructing a bridge. And the same points are recognizable in the line along which any scientific investigator moves when he scents a problem that interests him, goes energetically to work to solve it, and finally meets with success. There is only one satisfactory method for solving problems, no matter what the domain, and that method is the method of deliberative thinking, commonly known as the "method of science."

Nowadays a modest internist makes no claim to powers of diagnosis *von Gottes Gnaden;* instead, he recognizes the necessity of subjecting himself gracefully to the laws of logic that must be obeyed not only by him but also by his fellow-workers in the higher branches of human endeavor. The clinician who sees and hears will often greatly wonder; he will then feed himself with questionings in order that reason may diminish his wonder. He will observe and experiment; he will brood over and speculate upon his findings; his thick-coming fancies will keep him from rest until he has tested them rigidly as to their validity in all their implications; he may even distrust his eyes and will wrangle with his reason until he has convinced himself that the evidence in favor of one set of conclusions, and of one only, is good and satisfying. He will observe so accurately, he will experiment so appropriately, he will imagine so vividly, and he will verify so conscientiously that his diagnostic conclusions will be readily defensible and will be concurred in by such other diagnosticians as are keen and honest observers, skillful experimenters, and right reasoners. Feeling a difficulty, observing and experimenting to define and localize it, harboring hypotheses that may solve it, reasoning about the implications of these hypotheses, and finally verifying those that are valid, are the successive steps in the stairway of the process of diagnosis. Clinical diagnosis is, then, an arduous and composite process; its complexities and intricacies are unavoidable. But practice in the use of the scientific method gives strength, speed, and insight to him who employs it. Though the road followed by the reflective thinker may seem long, steep and involved, it is the only safe way to as much of certainty in diagnosis as the knowledge and technique of a given time will permit.

Stage I: The Recognition of a Problem to be Solved; Feeling a Diagnostic Difficulty

It seems worth while to make the feeling of a diagnostic difficulty a definite stage in the actual process of clinical diagnosis. Formerly, more often than now, a common cause of incomplete diagnostic study was a lack of realization of the difficulties that lie in the way of accurate diagnosis. This was true especially in the times when dogmas prevailed among physicians. In those times a single symptom, say the complaint of the patient, often sufficed for the making of a diagnosis. Thus a headache, a cough, a palpitation, or a pain in the epigastrium, gave rise to no diagnostic perplexity, for the symptom itself was regarded as a diagnosis and the treatment could at once be undertaken, for the universal principle or dogma left no doubt as to the course of action to be pursued. If, nowadays, a patient complain of a headache, we at least make an effort to discover the cause of the headache in the hope that we may be able to apply a rational treatment; we are not content with any single prescription to be used in all cases of headache. Similarly, if a man complain of a backache, the scientific practitioner of to-day will not resort at once to manipulative or other therapy, but will first undertake a thorough investigation of the case; he will try to understand the pathogenesis of the condition before he decides upon the form of treatment to be applied. Thus, a realization of the difficulties of diagnosis protects one from the extreme naïvety in therapy that formerly prevailed.

Even those who have been educated in the best medical schools sometimes fail to apprehend clearly the extent of the diagnostic study that is necessary in certain cases to insure the patient that he shall receive the full benefit derivable from the diagnostic and therapeutic methods that are available. A practitioner may be tempted at times to make a "snap-shot" diagnosis and to be content with it, but if he yield to this temptation often and curtail his diagnostic studies correspondingly, he will have occasion sooner or later to rue some of his hasty conclusions. The larger the experience one has had in diagnosis the more often has he demonstrated that clinical conditions that at first seem exceedingly simple may turn out to be very complex. In many cases it is only after numerous data have been collected that the real nature of the physician's problem becomes apparent. In order, then, that the diagnostic study of a given patient shall be sufficiently comprehensive, the physician must have an adequate appreciation of the diagnostic difficulty that confronts him.

One of the principal causes of detrimental curtailment of diagnostic study probably lies in feeble curiosity. The instinct of curiosity is, of course, a part of our common endowment. When we see, or hear, something that we do not fully understand, this instinct should come into function. We should have a feeling of wonder and we should be driven by an impulse to approach and examine carefully the object that excites our wonder. Different persons are doubtless endowed in variable degree with this inborn impulse closely to examine objects that excite their wonder. The impulse grows stronger through exercise, weaker through neglect. It is probable that many persons endowed with an instinct of curiosity of normal strength fail to profit by it as they should owing to faulty education. A normal child exhibits regularly the workings of the instinct, and the medical student and the physician should, to a certain extent, try to remain childlike in this respect. In clinical diagnosis, especially, the mind should be kept ever on the alert, ever sensitive to anything out of the ordinary, ever eager for new experience. The diagnostician should be always exploring, continually seeking new materials for thought. If he cultivate a healthy curiosity, if he foster the emotion of wonder, and if he keep strong the will to investigate in order that wonder may diminish, he will have provided the fundamental conditions that protect from one-sided and incomplete diagnostic studies and that insure the comprehensive survey, the accurate observation, the suitable experimentation, and the careful reasoning that lead to valid diagnostic conclusions.

Stage II: The Accumulation of Data That Help to Localize and Define the Diagnostic Problem

Once having realized that we are confronted by a diagnostic difficulty, that we face a problematic situation, we enter upon the second stage of the diagnostic procedure and begin to accumulate the data that will permit us more accurately to define and to localize the diagnostic problem. In other words, we avoid any immediate attempt at solution of the problem because we desire first to get a better idea of the nature of the difficulty before us. At this stage, therefore, restraint of inference and suspension of judgment are desirable. Even though suggestions of solution of the diagnostic problem arise in our minds as we proceed, it is best not to yield assent to them at this stage, even when they seem plausible, though it may be justifiable to pay as much attention to them as will help us to decide upon certain directions in which the investigation may be intensively undertaken, or to conclude that, in the particular instance, certain tests often made in clinical studies may safely be omitted. At this stage we must be sure that we drag our net over an area large enough to insure the enclosure of enough facts regarding the physical, psychical and social status of our patient to make the diagnostic problem precise in localization and definition.

The accumulation of the data necessary for this purpose is greatly facilitated by the following of some systematic plan. Thus it is customary to train medical students to collect the more important facts regarding a patient in a certain regular way. The following of a routine method of procedure here has both advantages and disadvantages. Among the advantages are (1) speed in the performance of an habitual process, (2) comprehensiveness, and (3) convenience of arrangement after the facts have been collected. Among the disadvantages may be mentioned (1) the danger of stifling curiosity by too rigid adherence to a routine program and (2) the danger that routine may not be varied from time to time as knowledge grows, as methods become elaborated, and as changes of emphasis are seen to be important. However, the intelligent and experienced diagnostician should know not only when to deviate from a regular routine in a given case, but also how to modify his routine from month to month and from year to year in order that his practice may keep pace with the advances of his science and his art. The beginner in diagnosis does well, nevertheless, to adhere rather closely to a well-thought-out scheme for the collection of data regarding patients; after he has attained to accuracy and celerity in applying this routine scheme, he may begin to consider the occasions when he is justified in modifying it or in diverging from it. A systematic plan of collecting data is helpful both to the experienced and the inexperienced diagnostician.

We may, for convenience, deal with the systematic accumulation of data regarding a patient in five different parts:

1. The recording of the anamnesis.
2. The recording of the results of a general physical and psychical examination.
3. The recording of the results of the application of laboratory tests.
4. The recording of the results of X-ray examinations.
5. The recording of the results of more intensive examinations of special domains.

ad 1.—*The Recording of the Anamnesis.* In collecting the data obtainable as answers to questions put to the patient or to his friends one must make sure that the questionnaire covers (1) the main complaints of the patient, (2) his family history, (3) his personal history, and (4) the history of the illness for which he consults the practitioner, including the symptoms existing at the time. It does not matter, as a rule, in what order these several parts of the history are taken. Some physicians, after ascertaining the main complaint of the patient, prefer to begin with the family history, to follow this with the personal history, and to end up with a history of the present illness. Others prefer to take the history of the present illness first, and, later, to secure the family history and the personal history of the patient. The latter method has some advantages, for the patient is always more interested in talking about his present illness than in giving the details of the history of his family and of his earlier experiences. Thus sick people often exhibit a certain impatience if one begin with the family history rather than with the history of the illness itself, though after the latter has been given in detail, they will willingly respond to inquiries regarding their family histories and their earlier personal histories. In the accompanying table a general outline is given of the principal points to be covered by the ordinary anamnesis:

A. Main complaints of the patient and their duration.
B. Family history (parents; brothers, and sisters; consort; children; other relatives).
C. Personal history (habits of work, eating, drinking, smoking, exercising, resting, sleeping, relaxing, etc.); education; experience; diseases; operations; traumata; mental conflicts; social adaptations.
D. Present illness (onset; supposed causes; course; previous treatment; epitome of symptoms referable to different anatomical-physiological domains).

It is important when recording the anamnesis to ask questions that bear upon the presence or absence of certain prominent symptoms referable to definite domains of the body; such inquiries are best made also in systematic sequence. After one has formed the habit of such questioning, a catalogue of the more important indications can be easily held in the mind. But the beginner will do well, while recording the anamnesis, to have before him a list of these symptoms, to make sure that he overlook no inquiry that could be pertinent. In this connection, the following list of betokening symptoms is a serviceable one:

Prominent Symptoms.

Pain (topography; time relations; severity; quality; radiations; modifying influences; associated phenomena).
Headaches.
Dizziness.
Tinnitus.
Otorrhea.
Nasal catarrh.
Sore throat; hoarseness.
Cough; sputum, including hemoptysis.
Dyspnea.
Palpitation; irregular action of heart.
Retrosternal or precordial oppression or pain (relation to effort; radiation).
Swelling of ankles or face; varicose veins.
Ingesta (quality; quantity). Disturbances of appetite and of deglutition; trouble with teeth and gums.
Nausea; vomiting, including hematemesis.
Gaseous eructations; flatulence.
Constipation; diarrhea; blood or mucus in stools; hemorrhoids; fistulae.
Herniae.
Pollakiuria; dysuria; polyuria; nocturia; hematuria; pyuria.
Disturbance of sexual functions (male; female).
Symptoms referable to muscles, bones, or joints, including the spine.
Skin eruptions; pigmentations; pruritus; loss of hair or nails.
Disturbances of motility (paralysis; weakness; wasting; rigidity; twitching; tremor; spasms; cramps; fits; ataxias; dysarthria; aphonia; aphasia; apraxia).
Disturbances of sensibility (anesthesia; hyperesthesia; paresthesia, especially tingling in the fingers and toes; defects of smell, taste, sight, and hearing).
Mental disturbances (nervousness; insomnia; amnesia; "fainting spells" or other losses of consciousness; delusions [hypochondriacal, melancholic, or paranoid]; exaltation; depression; loss of interests; fears; indecision; inability to concentrate; feelings of unreality; social maladjustments).
Obesity; emaciation; changes in weight.
Signs of infection (fever; chills; sweats; petechiae; etc.).

The experience and common sense of the examiner must guide him in the application of his questionnaire in any given case. There may often be a temptation to try to make short cuts and to limit the questionnaire unduly. Such abbreviation should be permitted only most cautiously, for even an experienced physician may easily overlook important clues if he deviate too far from his definite systematic plan of inquiry, or if he reduce too much the number of inquiries he makes. A special warning to the beginner regarding interrogations concerning sexual, psychical, and social details may be in place. It is often difficult to judge how far one ought to go in his inquiry at the first interview when such details seem to be of importance. The most sagacious and adroit inquirer will here sometimes make mistakes. It is, therefore, important for a beginner to go slowly and cautiously when he approaches this part of the anamnesis. He should try to elicit the facts in an easy, conversational way, and he should especially avoid giving the impression that he is unnecessarily curious or offensively prying. It is only in certain cases that the details of the sexual life must be inquired into, and even then the mode and extent of the inquiry will necessarily be influenced by many circumstances, among which are the age, intelligence, character, and experience of the patient. In determining the mental status of the applicant, too, good judgment must be used in deciding upon the nature and extent of the questions to be asked. One never asks a patient, for example, whether he has delusions! But if there be reason to suspect the existence of pathological ideas in the patient's mind, his answers to the four questions (1) Are you sick? (2) Have you been sad, blue, gloomy, depressed? (3) Do you blame yourself at all, or anyone else, for your trouble? and (4) Has everyone treated you well? will usually reveal the presence or absence of hypochondriacal, melancholic, and paranoid ideas and will afford sufficient clues for the further prosecution, or for the suspension, of investigation in these directions. Psychoneurotic patients in whom it is often desirable to hunt carefully for so-called "psychogenic data" are often especially sensitive to inquiries regarding their personal lives and their adaptation to the social environment. If on cautious approach to this domain the patient be found unwilling to talk at the first interview, it may be wise to postpone this part of the inquiry for a time. A little later, after the confidence of the patient has been established by the thorough physical examination made and by the sympathetic attitude of the physician, it will be more easily possible to secure, should it be deemed important, the full avowal of the patient regarding his more intimate life. The reticence of patients regarding abnormal feelings and emotions, moods, ideas, and experiences is easily understandable, and even though questions relating to these necessarily form a part of the daily work of the medical practitioner, it can scarcely be expected that all the patients will willingly, and immediately, place their hearts upon their sleeves for his inspection. The larger the world-experience of the physician, the greater his acquaintance with abnormal, nervous, and mental states, the wider his sympathies, and the more winsome his personality, the easier it will be for him quickly to acquire the confidence of patients and an avowal of the sort referred to when it is desired for the purposes of diagnosis. When the account given by the patient suggests the existence of abnormalities of the intellect, of the emotions, or of the will, it may be helpful also to interview, privately, members of the patient's family or his business associates, in order to learn what impressions they may have formed of the patient's nervous and mental state and what alterations, if any, in his personality they have observed. By the prudent application of measures such as those described, the psychical, social, and, when necessary, the sexual status, of the patient can nearly always be satisfactorily estimated and recorded.

Besides the general features of the anamnesis above referred to there are certain special points that are worthy, perhaps, of particular mention. One of these is the significance that sometimes pertains to recording the precise time-relations of the appearance of different symptoms. Thus when a tumor of the acoustic nerve developing in the cerebello-pontine angle is present, the exact chronology of the appearance of the different symptoms may be very helpful for the diagnosis. And in other diseases (typhoid fever, malaria, syphilis) the temporal relations of the symptoms may be informative. A second special point in the anamnesis worthy of attention is the interpretation given by the patient himself of his illness as a whole, or of any single symptom. It is desirable to put such an interpretation down no matter how improbable or how erroneous it may seem to the examiner. Every practitioner must have been impressed by the remarkable interpretation-delusions that patients sometimes harbor. But when the patient's explanation of his condition is obviously delusional, some care must be taken to avoid too brusque a refusal of acceptance of his pathological interpretative ideas. Only after confidence has been gained through a thorough investigation and through the establishment of a sympathetic relationship dare the practitioner hope to change such firmly set opinions. Even then the bringing of conviction to the patient may not be possible except through a somewhat prolonged reëducative process. A third matter that may well be again emphasized in the recording of the anamnesis is the extension of the questionnaire so that it shall certainly cover the marks of disturbances of the several anatomical-physiological systems of the body. If the several prominent symptoms mentioned in the above table be inquired about and the answers recorded, it is not likely that many of the pathological phenomena self-observed by the patient will be omitted from the record and the examiner can be confident that he has at hand the data necessary for his guidance in the further progress of the diagnostic investigation; these particulars are helpful for the making of decisions regarding the necessity of more intensive explorations in certain domains. Attention to the exact chronology of the appearance of symptoms, the appropriate management of the patient's interpretative delusions when such exist, and a search for the subjective marks of systemic disturbances are, therefore, especially serviceable to the physician who is recording a patient's recollections.

The totality of facts that the anamnesis can yield when it is skillfully elicited and recorded, has an importance to the diagnostician in his appraisement of the physical, psychical, and social status of the patient under study that can scarcely be overestimated. Both the anamnesis and the general physical and psychical examination are, of course, essential for clinical diagnosis, and neither should be neglected. I have heard more than one good clinician, however, state that if they had to be guided by one or the other alone, they would prefer to follow the path shown by anamnestic records that they had elicited rather than by the results of other examinations. These were men, however, who through long experience had learned better how to assess the value of single subjective symptoms and groups of such symptoms than any beginner could hope to do. Fortunately, we do not have to be guided by the anamnesis alone or by the physical examination alone; we utilize both to supply us with the symptoms and signs that clarify for us the diagnostic problem by which we are confronted. But the point that I would emphasize here is that the facts obtained by recording the recollections of the patient form an indispensable part of the data we accumulate before we allow ourselves to consider the solution of any problem in clinical diagnosis.

ad 2.—*Recording of the Results of a General Physical and Psychical Examination.* On making the general physical and psychical examination it is desirable to dictate the findings to a stenographer, or to a stenotypist, familiar with medical terms, item by item as the examination proceeds, for in this way only can a full objective record be obtained. It is not safe to trust the results of such an examination even in so far as to attempt writing or dictating a report immediately after the examination has been made. The examination involves so many details that one who attempts to make his records subsequently will often forget points of importance. Moreover, the record made later is pretty sure to be colored by the examiner's total impression derived from the examination, and at this stage of the diagnostic study any such coloring is undesirable. The examiner should make an unprejudiced record of the findings in each region quite independent of any idea of what the ultimate diagnostic decisions are to be.

Before undertaking the general physical examination the patient should be completely undressed and placed between sheets with a towel across the breasts, and the lighting arrangements should be such as to permit of satisfactory inspection. How many errors in diagnosis would be avoided if practitioners always insisted upon the undressing of the patient before the examination is made! Many an aortic aneurysm, many a breast tumor, many a hernia, many a bubo, and many a gibbus go unrecognized because of disobedience to this fundamental rule. Where on account of prudery of the patient, or of great nervousness, or of other cause, a complete disrobing is not practicable, a note of this should be made in the record in order to call attention to the fact that the examination has been made under hindering conditions; later on, another examination can, perhaps, be made under more favorable conditions, if it be thought desirable. The patient should be under observation in good daylight, the source of the light preferably being on the side of the patient opposite to that of the examiner. For the valuation of pigmentations of the skin and of the conjunctiva, daylight is essential; for the rest of the examination, good artificial light is permissible if daylight be unavailable. Only when the patient's body is uncovered and adequately illuminated can one expect to make a satisfactory physical examination.

When recording the results of the general physical and psychical examination, it will be found convenient to subdivide the record into three parts: A. General points; B. Regional examinations; and C. General examination of the nervous system and sense organs. Thus the general points summarized in the accompanying table should first be recorded:

A. General Points.

1. Body temperature; pulse at both wrists; respiration.
2. Height; weight; calculated ideal weight; build or habitus; acra; nutrition; musculature.
3. Posture; gait; behavior.
4. Skin (color; thickness; moisture; eruptions; ulcers; pigmentation; scars; striae; nodules; tumors; superficial blood vessels; edema).
5. Lymph glands (epitrochlear; superficial and deep cervical; occipital; posterior auricular; anterior auricular; submaxillary; axillary; pectoral; inguinal; subinguinal; popliteal).
6. Blood pressure (systolic; diastolic).

Passing on to the exploration by regions, one examines, successively, the upper extremities, the head, the neck, the thorax, the abdomen and pelvis, and the lower extremities. There is a special reason for making the examination first mainly by regions rather than according to anatomical-physiological systems, for regional examinations better permit one to accumulate facts without too much regard, at the moment, to their bearings upon the conclusion toward which the whole examination is aimed; diagnostic inferences are to be avoided at this stage of the inquiry; suspension of judgment regarding the nature of the patient's ailment is at this time desirable. One can scarcely, with beginners in diagnosis, emphasize too strongly this restraint of inference and suspension of judgment while the facts are being accumulated. There is a great tendency among those who have never learned the importance and value of a general diagnostic survey to seize hold of some salient feature in the anamnesis or physical examination, to allow it to dominate all of the further investigations, and to permit it detrimentally to curtail the study of the patient as a whole. Points of importance to be noted in the regional examinations are summarized in the accompanying table:

B. Regional Examinations.

1. *Head* (skull; face; eyes; ears; nose; mouth; throat; glands).
2. *Neck* (form; thyroid; tracheal tug; esophagus; blood vessels; lymph glands; cervical spine; cervical ribs; tumors; wryneck).
3. *Thorax* (form; bones; coverings; breasts; axillary hirci and glands; lungs; pleurae and mediastinum; heart and aorta).
4. *Abdomen and pelvis* (inspection, percussion, and auscultation of abdomen and abdominal viscera; examination of rectum and of urogenital apparatus).
5. *Extremities* (skin; bones; joints; muscles; nerves).

After having made a record of the general points and of the points noted under regional examinations, it is well even at this stage to make at least a general examination of the nervous system and sense organs, in order that the data referable to the nervous system accumulated during the regional examination may be supplemented sufficiently to prevent us from overlooking data that point to lesions, or to disturbances of function, of the nervous system. Points to be noted in this preliminary examination of the nervous system are summarized in the following table:

C. General Examination of the Nervous System.

1. *Sensory functions* (cutaneous, and deep sensibility; stereognosis; special senses, including vision, hearing, smell, and taste).
2. *Motor functions* (muscular power; finer movements, including speech and writing; coördination; tonus).
3. *Reflexes* (pupils; deep reflexes of extremities; superficial reflexes, plantar and abdominal; sphincters).
4. *Autonomic functions* (vasomotor; secretory; trophic).
5. *Mental state* * (orientation; memory; calculation; attention; sense deceptions; pathological ideas; mood; psychogenic data; etc.).

* If the exploration in this direction has been full enough and systematic enough in the recording of the anamnesis, it may be omitted here.

In making such a general physical and psychical examination we call upon our powers of clinical observation and of clinical experimentation and these functions should be exercised in an orderly and balanced manner. In simple observation we note and record conditions that we do not alter. In an experiment we exert some influence upon the character of the event that we observe, that is, our observations are then made under altered conditions. Every clinical examination includes these two modes of experience long ago referred to by Herschel, the astronomer, as "passive and active observation." The technique of clinical observation and experimentation has to be learned slowly. In our better medical schools the students are drilled in one method after another until a certain amount of skill is acquired. But the practitioner goes on increasing his skill as his experience grows. The well-trained and experienced practitioner can make a general physical and psychical examination, such as that outlined above, very quickly and accurately. But even the well-trained man should examine himself from time to time for tendencies to error. One's methods of examination by observation and experiment are undoubtedly easily influenced by his special interests. The making of an objective record of facts without bias is not easy, especially if they come into conflict with one's own peculiar views. It is surprising how some men will always find tenderness at McBurney's point, or in the right hypochondrium, how others will always find a few crackles in one interscapular space, how others will nearly always find a vertebral spine out of alignment, how others will suspect the existence of a stricture of the ureter, and how others will always regard a patient's feelings and behavior as psychoneurotic in type. Men are very prone to find what they are looking for and it is easy to decide that very slight deviations from normal are worthy of being regarded as pathological findings if they be in the line of one's special clinical interests. Minute and accurate observations are of course desirable, but one must remember that the accurate recording of very minute deviations in one domain (the domain of one's special interest) if accompanied by failure of observation of grosser deviations from normal in other domains may result in an unbalanced study and in fallacious diagnostic inferences. When several special examiners have coöperated with an internist in the clinical study of a patient it is of interest, when going over all the findings, to see how often the special interests of the several collaborators have colored the record. The observations and experiments made upon a patient should always be conducted with proper regard to a sense of symmetry and proportion, for there should be, in the clinical record, a "due and harmonious admeasurement of the parts to each other and to the whole."

The report of the general physical and psychical examination, after it has been typewritten, is placed along with the record of the anamnesis, pending the arrival of the records of results of laboratory examinations, of X-ray examinations, and of examinations in special domains. It is best to accumulate all this material beforc attempting to summarize the data and to rearrange them according to the anatomical-physiological systems to which they may be especially related.

ad 3.—*Recording of the Results of the Application of Laboratory Tests.* The methods of the clinical laboratory, as developed in recent years, yield data of real importance for clinical diagnosis. When making a general diagnostic survey of a patient, suffering from some obscure malady, certain routine tests are now commonly made in hospitals and in the offices of consultants. These include examinations of the blood, of the sputum, of the stomach contents, of the feces, and of the urine. Just how much laboratory work shall be decided upon as a minimum routine requirement in every general diagnostic survey will vary with different clinicians. There is a general tendency at present to have made as a routine in every case that is at all obscure, unless for some reason one or more of them is contraindicated, the laboratory tests mentioned in the following table:

A. Routine Laboratory Tests.

1. *Examination of blood.*
   - Red blood corpuscles; count, with notes on size and form.
   - White blood corpuscles; count.
   - Differential count of white blood corpuscles in stained smears.
   - Platelets.
   - Search for parasites.
   - Wassermann reaction.
2. *Examination of sputum* (especially for (1) tubercle bacilli and other bacteria and parasites, (2) tissue fragments, (3) spirals, (4) elastic fibers, (5) cells, and (6) crystals).
3. *Examination of stomach contents.*
   - Free HCl, combined HCl, and total acidity.
   - Occult blood.
   - Lactic acid.
   - Oppler-Boas bacilli.
4. *Examination of feces.*
   - Macroscopic and microscopic appearances.
   - Undigested food (meat; fats; starch).
   - Occult blood.
   - Bile.
   - Parasites, or their eggs.
5. *Examination of urine* (night and day specimens).
   - Physical (color; reaction; specific gravity).
   - Chemical (albumin; sugar; bile; indican; diacetic acid).
   - Microscopical (red blood corpuscles; white blood corpuscles; casts).

Some clinicians will be satisfied with a less comprehensive routine requirement and there are others who will desire a more extensive series of laboratory tests in every case. But no matter what routine requirement one decides upon, it is often desirable, in special cases, to have certain other laboratory tests made. Thus when there are signs of infection with continuous fever of unknown origin a blood culture will be made, but it is quite unnecessary to make a blood culture as a routine examination in every patient who presents himself. A lumbar puncture with examination of the cerebrospinal fluid may seem desirable if a patient who has had lues years before presents nervous symptoms suggestive of involvement of the cerebrospinal nervous system, or if in any patient there be signs of meningeal irritation, or if one suspect the existence of an epidemic encephalitis or of a Heine-Medin infection; but it would be an unnecessary procedure to examine the cerebrospinal fluid as a routine measure in every patient who comes for examination. Again, if a peculiar arrhythmia present itself in the course of the regional examination, it may seem desirable to have polygraphic tracings of the radial and jugular pulse and of the movements of the heart's apex, or an electrographic study, though to apply the polygraph and the electrocardiograph to every patient in practice would be a waste of time and energy. Laboratory tests in great variety have been devised, but our clinical laboratories are gradually sifting out the less important ones, and we are slowly becoming familiar with the best methods for securing the different kinds of valuable information that the clinical laboratory can yield. Among the special laboratory tests occasionally required may be mentioned the following:

B. Special Laboratory Tests (to be made in certain cases).

1. Cerebrospinal fluid (lumbar puncture).
2. Tuberculin tests.
3. Excision of a gland, a piece of muscle, or a nodule, or making uterine scrapings, for histological examination.
4. Bacteriological smears and cultures (blood; sputum; urine; pus; prostatic milkings; cerebrospinal fluid, etc.).
5. Blood chemistry; and other special blood examinations (agglutinins; lysins; opsonins; coagulation-time; bleeding-time; content in coagulation-factors; etc.)
6. Renal function tests.
7. Metabolic studies
8. Protein sensitization tests.
9. Pharmacodynamic tests (with epinephrin, pilocarpin, or atropin).
10. Electrocardiography.
11. Sphygmography.
12. Exploratory punctures.
13. Animal inoculations.

Some practitioners, especially young men recently trained in the medical schools, make all of the laboratory tests required themselves. Others make only their routine laboratory tests and depend upon special laboratory workers for the performance of the special tests. Still others have all their laboratory tests made for them by assistants, or by special clinical laboratory workers.

Since the results of laboratory tests have come to be so highly valued in diagnosis, clinical laboratories have been so greatly multiplied and the number of persons professing to do expert clinical laboratory work has so greatly grown, that it may be in place to sound a note of caution. Unfortunately the sudden demand for laboratory tests has occasioned a supply of laboratories and of laboratory workers that contribute results of variable value. Too often the work done is unsatisfactory. Much harm can result from inaccurate reports emanating from unreliable laboratory workers. Even the well-trained worker in the best clinical laboratory will make a mistake occasionally in the performance of some test. Especially is this true of the Wassermann reaction. Every effort should therefore be made to insure the avoidance of erroneous, or inaccurate, laboratory reports. The value of a general diagnostic survey is not infrequently vitiated by an unwarranted credence in a laboratory report.

It should further be emphasized that when practitioners call upon their co-workers in the clinical laboratories for the making of special tests, they should not expect the laboratory men to make their diagnoses for them. They should ask for, and expect, only reports upon the particular laboratory tests mentioned. The results of these tests should be valued in association with the results obtained by other methods of examination. It is only occasionally that a laboratory can report a result that is pathognomonic for diagnosis (positive Wassermann; positive streptococcus culture or typhoid culture from the blood; meningococcus, or tubercle bacilli, from the cerebrospinal fluid, etc.). One must remember, too, that even a pathognomonic finding by means of a laboratory test, though it reveal the existence of a certain disease in a patient, may not point to the pathological condition that is most important when the patient's whole state is considered. A man may have syphilis and a glioma of his brain at the same time. Another man may suffer from amebic dysentery and from leukemia at the same time. The report of a positive Wassermann reaction in the blood in the one instance, and the demonstration of the presence of amebae in the stools in the other, though not to be underestimated in value, would not point to the pathological conditions of paramount importance for the two patients mentioned. Our diagnostic study in any given case should be comprehensive enough to include, in the final summing-up, all the important deviations from the normal presented by the patient, arranged in the order of their relative importance. But no attempt at the ultimate diagnosis of the case should be permitted at the stage of examination now under description. The restraint of inference and the suspension of judgment that have been repeatedly emphasized should be continued until all of the data of our schema have been accumulated, including those already referred to and those obtainable by X-ray examinations and by intensive examinations in special domains.

ad 4.—*The Recording of the Results of X-ray Examinations.* The X-ray laboratory, like the clinical laboratory, has, in recent times, made important contributions to the methods of clinical diagnosis and is, accordingly, now much appealed to for help in accumulating data regarding patients undergoing diagnostic study. At first employed chiefly in surgical diagnosis, the X-ray laboratories to-day are utilized even more by internists than by surgeons. Many practitioners install a roentgenological department in their own office and do X-ray work themselves, or arrange for a roentgenological assistant. Others send their patients to X-ray laboratories conducted by physicians who limit their work to roentgenology. The great improvements that have been made in the manufacture of roentgenological apparatus have rendered the technique of X-ray examinations much more simple than formerly, so that any intelligent person can be trained to make good roentgenograms of the bones, joints, teeth, lungs, heart and aorta, and alimentary canal. The accurate interpretation of the roentgenogram is, however, not such an easy matter. In the first place, no one but a medical man trained in anatomy, pathology, and the clinics can be expected adequately to interpret what can be seen in a roentgenogram, or what is visible on roentgenoscopic examination. Even among medical men who devote their whole time and energy to roentgenological work the interpretative powers vary greatly, depending partly upon native endowment and partly upon length and intensity of experience. There can be no doubt that roentgenoscopic examinations and roentgenograms carefully made and properly interpreted are valuable contributions to the data with which the modern diagnostician should be supplied when he is studying obscure conditions.

The importance of close coöperation between internists and roentgenologists is growing every day clearer. An internist who to-day is unable, himself, to interpret roentgenoscopic and roentgenographic findings is decidedly handicapped in his diagnostic work, for even though he receive objective reports from competent roentgenological experts it will be hard for him to value these reports in a proportionate way. Any clinician who has made an extensive study of X-ray plates and who has familiarized himself with what can be seen on a fluoroscopic screen will testify to the great autodidactic advantage that results from combining personal roentgenological interpretation with the results obtainable by other clinical methods. Not that the hard-working internist can expect to become as proficient in the interpretation of plates and screen views as are professional roentgenologists who give their whole time and energy to roentgenological work. The close association of the expert internist with the expert roentgenologist is essential to the highest quality of work of each. The diagnostician who does not see the X-ray plates on his own patients misses a great deal and the roentgenologist who is never able to control the results of his X-ray examinations by the clinical history of the patient or by the physical examination made by the internist will fall into serious errors and will not grow as rapidly in X-ray interpretation as he should. Regular conferences should, therefore, be arranged between internists and associated roentgenologists.

Altogether too much reliance is placed at present by many practitioners upon the reports in the form of diagnoses rather than in the form of concrete objective descriptions of their actual findings that are made by some roentgenologists. The latter are perhaps not so much to blame for this as are the practitioners who pressingly solicit them to give specific diagnostic judgments based upon their X-ray plates. It may be very helpful, of course, to have the diagnostic impression of the experienced roentgenologist in addition to the objective description of his findings. But the diagnostician making the general survey of the patient should be on his guard against accepting too readily the diagnostic impression of the roentgenologist. The internist should pay much more attention to the objective description of the findings discovered by X-ray methods than to such diagnostic impressions, and should utilize these objective reports in connection with the data collected by all other methods in arriving at his diagnostic conclusion; otherwise he will, at times, be led astray by a positive diagnosis ventured by the roentgenologist.

General diagnosticians can, in turn, be very helpful to roentgenologists if they will report to the latter (1) the ultimate diagnostic conclusions to which they arrive after the study has been completed, and (2) a summary of the data upon which the complete diagnosis is based. We must gradually work out the methods by which roentgenology and internal medicine can be reciprocally most helpful. If the internist and the roentgenologist will each give his best and if arrangements can be made for frequent conferences and discussions regarding the findings in concrete cases, the accuracy of diagnostic studies requiring the coöperation of internists and roentgenologists will be rapidly advanced.

When one is making a general diagnostic survey of an obscure case it is a real comfort to be supplied with the data that roentgenology can yield regarding the structures mentioned in the following table:

Commoner Medical X-ray Examinations.

1. The paranasal sinuses.
2. Dead teeth and unerupted teeth.
3. The contents of the thorax (form; size; opacity or transparency).
4. The digestive tract as revealed in X-rays during and after ingestion of barium (deglutition: form, size, and motility of stomach and of different parts of intestine).

Roentgenograms of the paranasal sinuses and of suspicious teeth together with a roentgenoscopic report on the thorax and abdomen if made in the practitioner's own office can be done at very small expense, so small that many practitioners could include the charge for such reports, when made as a routine measure, in the general consultation fee. Only if the symptoms or physical signs point definitely to marked disturbance of the digestive functions, or if in the absence of such symptoms and signs the roentgenoscopic examination done for eliminative purposes reveal suspicious findings, need the more expensive serial roentgenograms of the gastrointestinal tract be made. The data obtainable by the simple and commoner X-ray examinations enumerated in the above table go far toward protecting the physician who is making a general diagnostic survey of a patient from making certain sins of omission and commission that are frequent.

In addition to such routine roentgenological examinations, certain special X-ray examinations may be indicated by the records of the anamnesis, by the results of the general physical examination, or by the preliminary roentgenological survey of the thorax and abdomen. A list of the roentgenological examinations most often used is included in the following table:

Special X-ray Examinations (to be made when indicated).

1. Stereoscopic roentgenogram of skull, of sella turcica, or of mastoid portion of temporal bone.
2. Stereoscopic roentgenograms of lungs and pleurae.
3. Teleroentgenogram of the heart.
4. Serial roentgenograms of the gastrointestinal tract.
5. Roentgenograms of the gall-bladder area.
6. Roentgenograms of bones, joints, and spine.
7. Roentgenograms for renal, ureteral, and vesical calculi.
8. Pyelograms and ureterograms after thorium injection.
9. Ventriculograms after trephining and injecting air into the cerebral ventricles.
10. Bronchiograms after insufflation of a bronchus with bismuth subcarbonate through the bronchoscope.

One files the records of the results of any X-ray examinations made, along with the other reports, pending the collection of data derived from the intensive examinations of special domains that have become suspect from a consideration of the anamnestic and physical study.

ad 5.—*The Recording of the Results of Intensive Examinations of Special Domains.* In making a general diagnostic survey, an internist must ask himself what systems of the body of the patient require an especially intensive study and how the intensive study shall be conducted. While taking the anamnesis and dictating notes on the physical and the psychical status of his patient, the examiner will have had his attention arrested at intervals by the discovery of symptoms or signs that his experience has taught him are most frequently referable to disturbances of function in particular anatomical-physiological domains. Though in general restraining inference and suspending judgment regarding the final outcome of his study the positively abnormal findings that have thus arrested his attention will serve as clues to suggest certain special lines of inquiry; they guide him to the domains that, in the particular case, merit a more thorough study than that made in the course of a general routine examination. Thus the complaint of oppression in the chest on exertion or the observation of an increased blood pressure, of an arcus senilis or of a cardiac arrhythmia, may point to the desirability of an especially thorough study of the cardio-vascular system. In another case, a history of recurring epigastralgia, of gaseous eructations, or of persistent constipation will lead the examiner to undertake a special study of the digestive apparatus. In another, the history of frequent micturition during the night, of difficulty in starting the flow of urine, or of hematuria, may make an examination of the urogenital system by special methods imperative. Or again, the presence of a polyarthritis will suggest to the examiner the importance of studying intensively all those domains of the body in which focal infections that may give rise to metastatic infections of the joints occur. In such cases the question arises, How shall this intensive study of special domains to which certain symptoms or signs point be undertaken? How can the data pertaining to these particular domains be most accurately, most quickly, and most inexpensively collected?

During the past fifty years the technical methods of diagnosis and therapy have been greatly enriched through that process of division of labor among medical men that we know as the rise of specialism in medicine. Physicians and surgeons interested in special domains have devised a whole series of new methods of observation and of experiment, some of them involving the skillful use of instruments of a greater or less degree of complexity. The technique of ophthalmoscopy, of refraction, of otoscopy, of laryngoscopy, of esophagoscopy, of sigmoidoscopy, of cystoscopy, of ureteral catheterization, and the like, can be learned by any medical man of intelligence, but mastership in these practical-technical procedures is not easy and requires a practical experience extending over a considerable time for its acquisition. The result has been that many men have decided to "specialize" in order that they may acquire extraordinary skill in the diagnosis and treatment of disease in certain regions or systems of the body. Thus, to-day, besides the general practitioner, general internist, and surgeon, we see professional men who are known as specialists in diseases of children, in diseases of the eyes, in diseases of the ears, nose, and throat, in tuberculosis, in cardio-vascular diseases, in diseases of the blood, in dentistry, in diseases of the digestive tract, in gynecology, in urology, in orthopedics, in neurology, in psychiatry, in dermatology, in endocrinology, in roentgenology, and in clinical chemistry. No single person can therefore hope to be equally familiar with the facts and principles and equally skillful in applying the practical-technical methods of all these specialties; indeed, few men pretend to mastery of more than two or three of them. If the internist is to avail himself, then, of all the diagnostic methods that are helpful, he must, in certain cases at least, call specialists in particular domains to aid him by sharing in the labor of accumulating clinical data.

Among the pressing problems that medical educators of the present time have to solve are those concerned with the training of both general practitioners and specialists, and with the making of arrangements that will insure the mutual helpfulness of these two groups in the diagnosis of disease and the treatment of the sick. The ordinary curriculum of the medical school is now so crowded that the medical student in his undergraduate course, though he receives a thorough training in history taking and in the general methods of physical and psychical diagnosis, can scarcely be expected to do more in addition than to learn the main facts and principles of the several medical and surgical specialties and to acquire enough first-hand experience with special instruments like the ophthalmoscope, the nasopharyngoscope, the bronchoscope, the cystoscope, the ureteral catheter, the polygraph, and the electrocardiograph to permit him to understand their uses and to make clear to him the importance of their application as aids to diagnosis in certain special cases. There is not time in the undergraduate medical course for the student to obtain the experience in any special domain that justifies him in regarding himself as a medical or surgical specialist. To become an expert ophthalmologist, urologist, orthopedist, neurologist, or dermatologist, he must undertake special work extending over a considerable period after his graduation. The post-graduate schools are attempting to supply opportunities for quickly gaining the experience in specialistic work that will make men competent, but as yet only a beginning in this direction has been made. There is urgent need for the endowment of post-graduate schools with suitable hospitals attached in which men may be adequately trained in the work of the several specialties. At present a young physician who desires to specialize in some one branch does best to attach himself as an assistant to a real expert in the subject that interests him. Opportunities of this sort are, of necessity, limited in number. It is owing to the paucity of such opportunities for intensive post-graduate studies in the special branches, despite the growing demand for specialists in practice, that so much pseudo-specialism now exists. For the sake of the suffering public as well as for the advancement of scientific medicine this situation must be squarely faced by medical educators, by philanthropists, and by the state, its defects recognized and the remedy sought and applied.

The sick should reap the advantages that can be derived from the division of labor in medicine. Laymen have discovered that some expert specialists exist, but they are unable often to distinguish the true expert from the pseudo-expert. Having found that the general practitioner is not always wise enough to seek the aid of a true specialist when his help is needed, laymen have tended more and more to apply directly to medical or surgical specialists when they themselves believe that their malady pertains to a special domain. This tendency can only be harmful not only to the patients themselves but also to the general practitioners and, in the long run, to the specialists. In order that the best work shall be done in diagnosis and therapy, some means of coördinating the activities of general practitioners and specialists so that the best results will be obtained for all must be found. A general practitioner or an internist, who works alone and who does not call to his aid, at least in an obscure case, men who have had special training in particular domains will be sure to miss facts that are highly important for a complete understanding of his patient's condition. On the other hand, the specialist who works by himself, taking care of all patients who apply to him, whether or not they are referred to him by a general practitioner or an internist, is in danger of forgetting that he studies only one part of the body and that, though he may find abnormalities in his special domain, these may be less important for the patient's whole state than are other abnormalities that exist unknown to him in other domains. Some way or another must be found by which patients may profit by the division of medicine into specialties while at the same time they are protected from the dangers of a one-sided study.

The medical profession is now trying to solve the problem just stated by means of "group work" or "coöperative diagnosis." Diagnostic groups are being formed in which each member of the group possesses special skill in some particular kind of work and one member, who acts as integrator, tries to combine the single parts into a properly proportioned whole. In this connection I can perhaps not do better than to quote from an address given before the New York Academy of Medicine in 1917, in which I briefly discussed this topic of coöperative diagnosis in obscure cases requiring the intensive exploration of several special domains:

"The integrator should preferably be a person who, though perhaps especially skilled in some one branch, is rather encyclopedic in training and comprehension, sympathetic and tolerably familiar with work in all the divisions of modern medicine and surgery, free from prejudices, disciplined by sufficient experience in hospital wards, in clinical laboratories, and in the autopsy room, and blessed with that common sense that is, in the last analysis, largely a sense of proportion.

"Specialism, thus resulting in the orderly coöperation of the members of a group, instead of acting as a disintegrating force, may be made to contribute to a higher unity, most helpful both to the public and to the profession. With organization in groups of the kind mentioned, it would matter but little to whom the patient applied for diagnosis; if the integrator be applied to first, he will secure the reports from other members of the group before undertaking the integration; if a specialist in some single anatomical domain be applied to first, he may make his own examination, refer the patient to the integrator for the conduct of the rest of the study, and receive from the latter the full and proportionate diagnostic report upon which a rational therapy can be planned. Obviously, mutual confidence and good-will must prevail among the members of such a group. Such groups already exist and the number of them is, I believe, destined rapidly to increase. The older competitive methods must give way to the newer coöperative methods in medicine as in all other walks of life. Nothing could be more unfortunate, however, than the formation of cliques when arranging for group work in diagnosis, and I would warn emphatically against this danger. It is obvious, I think, that such a system as I am referring to does not restrict any specialist or any integrator to activity in a single group; there is no reason why either should not participate in the activities of several different or overlapping coöperating groups, the important points being that the group at work on any single case shall be so constituted as to insure, first, expert study in each of the several bodily domains in which there is an indication of the need of special study, and, secondly, a combination of the parts of the study into a well-balanced whole, the systematic analysis being followed by an adequate synthesis.

"Now, in most cases, there is, of course, no necessity of examination by every member of a large group of specialists. In addition to the anamnesis, the general physical and psychical examination, the routine laboratory tests and X-ray tests already mentioned, there may be required special examinations in only one or two anatomical domains. In obscure cases, however, and especially in instances of chronic infections necessitating the search for hidden foci, we may feel the need of calling upon a number of experts for aid. How many cases of chronic infectious arthritis, for example, progress for months because the diagnostic studies have been limited to too few domains, when more complete studies might have located the primary foci that were responsible? No one can lay down hard and fast rules as to how extensive a study should be. The judgment and experience of the one who has the general conduct of the study in charge must decide after the anamnesis has been recorded and the general physical and psychical examination has been made. The main thing is that he who conducts the study shall be sensitive to the problems that confront him and know how to apply the best skill in attacking and solving them. The greater the talents and experience of the integrator, the better his insight and discernment, the more likely he will be to have a proper sense of the indicative importance of the various features of a puzzling case. The greater his familiarity with the making of general diagnostic surveys, the more he will avoid requesting examinations that are wholly superfluous, the less likely he will be to neglect a test that is essential in any single case. The taking of too much pains in one case may be foolish; the taking of too little in another may be disastrous."

Just how such coöperative diagnosis will ultimately be carried out is, as yet, somewhat doubtful. The general hospitals have been gradually working toward it, but there must be much reorganization of these hospitals if the best results of coöperative diagnosis are to be obtained and, especially, the men working in such hospitals must be brought to an understanding of the advantages of such group work and must be taught how to organize for it and how the organization must be managed in order that it may be efficient. Aside from the work of the general hospitals, coöperative diagnostic clinics have already arisen in different places in the United States. The Mayo Clinic at Rochester, Minnesota, and the "Pay Diagnostic Clinics" of Boston and of San Francisco are notable examples. In many places, group diagnosis is carried on in office buildings by coöperating physicians, surgeons, and specialists. In most places, however, the physician making a general diagnostic survey still has to send his patients to specialists in his own town or, even to those in more distant places for reports of intensive studies in special domains. A general practitioner when isolated in the country has to do the best he can without such coöperative work, and it has been matter of surprise and pleasure to me to see how successful some men so situated are in the general diagnostic surveys that they make. Certainly recent medical graduates, who have had a thorough training in general medicine, surgery, and the more important medical specialties, as well as in laboratory work and in X-ray work, may, single-handed, do general diagnostic work of a very high order before they become too busy, though even these men could do still better work if they were members of groups in which a division of labor was arranged for. It seems to me possible that, in country districts, county hospitals, in which the work of coöperative diagnosis by a differentiated staff will be undertaken and be supported in part by public funds, may ultimately be organized. Great convenience for patients and for physicians results from arranging for the combination of the differentiated diagnostic activities under a single roof. Centers in which coöperative diagnostic groups can work effectively seem destined to grow in numbers and in public esteem.

The cost of making a complete diagnostic survey in an obscure case requiring the coöperative activities of a general internist and a group of specialists is an item that merits special comment. Unless ways can be devised for bringing the cost of such an examination comfortably within the means of all that require it, many who would benefit by it will be compelled to do without it. It must, of course, be borne in mind that the great bulk of medical practice as done at present is carried on without the making of a general diagnostic survey of the patients in the sense of this discussion. Indeed, for the host of minor ailments from which patients suffer, it would be superfluous to undertake the kind of general diagnostic survey here described. An elaborate investigation of every minor ailment would be a waste of the patient's time and money and of the physician's time and energy. Among his patients the physician of good judgment will have but little difficulty, however, in selecting a certain number that, for their own sake as well as for the reputation of the practitioner, should be advised to undergo a general diagnostic survey. Those selected would include the class of patients ordinarily referred to internists, surgeons, and medical and surgical specialists for consultation. For this group of cases it is desirable that methods for making quickly, efficiently and inexpensively a general diagnostic survey shall be evolved. Thus far the well-to-do are becoming provided for in the private wards of general hospitals and in private group-clinics, and the poor are also being very well looked after in the public wards of those general hospitals in which the method of group diagnosis has been introduced. Provision has yet to be made, however, for satisfactory group diagnosis for those patients whose incomes preclude the use of free dispensaries or of the public wards of hospitals, but are not sufficiently large to permit them to pay the usual fees for the more expensive diagnostic survey carried on in private wards of hospitals or in private clinics by an expert integrator coöperating with a group of consulting specialists. Though groups of the latter sort study a certain number of patients of small or of moderate means, reducing the fees charged for the whole study to an amount that is no hardship or inconvenience to the patients, no matter what their incomes are, still the amount of such work that can be done by the groups thus far organized is relatively small in proportion to the public need. Moreover, many patients who would benefit by a general diagnostic survey hesitate to avail themselves of an organization in which the ordinary charge for a general study is beyond their means, even though the total charge be willingly reduced to a merely nominal sum. In Boston and in San Francisco an effort has been made to provide for this class of patients in the "Pay Clinics" that have there been organized, and at the Mayo Clinic the cost of an elaborate general diagnostic study has been kept low. There would seem to be room in all large cities for organizations of young men who are gradually making their reputations to be of service in this connection. This is work, too, for which community funds justifiably might be expended. Industrial establishments, towns, cities, counties and states might do well to foster organizations for group diagnosis, making financial appropriations to aid them, and providing for regulation and supervision that would insure efficient and ethical conduct. The methods of the business organizer and business manager might well be adopted here, not for exploitation, but for the welfare and protection of the sick.

The filing of reports of the results of intensive examinations of special domains completes the preliminary collection of data necessary for the localization and definition of the diagnostic problem. The facts accumulated include the records of the anamnesis, of the general physical and psychical examination, of the laboratory tests made, of the X-ray tests made, and of the intensive examinations made in special domains. These facts may now be summarized and arranged in groups, according to the anatomical-physiological systems to which they pertain. The time will then have arrived for brooding over the data gathered and for allowing the things that we have observed to bring into our minds things that we have not observed. Suggestions of solution of the diagnostic problem ought to begin to occur to us. We are ready, therefore, to enter upon the third stage of the diagnostic procedure.

Stage III: Summarizing and Arranging the Data Accumulated, Pondering Them and Recording the Diagnostic Suggestions That Occur to the Mind

In order that suggestions of possible solution of our diagnostic problem may occur to our minds, we must weigh mentally the facts that we have accumulated in recording the anamnesis, in making the general physical and psychical examination, in the making of laboratory tests and of X-ray tests, and on intensive examination of special domains. We stop observing and experimenting for a time in order that there may occur to us ideas of what the things already observed may mean. We begin to draw inferences from the facts.

Consideration of the facts with this purpose in view is greatly facilitated, however, (1) by making a preliminary summary and (2) by rearranging the facts in a systematic way.

Thus, in order that one may take in at a glance the positive abnormal findings in the case, it will be found convenient, first, to summarize these findings under the general headings that correspond to their mode of accumulation.

Summary of Abnormal Findings.

1. Anamnesis.
2. General physical and psychical examination.
3. Laboratory tests.
4. Roentgenological examinations.
5. Intensive examinations in special domains.

From the large mass of data accumulated one selects for this preliminary summary only the points that represent definite deviations from normal conditions. This makes for brevity and for ease of survey, and the summary serves as a valuable control of the fact accumulation, for one can, from looking over it quickly, discover whether any important method of examination suggested by the results of the anamnesis and of the general physical and psychical examination has been omitted in the study as carried on up to this point. Furthermore, when the more important facts are thus closely crowded together in a summary, defects in the reports of suggestive symptoms or of physical findings or of special examinations may be easily recognized and remedied before one entertains ideas of interpretation. One may find, for example, that the report of a dental consultation, or of an X-ray examination that has been requested, has not been sent in; or one may, on this quick review, become cognizant that he has neglected, on outlining the course of the study, to include the making of some observation, or of some special test, the necessity for which was clearly pointed to by one of the symptoms of which the patient complained or by one of the signs recorded at the first physical examination.

The data accumulated may next be rearranged according to the anatomical-physiological domains to which they reasonably may be supposed to be related. This is another method of finding out whether our observations and experiments have been sufficiently inclusive. For this rearrangement of the facts in a systematic way I, myself, make use of a single sheet upon which the following form is printed, sufficient space being provided for the inclusion of the various symptoms and signs that are likely to be met with in any case in connection with any one of the anatomical-physiological systems:

Data Rearranged According to the Systems to Which They May Be Related.

Name: Age: Body Temperature:
Chief Complaints:
Time and Mode of Onset:
Habits:
Infections:
Operations; Traumata:
Respiratory System:
Circulatory System:
Blood and Hematopoietic System: R. B. C. Hb. W. B. C. WaR.
PMN. PME. SM. LM. Tr.
Platelets Bacteria Parasites
Digestive System: Free HCl Total Acidity Occ. Blood Stool
Urine and Urogenital System: Urine: Sp. gr. Alba Sugar Cyla.
W. B. C. R. B. C. Phthalein Output
Locomotor System:
Nervous System and Sense Organs:
Metabolism and Endocrine System:
Remarks:

In this systematic rearrangement of the more important data, we include both positive and negative findings, jotting them down in as brief form as is compatible with quick apprehension, use being made of various symbols for purposes of abbreviation. Thus under the heading "Circulatory System" will be placed symptoms such as dyspnea, palpitation, precordial pain, and retrosternal oppression, should they be complained of, any physical signs referable to the heart and blood vessels (e.g. pulse rate, arrhythmias, systolic and diastolic blood pressure, position and character of apex beat, abnormal pulsations, heart murmurs, cyanosis, thickened vessels, arcus senilis, or edema), teleroentgenographic measurements and electrocardiagraphic results, if they have been recorded. Under the heading "Metabolism and Endocrine System" will be placed deviations from calculated ideal weight, notes from the anamnesis regarding gouty attacks or a gouty family history, diabetic symptoms, struma, tachycardia, fine tremor, eye signs common in the thyreopathies, abnormalities in the distribution of hair, pigmentations, condition of the acra, and the like. When placing a symptom like dyspnea, it may be well to include it not only under "Respiratory System" but also under "Circulatory System" and under "Metabolism" unless it has already become clear to what division the symptom predominantly belongs. Each integrator in rearranging the data will adopt or devise symbols and abbreviations that, though they are immediately intelligible, save space.

It will have been observed that, in making such a systematic rearrangement of the findings, the integrator has already begun to draw certain inferences and to make a series of particular judgments, for the assignment of given symptoms or signs to definite anatomical-physiological domains is based upon knowledge, or prior experience, concerning the possible meanings of those symptoms or signs. The actual process of clinical diagnosis includes a search for clues, or marks, and the formation of judgments regarding the meaning of such clues, or marks as are discovered. The rearrangement of these clinical marks in groups according to the several anatomical-physiological systems to which they presumably pertain takes the facts out of the quarantine hitherto imposed upon them; isolation of the single facts gives way to association in groups as the integrator works at this stage of the diagnostic procedure. The materials thus dealt with prepare the way for the perception of further relations that may exist among the facts. Thus, the data pertaining to each anatomical-physiological domain may next be considered as a whole and judgments formed concerning their meaning and origin; later on, the relationship of the disturbances discovered in one anatomical-physiological domain to those found to exist in other domains may be sought for, with the idea of uniting two things in a third that is the foundation of the relationship (*fundamentum relationis* of the schoolmen). Such partial considerations as those just mentioned are necessary preliminaries to the localization of disease processes, and the assignment of place to the pathological phenomena is, in turn, necessarily antecedent to a proper understanding of the nature and cause of these phenomena; reflection upon the state of the patient as a whole, which we depend upon for supplying us with suggestions regarding the ultimate solution of our total diagnostic problem, can be advantageously entered upon only after we have made a long series of partial considerations and particular judgments and have already surmounted a number of local and minor diagnostic difficulties.

It may be worth while to advert for a moment to the kind of mental process we make use of when we have reached the stage of our diagnostic investigation in which we allow ourselves to entertain suggestions of explanation of the data that we have gathered, summarized and systematically rearranged. We begin now to draw larger inferences, to form diagnostic hypotheses, to harbor interpretative ideas. Observation and experimentation, hitherto our main tasks, are now temporarily stopped. We begin to think and to make use of the creative imagination. With feet firmly fixed upon a basis of the facts observed, we try to pass by induction, or by deduction, to inference. We brood over the materials that we have selected and prepared in the hope that things that we have observed will lead us to ideas of things that cannot be observed. Contemplating the contents of our experience with the patient before us, we try to assimilate them with the contents of our own past experience (gained by studying patients and the medical sciences) and of the experience of other physicians as reported to us in medical literature, believing that, on such assimilation, suggestions will arise in our minds that we may tentatively entertain concerning things that our own present experience, by itself, does not hold. In other words, we now call upon our powers of reflection to make contributions beyond what our sense organs are able to yield to us. Were it not for this capacity of the mind to make leaps from facts to ideas, we should never go far in the process of clinical diagnosis. The mind of the diagnostician must bound forward by a leap, or by a succession of leaps, from the observed clinical facts to ideas of what these facts may mean. Thus, the integrating internist must be a mental gymnast; and he has to learn that expertness in the form of intellectual activity here described can scarcely be expected except after long experience, carefully directed. The regulation of the conditions under which the function of suggestion is allowed to take place is of the highest importance. Unless due care and attention have been exercised in the accumulation, selection, and arrangement of the facts from the consideration of which the diagnostic suggestions are to emerge, the conditions under which the creative imagination has to work will be faulty. Even when the conditions have been adequately regulated, a proper use of the function of suggestion implies the cultivation of both courage and caution as habits of mind. We should be bold enough to entertain several rival diagnostic conjectures that we test for validity, but we must be cautious enough to make sure that only hypotheses that are found, on testing them, to be valid are accepted as diagnostic conclusions. One sometimes hears medical men, well-meaning enough but innocent of any real acquaintance with the manner of working of the mind of the scientist, declare that "there is no place for imagination, or for hypothesis, in diagnostic work" and that "the real diagnostician should content himself with facts." But the truth is that everyone who does good work in clinical diagnosis is compelled, whether he is cognizant of it or not, to form hypotheses before he arrives at satisfactory diagnostic conclusions. A study of the conditions under which hypotheses should be permitted to arise and a knowledge of how to deal with these hypotheses once they have arisen in the mind would seem, then, to be indispensable for the higher walks of clinical diagnosis.

Returning now to the actual occurrence of diagnostic suggestions to the mind when studying given cases, we may illustrate, by citing a few examples, how suggestions of meaning begin to arise on looking over the groups of symptoms and signs after their systematic tabulation in groups corresponding to single domains. Thus, if one finds recorded under the "Digestive System" morning diarrhea and the absence of free hydrochloric acid in the stomach juice, he will at once think of an achylia gastrica and of its possible relationship to a chronic gastritis, to an oral sepsis, or to a pernicious anemia. Or, if under the same system, one finds recorded a gastric hyperacidity, tenderness in the right lower quadrant, displacement of the stomach, markedly downward and to the right in the roentgenogram, and the history of recurring attacks of indigestion, he will think of the possible existence of some lesion in the right lower quadrant of the abdomen, say a chronic appendix. Or if there be recorded, in an obese person above the age of 40, a gastric subacidity, a history of pain in the right upper quadrant of the abdomen (especially after riding horseback, after a night's ride in a sleeper, or after an automobile tour), of transitory attacks of jaundice, and of an earlier attack of typhoid fever, the idea of some gall-bladder trouble, probably gall-stones, will occur to the mind. Or, if one find recorded anorexia, an absence of free hydrochloric acid in the stomach juice, occult blood in the stool, and a definite filling defect in the roentgenogram of the stomach, the existence of carcinoma ventriculi will at once be suspected. Or, again, if under the "Circulatory System," one sees noted a retromanubrial dullness, a systolic blood pressure of 170, a diastolic pressure of 90, thickened radial arteries, an arcus senilis, a widened aorta or a transverse position of the heart in the X-ray, he will think at once of an arteriosclerotic process; or, if a definite thrill be palpable in the region of the apex of the heart and an asynchronism of the second sounds be audible in the pulmonic area, the first sound at the apex being abrupt, the existence of a mitral stenosis due to an earlier thrombo-endocarditis will no doubt suggest itself as a diagnostic idea. Or, if at the wrist a perpetually irregular pulse be felt and the record of the electrocardiogram shows a good many small waves arising in the atrium for every ventricular complex, the existence of atrial fibrillation will at once be thought of and a search for its etiology suggested. Or, if the pulse rate be 120 and there be no heart murmurs or marked enlargement of the heart, one will think at once of the possibility of a thyreopathy as an explanation and seek for corroborative data. Or, if, again, the pulse rate be 48, one would leap to the idea of the existence of a conduction-disturbance in the atrioventricular bundle of the heart and would also find himself wondering whether this disturbance had its origin in some organic lesion within the heart itself, or had been due to a depression of the function of the bundle through vagus influences excited from a distance (intestinal irritation; increased intracranial pressure).

If, to take another example, under the "Urogenital System," in a woman of forty-two, one find recorded a prolonged metrorrhagia, say a flow of ten days each month, along with enlargement of the uterus, he will probably think of myomatosis with endometritis, and of carcinoma uteri, as rival explanatory hypotheses, each of which is rigorously to be tested for validity. If, under the "Nervous System," the data include nystagmus, loss of abdominal reflexes, and scanning speech, the integrator will think at once of lesions disseminated through the nervous system, the exact topography and nature of which he may try to determine. Or, if under the "Hemapoietic System," he finds jotted down a profound anemia with leukopenia, with a differential count of the white corpuscles showing a relative lymphocytosis of 94 per cent., along with enlargement of the spleen and with slight enlargement of the cervical lymph glands, the experienced internist may think of the possible existence of an aleukemic lymphadenosis, of a pernicious anemia, or of an anemia occurring in the course of a syphilis. As these examples illustrate, we deal at this stage separately with the symptoms and signs that pertain to each one of the several anatomical-physiological domains, cudgeling our brains for cues of possible meaning. When a group of signs and symptoms are present in a single domain, one should not be too easily satisfied with the occurrence to the mind of a single descriptive or explanatory hypothesis. Several possible hypotheses should be allowed to present themselves if they will and these should be pitted against one another as lusty rivals that are to be given opportunity to fight for supremacy. Hundreds of examples of syndromes might easily be given, were there need, but those mentioned will doubtless suffice to illustrate the mode of occurrence of diagnostic ideas to a mind that is pondering the symptoms and signs that have been referred to a given anatomical-physiological system.

As has been repeatedly emphasized in this article, on encouraging diagnostic suggestions to which a consideration of the facts as summarized and rearranged is to give rise, one tries to make scientific use of the imagination, a process that makes demands not only upon the intellect but also upon the affective-conative functions (the feelings and the will). From one's previous knowledge and experience he attempts to recognize in the group of facts before him either some well-known uniformity of sequence or some easily identifiable uniformity of coexistence; only when no well-known one can be discovered by him, does he permit himself to think that he may be dealing with some new, or hitherto undescribed, syndrome. The aim of every scientific worker is to discover scientific laws to which the facts that he accumulates will conform. The scientific diagnostician desires also to summarize in a single statement, or in some brief formula, the disease process by which he is confronted and from which the whole group of facts that he has collected regarding the patient can be seen to flow. Out of a vast complexity of anamnestic data, of physical signs, of chemical reactions, and of biological tests, he strives to derive a unity, to detect the "one in the many"; by means of a disciplined imagination he attempts to formulate conceptions in which the whole range of facts may be resumed. He sets up groups of tentative or hypothetical conclusions that he is to scrutinize thoroughly and to examine adversely before admitting their validity. In order that a clinician may make a diagnosis as complete and as satisfactory as is possible in the state of medical knowledge that exists in his time, he must obviously, in addition to native ability, have a wide acquaintance with the main facts of all the medical sciences and he must have already become familiar with the classifications of groups of facts and with the descriptive formulae that have hitherto been made use of by other clinical workers. A certain esthetic element doubtless enters into the experience. The brief statement under which a large number of facts, or of perceptions and conceptions, is resumed must be felt to be adequate.

It was Karl Pearson, I believe, who emphasized that the continual gratification of the esthetic judgment is one of the chief delights of the pursuit of science. That this is true in the science of diagnosis, will be admitted by every advanced worker. The more comprehensive the diagnostic study made, and the more complete the understanding of the relationships of alterations of form and function to causes arrived at, the greater the esthetic appeal to the mind of the diagnostician of philosophic turn. This is why he, in making a clinical diagnosis, strives to arouse satisfactory suggestions of solution of his diagnostic problems by thinking systematically, first, of the possible pathological-physiological significance, secondly, of the possible pathological-anatomical basis, and thirdly, of the possible etiological and pathogenetic relationships of a given fact or group of facts. He thus secures his ideas of syndromes made up of functional disturbances, of the lesions present and their topographical relationships, of the nature of the disease processes that are going on in his patients and of their etiology. The several ideas that thus occur to him must, he knows, be subjected to such rigid criticism that the conclusions he finally arrives at will be equally valid for the minds of other clinicians who work in the same way. Intellect, emotion, and will,—all contribute, then, their share to the mental operations of this stage of the diagnostic inquiry.

One may ask the question, What reason have we to believe that different physicians, even when using the method of science, will, in studying a given case, arrive at similar, or identical, diagnostic conclusions? The reason why there can be, and often is, agreement in opinion among diagnosticians lies, one must believe, in a similarity of behavior of normally constituted minds. To the normal mind, the world outside—the world of phenomena—presents itself in a certain way. The perceptive powers of normal minds must be very similar to one another. The same must be true of the reflective activities of the mind in normal persons. The mechanisms of association and of logical inference work similarly in different healthy people with the result that the mental contents of stored sense-impressions and of conceptions will be sufficiently similar to yield almost identical results in the same circumstances. The normal mind, when bombarded by a series of sense-impressions or perceptions, associates them with sense-impressions that have been stored in the memory; it combines these into conceptions or constructs; a train of thought is set up through association and the recognition of relationships; conceptions are formed and inferences begin to be drawn. Were it not that normal human beings perceive the same phenomena and reflect upon them in very similar manner, there could be no agreement regarding diagnostic conclusions, indeed there could be no such thing as science of any sort. As Pearson has well put it, "Human minds are, within limits, all receiving and sifting machines of one type." Minds that in their activities deviate too much from this normal type, we call disordered or insane. Within the range of normality, however, there is opportunity for considerable variation in activity. Minds that we call normal, though very similar in their activity, are by no means identical. We have abundant proof of this in the diagnostic suggestions that occur to different physicians who have had similar training and equality of opportunity for acquiring experience. To one mind, ideas of meaning may come easily and promptly, to another they come slowly and with difficulty. To one mind, a group of facts may quickly give rise to several ideas of possible meaning; to another mind, the stimulation by the same group of facts is barren of response. It is desirable of course that the number and range of ideas excited by the facts accumulated will suffice for the purpose of the study; there should not be too few of them and there should not be too many. Moreover, the quality of the ideas of solution that are aroused is even more significant than the promptness with which they come, or the abundance of the supply. One physician's mind may respond speedily with an abundance of suggestions and yet these suggestions may be inferior for the purpose in hand to those that arise in a mind whose response is slower but more profound. Rapidity of response is of course good in itself, but mere quickness will not compensate for either excessive prolificity or superficiality. A physician should, as far as possible, train his mind to make quick, balanced, and deep responses when he contemplates groups of clinical facts, in order that he may be supplied with enough worthy and substantial diagnostic ideas to test systematically for validity. Good native ability and prolonged training are essential for the best kind of diagnostic work. Though minds differ, the differences within normal limits are less important than the resemblances. Normally constituted minds are so nearly alike in their workings that diagnosticians of normal mental endowment who are well-educated in the contents and methods of the medical sciences, on studying similar pathological conditions, will, we may feel sure, arrive at similar conclusions.

In making a general diagnostic survey of a patient, the aim is to get as complete an understanding as possible of the functioning of the whole man in his physical, psychical, and social aspects with the object of being of real help to him in improving his condition. As has been pointed out, the group of facts pertaining to each of the bodily domains (respiratory, circulatory, digestive, etc.) is first appealed to for suggestions of meaning and for calling forth in our mind ideas of similarity, of coexistence, or of sequence. We should not stop, however, with the recording of suggestions based upon the consideration of the data pertaining to these several systems, but should next turn to a survey of the whole series of suggestions that have thus arisen. For after testing systemic ideas for their validity, we want to know the relative importance of the several partial diagnoses that are found to be valid for an understanding of the condition of the patient as a whole. Until this general survey has been undertaken and completed, no final unified diagnostic conclusion with suitable ordination of all the factors in the case can be arrived at. By keeping the purpose of the diagnostic study vividly in mind, namely, the desire to find out what is wrong with the patient, in order to direct him how best to act, we shall find a suitable guide to the whole diagnostic procedure; this directing principle will enforce orderliness in the application of our methods, and it will give steadiness and continuity to our thinking as it moves toward its goal.

Stage IV: The Elaboration by Reasoning of the Implications of Each Diagnostic Suggestion or Inference

Before yielding assent to any suggestion that has issued from a consideration of the facts after they have been summarized and arranged, no matter how plausible such a suggestion may seem, it should have been traced to its full consequences and its validity carefully tested. The acceptance of an idea as valid before it has been elaborated so that its full bearings may be clearly seen and compared with the facts that exist is the mark of an uncritical thinker. There is no room in clinical diagnosis for light-hearted and over-ready belief. Any tendency to infer wildly, rashly, or fallaciously must be vigorously combated. One should familiarize himself with the canons of legitimate inference and make sure that he is governed by them. When resorting to this reasoning process in which all the implications of each suggestion deemed worthy of testing are developed and are compared with the facts that have been accumulated regarding the patient, it will frequently occur that the diagnostician will discover the need of supplementing his first store of facts by further observation or by further experiment. It may even be necessary to apply methods other than those that have been used in a search for new materials to support, or to render untenable, an idea of interpretation that has occurred to the mind. It is only after we have entirely unfolded a diagnostic idea in detail that we can compare the several particulars that compose it with the facts as we have observed them and decide whether or not sameness can be recognized and identity established. When the facts observed are found to be in accord with the implications of a diagnostic suggestion as fully reasoned out, we accept the suggestion as valid and have a feeling of belief in it.

This process of developing the implications of diagnostic suggestions by reasoning may be illustrated by considering, as examples, the diagnostic suggestions that occur to us as solutions of the diagnostic problem presented by a patient who exhibits an acute febrile process with leukopenia. The patient, let us say, has complained of headache, of pain in his back, of loss of appetite, and of disinclination for exertion. The temperature of his body has been found to be 102.5° Fahrenheit, his pulse rate is 84 and the pulse is slightly dicrotic. A few rhonchi are audible over the lungs, the spleen is palpable, and the white-cell count of the blood is 4,800. When confronted by this group of facts, the diagnostician will at once think of infectious processes associated with splenomegaly and leukopenia, and he will recall that two of the commoner infections of this sort are typhoid fever and malaria. His next step will be to develop the implications of each of these two diagnostic suggestions by reasoning. He will say to himself, "If the suggestion of typhoid fever be correct, we should find in studying the history of this patient's illness an insidious onset of the symptoms, a characteristic temperature curve, a relative bradycardia, an initial bronchitis, headache, anorexia, palpable spleen, perhaps rose spots, a leukopenia, an early bacillaemia, an absence of coryza and herpes, an epidemiological record that gives the clue to the source of a bacillus typhosus in the case, the presence of the typhoid bacillus in plate-cultures made from the feces on the Drigalski-Conradi medium, or on Endo's fuchsin agar, the presence of specific agglutinins in the blood after the disease has lasted for a certain length of time, etc." He will also elaborate the suggestion of malarial fever and will say to himself, "If this patient has malaria, his temperature-chart should be that of either an intermittent fever (if it be a tertian or a quartan case), or a continuous or remittent fever (if it be an estivo-autumnal case); the patient will have had chills, sweats, headaches, anorexia, palpable spleen, herpes labialis, leukopenia, anemia, a history of exposure to the bite of an *Anopheles* mosquito, and perhaps neuralgic pains; in his blood, the presence of malarial parasites should be demonstrable, and pigment containing leukocytes may also be discernible; marked amelioration of the symptoms will follow the administration of quinine, etc." If the diagnostician be a careful and experienced worker, he will have thought not only of the commoner infections associated with leukopenia, such as typhoid fever and malaria, but also of the somewhat less common conditions so associated, such as paratyphoid fever, measles, mumps, glanders, and dengue. It will have occurred to him still further that leukopenia is sometimes met with in certain very severe forms of infection, like pneumonia and septicemia, that in ordinary circumstances are associated with leukocytosis. He will then develop the full implications of these diagnostic ideas also. These several diagnostic suggestions, thus fully developed as to their implications, will be looked upon by him as so many intellectual keys with which he will successively try to fit the lock.

If none of the keys he has forged is found to fit, he must try some modification of one of them or make still other keys to try. It may be that some complicating process of a secondary nature is changing the clinical picture so that it deviates from type. When, in a case, a survey of the data as a whole suggests the existence of a certain disease-process, one should give this process careful consideration, even though some of the data recorded seem to be inconsistent with it. Thus, if the symptoms and signs on the whole suggest the existence of typhoid fever, one should not throw this diagnostic suggestion into the discard simply because a leukocytosis is present, for, although leukopenia is the rule in typhoid fever, we do sometimes find a leukocytosis in that disease, owing to a complicating pyogenic process (phlebitis, pneumonia, cholecystitis, etc.). Or, to take another example, if the knee-jerks and ankle-jerks are absent in a patient, and anesthesias and paresthesias of his lower extremities have been recorded, the diagnostician will not rule out the idea of tabes dorsalis, at once, simply because an Argyll-Robertson pupil is not present, but will still keep this diagnostic suggestion in mind along with other conjectures of possible solutions of the diagnostic problem (funicular myelitis; polyneuritis; etc.). He will then reason each of the suggestions out fully as to its implications, and, if necessary, will make further observations or experiments that will decide whether identity exists. He may require to extend the blood examination, to undertake the examination of the cerebrospinal fluid, or to map out the exact topography of the sensory disturbances. It may even be necessary considerably to enlarge the anamnestic record in the case. If there be no anemia, if the cerebrospinal fluid yield a positive Wassermann reaction and contain many lymphocytes and more globulin than normal, if the topography of the sensory disturbance be segmental in type, and if the revised anamnesis reveal the history of luetic infection, of periods when lancinating pains occurred and show the absence of any abuse of alcohol and of any poisoning by lead, arsenic, or other substances that cause neuritis, the idea of tabes dorsalis as a satisfactory diagnosis may be accepted as valid even though no Argyll-Robertson pupil be demonstrable. Thus a diagnostic suggestion that, on elaboration, seems to be inconsistent with some of the data present, may, on modification, be found to be adequate as a solution of a diagnostic problem.

The original diagnostic suggestions that come up in our minds are always inchoate; they require to be developed. From principles that have already been established in medicine and with which we have become familiar through our earlier clinical experience and through our study of medical books and journals, we deduce the fullness and completeness of their meaning. The data accumulated by the analytical processes of the anamnesis, and by means of the general physical and psychical examination, the laboratory tests, the X-ray tests, and the special tests, suggest to us, when we brood over them, wholes into which they may be synthesized. Such suggested wholes are then again disintegrated by a reasoning process of deduction into their known constituent parts. Further observation and experimentation may then be required before identity can be established between one of these suggested wholes with its constituent elements and the actual whole to which the symptoms and signs in our patient really belong. Indeed, one of the great advantages of the consideration of all the possible bearings of the general diagnostic notions that we tentatively harbor is that it often leads us to expand substantially our collection of particular data. The full development, by reasoning, of all the implications of the diagnostic suggestions that occur to us is, then, an essential part of the diagnostic procedure.

Stage V: The Testing of Diagnostic Suggestions (Elaborated by Reasoning) for Their Validity and Arriving at Diagnostic Conclusions or Beliefs

It has been repeatedly emphasized that before we accept a diagnostic suggestion, inference, or hypothesis, after developing its bearings and implications, as a true explanation or description of the facts in a case, we must test it carefully for its validity. Having found out by a process of deductive reasoning precisely what it implies, we must demonstrate that there is identity between its implications and the actual data that we have accumulated, or can accumulate, regarding the patient. If the diagnostic suggestion as developed by ratiocination be found to be out of accord with the facts collectable we dare not give credence to it. Accordance in composition with what has been, or can be, observed is the sole real test for the validity of a diagnostic suggestion.

If, on looking over our amassed data, we find some single fact that seems to be in absolute conflict with some implication of our reasoned-out suggestion, though the other facts are in entire conformity, we shall do well to question the accuracy of our observation on the one hand and the flawlessness of our reasoning on the other. If the discordant fact be confirmed by a second observation and if it can be shown that there has been no fallacy in reasoning out the implications of a diagnostic suggestion, the latter, unless it can be so modified as to do away with the discrepancy, must be regarded as untenable. Any absolute conflict between clinical facts and diagnostic suggestion is fatal to the suggestion as a whole, for in the phrase of the logicians, "*falsus in uno, falsus in omni.*" It must surely be quite clear that what is true of one thing must be true also of its equivalent.

In this last, or fifth stage, of the diagnostic procedure we have to deal, then, with the verification, or corroboration, of our conjectural ideas. It will be recalled that in the third stage of our inquiry we allowed the particular facts that we had accumulated regarding the patient to call forth in our minds suggestions of a general nature that might explain these facts, or that might at least classify them under a common head; we there tried, by an inductive process, to pass from certain results or consequences (our collected data) to some general conceptions from which they might be presumed to flow. It will also be remembered that in the fourth stage of our study these suppositional general conceptions were, by a process of deduction, reasoned out fully as to their bearings and implications; through ratiocination we determined what particular clinical facts or consequences ought to be present in the patient if the general ideas were valid. Now we come to the last stage of the diagnostic inquiry, in which our task consists in comparing the whole meaning embodied in the diagnostic suggestion, that is, the whole of the consequences that flow from it, with the actual clinical facts that we have gathered, or that we can gather by further observation and experimentation. We have, at this stage, to trace out fully the degree of similarity that obtains between the facts that exist and the facts that should exist if the ideas that have occurred to us are true. We must ascertain whether there is a sufficient degree of likeness or sameness to justify the acceptance of the idea that we have tentatively entertained and rationally elaborated; and if we have provisionally considered other diagnostic ideas as rivals to it, we must demonstrate that the distinguishing criteria of these rivals are absent. Unless a diagnostic idea as fully reasoned out can be verified we dare not believe it to be true.

The secondary observation and experimentation stimulated by our attempt to establish identity between observable particulars and the implications of a tentative idea may strengthen or weaken the diagnostic conjecture and result in corroborating it, or in refuting it. Thus in the case of infection with fever, leukopenia, and palpable spleen to which we have referred, it may be found possible on reëxamination of the patient to discover that we had previously overlooked a roseola; or we may find on the patient's lip a slight herpes that had not been noticed at the first examination or that had been passed over as insignificant; or in a blood culture made in bile-bouillon we may be able to grow a motile bacillus which, on being tested, turns out to be the bacillus paratyphosus; or again, on making another careful search of a stained smear of the blood, we may find a single crescent-shaped malarial parasite, or some small intracorpuscular forms that earlier had escaped observation; or, a week or two after the first examination, during which time the diagnosis has remained in doubt, we may become able to demonstrate specific agglutinins for bacillus typhosus in the blood, though the Widal reaction had been negative at the first examination. Thus, where neither corroboration nor entire rejection may be justifiable on comparison of the facts originally collected with the implications of the conjectural idea of diagnosis entertained, additions that will bring a decision may sometimes be made to the clinical data.

As long as the data are insufficient for the determination of identity between the facts of experience and the reasoned-out implications of a diagnostic idea, the scientific diagnostician will reserve his judgment. And though doubt as to diagnosis will seem intolerable to him as long as a chance of a justifiable decision remains open, he will nevertheless often be compelled to suspend a conclusion when a more ignorant, or a less cautious, mind, unwilling to bear a painful feeling of incapacity, will indulge in a positive decision and advance in a wrong direction. The only safe way to arrive at accurate diagnostic conclusions or beliefs is to follow the slow process that has been indicated, namely, fact accumulation by observation and experiment, lying with the facts that tentative ideas of solution may be engendered, reasoning these out fully as to their implications, comparing these implications with the facts to see whether or not identity can be established, if necessary making further observations or experiments to extend the facts, and testing one suggestion after another until at least some one of them can be corroborated and accepted as valid; then, and not until then, should a diagnostician permit himself to feel that his problem has been solved.

The best diagnostic brain, fortified by a large experience, will sometimes make mistakes in diagnosis, even when all the precautions that have been referred to have been observed. Indeed, it has been among the highest type of clinicians, from the earliest times on, that can be found most often the evidences of willingness to acknowledge that "experience is fallacious and judgment difficult." No medical man is so expert or so careful that he never arrives at diagnostic conclusions that, later on, have to be revised. Exploratory operations on the living and complete autopsies upon fatal cases, are most salutary correctives of diagnostic jauntiness. The diagnostician who follows his patients to the operating room, or their bodies, should they die, to the morgue, learns lessons in modesty and takes the best course for the avoidance of presumption on the one hand and undue diffidence on the other. The physician who conscientiously applies the method of science to clinical diagnosis, who recognizes how difficult diagnosis in a given case may be, who tries to make accurate observations himself, who is willing sometimes to enlist the aid of expert observers in special domains in the collection of data, who deduces fully the consequences that flow from any diagnostic suggestions that occur to him, and who insists upon accordance between these reasoned consequences and the clinical facts before he permits himself to arrive at a diagnostic conclusion, can feel sure that he is working in the right way and can know that, as he grows in knowledge and experience, he will become an ever more expert diagnostician.

The extent to which a diagnostic study is carried will depend partly upon the purpose for which the study is made and partly upon the natural endowment and the experience of the man making it. The purpose of the general practitioner varies somewhat from that of the consulting physician, and the purpose of the latter is different to a certain extent from that of the man who devotes his life to original investigation. The particular aim that the diagnostician has in view (welfare of the single patient; or additions to knowledge that may contribute to the welfare of future generations) will, in some degree, determine the methods of clinical investigation employed and the scope of the diagnostic inquiry.

The natural capacity, the experience, and the ideals of the diagnostician will have their influence upon the work that he does. They will reveal themselves in problem recognition, in the practical technique of fact accumulation, in creative imagination, in reasoning power, in verification, in philosophic grasp, and in esthetic appreciation. It is well, now and then, perhaps to take stock of the personal qualities that make for success in diagnosis. What Faraday said of the philosopher is very applicable to the diagnostician of the higher type. He " should be a man willing to listen to every suggestion, but determined to judge for himself. He should not be biased by appearances; have no favorite hypothesis; be of no school; and in doctrine have no master. He should not be a respecter of persons, but of things. Truth should be his primary object. If to these qualities be added industry, he may indeed hope to walk within the veil of the temple of nature."

BIBLIOGRAPHY

ANGELL, J. R.: Psychology: An Introductory Study of the Structure and Function of Human Consciousness. 4th ed. New York: Henry Holt & Co., 1908.

BALDWIN, J. M.: Thought and Things. 3 vols. New York: The Macmillan Company.

BARKER, L. F.: The General Diagnostic Study by the Internist, etc. N. Y. Med. J., 1918.

BOSANQUET, B.: The Essentials of Logic. New York: The Macmillan Company, 1895.

BRADLEY, F. H.: The Principles of Logic (Anastatic Reprint). New York: G. E. Stechert & Co., 1912.

CABOT, R. C.: Differential Diagnosis. Philadelphia: W. B. Saunders Company, 1911.

DAVIS, M. M.: Group Medicine, Am. Jour. Public Health, Boston, 1919.

DEWEY, J.: How We Think. Boston: D. C. Heath & Co., 1916.

FOLLETT, M. P.: The New State: Group Organization the Solution of Popular Government. London: Longmans, Green & Co., 1918.

FRENCH, H.: Index of Differential Diagnosis. New York: Wm. Wood & Co., 1917.

HORNE, H. H.: Psychological Principles of Education: A Study in the Science of Education. New York: The Macmillan Company, 1906.

JAMES, W.: The Principles of Psychology. 2 vols. New York: Henry Holt & Co., 1890.

JEVONS, W. S.: The Principles of Science: A Treatise on Logic and Scientific Method. New York: The Macmillan Company, 1900.

JONES, BENCE: The Life and Letters of Faraday. 2 vols. London: Longmans, Green & Co., 1870.

LASÉGUE, C.: De la logique scientifique et de ses applications médicales. Paris: Arch. gén. de med., 1868, 6. s., XI, 715-732.

McDOUGALL, W.: An Introduction to Social Psychology. 9th ed. London: Methuen & Co., 1915.

MACKENZIE, J.: Symptoms and Their Interpretation. New York: P. B. Hoeber, 1914.

MILL, J. S.: System of Logic, Ratiocinative and Inductive. 8th ed. New York: Harper & Brothers, 1900.

MILLER, J. E.: The Psychology of Thinking. New York: The Macmillan Company, 1917.

MINTON, W.: Logic: Inductive and Deductive. New York: Charles Scribner's Sons, 1905.

MÜLLER, F.: Der Ausbau der klinischen Untersuchungsmethoden. Ztschr. f. ärzt. Fortbild., Jena, 1906, III, 433.

OESTERLEN, F.: Medical Logic. Transl. and edited by G. Whitley, M.D. London: Sydenham Society, 1855.

O'SHEA, M. V.: Social Development and Education. Boston: Houghton Mifflin & Co, 1909.

OSLER, SIR W.: Internal Medicine as a Vocation. In: Æquanimitas and Other Essays. Philadelphia, 1904.

PEARSON, K.: The Grammar of Science. 2nd ed. London: A. & C. Black, 1900.

PRATT, J. H.: The Method of Science in Clinical Training. Boston Med. and Surg. Jour., 1912, CXLVI, 835.

RICHMOND, MARY E.: Social Diagnosis. New York: Russell Sage Foundation, 1917.

SIDGWICK, A.: The Application of Logic. London: The Macmillan Company, 1910.

SOUTHARD, E. E.: Diagnosis per exclusionem in ordine: general and psychiatric remarks. Trans. Ass. Am. Physicians. Philadelphia, 1918, XXXIII, 267.

THAYER, W. S.: On the Importance of Fundamental Methods of Physical Examination in the Practice of Medicine. Mobile: South. M. J., 1914, VII, 933-942.

THOMPSON, J. A.: Introduction to Science. New York: Henry Holt & Co., 1911.

CHAPTER XVI

TESTS OF FUNCTION IN INTERNAL MEDICINE

By HENRY A. CHRISTIAN

Table of Contents

Introduction

When body structures function within the limits of what is considered normal variation, and when the function of each structure is correlated with that of all the other structures in the body, so that these structures are coordinated in their activities to produce an harmonious total activity, we consider the result to be what we term health. In contrast, dysfunction of any structure or structures of the body, not compensated by that of other structures, results in what we term sickness or disease. Such dysfunctions of body structures are of primal importance in clinical internal medicine or the study of medical patients who have the symptoms or signs of sickness or disease.

Body dysfunctions, as referred to in the preceding paragraph, express themselves in symptoms and signs of sickness or disease, and their recognition and evaluation are necessary to diagnosis and treatment. For an adequate understanding and evaluation of such symptoms and signs knowledge of the function of the various body structures is needed, so that the internist may know which are and which are not functioning within normal limits as determined from the accumulated recordings of many studies. Many methods for such studies or, as we term them, tests of function have been developed and applied to human beings, both well and sick. Repetition has determined for each test what we regard as the limits of normality. In drawing conclusions for the individual it needs to be recognized that one form of decrease in function often can and is compensated for by an increased functional activity of some other body structure, so that not one but several tests of function are needed to evaluate what seem to be departures from normal limits of function affecting significantly the individual.

In the period of early editions of Oxford Medicine many tests of function were so new that they had not been incorporated in easily available descriptions of many diseases. Consequently it seemed desirable to describe in some detail in one place numerous tests of function, which had been recognized as useful in the examination of individual patients. Their use then constituted something new in internal medicine; the results obtained from them were yielding important data, not otherwise readily attainable, applicable to diagnosis and treatment. At present tests of function have become so generally used and the figures and other data obtained from them so well known, that no longer is a separate consideration of them needed. Descriptions of many tests of function and their interpretation now are incorporated in the chapters in Oxford Medicine on different diseases. Also there are available excellent books on diagnosis and diagnostic technics where descriptions of tests of function and their interpretation will be found. The reader, seeking information about different tests of function, is referred to other chapters in Oxford Medicine and to the books just cited. There he will find tests of the function of almost every structure in the body described and interpreted with advice as to which tests to use and when.

It has seemed worth while, however, to record in this chapter a considerable number of the normals for various laboratory tests, many of which are needed for an appreciation of departures from normal encountered and noted in various places in the chapters in Oxford Medicine. Such a table follows.

TABLE OF NORMAL LABORATORY VALUES *

BLOOD, PLASMA OR SERUM VALUES

DETERMINATION	MATERIAL ANALYZED	MINIMUM QUANTITY REQUIRED cc.	NORMAL VALUE	METHOD
Amino acids (CO_2 of carboxyl carbon)	Plasma	2	3.4–5.5 mg. per 100 cc.	Hamilton and Van Slyke: *J. Biol. Chem.* **150**:231, 1943.
Amylase	Serum	2	15–35 units per 100 cc.	Adapted from Somogyi: *Biol. Chem.* **125**:399, 1938.

* From Case Records of the Massachusetts General Hospital, *New England Journal of Medicine*, Vol. **234**, pages 24–28, 1946.

Determination	Material Analyzed	Minimum Quantity Required cc.	Normal Value	Method
Ascorbic acid (vitamin C)	Plasma	0.5	0.4–1.0 mg. per 100 cc. (fasting)	Butler, Cushman and MacLachlan: *J. Biol. Chem.* **150**: 453, 1943.
Ascorbic acid	White cells	8 (whole blood)	25–40 mg. per 100 cc.	*Ibid.*
Bilirubin (van den Bergh test)	Serum	2	Direct, 0.4 mg. per 100 cc.; indirect (total) 0.7 mg. per 100 cc.	Malloy and Evelyn: *J. Biol. Chem.* **119**:481, 1937.
Calcium	Serum	2	9.0–10.5 mg. per 100 cc.	Fiske and Logan: *J. Biol. Chem.* **93**:211, 1931; Folin: *Lab. Manual Biol. Chem.*, 5th ed., p. 351.
Carbon dioxide (content)	Serum	0.5	26–28 meq. per liter	Van Slyke and Neill: *J. Biol. Chem.* **61**:523, 1924; Peters and Van Slyke: *Quant. Clin. Chem.*, Vol. II (Methods), p. 283.
Carotenoids: (total)	Serum	2	100–300 int. units per 100 cc.	Josephs: *Bull. Johns Hopkins Hosp.* **65**:112, 1939 (modified for photocolorimeter and calibrated with haliver oil of specified vitamin A content).
Vitamin A	Serum	2	40–100 int. units per 100 cc.	
Chloride	Serum	0.5	100–106 meq. per liter	Wilson and Ball: *J. Biol. Chem.* **79**:221, 1928.
Cholesterol	Serum	0.5	150–230 mg. per 100 cc.	Bloor: *J. Biol. Chem.* **24**:227, 1916.
Cholesterol esters	Serum	0.5	65 per cent of total cholesterol	Bloor and Knudson: *J. Biol. Chem.* **27**:107, 1916.
Glucose	Blood	0.1	70–100 mg. per 100 cc. (fasting)	Folin: *Lab. Manual Biol. Chem.*, 5th ed., p. 307; Folin: *New Eng. J. Med.* **206**:727, 1932.

Determination	Material Analyzed	Minimum Quantity Required cc.	Normal Value	Method
Hemoglobin	Blood	0.05	14–16 gm. per 100 cc.	Evelyn: *J. Biol. Chem.* **115**: 63, 1936.
Iodine, protein-bound (thyroid hormone)	Serum	4	4–8 microgm. per 100 cc.	Talbot, Butler, Saltzman and Rodriguez: *J. Biol. Chem.* **153**:479, 1944.
Magnesium	Serum	2	1–2 meq. per liter	Briggs: *J. Biol. Chem.* **59**:255, 1924.
Nonprotein nitrogen	Serum	0.5	15–35 mg. per 100 cc.	Folin: *Lab. Manual Biol. Chem.*, 5th ed., p. 265.
Oxygen: Capacity	Blood	3	19–22 vol. per cent.	Van Slyke and Neill: *J. Biol. Chem.* **61**:523, 1924; Peters and Van Slyke: *Quant. Clin. Chem.*, Vol. II (Methods), p. 321.
Arterial content	Blood	3	18–21 vol. per cent.	*Ibid.*
Arterial percentage saturation	—		94–96 per cent.	(Arterial content x 100) ÷ capacity.
Venous content	Blood		10–16 vol. per cent.	*Ibid.*
Venous percentage saturation	—		60–85 per cent.	(Venous content × 100) ÷ capacity.
pH (reaction)	Serum	0.2	7.35–7.45	Hastings and Sendroy: *J. Biol. Chem.* **61**:695, 1924; Peters and Van Slyke: *Quant. Clin. Chem.*, Vol. II (Methods), p. 796.
Phosphatase, acid	Serum	1	0.5–2.0 units per 100 cc.	Gutman and Gutman: *J. Biol. Chem.* **136**:201, 1940.
Phosphatase, alkaline	Serum	0.5	2.0–4.5 units per 100 cc.*	Bodansky: *J. Biol. Chem.* **101**:93, 1933 (using the method for determining inorganic phosphorus).

* In the newborn infant values may be as high as 6 mg. per 100 cc., which then diminish during the first year; in childhood they approach the normal adult average value of 3.5 mg.

Determination	Material Analyzed	Minimum Quantity Required cc.	Normal Value	Method
Phosphorus, inorganic	Serum	0.2	3.0–4.5 mg. per 100 cc.*	Fiske and Subbarow: *J. Biol. Chem.* 66:375, 1925; Folin: *Lab. Manual Biol. Chem.*, 5th ed., p. 341 (modified for photocolorimeter).
Potassium	Serum	3–4	3.5–5.0 meq. per liter	Fiske and Litarczek in Folin: *Lab. Manual Biol. Chem.*, 5th ed., p. 353.
Protein: Total	Serum	0.5(macro) 0.05(micro)	6.5–8.0 gm. per 100 cc.	Macro: Peters and Van Slyke: *Quant. Clin. Chem.*, Vol. II (Methods), p. 691. Micro: Lowry and Hastings: *J. Biol. Chem.* **143**:257, 1942.
Albumin	Serum	0.5	4.5–5.5 gm. per 100 cc.	*Ibid.*
Globulin	Serum	0.5	1.5–3.0 gm. per 100 cc.	*Ibid.*
Prothrombin clotting time	Plasma	0.3	By control	Quick: *J. A. M. A.* **110**:1658, 1938.
Pyruvic acid	Blood	2	0.7–1.2 mg. per 100 cc. (fasting)	Friedemann and Haugen: *J. Biol. Chem.* **147**:415, 1943; Bueding and Wortis. *Ibid.* **133**:585, 1940.
Sodium	Serum	0.5	136–145 meq. per liter	Butler and Tuthill: *J. Biol. Chem.* **93**:171, 1931.
Urea nitrogen	Serum	1	10–28 mg. per 100 cc.	Van Slyke: *J. Biol. Chem.* **73**:695, 1927; Peters and Van Slyke: *Quant. Clin. Chem.*, Vol. II (Methods), p. 372.
Uric acid	Serum	1	3–5 mg. per 100 cc.	Folin: *J. Biol. Chem.* **101**:111, 1933.

* The value parallels the rate of growth, diminishing from approximately 14 units per 100 cc. in infancy to 5 units in adolescence and thereafter being maintained at approximately 3.5 units.

Urine Values

Determination	Minimum Quantity Required cc.	Normal Value	Method
Albumin (quantitative)	10	0	Folin: *Lab. Manual Biol. Chem.*, 5th ed., p. 225.
Creatine	24-hour sample	Less than 100 mg. per 24 hr.*	Folin: *Lab. Manual Biol. Chem.*, 5th ed., p. 163.
Creatinine	24-hour sample	15–25 mg. per kg.†	*Ibid.*, p. 159 (modified for photocolorimeter).
Diastase	2	Dilution of 1:4 to 1:16	Stitt: *Pract. Bact. Hæm. & Parasitol.*, 9th ed., p. 731.
Follicle stimulating hormone	24-hour sample	Before puberty, less than 6.5 mouse units per 24 hr.; after puberty 6.5–52 mouse units per 24 hr.; after menopause 104–600 mouse units per 24 hr.	Klinefelter, Albright and Griswold: *J. Clin. Endocrinol.* 3:529, 1943.
Sugar:			
Total (quantitative)	5		Benedict: *J. A. M. A.* **57**:1193, 1911.
Total (roughly quantitative)	0.5	0	Somogyi: *J. Lab. Clin. Med.* **26**:1220, 1941.
Fermentable			Hawk and Bergheim: *Pract. Physiol. Chem.*, 10th ed., p. 750.
Fructose			*Ibid.*, p. 772.
Galactose or lactose	6		(Total sugar × 1.24) minus fermentable sugar.

* Per kilogram of body weight, the excretion is higher in women and children than in men, and still higher in infants.

† The value depends on the ratio of muscle to fat in the body mass of the patient. The higher the ratio, the greater the creatinine excretion per kilogram of total body weight. Because this ratio is low in infants, the excretion per kilogram is low.

Determination	Minimum Quantity Required cc.	Normal Value	Method
Osazone, differentiation of	5	0	*Ibid.*, p. 50.
Urobilinogen	10	Dilution of 1:4 to 1:30	Wallace and Diamond: *Arch. Int. Med.* **35**:698, 1925.
17-ketosteroids	12-hour	Under 8 yr., 0–2 mg. per 24 hr.; adolescents, 2–20 mg. per 24 hr.; males, 8–20 mg. per 24 hr.; females, 5–14 mg. per 24 hr.	Talbot, Butler, MacLachlan and Jones: *J. Biol. Chem.* **136**:365, 1940; Fraser, Forbes, Albright, Sulkowitch and Reifenstein: *J. Clin. Endocrinol.* **1**:234, 1941.

Liver Function Tests

Determination	Amount Administered	Material Analyzed	Minimum Quantity Required cc.	Normal Value	Method
Bromsulfalein	2 mg. per kg. intravenously	Serum (30 min. after injection)	2	Less than 5 per cent. retention	Rosenthal and White: *J. A. M. A.* **84**:1112, 1925; Peters and Van Slyke: *Quant. Clin. Chem.*, Vol. II (Methods), p. 910.
Bromsulfalein *	5 mg. per kg. intravenously	Serum (45 min. after injection)	2	Less than 5 per cent. retention	*Ibid.* (modified, *i.e.*, result ÷ 2.5)
Cephalin flocculation		Serum	0.2	Up to ++ in 48 hr.	Hanger: *J. Clin. Investigation* **18**:261, 1939.
Galactose tolerance	0.5 gm. per kg. intravenously	Blood	1	Less than 5 mg. at 75 min.	Basset, Althausen and Coltrin: *Am. J. Digest. Dis. & Nutrition* **8**:432, 1941.

* The 2-mg. method is used in patients with slight jaundice, and the 5-mg. method in patients without jaundice; the method is valueless in patients with obvious jaundice.

Determination	Amount Administered	Material Analyzed	Minimum Quantity Required cc.	Normal Value	Method
Hippuric acid	1.77 gm. sodium benzoate intravenously	Urine	1-hr. sample	Greater than 1 gm.	Quick, Ottenstein and Weltchek: *Proc. Soc. Exper. Biol. & Med.* **38**:77, 1938; Moser, Rosenak and Hasterlik: *Am. J. Digest. Dis. & Nutrition* **9**:183, 1942.

Renal Function Tests

Determination	Amount Administered	Material Analyzed	Minimum Quantity Required cc.	Normal Value	Method
Phenolsulfonphthalein	1 cc. intravenously	Urine	Total output	25 per cent. or more in first 15 min.; 40 per cent. or more in 30 min.; 55 per cent. or more in 2 hr.	Chapman: *New Eng. J. Med.* **214**:16, 1936.
Urea clearance		Blood and urine	Blood, 1 cc.; urine, two 1-hr. samples	75 to 125 per cent. of normal	Peters and Van Slyke: *Quant. Clin. Chem.*, Vol. II (Methods), p. 564.

HEMATOLOGIC VALUES

DETERMINATION	MINIMUM QUANTITY REQUIRE CC.	NORMAL VALUE	METHOD
Bleeding time	—	Below $4\frac{1}{2}$ min.	Lee and White in Todd and Sanford: *Clin. Diag. by Lab. Methods,* 10th ed., p. 199.
Clotting time	10	Below 20 min.	Duke: *J. A. M. A.* **55**:1185, 1910.
Sedimentation rate (two methods)	4	Less than 0.35 mm. per min.	Rourke and Ernstene: *J. Clin. Investigation* **8**:545, 1930.
	4	Less than 15 mm. per hr.	Modification* of Wintrobe and Landsberg: *Am. J. M. Sc.* **189**:102, 1935.
Hematocrit reading (percentage volume of packed red cells)	2	Male, 40–54 per cent; female, 37–47 per cent.	*Ibid.*
Hemoglobin	0.05	14–16 gm. per 100 cc.	Evelyn: *J. Biol. Chem.* **115**:63, 1936.
Mean corpuscular volume	—	80–94 cu. microns	(Hematocrit × 10) ÷ red cells (in millions).
Mean corpuscular hemoglobin	—	27–32 micromicrogm.	(Gm. of hemoglobin × 10) ÷ red cells (in millions)
Mean corpuscular hemoglobin concentration	—	33–38 per cent.	(Gm. of hemoglobin × 100) ÷ hematocrit.

* Internal diameter of tube should be 4 mm. instead of 2.5 mm.

SPINAL FLUID VALUES

DETERMINATION	MINIMUM QUANTITY REQUIRED CC.	NORMAL VALUE	METHOD
Initial pressure	—	70–180 mm. of water	
Cell count	0.2	0–5 mononuclear cells (lymphocytes)	

Determination	Minimum Quantity Required cc.	Normal Value	Method
Chloride	2	120–130 meq. per liter	Wilson and Ball: *J. Biol. Chem.* **79**:221, 1928.
Protein	0.6	15–45 mg. per 100 cc.	Ayer, Dailey and Fremont-Smith: *Arch. Neurol. & Psychiat.* **26**:1038, 1931.
Glucose	1	50–75 mg. per 100 cc.	Same as that for blood (see above).
Colloidal gold	0.1	0000000000	Wuth and Faupel; *Bull. Johns Hopkins Hosp.* **40**:297, 1927.

Miscellaneous Values

Determination	Material Analyzed	Minimum Quantity Required cc.	Normal Value	Method
Stool fat		Representative sample	Less than 30 per cent. dry wt.	Tidwell and Holt: *J. Biol. Chem.* **112**:605, 1936.
Calculi		Representative sample		McIntosh and Salter: *J. Clin. Investigation* **21**:751, 1942.
Congo red test	Serum	2	More than 60 per cent. retention in serum after 1 hr.	Bennhold: *Deutsches Arch. f. klin. Med.* **142**:32, 1923.

September 1, 1947.

CHAPTER XVII

THE TREATMENT OF DISEASE

By SIR WILLIAM OSLER

As true today as when Celsus made the remark, "The dominant view of the nature of disease controls its treatment." As is our pathology so is our practice; what the pathologist thinks today the physician does tomorrow. Roughly grouped, there have been three great conceptions of the nature and treatment of disease.

A. For long centuries it was believed to be the direct outcome of sin, "flagellum Dei pro peccatis mundi," to use Cotton Mather's phrase, and the treatment was simple—a readjustment in some way of man's relation with the invisible powers, malign or benign, which had inflicted the scourge. From the thrall of this "sin and sickness" view man has escaped so far as no longer, at least in Anglo-Saxon communities, to have a proper saint for each infirmity. Against this strong bias towards the supernatural even the wisdom of Solomon could not prevail; was not the great book of his writings which contained medicine for all manner of diseases and lay open for the people to read as they came into the temple removed by Hezekiah lest out of confidence in remedies they should neglect their duty in calling and relying upon God? And the modern book of reason, which lies open to all, is read only by a few in the more civilized countries. The vast majority are happy in the childlike faith of the childhood of the world. I am told that annually more people seek help at the shrine of St. Anne de Beaupré, in the Province of Quebec, than at all the hospitals of the Dominion of Canada. How touching at Rome to see the simple trust of the poor in some popular Madonna, such as the Madonna del Parto! It lends a glow to the cold and repellent formalism of the churches. In all matters relating to disease credulity remains a permanent fact, uninfluenced by civilization or education.

B. From Hippocrates to Hunter the treatment of disease was one long traffic in hypotheses; variants at different periods of the doctrine of the four humors, as dominated by some strong mind in active revolt it would undergo temporary alteration. The peccant humors were removed by purging, bleeding, or sweating, and until the early years of the nineteenth century there was very little change in the details. To a very definite but entirely erroneous pathology was added a treatment most rational in every respect, had the pathology been correct! The practice of the early part of the last century differed very little from that which prevailed in the days of Sydenham, except, perhaps, that our grandfathers were, if possible, more ardent believers in the lancet.

C. In the past fifty years our conception of the nature of disease has been revolutionized, and with a recognition that its ultimate processes, whether produced by external agents or the result of modifications in the normal metabolism, are chemico-physical, we have reached a standpoint from which to approach the problems of prevention and cure in a rational way. Let me indicate briefly the directions in which the new science has transformed the old art.

In the first place, the discovery of the cause of many of the great scourges has changed not only its whole aspect, but, indeed, we may say, the very outlook of humanity. No longer is our highest aim to cure, but to prevent disease; and in its career of usefulness the profession has never before had a triumph such as we have witnessed in the abolition of many fearful scourges. Great as have been the Listerian victories in surgery, they are but guerrilla skirmishes, so to speak, in comparison with the Napoleonic campaigns which medicine is waging against the acute infections. These are glorious days for the race. Nothing has been seen like it on this old earth since the destroying angel stayed his hand on the threshing-floor of Araunah the Jebusite. For seventeen years Cuba, once a pest-house of the tropics, has been free from a scourge which has left an indelible mark in the history of the Englishman, Spaniard, and American of the New World. Today the Canal Zone of Panama, for years the graveyard of the white man, has a death rate as low as that in any city of the United States. In the island of Porto Rico, where many thousands have died annually of tropical anemia, the death rate has been cut in half by the work of Ashford and others. But, above all, the problem of life in the tropics for the white man has been solved, since malaria may now be prevented by very simple measures. These are some of the recent results of laboratory studies which have placed in our hands a power for good never before wielded by man.

Secondly, a fuller knowledge of etiology has led to a return to methods which have for their object, not so much the combating of the disease germ or of its products, as the rendering of conditions in the body unfavorable for its propagation and action. How fruitful in practical results, for example, have been the new views on tuberculosis! Not that the discovery of the bacillus itself modified immediately our treatment of the disease, but, as so often happens, a combination of circumstances was responsible for the happy revolution—the recognition of the widespread prevalence of the infection, the great frequency with which healed lesions were found, and the knowledge of the importance of the character of the tissue soil, led to the substitution of the open-air and dietetic treatment for the nauseous mixtures with which our patients were formerly drenched. We scarcely appreciate the radical change which has occurred in our views even within a few years. Contrast with a recent work on tuberculosis one published thirty-five or forty years ago. In the latter the drug treatment takes up the larger share, while in the former it is reduced to a page or two. And it is not only in the acute infections that the use of the "non-naturals," as the old writers called them, has replaced other forms of treatment, but in diet, exercise, massage, and hydrotherapy, we are every day finding out the enormous importance of measures which too often have been used with greatest skill by those outside or on the edge of the profession.

Thirdly, the study of morbid anatomy combined with careful clinical observations has taught us to recognize our limitations, and to accept the fact that a disease itself may be incurable, and that the best we can do is to relieve symptoms and to make the patient comfortable. The relation of the profession to this group, particularly to certain chronic maladies of the nervous system, is a very delicate one. It is a hard matter, and really not often necessary (since Nature usually does it quietly and in good time), to tell a patient that he is past all hope. As Sir Thomas Browne says, "It is the hardest stone you can throw at a man to tell him that he is at the end of his tether," and yet, put in the right way to an intelligent man it is not always cruel. Let us remember that we are the teachers, not the servants, of our patients, and we should be ready to make personal sacrifices in the cause of truth, and of loyalty to the profession. Our inconsistent attitude is, as a rule, the outcome of the circumstances that of the three factors in practice, heart, head and pocket, to our credit, be it said, the first named is most potent. How often does the consultant find the attending physician resentful or aggrieved when told the honest truth that there is nothing further to be done for the cure of his patient! To accept a great group of maladies, against which we have never had and can scarcely ever hope to have curative measures, makes some men as sensitive as though we were ourselves responsible for their existence. These very cases are "rocks of offense" to many good fellows whose moral decline dates from the rash promise to cure. We work by wit and not by witchcraft, and while these patients have our tenderest care, and we must do what is best for the relief of their sufferings, we should not bring the art of medicine into disrepute by quack-like promises to heal, or by wire-drawn attempts to cure in what old Burton calls "continuate and inexorable maladies."

Fourthly, the new studies on the functions of organs and their perversions have led to most astonishing results in the use of the products of metabolism, which time out of mind physicians have employed as medicines. Pliny's "Natural History" (Bohn, London, 1855-57, vol. ii, 291) is a storehouse of information on the medicinal use of parts of animals or of various secretions and excretions. Much of the humbuggery and quackery inside and outside of the profession has been concerned with the use of the most unsavory of these materials. The seventeenth century pharmacopeias were full of them, and in his oration at the Hunterian Society, 1902, Dr. Arthur T. Davies has given an interesting historical sketch of their use in practice. Modern metabolic therapy represents one of the greatest triumphs of science. The demonstration of insufficiency of the thyroid gland is a brilliant example of successful experimental inquiry, and as time has passed the good results of treatment in suitable cases have become more and more evident. Before long, no doubt, we shall be able to meet, in the same happy way, the perverted functions which lead to such diseases as exophthalmic goitre, Addison's disease, and acromegaly; and as our knowledge of the pancreatic function and carbohydrate metabolism becomes more accurate we shall probably be able to place the treatment of diabetes on a sure foundation. And it is not only on the organic side that progress has been made. Important discoveries relating to the metabolism of the inorganic constituents, such as those relative to acidosis, have opened a new and most hopeful chapter in scientific medicine.

But the best of human effort is flecked and stained with weakness, and even the casual observer may note dark shadows in the bright picture. Organotherapy illustrates at once one of the great triumphs of science and the very apotheosis of charlatanry. One is almost ashamed to speak in the same breath of the credulousness and cupidity by which even the strong in intellect and the rich in experience have been carried off in a flood of pseudo-science. This has ever been a difficulty in the profession. The art is very apt to outrun or override the science, and play the master where the true rôle is that of the servant.

And; lastly, we have advanced firmly along a new road in the treatment of diseases due to specific microorganisms, with the toxic products of which we are learning to cope successfully. The treatment with antitoxins and bacterial vaccines, so successfully started, bears out the truth of that keen comment of Celsus: "He will treat the disease properly whom the first origin of the cause has not deceived." We are still far from the goal in some of the most important and fatal infections, but anyone acquainted in even slight measure with the progress of the past twenty year's cannot but have confidence in the future. Considering that the generation is still active which opened the whole question, we cannot but feel hopeful in spite of disappointments here and failures there. But in our pride of progress let us remember cancer and pneumonia. The history of the latter disease affords a good illustration of the truth of the remark of Celsus with which I began. Year by year the lesson of pneumonia is a lesson of humility. For purposes of comparison statistics are not available, but it is not likely that the great masters from Galen to Grisolle lost a larger number of cases than we do. Pneumonia has always been, as today, a dreaded and a fatal disease. For one thing let us be thankful. We have had the courage to abandon the expectorant mixtures, the depressants, the cardiac sedatives, the blisters, the emetics, the resulsives, the purges, the poultices, and, to a great extent, the bleedings. Surely our forefathers must have killed some patients by the appalling ferocity of their treatment, or to have stood it the constitutions of those days must have been more robust. We still await, but await in hope, the work that will remove the reproach of the mortality bills in this disease. I say reproach because we really feel it, and yet act justly, for who made us responsible for its benign or malignant nature? We can relieve symptoms, but we must find the means which will, on the one hand, limit the extension of the process, loosen the exudate, minimize the fluxion, control the alveolar diapedesis, and, on the other hand, diminish the output of the toxins, neutralize those in circulation, or strengthen the opsonic power of the blood. But someone will say, Is this all your science has to tell us? Is this the outcome of decades of good clinical work, of patient study of the disease, of anxious trial in such good faith of so many drugs? Give us back the childlike trust of the fathers in antimony and in the lancet rather than this cold nihilism. Not at all! Let us accept the truth, however unpleasant it may be, and with the death rate staring us in the face, let us not be deceived with vain fancies. Not alone in pneumonia, but in the treatment of certain other diseases, do we need a stern, iconoclastic spirit which leads, not to nihilism, but to an active skepticism—not the passive skepticism born of despair, but the active skepticism born of a knowledge that recognizes its limitations and knows full well that only in this attitude of mind can true progress be made. I hope to live to see a true treatment of pneumonia. Before long we should be able to cope with the products of the pneumococci; it may indeed come within the list of preventable diseases.

II

Along these five lines the modern conception of the nature of disease has radically altered our practice. The personal interest which we take in our fellow creatures is apt to breed a sense of superiority to their failings, and we are ready to forget that we ourselves, singularly human, illustrate many of the common weaknesses which we condemn in them. In no way is this more striking than in the careless credulity we display in some matters relating to the treatment of disease. Recently the *Times* had an editorial upon a remark of Bernard Shaw that the cleverest man will believe anything he wishes to believe, in spite of all the facts and textbooks in the world. We are at the mercy of our wills much more than of our reason in the formation of our beliefs, which we adopt in a lazy, haphazard way, without taking much trouble to inquire into their foundation. But I am not going to discuss, were I able, this Shavian philosophy; but it will serve as an introduction to a few remarks on the Nemesis of Faith which in all ages readily overtakes doctors and the public alike. Without trust, without confidence, without faith in himself, in his tools, in his fellowmen, no man works successfully or happily. For us, however, it must never be the blind unquestioning trust of the devotee, but the confidence of the inquiring spirit that would prove all things. But it is so much easier to believe than to doubt, for doubt connotes thinking and the expenditure of energy, and often the disruption of the *status quo*. And then we doctors have always been a simple, trusting folk! Did we not believe Galen implicitly for 1,500 years and Hippocrates for more than 2,000? In the matter of treatment the placid faith of the simple believer, not the fighting faith of the aggressive doubter, has ever been our besetting sin.

In the progress of knowledge each generation has a double labor—to escape from the intellectual thralls of the one from which it has emerged and to forge anew its own fetters. Upon us whose work lay in the last quarter of the nineteenth century fell the great struggle with that many-headed monster, Polypharmacy—not the true polypharmacy which is the skillful combination of remedies, but the giving of many—the practice of at once discharging a heavily loaded prescription at every malady, or at every symptom of it. Much has been done and an extraordinary change has come over the profession, but it has not been a fight to the finish. Many were lukewarm; others found it difficult to speak without giving offense in quarters where on other grounds respect and esteem were due. As an enemy to indiscriminate drugging, I have often been branded as a therapeutic nihilist. That I should even venture to speak on the subject calls to mind what Professor Peabody of Harvard remarked about Jacob Bigelow, that, "for his professorship of Materia Medica he had very much the same qualifications that a learned unbeliever might have for a professorship of Christian theology. No other man of his time had so little faith in drugs." I bore this reproach cheerfully, coming, as I knew it did, from men who did not appreciate the difference between the giving of medicines and the treatment of disease; moreover it was for the galled jade to wince, my withers were unwrung. The heavy hands of the great Arabians grow lighter in each generation. Though dead, Rhazes and Avicenna still speak, not only in the Arabic signs which we use, but in the combinations and multiplicity of the constituents of too many of our prescriptions. We are fortunately getting rid of routine practice in the use of drugs. How many of us now prescribe an emetic? And yet that shrewd old man, Nathanial Chapman, who graced the profession of Philadelphia for so long, used to say, "Everything else I have written may disappear, but my chapter on emetics will last!" How much less now does habit control our practice in the use of expectorants? The blind faith which some men have in medicines illustrates too often the greatest of all human capacities—the capacity for self-deception. One special advantage of the skeptical attitude of mind is that a man is never vexed to find that after all he has been in the wrong. It is an old story that a man may practice medicine successfully with a very few drugs. Locke had noticed this, probably in the hands of his friend Sydenham, since he says, "You cannot imagine how far a little observation carefully made by a man not tied up to the four humors . . . would carry a man in the curing of diseases, though very stubborn and dangerous, and that with very little and common things and almost no medicine at all." Boerhaave commented upon this truth in a remark of Sydenham "that a person well skilled in cases seldom needs remedies." The study of the action of drugs, always beset with difficulties, is rapidly passing from the empirical stage, and this generation may expect to see the results of studies which have already been most promising. It is very important that our young men should get oriented early in this matter of drug treatment. Our teachers used to send us to the works of John Forbes ("Nature and Art in the Cure of Disease," J. Churchill, London, 1857), and to Jacob Bigelow ("Nature in Disease," Ticknor and Fields, Boston, 1854), for clear views of the subject. A book has been written by Dr. Harrington Sainsbury, the well-known London physician and teacher ("Principia Therapeutica," E. P. Dutton & Company, New York, 1907), which deals with these problems in the same philosophic manner. It opens with a delightful dialogue between the pathologist and the physician. He lays his finger on the weak point of the pure morbid anatomist who thinks of the lesion only, and not enough of the function which even a seriously damaged organ may be able to carry on. The book should be in the hands of every practitioner and senior student. Some of you may have heard of the lecture-room motto of that distinguished pathologist and surgeon, and the first systematic writer on morbid anatomy in the United States, S. D. Gross: "Principles, gentlemen, principles! principles!!" And it is upon these fundamental aspects that Dr. Sainsbury dwells in his most suggestive work, which I would like to see adopted as a textbook in every medical school in the land.

And we are yet far too credulous and supine in another very important matter. Each generation has its therapeutic vagaries, the outcome, as a rule, of attempts to put prematurely into practice theoretical conceptions of disease. As members of a free profession we are expected to do our own thinking; and yet the literature that comes to us daily indicates a thraldom not less dangerous than the polypharmacy from which we are escaping. I allude to the specious and seductive pamphlets and reports sent out by the pharmaceutical houses, large and small. We owe a deep debt to the modern manufacturing pharmacist, who has given us pleasant and potent medicines in the place of the nauseous and weak mixtures; and such firms as Parke, Davis & Company, of the United States, and Burroughs & Wellcome, of England, have been pioneers in the science of pharmacology. But even the best are not guiltless of exploiting in the profession the products of a pseudo-science. Let me specify three items in which I think the manufacturing pharmacists have gone beyond their limit and are trading on the credulity of the profession to the great detriment of the public. The length to which organotherapy has extended (not so much on the American side of the water as on the European continent) beyond the legitimate use of certain preparations is a notorious illustration of the ease with which theoretical views place us in a false position. Because thyroid extract cures myxedema and adrenalin has a powerful action, it has been taken almost for granted that the extract of every organ is a specific against the diseases that affect it. This forcing of a scientific position is most hurtful, and I have known an investigator hestitate to publish results lest they should be misapplied in practice. The literature on the subject issued by reputable houses indicates, on the one hand, the pseudo-science upon which a business may be built up, and, on the other, the weak-minded state of the profession on whose credulity these firms trade. A second most reprehensible feature is the laudatory character of literature describing the preparations which they manufacture. Foisted upon an innocent practitioner by a traveling Autolycus, the preparation is used successfully, say, in six cases of amenorrhea; very soon a report appears in a medical journal, and a few weeks later this report is sent broadcast with the auriferous leaflets of the firm. Some time ago a pamphlet came from X and Company, characterized by brazen therapeutic impudence, and indicating a supreme indifference to anything that could be called intelligence on the part of the recipients. That these firms have the audacity to issue such trash indicates the state of thraldom in which they regard us. And I would protest against the usurpation on the part of these men of our function as teachers. Why, for example, should Y and Company write as if they were directors of large genitourinary clinics instead of manufacturing pharmacists? It is none of their business what is the best treatment for gonorrhea—by what possibility could they ever know it, and why should their literature pretend to the combined wisdom of Neisser and Guyon? What right have Z and Company to send on a card directions for the treatment of anemia and dyspepsia, about which subjects they know as much as an unborn babe, and, if they stick to their legitimate business, about the same opportunity of getting information? For years the profession has been exploited in this way, until the evil has become unbearable, and we need as active a crusade against pseudo-science in the profession as has been waged of late against the use of quack medicines by the public. We have been altogether too submissive, and have gradually allowed those who should be our willing helpers to dictate terms and to play the rôle of masters. Far too large a section of the treatment of disease is today controlled by the big manufacturing pharmacists, who have enslaved us in a plausible pseudo-science. The remedy is obvious: give our students a first-hand acquaintance with disease, and give them a thorough practical knowledge of the great drugs, and we will send out independent, clear-headed, cautious practitioners who will do their own thinking and be no longer at the mercy of a meretricious literature which has sapped our independence.

Having confessed some of our weaknesses, I may with better grace approach the burning question of the day in the matter of treatment. An influenza-like outbreak of faith-healing seems to have the public of both continents in its grip. It is an old story—the oldest, indeed, in our history—and one in which we have a strong hereditary interest, since scientific medicine took its origin in a system of faith-healing beside which all our modern attempts are feeble imitations. Lincoln's favorite poem, beginning "We think the same thoughts that our fathers have thought," expresses a tendency in the human mind to run in circles. Once or twice in each century the serpent entwining the staff of Æsculapius gets restless, untwists, and in his gambols swallows his tail, and at once in full circle back upon us come old thoughts and old practices, which for a time dominate alike doctors and laity. As a profession we took origin in the cult of Æsculapius, the gracious son of Apollo, whose temples, widespread over the Greek and Roman world, were at once magnificent shrines and hospitals, with which in beauty and extent our modern institutions are not to be compared. Amid lovely surroundings, chosen for their salubrity, connected usually with famous springs, they were the sanatoriums of the ancient world. The ritual of the cure is well known, and has been beautifully described by Walter H. Pater in "Marius the Epicurean" (Macmillan, New York, 1907). Faith in the god, suggestion, the temple sleep and the interpretation of its dream were the important factors. Hygienic and other measures were also used, and in the guild of secular physicians which grew up about the temples scientific medicine took its origin. No cult resisted so long the progress of Christianity; and so imbued were the people with its value, that many of the practices of the temple were carried on into the Christian ritual. The temple sleep and the interpretation of its dreams were continued long into the Middle Ages, and, indeed, have not yet disappeared. The popular shrines of the Catholic Church today are in some ways the direct descendants of this Æsculapian cult, and the cures and votive offerings at Lourdes and St. Anne are in every way analogous to those of Epidaurus.

As I before remarked, credulity in matters relating to disease remains a permanent fact in our history, uninfluenced by education. But let us not be too hard on poor human nature. Even Pericles, most sensible of men, when on his deathbed, allowed the women to put an amulet about his neck. And which one of us, brought up from childhood to invoke the aid of the saints and seek their help—which one of us under these circumstances, living today in or near Rome, if a dear child were sick unto death, would not send for the Santo Bambino, the Holy Doll of the Church of Ara Coeli? Has it not been working miracles these four hundred years? The votive offerings of gold and of gems from the happy parents cover it completely, and about it are grateful letters from its patients in all parts of the world. No doll so famous, no doll so precious! No wonder it goes upon its ministry of healing in a carriage and pair, and with two priests as its companions! Precious perquisite of the race, as it has been called, with all its dark and terrible record, credulity has perhaps the credit balance on its side and in the consolation afforded the pious souls of all ages and of all climes, who have let down anchors of faith into the vast sea of superstition. We drink it in with our mother's milk, and that is indeed an even-balanced soul without some tincture. We must acknowledge its potency today as effective among the most civilized people, the people with whom education is the most widely spread, yet who absorb with wholesale credulity delusions as childish as any that have ever enslaved the mind of man.

Having recently had to look over a large literature on the subject of mental healing, ancient and modern, I have tried to put the matter as succinctly as possible. In all ages and in all climes the prayer of faith has saved a certain number of the sick. The essentials are first a strong and hopeful belief in a dominant personality, who has varied naturally in different countries and in different ages. Buddha in India, and in Japan, where there are cults to match every recent vagary; Æsculapius in ancient Greece and Rome; our Saviour and a host of saints in Christian communities; and lastly, an ordinary doctor has served the purpose of common humanity very well. Faith is the most precious asset in our stock-in-trade. Once lost, how long does a doctor keep his *clientèle?* Secondly, certain accessories—a shrine, a grotto, a church, a temple, a hospital, a sanatorium—surroundings that will impress favorably the imagination of the patient. Thirdly, suggestion in one of its varied forms—whether the negation of disease and pain, the simple trust in Christ of the Peculiar People, of the sweet reasonableness of the psychotherapeutist. But there must be the will-to-believe attitude of mind, the mental receptiveness—in a word, the *faith* which has made bread pills famous in the history of medicine. We must, however, recognize the limitations of mental healing. Potent as is the influence of the mind on the body, and many as are the miracle-like cures which may be worked, all are in functional disorders, and we know only too well that nowadays the prayer of faith neither sets a broken thigh nor checks an epidemic of typhoid fever.

What should be the attitude of the clergy, many of whom have been drawn into the vortex of this movement? I feel it would be very much safer to hand over this problem to us. It is not a burden which we should ask a hard-working and already overwrought profession to undertake or to share. It might be a different matter if it were really a gift of healing in the apostolic sense, but we know this was associated with other signs and wonders at present conspicuous by their absence. Then think of the possibilities of self-deception—of the saintly Edward Irving and the gift of tongues; of Monsieur de Paris, the French priest, and the miracles at his tomb, to the truth of which two fine quarto volumes, with "before and after" pictures, attest! The less the clergy have to do with the bodily complaints of neurasthenic and hysterical persons the better for their peace of mind and for the reputation of the Cloth. As wise old Fuller remarked, Circe and Æsculapius were brother and sister, and the wiles of the one are very apt to entrap the wisdom of the other.

III

It adds immensely to the interest in life to live in the midst of these problems which concern us so closely. We must meet them with an intelligent cheerfulness, in the full confidence that the Angel of Bethesda never stirred the waters without happy results. It is for us to see that the soldiers we are training for the fight against disease, bodily and mental, are well equipped for the battle; and let me briefly, in conclusion, indicate how I believe we should teach the art—the management of patients and the cure of disease. To know how to deal with disease is the final goal, to reach which the whole energies of the student should be directed. We all recognize that it is in the out-patient departments and in the wards—I wish I could add in the homes of the general practitioners—that he must get this part of his training, not in an elaborate course of lectures on the properties and action of drugs. In the congested curriculum it is by no means easy to find the proper amount of time for this, the most essential part of his education. But as we learn the futility of the lecture room as an instrument of teaching men the Art, so, I think, we shall gradually be able to adapt the courses so that plenty of time may be given to the practical study of the treatment of cases under skilled direction. We should take over to the hospital of the school the whole subject known in the curriculum as therapeutics. The composition of drugs, the method of their preparation, and the study of their physiological action should be taught in practical classes in the pharmaceutical laboratories. In the out-patient departments and in the wards much more systematic practical instruction should be given how to treat disease and how to manage patients. If we could only get the students for a sufficiently long period in the hospital, what helpful courses could be arranged in the senior years! Certain aspects of the subject must be ever kept before the assistants * and the students, considered, perhaps, by different men associated with the clinic according to the special capacity of each one. The fundamental law should be ingrained that the starting-point of all treatment is in the knowledge of the natural history of a disease. Typhoid fever, tuberculosis, pneumonia, and, where possible, malaria, should be used for this important lesson, and in the everyday routine observation of cases the student would learn to know the course of the disease, its obvious features, the

* A post-graduate course in medical pedagogy would be most helpful organized by five or six of the large colleges and conducted by them in rotation with teachers selected from the different schools. Many able young fellows take years to acquire methods to which they might be introduced in a six months' course.

complications likely to arise; and he would be taught how to discriminate between the important and the unimportant symptoms of a case. This work should form the very basis of his course in medicine, and it should be accompanied by a *seminar* to take the place of set lectures, in which the features of all the common diseases would be discussed.

The hygienic and dietetic management of patients has now come to be such a prominent part of the work of our hospitals that the student may become acquainted with the open-air treatment, the various modifications of diet suitable to different diseases, and the use of massage, electricity, and other physical agents. But too often he is allowed to pick up this information in a haphazard, irregular fashion. One assistant of the clinic should be detailed to see that every member of the class knows, for example, how to arrange the open-air treatment for a tuberculous patient, and how to supervise the diet of a diabetic case. The student should prepare personally the various nutritive enemata, and be able to give the different kinds of massage, and I would have him thoroughly versed in all branches of hydrotherapy. A serious difficulty is that nowadays the nurse does a great many things that it is essential the medical student should know how to do—the administration of hypodermics, the giving of a cold pack, etc.

Much more attention should be paid to the important subject of psychotherapy. It is not every teacher who has a special gift for this work, but if the professor himself does not possess it, he should, at any rate, have sense enough to have an assistant familiar with and interested in the modern methods. How many of our graduates have been shown how to carry out a Weir-Mitchell treatment or to treat a patient by suggestion? The student should be taught that the very environment of a well-managed clinic is in itself an important factor in psychical treatment. A Philadelphia friend once jokingly defined my practice at the Johns Hopkins Hospital as a mixture of hope and nux vomica, and the grain of truth in this statement lies in the fact that with many hospital patients once we gain their confidence and inspire them with hope, the battle is won.

And lastly, from the day the student enters the hospital until graduation, he should study under skilled supervision the action of the few great drugs. Which are they? I am not going to give away my list. A story is told that James Jackson, when asked which he considered the greatest drugs, replied: "Opium, mercury, antimony and Jesuit's bark; they were those of my teacher, Jacob Holyoke." "Yes," replied his interlocutor, "and they were those of Holyoke's master, James Douglas, in the early part of the eighteenth century." Mine is a much longer one! The student should follow most carefully the action of those drugs the pharmacology of which he has worked out in the laboratory. He should be sent out from the hospital knowing thoroughly how to administer ether and chloroform. He should know how to handle the various preparations of opium.* Each ward should have its little case with the various preparations of the ten or twelve great drugs, and when the teacher talks about them he should be able to show the preparations. He should study with special care the action of digitalis on the circulation in cases of heart disease. He should know its literature, from Withering to Cushney. It should be taken as the typical drug for the study of the history of therapeutics—the popular phase, as illustrated by the old woman who with it cured the Principal of Brasenose; the empirical stage, introduced by Withering in his splendid contribution, a model of careful work of which every senior student should know; and the last stage, the scientific study of the drug, which he will already have made in the pharmacological laboratory. He should day after day personally give a syphilitic baby inunctions of mercury; he should give deep injections of calomel and he should learn the history of the drug from Paracelsus to Fournier. He should know everything relating to the iodides and the bromides, and should present definite reports on cases in which he has used them. He must know the use of the important purgatives, and he should have a thorough acquaintance with all forms of enemata. He should know cinchona historically, its derivatives chemically, and its action practically. He should study the action of the nitrites with the blood pressure apparatus, and he should over and over again have tested for himself the action, or the absence of action, of strychnine, alcohol, and other drugs supposed to have a stimulating action on the heart and blood vessels. While I would, on the one hand, imbue him with the firmest faith in a few drugs, "the friends he has and their adoption tried," on the other hand, I would encourage him in a keenly skeptical attitude towards the pharmacopeia as a whole, ever remembering Benjamin's Franklin's shrewd remark that "he is the best doctor who knows the worthlessness of the most medicines." You may well say this is a heavy contract, and one which it is impossible to carry out. Perhaps it is with our present arrangements, but this is the sort of work which the medical student has a right to expect, and this is what we shall be able to give him when in his senior years we give up lecturing him to death, and when we stop trying to teach him too many subjects.

* Sydenham obtained the appellation "Opiophilos" (Ogle); and the best practitioner is the man who knows best how to use "God's own medicine," as it has been called.

CHAPTER XVIII

THE PREVENTION AND CONTROL OF ACUTE RESPIRATORY INFECTIONS

By JOSEPH A. CAPPS

TABLE OF CONTENTS

INTRODUCTION

RESPIRATORY infections and their prevention have assumed a place of first importance in medicine as a result of the vast epidemics in the World War. The medical history of the war will bring out two surprising facts: first, the rarity of gastrointestinal infections; second, the frequency of respiratory infections. In former wars infections of the alimentary tract, such as typhoid and dysentery, were responsible for the great epidemics. In our military camps of today typhoid and paratyphoid are curiosities and dysentery is an exceptional occurrence. The disappearance of this formidable group of diseases can be attributed in part to the general use of typhoid inoculation and in large measure to the safeguarding of the drinking water from contamination. During the Spanish-American War the danger arising from polluted water was well known, but nevertheless careful and comprehensive methods of protection were not carried out. Today an army digs its own wells, builds reservoirs, subjects the water to frequent bacteriological tests, and in other ways rigidly and scientifically applies this knowledge. No expense is too lavish, no effort too great to provide this assurance of soldiers against water-borne infections, and the results abundantly justify the expenditure. The campaign against insect-borne diseases has been prosecuted with similar intelligence and diligence. The destruction of flies and mosquitoes, and their breeding-places, and the persistent warfare against the body louse, has almost rid the army of malaria, yellow fever, and trench fever.

Contrast these brilliant results with our experience in the management of respiratory infections. Influenza, measles, pneumonia and streptococcus infections flourish and spread without let or hindrance, both in military and civil communities. A multitude of precautions are employed and enforced with laxity or strictness according to the individual bias of officials, but apparently these diseases are checked only by the exhaustion of susceptible human material.

The history of successful control of any infection reveals the important truth that the manner in which the virus gains entrance into the body must be known. The causative germ need not be identified in order to work out efficient prevention. The attack on yellow fever was most complicated and quite unavailing until it was discovered that the virus entered the body only through the bite of the mosquito. After this knowledge was obtained, although the germ was still unknown, the methods of prevention became direct, simple and effective.

Therefore, the most intensive study should be directed to definite understanding of the portals of entry and the means of conveyance of the virus of infection in order to insure success in its control or prevention.

So-called Acute Respiratory Infections

The classification of this group is somewhat arbitrary and provisional and includes the majority of the contagious diseases; namely, influenza, pneumonia, measles, whooping cough, mumps, meningitis, diphtheria, scarlet fever, septic sore throat, acute pulmonary tuberculosis as well as ordinary colds and bronchitis. Some of these infections are, strictly speaking, not in the respiratory tract. Thus mumps affects the ducts leading from the mouth to the salivary glands. Septic sore throat affects tonsils and pharynx, which form, as it were, a crossing of the respiratory and digestive highways. But it is supposed that these infections are governed by the same laws of transmission as the true respiratory infections and until proof to the contrary is offered they are included. It is worthy of note that the specific germs of all these diseases have been identified with the exception of scarlet fever, measles, influenza, and perhaps the ordinary colds and bronchitis.

Transmission of Respiratory Diseases

Our notions concerning the transmission of the acute respiratory infections are founded too much on traditional ideas and too little on experimental evidence. We are warranted in assuming that the germs pass from the infected to the healthy individual; but in what way? Are they carried by the droplets of sputum; by the expired air; by particles of dried sputum in the dust; by contact of hands and dishes; by food and drink; by kissing; by drinking cups? If the germs can travel by all these routes, then it is important to determine the route that is most common, in order that our efforts at control may be well balanced.

Tuberculosis has been the subject of more intensive study than any other infection. Koch's discovery of the tubercle bacillus and the universal prevalence of the disease have been stimuli to a legion of investigators, both clinical and experimental. It is generally regarded as a respiratory infection, but the ordinary chronic cases may well be excluded from the group of acute diseases under discussion. The chronicity of tuberculosis, the absence of any definite incubation period, the latency of its lesions and the resistance of the bacillus to destructive influences outside the body, all these factors render the study of transmission more difficult than in the acute respiratory infections. They likewise greatly complicate preventive measures, because any precautions to be effective must be continued over a long period of time. Nevertheless there is much to be learned in reviewing the methods and conclusions of the great scientists who for years have endeavored to solve the riddle of the transmission of the bacilli of tuberculosis ([1]).

The chief source of infection is the sputum of tuberculous human beings, but man may become infected also with bovine bacilli from the meat and milk of tuberculous cows. The principal modes of infection that have been championed can here be only summarized:

1. The theory of ingestion was advocated by Chauveau and Gerlach, who demonstrated that both contaminated meat and milk were capable of infecting man. The universal custom of cooking meat almost eliminates this source. Further investigations have shown that fifteen to twenty per cent. of tuberculosis in childhood are of bovine origin and may be attributed in large part to the use of infected milk.

2. The theory of inhalation of dried dust was put forward by Cornet and his associates, and was made plausible by the finding of living bacilli in the dust on floors, walls and furniture. When, however, it was shown that sunlight destroys even the hardy tubercle bacillus in a state of pulverization, this mode of transmission seemed less probable.

3. The theory of droplet infection was offered by Flügge, who succeeded in infecting animals by direct exposure to the coughing of consumptives. Koch endorsed this hypothesis and considered that the tuberculous virus is communicated from phthisical patients to the healthy by means of particles of sputum expelled in coughing.

4. The theory of mouth and throat infection combines and includes both the ingestion and inhalation methods. It differs from both in that

it lays great stress on the transmission of sputum to the mouth by the hands, eating and drinking utensils, etc. Also it emphasizes the frequency of primary invasion of the tonsils and throat in distinction to primary invasion of lungs or intestines. Krause favors this theory above the others. He believes the spraying experiments of Flügge were not rigidly controlled, since the mouth was sprayed as well as the nose. Recently, however, Rogers ([2]) has wrapped guinea pigs completely in cloth, including the mouth, and subjected them to a spray of finely divided particles of sputum. Invariably they contracted pulmonary tuberculosis in a few weeks.

From a review of these investigations we may conclude that: many persons are infected in childhood through the milk of tuberculous cows; many by means of sputum droplets coughed into the mouth and nose; a small number by inhalation of dry contaminated dust; an unknown number by means of mouth infection through the medium of contaminated hands and utensils. The factors concerned in the transmission of tuberculosis must all receive due consideration in any study of the acute respiratory infections.

Sources of Infection in Acute Respiratory Diseases

The infective virus is known to be in the mucous secretions of the mouth, throat, bronchial tubes or nose in all of the so-called acute respiratory infections; namely, pneumonia, influenza, measles, mumps, streptococcus infections, diphtheria, scarlet fever, septic sore throat, whooping cough, and the common colds. This affords a safe starting-point for the study of transmission. The blood in a few diseases may also contain the pathogenic germs; e.g. in pneumonia and streptococcus infections, but there is no evidence that these infections are ever communicated through the medium of the blood except possibly by invasion of wounds. Open wounds or mustard gas burns invaded by diphtheria were believed to be an active source of throat diphtheria in hospitals near the front in France, but in civil life such occurrences are probably rare. Food and drink are also potential dangers, but the virus usually reaches them through the medium of infected sputum.

It is safe to assume that the ultimate source of infection, however transmitted, usually lies in the sputum or nasal secretions. The portals of entry with few exceptions are the mouth, throat, nose, and perhaps the eyes. These assumptions are tenable regardless of the different theories of the modes of communicability.

Routes of Transmission

The possible routes of travel of infected mucus from sick to healthy are numerous and much discussion has arisen over their relative importance. They may be classed as follows:

(1) *The Direct Routes.*—(a) Transmission by the spray of mucus droplets from the mouth and nose of the diseased to the healthy during the act of talking, coughing and sneezing. Flügge ([3]) found that the expired breath carried no bacteria, that talking expelled occasional particles of mucus, while sneezing and coughing projected a spray to a distance of a meter. Doust and Lyon ([4]) recovered bacteria on a Petri dish at a distance of ten feet from the person coughing.

(b) Similar transmission of droplets from a "carrier" to a healthy individual. The importance of the carrier as a disseminator of contagion has been more and more emphasized in recent years.

(c) Transmission by kissing.

(2) *The Indirect Routes.*—(a) Inhalation of sputum in the form of dust, especially after dry sweeping of floors, walks and streets. In the southern camps an increase in measles and streptococcus infections was noted following dust storms. Most bacteria die rapidly after drying and exposure to sunlight, so that this danger may be more apparent than real.

(b) Hand to mouth infection. The patient coughs in his hand and soils door knobs, pens, furniture, or transmits the mucus to others in handshaking. This virus, collected on the hands of the healthy, reaches the mouth while wetting the fingers or eating and thus gains entrance to the body.

(c) The use of contaminated canteens, drinking cups and eating utensils. According to Lynch and Cummins ([5]) the custom of soldiers washing the mess kits in a common can of lukewarm water disseminates infection, partly by contaminating the kits but more particularly by transplanting germs from the water to the hands, which eventually find their way to the mouth.

(d) Use of a common wash basin or bowl. In hotels or camps the wash basin is often used for brushing the teeth or washing the mouth, thus opening the way for infection of the next person who washes his face in the same receptacle.

(e) Exchange of pipes and cigarettes, a habit prevalent among soldiers.

(f) Food contaminated by diseased individuals and by carriers.

(g) Milk has long been recognized as a vehicle for transmission of infectious diseases to man. The first organisms found to be carried by milk were those of typhoid, dysentery and cholera. Later on it was repeatedly demonstrated that diphtheria, scarlet fever and septic sore throat were disseminated by milk. During the last decade formidable epidemics of septic sore throat in Boston, Baltimore, and Chicago have been definitely traced to the milk supply, as well as many smaller outbreaks.

The contamination of the milk supply with the organisms of diphtheria, scarlet fever and septic sore throat occurs in various ways, but some of the following conditions are usually associated with milk-borne epidemics: (a) Cases of active infection or of carriers are found among the milkers. (b) Cases of active infection or of carriers exist among the milk handlers. (c) Milk vessels, bottles, containers, etc., are infected. Sometimes the human agent is not discovered, but he may be on the farm, at the collecting station or employed as a distributor. (d) *Bovine mastitis* resulting from infection with human pathogenic germs is a source that is probably more common than formerly supposed. The evidence in favor of scarlet fever germs affecting the udders is discussed by Savage ([6]). Since the causative organism of scarlatina is unknown, the question is not capable of proof by experimentation and is supported only by the occurrence of garget and ulcerated teats in certain scarlatina outbreaks. Diphtheria bacilli of definite pathogenic character were found by Ashby ([7]) in ulcers on the teats of cows, during the investigation of a milk-borne epidemic of scarlet fever, but no instances of diphtheria mastitis have come to the attention of the writer.

Septic streptococcus sore throat has been traced to bovine mastitis. Strains of hemolytic streptococci, similar to those found in cultures from septic sore throat patients, have been identified in milk of gargety cows. Experiments ([8]) have shown that streptococci of human origin, injected by catheter into the udder of a healthy cow, will result in mastitis. After producing an abrasion of the teat and rubbing in a suspension of human streptococci an ascending infection of the ducts took place finally invading the udder. For several weeks thereafter pus cells and streptococci were present in large number in the milk.

Theobald Smith and his co-workers ([9]) believe that bovine mastitis due to infection with strains of human streptococci may explain the explosive nature of the outbreaks. It is probable that in bovine mastitis from human streptococci the ultimate source is the sputum of the milker, carried to the cow's teats by contaminated hands. Mastitis of this type is a massive infection, capable of provoking sudden and extensive outbreaks of sore throat, lasting several weeks. How frequently epidemics actually spring from this source can be determined only by further investigation.

Factors Influencing the Spread of Respiratory Infections

The analysis of the causes that are responsible for the spread of these diseases does not permit of arbitrary and dogmatic conclusions. Observers of a given epidemic will frequently place a very different value on the admitted facts of evidence. Much is gained by classifying causes into three groups: (1) factors concerned with proximity; (2) factors concerned with lowered resistance or increased susceptibility; (3) other factors.

The relative importance of the first two groups depends, to a degree not generally appreciated, on the nature of the disease in question. Thus Zinsser ([10]) points out that susceptibility is almost universal in certain infections; e.g. mumps, measles, influenza and streptococcus infections. Hence in these diseases proximity and contact are the primary etiological elements of the problem and susceptibility plays a secondary rôle.

On the other hand most individuals have a considerable resistance to pneumococcus pneumonia, meningitis and scarlet fever even though exposed to these diseases. Consequently conditions tending to lower resistance assume the greater importance, while proximity is of lesser moment.

No pretense is made that causes falling in both groups may not be operative and that often the two may not overlap, but the distinction here formulated will be found useful for a better valuation of factors and for more intelligent application of preventive measures.

One must remember also that the natural resistance of an individual to a disease such as pneumonia is quite broken down by another antecedent infection such as influenza or measles.

(1) *Factors Concerned with Proximity.*—These are most important in the diseases to which there is an almost universal susceptibility; namely, influenza, measles, streptococcus infection and mumps.

(a) *Overcrowding* in civilian life and in the military service is the bane of sanitarians. Overcrowding in camps, in hospitals, at ports of embarkation, in barracks, and on troop transports was, by common consent, the overwhelming factor in causing the great prevalence of respiratory diseases in our army. In barracks the bunks were close together, at the mess tables men sat on opposite sides with only three or four feet intervening; in reading and recreation rooms and about the stoves they gathered in compact groups; in hospital wards with the regulation provision of fifty beds there was a space of two feet between beds, but in wards with seventy to seventy-four beds, which were the rule in the American Expeditionary Force during the active period, only five inches separated the beds. On transports the men in crowded sleeping quarters suffered also from a lack of ventilation and air foul beyond description. The opportunities for direct and indirect dissemination were legion.

(b) Promiscuous *dissemination of sputum and nasal secretions* incident to crowding. This includes the contamination of drinking cups and dishes, the conveyance by soiled hands of secretions to cigarettes, pipes, or directly to the mouth, and the use of a common wash bowl. All of these details of personal hygiene and cleanliness are rendered difficult or impossible by living in crowded quarters.

(2) *Factors Concerned with Lowered Resistance.*—(a) Exhausting drills or long marches; (b) exposure to rain and cold; (c) inadequate bed covering; (d) poor ventilation; (e) racial susceptibility; (f) men from rural homes are more susceptible to infectious diseases than those from the city.

(3) *Other Factors.*—(a) The failure to recognize and isolate early cases of infection exposes others to contagion. Many army surgeons were culpable in this respect. (b) Failure to discover and isolate "carriers" of diphtheria bacilli and meningococci.

Emerson ([11]) attributes the unfavorable conditions responsible for the high rate of respiratory infections in the American Expeditionary Force partly to inevitable limitations of transportation on land and sea imposed by military operations and requirement of speed in troop movements; partly to lack of labor and materials for building shelters; partly to lack of discipline in matters of personal hygiene; and partly to lack of imagination on the part of medical officers who subordinate the protection of a community to the symptomatic treatment of the patient.

The Rôle of Carriers

In every epidemic there are many mild or atypical cases of infection that are not reported to the health authorities. There are also many "carriers" or healthy individuals who harbor pathogenic germs without being infected. Presumably the sick are more liable to infect others than the carriers, but the sick are quarantined while carriers are allowed their freedom. Thus carriers may become important factors in the spread of disease. Failure to control diphtheria and meningitis epidemics has been attributed to the neglect of carriers.

Since carriers are often very numerous it is not practicable to attempt universal cultures of a community or camp. But cultures of contacts in families, wards, or small military organizations are desirable, since the segregation of carriers has often been the means of ending an epidemic. The whole problem of carriers needs further investigation, which may lead to radical changes in preventive medicine.

The Importance of Cross Infections

In times of peace contagious hospitals have always been embarrassed by cross infections, especially of scarlet fever and diphtheria or of measles and diphtheria. Frequently these cross infections have been contracted in the hospital. But in our military camps the tremendous importance of cross or multiple infections in the respiratory tract has been for the first time brought home to the profession. Reports from our home camps indicate that measles uncomplicated was of little danger, but that the secondary invasion of streptococci causing pneumonia gave rise to a formidable mortality. Similarly in the American Expeditionary Force, influenza alone was rarely serious. Most clinicians and bacteriologists are of the opinion that the deadly pneumonia following in the wake of influenza was due to a secondary infection of streptococcus, pneumococcus or other germs. Multiple infections were the rule in fatal cases. This so-called "polybacterialism" finds its simplest explanation in promiscuous transfer of infected secretions from one individual to another. An initial attack of measles or influenza renders the mouth and air passages highly susceptible to other pathogenic organisms. Toxic gases likewise prepare the soil for bacterial growth.

Cross infections may occur anywhere, but there are certain places where the combination of close quarters and the presence of carriers of different organisms is highly favorable. Such places are: the hospital trains where gas, influenza, streptococcus, pneumococcus and wounded patients are herded together in sitting compartments or placed in adjacent bunks; the ambulances and the receiving wards where these men are again brought together with new contacts; and finally in the hospital wards. We have repeatedly observed the onset of pneumonia within forty-eight hours of the arrival of a convoy on these trains. In civil life cross infections are favored by the living conditions in charitable institutions, college dormitories and public schools. The probability that hospitalization is responsible for the dissemination of bacteria is pointed out by Cole ([12]), who found that the number of measles patients that on admission to a hospital harbored streptococcus hemolyticus was small, but that the majority of these patients acquired the organism during their residence in the hospital.

Levy and Alexander ([13]) recovered streptococci from the throats of 14.8 per cent. of 489 new recruits, whereas 95 men in one organization that had been in camp for months yielded 83 per cent. positive cultures. Still more significant is their observation that most of the "clean" cases in measles wards acquired streptococci within a week from neighboring streptococcus carriers. Bronchopneumonia following measles occurred exclusively in those patients who were carriers of streptococci. Careful studies of this kind on cross infections in influenza are not available, but would probably give similar results. It is not an overstatement to assert that, in the great epidemics of influenza and measles in the army and in civil hospitals, cross or secondary infections with streptococcus, pneumococcus and other organisms ushered in most of the pneumonias and were, therefore, responsible for a large percentage of deaths.

Preventive Measures

The campaign against the epidemics of respiratory infections so far has developed very little along offensive lines. It is essentially a series of defensive battles, designed to give protection to humans against the bacterial weapons and to minimize the effect of wounds thereby inflicted. The methods of proved value may be considered under the following classification: (1) early recognition of infection; (2) prophylactic vaccination; (3) destruction of pathogenic germs; (4) the aseptic method; (5) blocking transmission by physical means.

(1) *Early Recognition of Infection.*—The immediate discovery and identification of a case of infectious disease is the keynote of success in controlling an epidemic. Prompt isolation and quarantine of the first case during the contagious period is more efficacious in stamping out the disease than the most elaborate general measures later on, when the contagion has spread and become intrenched in many foci. Confinement of the patient to bed simplifies quarantine and renders it more effective, and at the same time secures to the individual his maximum power of resistance.

(2) *Prophylactic Vaccination.*—Antidiphtheria inoculation by the toxin-antitoxin method marks a great advance in the control of diphtheria. The immunizing process requires several weeks and is most advantageously employed among the children of the crowded cities where diphtheria is endemic. Zingher ([14]) advocates its more general use in young children as the best means of eliminating the existing prevalence of the disease. For the immediate protection of individuals exposed to infection the single dose of prophylactic antitoxin affords an immunity lasting several weeks and because of its quick action is the method of choice.

In prophylactic immunization against pneumonia, some progress has recently been made. Cecil and Austin ([15]) obtained encouraging results at Camp Upton, where 12,519 men were vaccinated with Types I, II and III pneumococcus. During an observation period of ten weeks none of these cases that had received two or more injections developed pneumonia of these three fixed types, whereas in a control of about 20,000 men unvaccinated there were 26 cases of pneumonia of Types I, II and III. Later, Cecil and Vaughan ([16]) used a lipovaccine in 13,460 men at Camp Wheeler for the same types of pneumococcus. Although considerable protection was conferred, the prevalence of influenza obscured the effects of the pneumococcic immunization and the results were not so favorable as at Upton. During measles, streptococcus and influenza epidemics Type IV pneumococcus pneumonias are numerous and up to the present time little has been accomplished in preventing this formidable group by vaccination. Influenza prophylactic vaccines have been tried with varying success (Rosenow ([17]), McCoy ([18]), but the treatment is still in the experimental stage. The other respiratory infections have so far proven refractory to immunizing measures.

(3) *Destruction of Pathogenic Germs.*—The use of antiseptic gargles and sprays has had many advocates. Sailer believes that the daily irrigation of the throat in hospital wards causes a marked diminution in cross infections. But the disappointing results of these methods in clearing up the throats of carriers of diphtheria bacilli and meningococci have undermined our confidence in their efficacy. The removal of diseased tonsils and adenoids in diphtheria and meningococcus carriers has given excellent results in the experience of Friedberg ([19]) and others and deserves further trial.

If the sputum and nasal discharges could be effectively collected on bits of cloth and in sputum cups and burned, a definite source of contagion would be eliminated. The enforcement of this precaution in carriers and ambulatory patients is extremely difficult. All dishes and drinking vessels should be sterilized in boiling water. Spitting about the wards, on the streets, and in public conveyances should be rigidly prevented. The danger from fomites in respiratory infections is greatly underrated in the opinion of no less an authority than Chapin ([20]), who states: that physicians rarely carry disease from the sick to the well; that infection by clothing is rare; and that fomites in a room occupied by scarlet fever or smallpox are not likely to convey contagion. Upon this general assumption the fumigation of rooms after occupancy by contagious cases has been limited or abandoned by many of our municipal health departments. The belief is strong that most germs die or lose their virulence soon after leaving the body.

(4) *The Aseptic Method.*—The aseptic method of "antisepsie médicale" was introduced by the French for the purpose of combating cross infections in hospitals. The method is based on the hypothesis that respiratory infections are transmitted chiefly by contact, dissemination by the air being neglected. At the Pasteur Hospital in Paris, isolation in the

ordinary sense is less emphasized than the aseptic details in the care of the sick. Patients with various contagious diseases are placed in adjoining rooms. The same nurse attends different diseases, but observes rigid precautions in wearing a gown that is left in the room and in washing the hands upon leaving the room. Similar methods have been successfully employed in the care of ward patients at the Monsell Hospital in Manchester ([21]), where a sheet-covered screen forms a barrier about each bed. The nurse is required to wear rubber gloves whenever a patient is handled and a gown that is always kept inside. Wherever this idea has been put in practice rigidly, cross infections have been very few. No one can question the success of the method.

But the conclusion that contact between patients and nurses is the essential and only means of transmission overcome by these precautions seems unwarranted. This technique demands most rigid isolation of patient from patient and the separation of patients by partitions or screens also prevents droplet infection by coughing. From a practical point of view the system is complicated and expensive as a nurse must be highly specialized in the technique by long training before she is competent to take charge of a ward. While freely admitting the efficiency of the "aseptic method," we will do well to inquire into ways and means of rendering it more simple and economical, at the same time retaining its essential features.

(5) *Blocking Transmission by Physical Means.*—Could it be proved that droplet infection and direct contact were the primary factors in transmission and that indirect contact with sputum, soiled hands and objects were secondary factors, then our attention would be focussed on blocking the germs in their course of travel from one person to another. The blocking method is accomplished principally by the following means:

(1) Cubicles or separate rooms. In hospital wards and especially in military hospitals where small rooms are often not available, the sheet cubicle, a sheet suspended on a wire seven feet above the floor and extending from the head to the foot of the bed, has given universal satisfaction.

(2) Face masks. The gauze face mask has long been employed by surgeons in the operating room to prevent droplet infection of wounds. Strong ([22]) and his associates worked with impunity among victims of the pneumonic plague in Manchuria by using masks made of gauze reinforced with cotton. Meltzer ([23]) urged the use of a fine net over the faces of patients with infantile paralysis and also over the faces of attendants. To Weaver ([24]) belongs the credit of demonstrating the value of the mask in protecting attendants and physicians from contracting infection. During a period of eighteen months he succeeded in eliminating scarlet fever among nurses, whereas in the preceding twenty-one

months eight per cent. had acquired the disease. At the same time the incidence of diphtheria carriers was reduced from twenty-six per cent. to about five per cent.

Weaver's method afforded such apparent protection to the doctors and nurses at the Base Hospital at Camp Grant that the author ([25]) undertook the experiment of using face masks on patients to protect them against cross infection. So long as a patient remains isolated in the cubicle, he is protected; when he leaves the cubicle he endangers others, and is himself exposed to cross infections. As a result of numerous cross infections, particularly scarlet fever, measles and streptococcus, we instituted the use of the mask on patients in all wards where respiratory infections were treated. Each patient was issued daily a clean mask which when not in use was pinned to his cubicle sheet.

Haller and Colwell ([26]) made a careful study of various qualities and thickness of gauze necessary to procure blocking of droplets. They advise the use of five layers of gauze with a 32 x 36 mesh when worn by the attendant only, and three layers when worn by both attendant and patient. The patients were told that the cubicle is like the dugout in a gassed area; as long as one remains inside the mask is superfluous, but it is dangerous to leave the cubicle unmasked.

Since many persons were exposed to both primary and cross infections before reaching the ward the following means were adopted. At the regimental infirmary every case with respiratory infection was masked as soon as recognized. Upon entering the ambulance every patient, sick or well, was masked. In the receiving ward every ambulatory patient who entered the hospital was masked at the door and all patients continued to wear the mask until they reached the shelter of their ward and cubicles.

Before the method of masking patients was introduced, and the cubicle alone was employed, we had ten instances of cross infection with scarlet fever in wards occupied by other diseases. In four instances, or forty per cent., there were subsequent cases of scarlet fever during the week of quarantine. In three wards where measles broke out as a cross infection there was one ward in which a subsequent case of measles developed during the two weeks of quarantine. After masks were used universally by patients and attendants, the results were as follows: in twenty-four wards where scarlet fever appeared as a cross infection, there was only one ward, or five per cent., in which a subsequent case developed; in twelve wards where measles occurred as a cross infection, there were two wards, or seventeen per cent., in which a subsequent case developed. To summarize: Before general masking, in thirteen wards with cross infection, there were five wards, or thirty-eight per cent. with subsequent cases. After masking, in thirty-six wards with cross infection, there were three wards, or 8.3 per cent., with subsequent cases. The statistics in streptococcus cross infections cannot be tabulated, because there was no period of quarantine after exposure. It may be significant, however, that only twenty cases of bronchopneumonia developed in over 900 cases of measles, although streptococcus infections were prevalent.

The Limitation of Isolation Measures

What measure of success can be expected of the isolation methods just described in preventing the spread of epidemics of influenza, measles and streptococcus infections in civil communities and in military camps? Can they be depended on to check the onward sweep of these infections? The experience of public health officers and epidemiologists in the army shows very definitely that these barriers cannot withstand the irresistible advance of such epidemics. Individuals, families, organizations may here and there secure protection, but the population as a whole is submerged. The reason for this failure is that universal enforcement of isolation among healthy people or healthy troops is impossible. Even the infected cannot be easily isolated since healthy "carriers" are always numerous and cannot be recognized without taking cultures of all. The attempts to rigidly isolate healthy people wherever they congregate in civil life; e.g. compulsory masking as practiced in San Francisco in the recent influenza outbreak, would seem doomed to failure as a general measure, although doubtless many individuals might thereby secure protection.

In army camps where it is possible to quarantine large organizations, the chances of success are far greater, but in practice they were often disappointing in the case of influenza and measles, diseases in which "carriers" cannot be identified because cultures are of no assistance. Isolation in meningitis and diphtheria yielded much better results because both sick and "carriers" can be recognized by cultures of the throat. The bald truth may as well be faced, that in the army, influenza, measles, mumps and streptococcus infections spread rapidly and freely in spite of all the efforts of sanitarians.

Isolation Methods in Control of Cross Infections

To stem the tide of a highly contagious disease is one thing; to protect healthy individuals from the disease and to protect the sick from cross infections is another. In the first situation the individuals are not under personal control and supervision; in the second situation the individuals are under the influence of personal discipline. Isolation methods are not at all effective in checking the spread of the most contagious diseases and only partly effective in the less contagious ones. On the

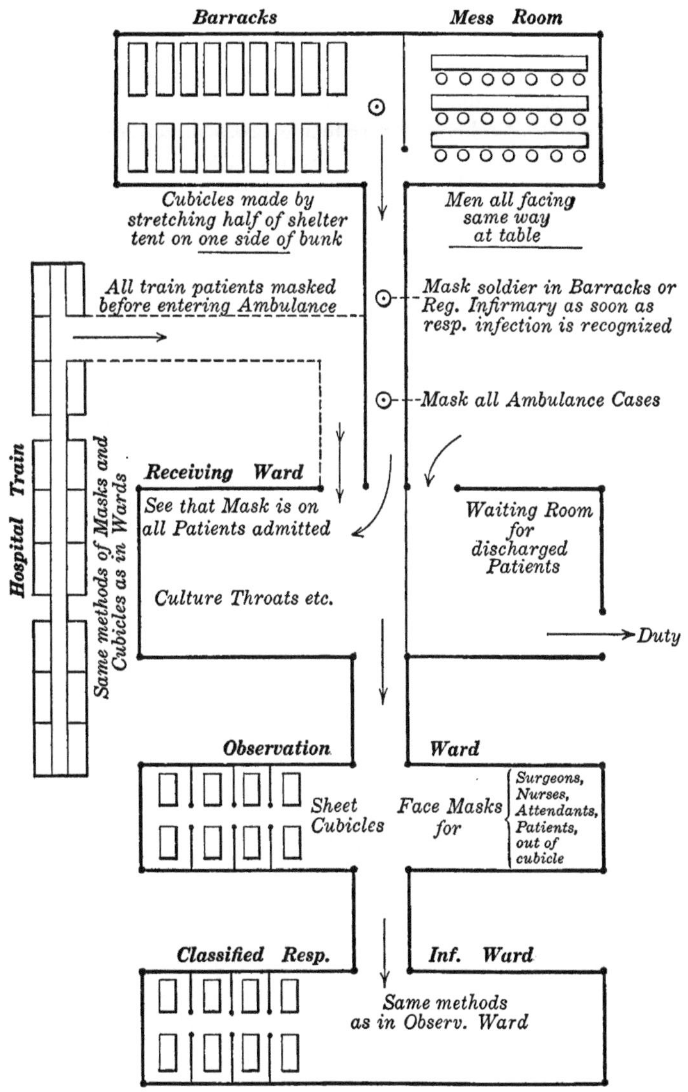

FIG. 1.—DIAGRAM OF THE TECHNIC FOR THE CONTROL OF RESPIRATORY CROSS-INFECTIONS IN MILITARY CAMPS

other hand, isolation is capable of greatly reducing the incidence of cross infections. At first blush the control of cross infections appears to be a comparatively insignificant phase of the problem, and it is when expressed in mere numbers. But its importance defined in terms of mortality is very great, for death usually follows in the wake of cross infections.

A comprehensive scheme for reducing cross infections in the army is outlined. (Fig. 1.) Most of these measures have been employed in the service, but not consistently and rigidly.

(1) In camps newly arrived troops should be segregated.

(2) In the triage every effort should be made to keep the gas and respiratory infections separated.

(3) In hospital trains the patients should be sorted as far as possible to segregate all respiratory infections. The proximity of such patients to gassed or wounded soldiers should be avoided. Since minor throat and bronchial infections and carriers are a menace, the stretcher cases should be separated by a sheet partition. The nursing personnel and surgeons should wear masks when on duty.

(4) In barracks overcrowding is to be avoided. The bunks should be separated by the half of a shelter tent or other partition. As soon as a case of respiratory infection is recognized he should be masked and sent to the hospital.

(5) In the mess seating soldiers at a narrow table all facing the same direction is a simple and useful expedient for limiting the danger of droplet infection, and has been tried with success.

(6) All patients traveling by ambulance should be masked.

(7) An orderly stationed at the entrance of the receiving ward should see that every patient admitted is masked, unless he is suffering from dyspnea. The mask should be worn until the patient reaches the shelter of his cubicle. Patients awaiting discharge should be kept separate from those awaiting admission.

(8) Separate wards are desirable for influenza, pneumonia and gassed cases as well as for those diseases ordinarily isolated, such as measles and meningitis.

The beds should be separated by sheet screens. The face masks should be worn by physicians, nurses, ward men and by all patients when out of their cubicles. Within the cubicle the mask may be removed and pinned to the sheet. The patient should wear the mask when leaving the cubicle at all times, except in the wash room, where only one person should enter at a time. Meals should be eaten in the cubicle, although the patient, if masked, may be allowed to carry his dishes from and to the kitchen. Smoking should be prohibited in these wards, as it necessitates removal of the mask and is also harmful to the inflamed air passages.

All eating utensils should be sterilized in boiling water after each meal. Physicians and attendants after examining or handling a patient should wash the hands with soap and water. Masks should be disinfected by soaking an hour in two per cent. cresol solution, then by boiling half an hour in soap and water. In practice the mask may owe much of its value to limiting the opportunities of hand-to-mouth infection as well as to direct droplet dissemination.

Control of Cross Infections in Civil Practice

The principles of prevention are the same in civil as in military practice, but their application is quite different owing to the loose organization and lack of discipline in civil communities. The immediate diagnosis and reporting of all contagious diseases is a fundamental procedure. The reportable diseases should include streptococcus sore throat, which is generally neglected by physicians.

In carrying out isolation measures in the home emphasis should be laid on the danger of secondary infection to the patient as well as on the spread of the patient's contagion to others. Especially in measles and influenza the patient needs this safeguarding, so easily afforded by masking the face of nurse and all others entering the sick room and the insistence on cleanliness of hands and eating utensils. In this way there is hope of minimizing the frequency of complicating pneumonia, otitis media, etc.

Hospitalization

For years our health departments have believed that the hospitalization of all contagious diseases would bring about a decided diminution of the morbidity rate. This has been the motive for building large municipal hospitals for contagious diseases. According to Chapin the results of the movement have been disappointing. He states that communities in which hospitalization of contagious diseases has been almost complete for years, show quite as high prevalence of these diseases as communities in which there is no attempt at hospitalization. The bringing together under one roof of many different infections may actually expose the patient to a new disease. Moreover, the healthy "carriers" of infection are not controlled by this method. In the light of this experience more attention should be given to the supervision of house quarantine, not only by city physicians, but by visiting nurses capable of instructing the family in preventive measures.

Closing of Public Places

During the epidemic of influenza the advisability of closing schools, theaters, and other places of assembly, was heatedly discussed by health officials. The danger of contagion was admitted. On the other hand it was urged that the discipline, regular hours, and good ventilation of the schoolroom afforded less exposure to disease than the uncontrolled mingling of children on the streets. The belief is firmly rooted among sanitarians that proximity out of doors where the air is in constant movement is far less liable to disseminate contagion than proximity indoors, where the air is often stagnant.

For sporadic cases of infectious disease the segregation of the patient, and if possible of carriers, is sufficient. When, however, an existing epidemic invades a school, it is often desirable to close its doors until the force of the infectious wave is spent. In theaters and churches much might be accomplished in checking transmission by direct appeal to the audience to always cover the mouth with a handkerchief during coughing and sneezing—a practice introduced by a noted evangelist. Teachers in the schools and parents in the home are under obligation to instruct children upon this matter of personal hygiene.

Good ventilation of assembly rooms materially lessens the liability of germ dissemination and should receive more attention. The air in public libraries, schoolrooms and lecture halls where the windows are closed to exclude noise and smoke is often oppressively stale, and in consequence favors the spread of contagion.

Special Measures

This chapter is intended to treat only of the general principles concerned in the control of respiratory infections, since specific therapy will be discussed under the separate diseases. Only a few applications of these principles to individual infections need special mention.

Pneumonia.—The promising work on vaccine prophylaxis has already been referred to. Individual isolation of different types of pneumococcus infection in pneumonia wards is advocated by Cole, but Zinsser considers this unessential. Isolation for the purpose of preventing cross infection with other germs, especially streptococcus, is, however, of undoubted value.

Measles is a dangerous disease in proportion to the incidence of secondary infections. Hence the importance of isolation measures. During the prevalence of streptococcus infections the separation of measles patients harboring streptococci in the throat from the clean cases is deserving of trial. Isolation in the home with rigid enforcement of masking and cleanliness on the part of attendants should diminish the frequency of pulmonary and other complications.

Influenza as a primary infection cannot be adequately controlled by isolation or any other measures now known. Still it is possible to give a large degree of individual protection to the sick in hospitals by rigid quarantine and by the prevention of secondary infections.

Meningitis and Diphtheria demand a search for carriers among contacts by means of throat cultures. The isolation of contacts leads to the questionable quarantine of many persons with positive cultures. There is need of discretion in avoiding promiscuous culturing of organizations beyond the immediate focus of the disease and also in releasing carriers of non-virulent diphtheria bacilli. Immunization of contacts yielding a positive Schick test is also a valuable means of restricting the contagion.

Streptococcus infections like influenza are at present most difficult of control. We must be content to check by isolation methods their invasion of other respiratory diseases. Preëminently in limiting secondary streptococcus infections the barriers of cubicle and mask should be efficacious. The appearance of a streptococcus outbreak should invariably lead to an investigation of the milk supply. Whether the evidence of milk contamination is obtained or not, pasteurization or boiling of the milk and milk products is advisable. All influences previously discussed that lower the resistance to infection should be avoided as far as possible, but they play a rôle in cross infections of less importance than factors of proximity.

BIBLIOGRAPHY

1. KRAUSE, A. K.: Jour. Outdoor Life, 1918, XV, 1.
2. ROGERS, J. B.: Am. Rev. of Tuberculosis, 1919, III, X, 238.
3. FLÜGGE, F.: Zeitsch. f. Hygiene, 1899, XXXI, 107.
4. DOUST, B. C., and LYON, A. B.: Jour. Am. Med. Assoc., 1918, LXXI, 1216.
5. LYNCH, C., and CUMMING, J. G.: Military Surgeon, 1918, XLIII, 597.
6. SAVAGE, W. G.: Milk and the Public Health. London, 1912, 114.
7. ASHBY, A.: Public Health, 1906-07, XIX, 145.
8. MATHERS, G.: Jour. Inf. Dis., 1916, XIX, 222.
9. SMITH, T., and BROWN, J. H.: Jour. Med. Res., 1914-15, XXXI, 455.
10. ZINSSER, H.: War Medicine, 1918, II, 316.
11. EMERSON, H.: War Medicine, 1918, II, 311.
12. COLE, R., and MacCALLUM, W. G.: Jour. Am. Med. Assoc., 1918, LXX, 1146.
13. LEVY, R. L., and ALEXANDER, H. C.: Jour. Am. Med. Assoc., 1918, LXX, 1827.
14. ZINGHER, A.: Am. Jour. Dis. of Child., 1918, XVI, 83.

15. CECIL, R. L., and AUSTIN, R. S.: Quoted by Cecil and Vaughan, loc. cit.
16. CECIL, R. L., and VAUGHAN, H. F.: Jour. Exper. Med., 1919, XXIX, 457.
17. ROSENOW, E. C.: Jour. Am. Med. Assoc., 1919, LXXII, 31.
18. McCOY, G. W.: Public Health Rep., 1919, XXXIV, 1193.
19. KEEFER, F. R., FRIEDBERG, S. A., and ARONSON, J. D.: Jour. Am. Med. Assoc., 1918, LXXI, 1206.
20. CHAPIN, C. V.: Sources and Modes of Infection. New York, 1912, 217.
21. Gordon Report on Health of Manchester, 1908, 1206.
22. STRONG, R., and TEAGUE, O.: Jour. Am. Med. Assoc., 1911, LVII, 1270.
23. MELTZER, S. J.: Med. Rec., 1916, XC, 292.
24. WEAVER, G. H.: Jour. Am. Med. Assoc., 1918, LXXI, 1405.
25. CAPPS, J. A.: Jour. Am. Med. Assoc., 1918, LXXI, 448.
26. HALLER, D. A., and COLWELL, R. C.: Jour. Am. Med. Assoc., 1918, LXXI, 1213.

CHAPTER XIX

ENVIRONMENT AND ITS RELATION TO HEALTH AND DISEASE

By LEWELLYS F. BARKER

TABLE OF CONTENTS

From the time of beginning as a fertilized egg-cell to the time of death each human individual is subjected to environmental influences that are ever changing. The intra-uterine, infantile, puerile, adolescent, mature and senescent periods of life have, each of them, to a varying degree, certain special surroundings that may be of significance both for health and for disease. In the formation of environments, physical, chemical, biological, psychological and social components participate in greatly differing combinations. (Some of these effects are described also in other chapters; reference to the index will show where these descriptions may be found.)

PHYSICAL COMPONENTS OF ENVIRONMENTS

Among the physical influences of environments are included those of temperature, light, electricity, x-rays and radium, air pressure and propagated motion.

Thermic Influences

These have been of great importance in influencing the development of human civilization as well as of personal hygiene. The world man lives in has great extremes of temperature; the mean yearly temperature of a climate may be as high as +30° C. or as low as −26° C., the mean monthly temperature as high as +39° C. or as low as −51° C., and the extreme single temperatures may be as high as +56° C. and as low as −63° C., and yet thanks to the heat-regulating mechanisms of the body and to the types of clothing and dwellings he has devised, man can continue to exist in such climates for he creates a "private climate" within the general thermal environment. The mechanisms within man's body for the regulation of his temperature are complex; chemical regulation with heat production depends largely upon (1) muscle contraction (as in shivering) and (2) more rapid combustion processes because of the increased rate of metabolism when the external temperature falls; physical regulation with heat dissipation depends upon the giving off of heat to the surroundings (1) by conduction and radiation and (2) by the evaporation of secreted sweat. These regulatory mechanisms are mediated by vegetative centres in the hypothalamus; afferent impulses to these centres are excited by stimulation of the warm-points in the skin by heat and of the cold-points by cold; efferent impulses from the same centres pass to the muscles, to the sweat glands and vasomotor apparatus of the skin, and to the structures mediating the metabolic rate. Though these heat-regulating mechanisms provide excellent physiological methods of defence to changes in the thermal environment, there are limits beyond which they are no longer capable of preventing local or general injury to either heat or cold.

Thus the local injuries ("burns") from excessive heat may vary in degree from erythema and blistering to necrosis and actual charring; if local burns be extensive, symptoms of general intoxication of the body will follow, and death has occurred as the result of a burn of approximately one-eighth of the body-surface.

When the human body as a whole becomes overheated, say because of strenuous muscular activity in a very hot environment, so-called "heat stroke" may occur of which several types have been observed, including (1) heat prostration, (2) hyperpyretic heat stroke and (3) forms with gastro-intestinal or psychic symptoms predominant. In the Great War there were many cases among the troops in Mesopotamia and other hot regions with a relatively high mortality. But even in temperate climates, heat stroke is frequently met with, sometimes in "epidemics" as in New York City in August 1896.

In "heat stroke" the blood of the body as a whole becomes overheated and causes overheating of the brain centres; in "sun-stroke" the same centres may become overheated through the direct over-heating of the head.

Excessive cold can cause local injury manifested as "frost-bite" or "freezing"; there may be every degree of injury from erythema to gangrene. During the World War there were many cases of so-called "trench foot", following exposure of the feet to melting snow in the trenches. It was found this snow water withdrew more heat from the feet than dry cold snow did. A milder form of local injury following exposure of predisposed persons to cold in our climate is that known as chilblains; here, however, the local tissue disposition is the most important factor, cold acting as a provocative cause.

The general effects of low temperatures upon the body have been studied both in man and in experimental animals. In insufficiently protected persons exposed to cold winds, cold water, or snow storms over too long a period, the temperature of the interior of the body may fall to so low a level that death results. Drunken men, Alpine tourists and shipwrecked sailors sometimes meet with death from cold. After the preliminary chilling, they are overpowered by a sense of fatigue, begin to yawn, become drowsy and enter into coma.

Of late years, much attention has been given to the "common cold" and to the nasal, pharyngeal, and pulmonary sequels of "catching cold". Both laymen and physicians are convinced that exposure to cold and damp may be an important etiological factor in "catching cold", though disposition (inherited or acquired) to colds seems to be just as important, and at least in many cases infection also plays a part. The effect of the cold may directly injure local tissues; many, however, are wedded to the hypothesis that the cold, through reflex action, changes the blood-supply of certain organs (nose, throat, lungs) in which the disease develops. Much progress has been made in lessening the susceptibility to colds through wiser methods of clothing, better ventilation of houses, practice of out-door sports and so-called "hardening" measures. Treatment of local infections of the nose, mouth, throat and paranasal sinuses seems also to be helpful in lessening disposition to "catching cold". Many persons have found by experience that when after exposure to cold they have observed the premonitory symptoms of a cold they can often abort it by provoking sweat and keeping warm afterwards.

Influence of Light

Sunlight, if allowed to act upon the skin, may cause erythema and dermatitis. The erythema produced may occur at once or shortly after exposure and disappear again in a few hours; this type is like any burn due simply to the heat action of the light rays and the ultra red rays. Another type of erythema, the so-called "photochemical exanthem", appears only after a latent period of several hours and is due to the action of the ultraviolet rays; this type is often met with among tourists in the high mountains and upon glaciers, since the sunlight at high altitudes is said to contain relatively more ultraviolet rays than the light at lower levels. The pigmentation that follows the dermatitis is an especial protection against the skin-harming effects of ultraviolet rays. It is said that the application of a 5 per cent. quinine paste to the exposed parts of the skin, when making a mountain or glacier tour, will protect from injury to the skin since this paste will absorb most of the ultraviolet rays.

Electrical Influences

About electrical influences in the environment aside from lightning stroke and accidental contact with strong electrical currents but little is known. Death due to being struck by lightning has decreased in houses, since lightning rods have been in use, but there has been but little if any change in the number struck in the open. Some five hundred persons yearly die from this cause in the United States.

With the great increase in the use of electricity in industrial establishments and in households, accidental contacts with powerful electric currents have become ever more common, so that now approximately ten persons per million of population are killed by such contacts each year in the United States. The majority of these accidents, though not all, have been due to contact with alternating currents. In case of contact, a person standing in rooms with dry floors, carpets or linoleum is safer than one standing in rooms with tiled, brick or cement floors. Many safety devices have been introduced that lessen the likelihood of electrical injury.

When a strong current enters the human body, violent muscular contractions occur. It is fortunate when such contractions remove the part, at which the current has entered, from contact with the conductor of the current. Sometimes, when the part entered is the hand, there is tetanic contraction of the muscles so that the conductor is firmly gripped and cannot be let go. On lightning stroke, the person struck may fall dead, or apparently dead, or he may cry out before losing consciousness.

When the current has not been too strong, death does not occur; even comatose patients may be revived, especially with artificial respiration. On recovery, evidences of the site of entry and of exit of the current may be seen on the skin (burns, epidermolysis, localized œdema, "lightning figures", necroses). Some patients after injury become hysterical or show other evidences of traumatic neurosis. Occasionally, there are sequels in the form of neuritis or of focal lesions within the central nervous system.

Influences of X-Rays and Radium

Roentgen rays and the gamma rays of radium have great capacity for penetrating the body because of their extremely short wave-lengths. The tissues of the body vary in their sensibility to the action of the rays, the lymphadenoid tissues and the gonadal tissues being perhaps most sensitive, the connective tissues, cartilage and bone least sensitive. Mild exposures, not too often repeated, appear to be harmless, whereas stronger and frequent exposures can cause severe damage, even death, of tissue cells.

Because of the sensitiveness of the skin, radiologists are careful in examining patients and especially when treating them with larger dosage to avoid the production of a dermatitis; hence at any one treatment a single area receives only a certain fraction of a "skin-erythema dose". Chronic dermatitis, with hyperkeratoses and changes in the finger nails, frequently develops among x-ray operators and should be avoided by better protective measures than those formerly used; all too many of our pioneer roentgenologists have succumbed to carcinomatous processes that developed upon the basis of skin injuries due to the x-rays.

With the increased use of radium and of x-rays for the treatment of leukæmias, hyperthyroidism and neoplasms, physicians have become ever better acquainted with the dangers of excessive dosage and have formulated rules of safety. The incautious application of these rays during pregnancy may cause abortion, or may injure the fœtus if it survive.

Influence of Air-Pressure

Many persons are sensitive to changes in the weather. Though these changes are associated with rise or fall of the barometer, it is not believed that it is the mere oscillations in the air pressure that are directly responsible for the weather sensitiveness complained of. It is, apparently, only in very rarefied air or very highly compressed air that the changes in pressure cause functional disturbances.

When the body is exposed to very high pressures, disturbing symptoms, aside from those referable to the ears and paranasal sinuses, rarely occur unless there is too sudden diminution of the pressure. Bridge builders who work in large water-tight and air-tight cases, caissons, in laying foundations in deep water run the risk of developing "caisson disease", unless great care is taken to return only gradually to normal atmospheric pressures. They are prone to suffer from pains in the abdomen and in the joints of the extremities, "the bends", from pruritus, epistaxis and vomiting. In some instances, severer syndromes, spastic paraplegia, a Menière syndrôme, make their appearance; occasionally, especially if circulatory or pulmonary disease have pre-existed, fatalities occur.

The phenomena are explained through the fact that nitrogen is absorbed by the fluids and tissues of the body when the worker is exposed to high pressure, and when these are reduced too rapidly, nitrogen gas bubbles develop in the tissue spaces and in the blood and injure tissue elements by the pressure they exert, or cause gas embolism of smaller vessels with resulting local ischæmias. That is why laws have been passed requiring slow decompression, and by successive stages, of the workers.

The danger to deep water divers, who encased in water-tight and air-tight diving suits have to stay at times under pressures from five to seven times the normal atmospheric pressure, is still greater because of the difficulty or impossibility of providing for slow decompression. Prophylaxis here consists in shortening the period of exposure to high pressure in order that the body tissues and fluids do not absorb so much nitrogen.

When the body is exposed to very low pressures, the diminished partial pressure of oxygen makes itself felt; dyspnœa and cyanosis develop especially in those not trained, "acclimatized", to life at low pressures. Thus arise mountain-sickness among climbers, balloon sickness and aviators' sickness at high altitudes; some of the latter provide themselves with oxygen masks for prophylactic purposes.

The influences of weather and of climate in general depend largely upon physical components of environment. Thus, studies of the relationships of tuberculosis to the environment have indicated that hot climates, low altitudes and moist atmospheres are, in general, more unfavorable than their opposites.

Influence of Propagated Motion (Kinetic Influences)

Sudden acceleration of motion in any direction by irritation of the vestibular apparatus can cause dizziness and nausea, to which rapidly changing optical impressions may also contribute. Personal disposition plays a great rôle, some people being very sensitive, others very resistant to the influences of changes of propagated motion. Sea-sickness is the best example of a "kinetosis"; "car-sickness" and "elevator-sickness" are minor forms. In the production of sea-sickness, except in the cases due to auto-suggestion, the pitch of a boat is more effective than the roll, though worst of all is the combined pitch and roll spoken of as "cork-screw-like motion". Susceptibility to sea-sickness is said to be absent in children under two years of age and only slight up to the sixth or eighth year of life. A few adults, perhaps 3 per cent., appear to be almost wholly immune to sea-sickness, but many, who have thought themselves immune, have found in extraordinary circumstances that they were really not so. Visceroptosis seems to be a predisposing factor. Many do not become ill, if they stay on deck in the open air, whereas in badly ventilated rooms they quickly succumb. Mild sedatives like phenobarbital or sodium bromide by lessening the sensitivity of the nerve centres are used by some as preventatives.

It is interesting that Bohec has reported that sailors with inborn or acquired immunity to sea-sickness sometimes develop "land-sickness" or "channel sickness" when at or near the end of a voyage! Though they do not have vertigo, they may complain of headache, feelings of anxiety, anorexia, nausea and insomnia, to be followed later by great drowsiness.

Chemical Components of Environment

Man lives in a chemical as well as a physical environment. Thus, in the open air, he is constantly inhaling oxygen, nitrogen, and other gases and particles, dusts of various sorts; and in houses and in industrial establishments the air may be contaminated by many different gaseous substances, some of which may be toxic to the respiratory passages, occasionally to the skin, and often, after absorption, to the organism as a whole by way of the blood.

Again, in food and drink, a vast number of chemical substances are ingested, most of them beneficial, some of them harmful when ingested in excessive quantities, or when food-stuffs have been improperly preserved or prepared.

In addition, human beings may, in certain environmental circumstances, be exposed to the action of chemical substances that through their chemical effects may provoke injury or disease, or even cause death. Such "poisons" may do harm by the local effects they produce upon the skin or mucous membranes by virtue of their concentration and their physico-chemical properties or through their general effects upon the bodily organs after absorption into the blood.

The amounts of chemical substances that act upon the body are very important from the standpoint of toxic injury. Thus very minute amounts of certain substances (like alkaloids, arsenic, or potassium cyanide) may be very harmful or fatal; doses of from 5 to 50 g. of potassium chlorate or potassium nitrate may kill; even ordinary foodstuffs may be toxic in large doses for we read in the literature even of "water-intoxication", and a favorite method of committing suicide among the Chinese has been to swallow large quantities of common salt (300 to 500 g.). It should be borne in mind, too, that certain persons may show outspoken symptoms after ingestion of much smaller amounts of certain chemical substances than those that are innocuous to the majority of people, owing to excessive sensitivity or so-called "idiosyncracy"; in this connexion, we have in recent years become familiar with a whole series of "allergic reactions" (see chapters on hay fever, asthma, and serum disease).

Toxic amounts of chemical substances may reach human beings either through ignorance, mistake, or intention. Thus, industrial workers may be subject to chronic poisoning inadvertently, neither they nor their employers being aware that dangers exist. Many persons become gradually addicted to the excessive use of alcohol, tobacco, coffee or tea, or to the morphine, cocaine, barbital or sodium amytal habit, scarcely realizing what they are drifting into. Physicians, pharmacists and nurses or their aids occasionally administer poisonous substances entirely by mistake. Criminals use poisons with murderous aims. Suicides are often due to either impulsive or deliberate self-poisoning.

Some poisons in small doses produce no evident immediate effects, but long continued exposure to them may result in slow changes in the body and give rise later on to symptoms or increase susceptibility to disease. Thus, persons exposed to benzol fumes may after weeks or months give rise to a progressive anæmia and to a hemorrhagic tendency. In factories for the manufacture of artificial silk and among certain varnish workers poisonings by organic chlorine preparations may lead to atrophy of the liver and to disturbances of the liver functions. The prophylaxis of acute and chronic intoxications has become, in recent years, one of the most important tasks of preventive medicine. In other parts of this treatise, the toxicology of the many inorganic poisons and of the organic poisons of industrial, plant and animal origin is discussed.

Biological Components of Environment

Human beings are surrounded not only by other persons but also by a host of other living organisms, many of them most helpful, others often highly detrimental. To these biological components of man's environment ever-increasing attention is being paid. Among the harmful members are certain of the bacteria, the ultra-filtrable viruses and the animal parasites.

Bacteria often cause intoxications through baneful alterations of food-stuffs; meat-poisonings, botulism, poisoning through fish, molluscs and crustacea, and intoxications from milk, cheese, eggs, potatoes and preserved foods of various sorts are notable examples.

The members of the great group of acute and chronic infectious diseases are, in large part, caused by bacterial and protozoan invaders of man from his surroundings; some are due definitely to ultra-filtrable viruses; some, again, are of unknown etiology but presumably are due to as yet undiscovered living infectious agents of some sort.

The proof that diphtheria, tetanus, epidemic cerebrospinal meningitis, cholera, bacillary dysentery, typhoid fever, typhus fever, erysipelas, the septic diseases, tuberculosis, leprosy, plague, undulant fever, tularæmia; gonorrhœa and syphilis are due to cocci, bacilli or spirochætes is one of the great triumphs of modern medicine. Malaria has been shown to be due to a protozoan parasite introduced by the bite of a special mosquito, and yellow fever is due to a living virus introduced by another type of mosquito. Acute anterior poliomyelitis and epidemic encephalitis have been proven to be due to invasions by neurotropic ultra-filtrable viruses. The etiological agents of many infectious diseases, among them the acute exanthemata, remain still to be discovered.

Psychological, Social, Economic and Political Components of Environment

The influence of psychological components of environments has received an increasing amount of attention during the past few decades. It has become ever more clear that the tendency of the layman to attribute mental disturbances to psychic traumata of various sorts is due in large part to a confusion of cause and effect. In the so-called "reactive melancholia" especially, the inherited tendency to depression is often of greater importance than the psychic influence from without to which it may be attributed. In Freud's theory of the origin of the psychoneuroses and some psychoses the "suppressed complexes" may have played a part in altering constitutional make-up so that in later life there is an abnormal readiness to react to psychic influences in a pathological way. Thus, hysterical manifestations are believed by many to be of psychogenic origin, in that certain persons expect to be ill in a certain way, or desire to appear to have a certain form of ailment; in conflicts, or in certain situations, they tend to "react" in a characteristic way. But, recently, psychiatrists seem inclined to accept the view that the abnormal mental pictures they see in the neuroses and psychoses that develop after strong psychic influences in the environment, such as in earthquakes, war, social upheavals, etc., depend more upon the personality make-up of the individuals concerned than upon the particular form of the external irritation.

Medical literature is full of reports of cases in which the psychic influences attendant upon earthquakes, shipwrecks, strikes, panics, explosions, fires, railway and motor accidents, economic crises, political upheavals and great religious movements have been regarded as precipitating causes of emotional upsets and of the insanities of various sorts. The psychic effects of homesickness, of estrangements, of isolation, of imprisonment, of legal entanglements, of conflicts in familial and social life, of spiritualistic seances and other special situations have been much commented upon. But writers have had great difficulty in determining in how far in any given case the psychic influences were responsible, and in how far the *anlage* has been responsible. Experiences in the Great War, especially, proved how dangerous it is to speak of pure psychic causal stimuli. To the surprise of everybody, it was found that the frightful conditions experienced, the horrible spectacles witnessed and the fears of injury or death that could not help but exist gave rise to far less psychopathic reaction than many had anticipated; indeed, not a few persons who before the war had manifested hypochondriacal and psychasthenic symptoms got rid of them instead of finding them increased! And since the war, some doubt has become prevalent regarding the etiological influence of fear in the production of the so-called "fright-psychoses". An analysis of many of them has made it clear that pre-existent states of somatic weakness on the one hand, or pre-existent desires of hysterical persons on the other, or mixtures of the two were largely responsible for the development of the profound feeling of physical and psychical impotence of those who manifested acute mental disturbances after emotional shocks in the war. Many of those who were affected were of hyperthyroid tendency or had exhibited vasomotor instability earlier.

Much has been written also about the "exhaustion-syndromes" or "fatigue syndromes" of the war, occurring after prolonged physical, intellectual or emotional strains. Even persons previously healthy might after such excessive fatigue enter a state of extreme lassitude accompanied by feelings of complete indifference, apathy or morose depression. During such fatigue-states, illusions and hallucinations were sometimes observed. The mechanical excitability of the muscles was increased, the pulse-rate became accelerated, the blood pressure sometimes rose, and there was a tendency to sweating and to paræsthesias. These otherwise healthy persons usually recovered completely, if they were able to secure a long period of sleep. A most striking thing during the war was the extraordinary capacity of the healthy brain to resist the deleterious influences of severe exhaustion combined with strong excitation of the emotions, often too with severe bodily injuries. In less healthy brains, exhaustion psychoses often appeared. Moreover, under the influence of great fatigue epilepsies sometimes developed and latent neurosyphilis or latent dementia paralytica tended to become manifest.

Recently, there has been ample opportunity to observe the mode of reaction of people both in Europe and in America to a most severe economic crisis. More astonishing perhaps than the suicides and the depressions reported has been the calmness and the brave willingness to adjust to the difficulties of the time; it has become in many circles "bad form" to complain.

In Russia, during the past decade, the influence of rapidly changing forms of social and political organization could be witnessed; in Italy the influence of fascism and in Germany and Austria, the influence of the change from a monarchical government to a republican form has been in evidence. In time, doubtless, we shall have reports of systematic studies of the effects of such influences.

Since the opening of the new century, the mental hygiene movement has developed rapidly, and the public has been ever better educated in the mental hygiene of childhood, of school life and of adulthood. It is hoped that through these mental influences, and especially through the early conditioning of reflexes and the establishment of desirable behaviour patterns, much may be accomplished for general welfare.

July 1, 1933.

CHAPTER XX

MEDICAL-SOCIAL SERVICE AS A FACTOR IN THE DIAGNOSIS AND TREATMENT OF DISEASE

By RICHARD C. CABOT

Both in the causation and the relief of disease, bacteria and their products, together with certain physical and chemical agents, play the chief parts. But they are not the whole. Psychological, industrial, and educational factors, for instance, are also of some importance. Medical-social service, a branch of social work in general, deals with these factors and is therefore a useful tool in the medical kit.

In war medicine, these factors are at their minimum and medical-social service is relatively unimportant there. On the other hand, in the hospitals of great cities, especially in Out-Patient work, the social, economic, racial, domestic, and other influences dealt with by medical-social workers are at their maximum. Hence good medical practice is there impossible, or at least improbable, without the social worker's aid.

In private practice and especially in the general practice of country districts and small towns, the successful doctor usually does the social work himself. He deals as best he can with the mental, emotional, and industrial life of his patients in its bearings on their diseases. He is his own social worker as he is his own surgeon, laboratory man, and radiologist. This is possible because he knows each patient (and often his family) individually. He can see how each sufferer's maladies are the joint product of physical, chemical, and bacterial agencies *and* of the worries, deprivations, work conditions, and home conditions under which he lives.

But in the organized medical work of a great hospital or a metropolitan public school it is impossible for the physician to know all the important facts about his patient, unless those facts lie on the surface. The cut finger, the diphtheritic membrane, the gonorrheal discharge he can see, but the root causes of the stomach troubles, backaches, debilitated states which bring nearly half the patients to the hospital he cannot see at once and has neither the time nor the means to investigate thoroughly. Yet without finding root causes, his treatment is bound to be a failure and his daily work a waste of time.

Whenever a person's sickness *arises out of the way he lives* (rather than out of some acute catastrophe like an explosion or a railway accident), the doctor must know how he lives. But in hospitals or public schools the doctor has no chance to grasp these essential factors. Hence the need of such help as a good social worker can give.

A child is pale, thin, listless in school work. Physical examination may show no clues for diagnosis. Questioning seldom helps. But a series of home visits by a woman who has the faculty of getting along pleasantly with school children and their families, who can investigate the details of diet, sleeping rooms and sleeping habits, the opportunities for contagion, the possible bearings of family income, family discord or paternal alcoholism on the children's health,—this, I say, may bring to light the facts on which rational diagnosis and treatment can be based.

So far I have written of social work chiefly in diagnosis and in etiology as a part of diagnosis. But social work bears also on prognosis and on treatment. If malnutrition, dyspepsia, headaches, gonorrheal vulvovaginitis, scabies, or rheumatism are based on home conditions which we are practically powerless to change, then the prognosis is a blind alley, no thoroughfare, and we can turn our energies elsewhere.

If, on the other hand, the causative conditions can be changed by social-service work, then that is the treatment indicated. Sometimes really brilliant therapeutics can be thus achieved.

II

I have already tried to show, as under a low power of the microscope, the field of medical-social work and the tools likely to be useful there. Seen in more detail, its place and methods are as follows:

In the neurological and psychiatric clinics of a hospital Out-Patient Department and in the pediatric clinic, almost every case needs study and treatment by a social worker acting under direction of the Clinic Chief. To feed babies, to get older children properly nourished and fit to resist the common infections with success, is a matter of multitudinous detail. An exact knowledge of how the child lives, eats, sleeps, works, and plays is essential. The doctor cannot get this knowledge satisfactorily by questioning the child or its mother. Still less can he be sure that his directions and prescriptions are carried out exactly and persistently. He is at arm's length from his case. He cannot handle it. The social worker, acting as his agent both in the clinic and in the child's home, can see what is going on and can get things done—or at least ascertain that they are not done and that no good results can therefore be looked for.

In the neurological clinic the hemiplegics, arteriosclerotics, paretics, and epileptics must be gotten into institutions or their home companions must be shown the little that can be done to ease and cheer their lives. By teaching and occupation the social worker can save them much suffering, though medicine and surgery are practically helpless.

The " functional " cases, the tics, stammerers, psychoneurotics need re-education of a type which no clinic physician has time and few have ability to give. A properly trained social worker, by intensive effort, can do wonders for a few patients and accomplish substantial good for many more.

Still more important is the social worker as a magnet or focal point to which are drawn the functional neuroses usually hidden in the gynecological or general medical clinics where they are maltreated under diagnoses like gastritis, constipation, ptosis (gastric, intestinal, or uterine), endometritis, " anemia," and debility. In the orthopedic, in the general medical clinic, and in the departments of dermatology, syphilis, and tuberculosis, social-service work is important but somewhat less essential than in pediatrics and neurology.

In the surgical and throat departments there is still less need of anything beyond what doctors and nurses can give.

III

What the social worker does for disease can be grouped under four headings: (*a*) Discovery, (*b*) prevention, (*c*) education, (*d*) disposition.

The **discovery** of concealed nests, foci, or cases of disease through visits to the patient's home, workshop, or school, can be carried out by health officers or public health nurses as well as by social workers, especially when the data sought for are obvious. Thus hidden nests of malaria, uncinariasis, pellagra, lead poisoning, and tuberculosis are now and then brought to light by public officials.

But in hospital work where the single case of phthisis, rickets, syphilis, or occupational disease is the natural starting-point and spur to the search for nests of cases like it, we need someone who can act as the doctor's and the hospital's agent, following a clue held there. Because the social worker is not a public official and comes from an institution which tries to assist rather than to discipline or check people, she * is in a good position psychologically to get the facts she is after. She is welcome. People are not afraid of her and are less likely to lie to her than to a public health official.

Besides the discovery of *new* cases of disease, the social worker, by her greater intimacy with the patient's family and by her chance to talk with him uninterrupted in his home and for a good while, may find *new features* in the cases already known and treated. Omissions in the history, new light on its interpretation, further links in the chain of causation may be brought out thus. Why cannot the doctor do this better? First, because under present conditions of hospital organization he has not the time for home visits; i.e. he is more useful to more people by spending his time on such diagnoses and treatments as he can offer in conjunction with the other elements of the hospital team-consultants, assistants, machines, and laboratories. This ties him down.

Moreover, he is not usually an expert in the give and take of intimate personal intercourse with people of the type who consult him at a free hospital. He cannot get at them as well, understand them as quickly or as far as a well-trained and sympathetic woman can.

Prevention through social worker's efforts springs from the discovery of incipient cases on home visits and through the detailed, hygienic explanations and therapeutic teaching presently to be referred to. She may thus prevent the relapses of mental disease, of peptic ulcer, of flat-foot, of industrial dermatitis, and to this extent prevent the existence of new cases of disease of "old" patients.

Education in the details of diet, sleeping arrangements, exercise, recreation, and the other departments of hygiene must be fitted to the individual like a suit of clothes if it is to be of use to him. General rules are of little value, especially if presented in printed circulars and in a hasty offhand way. The rules must be applied, reshaped, and modified to suit the individual's needs after these needs have been studied with care. Moreover, since these hygienic rules often call for the reform of tough old habit, one must use every effort to get a *dynamic* sufficient to make the patient put himself to so much trouble. The fear of disease and the doctor's authority can accomplish something towards making a man change his habits of diet, of work, or of thought. But usually we need also the persuasive force of someone who cares for the individual sufferer and is believed by him to understand his circumstances, his difficulties, and his point of view. The medical-social worker, acting for the doctor and transmitting his authority and his directions to a patient who believes that she under-

* Why a woman is preferable I will try to show later.

stands him and feels a genuine interest in him, can accomplish more therapeutic education than anyone else now in sight.

By the **disposition** of patients I mean here the process of getting them into institutions, of getting financial or other aid for them through coöperation with other charitable agencies or with private individuals; all of these which are available in her district the social worker first lists and sizes up, then learns to use.

Hospitals, special and general, sanitoria, convalescent homes, homes for the aged, special funds for vacations, for recreation, for pure milk, for trade training (as in the case of mutilated persons), exemplify the tools which the social worker learns to use more or less effectively for hospital patients.

IV

The social-service department of a hospital should function as the X-ray department does—not as an independent agent, but as part of a team under the direction of one guiding mind. The facts elicited by the social worker's studies, talks, and visits should (like X-ray data) be pooled with the data of physical examinations, the laboratory findings, etc. Then they are appreciated and of value; not otherwise.

So with her educational therapy. It will often go wide of the mark, unless *it* is supervised (like X-ray treatment or massage) by the doctor in charge of the case.

To turn a patient over to the social-service department once for all is a common but wholly mistaken practice.

Why has the work described here arisen only since 1905?

Because of the development of big Out-Patient Clinics where team work of many takes the place of one's doctor's attempt to do everything himself. The development of diagnostic and therapeutic teams and with this the stratification of medical jobs so that untrained people can do much of the job, leaving the doctor for his expert work, has helped to show us how many-sided is the task of helping a sick person towards recovery.

In the division of labor thus developed, place is found for one who deals in details, who knows the patient in his home, his work and his school, and who gradually becomes competent to trace out and record the mental elements present in all organic disease as well as in functional or neurotic maladies.

This is the most important point in the whole matter. Mental elements in the causation, in the symptomatology, in the prognosis and treatment of disease are recognized today more fully than ever before.

We know today more than we ever did before what worry, fear, grief, and other emotional strains can do in modifying and augmenting and prolonging disease. We also know something of what peace of mind, habits of concentration, recreative enjoyment, satisfaction in work, friendship or religion can do to banish or to alleviate disease.

No medical-social worker is an expert fit to succeed often in understanding or manipulating all these delicate and pervasive forces. But when she is born for her job and then trained on it, she can contribute perhaps as much to the hospital team work as any single person in it.

It is in organized medicine, then, as we have it in the best modern hospitals, sanitoria, schools, and factories that medical-social service has its chief function. Whenever medical organization takes a step forward, whenever group medicine in any form progresses, the sort of aid and technique here described will, I believe, find a part.

CHAPTER XX-A

PSYCHOSOMATIC MEDICINE

By EDWARD WEISS

Table of Contents

Introduction

Psychosomatic is a new term, but it describes an approach to medicine as old as the art of healing itself. It is not a speciality but rather a point of view which applies to all aspects of medicine and surgery. It does not mean to study the soma less; it only means to study the psyche more. Its subject matter is founded on the important advances in physical medicine as well as on the biologically oriented psychology of Freud without whose epochal discoveries no work on psychosomatic medicine could be attempted. Following these discoveries, Felix Deutsch, then of Vienna, and Jelliffe in America applied this new psychopathology to general medical problems. Later Alexander and his associates at the Chicago Institute of Psychoanalysis, Karl and William Menninger of Topeka, Halliday of Scotland and Dunbar and her associates at the Presbyterian Hospital in New York by their important researches added materially to our knowledge of this subject. In 1935 Dunbar in addition to her valuable studies performed the great service of collecting the widely scattered literature in this field under the title "Emotions and Bodily Changes[9]". The epochal discoveries of Freud, the researches mentioned, and the compilation of literature by Dunbar as well as the contributions of many others are all used freely in the following discussion.

Physicians have always known that the emotional life had something to do with illness, but the structural concepts introduced by Virchow led to the separation of illness from the psyche of man and to a consideration of disease as only a disorder of organs and cells. With this separation of diseases into many different ailments came the development of specialists to attend to all of these distinct diseases. With the specialists came the introduction of instruments of precision, and the mechanization of medicine began. Medicine now contented itself with the study of the organism as a physiological mechanism, impressed by blood chemistry, electrocardiography and other methods of physical investigation, but unimpressed by, and indeed often holding in contempt, the psychological background of the patient, which was considered not so scientific as the results of laboratory studies. This period may, in truth, be referred to as the "machine age in medicine". It is not to be denied that remarkable developments have occurred during this period of laboratory ascendancy, but it also must be admitted that the emotional side of illness has been almost entirely neglected.

Psychosomatic Problems in the Practice of Medicine

Defined as bodily disorders whose nature can be appreciated only when emotional factors are investigated in addition to physical factors, psychosomatic affections can be studied in the following manner.

(1) Between the small number of obviously psychotic persons whom a physician sees and the larger number of patients who are sick solely because of physical disease in which emotional factors play no part are a vast number of sick people who are not "out of their minds" and yet who do not have any definite bodily disease to account for their illness. Psychosomatic medicine is

much concerned with such patients. It is estimated reliably that about a third of the patients who consult a physician fall into this group. These are the so-called purely "functional" problems of medical practice.

(2) Another large group of patients, who consult a physician, have symptoms that are in part dependent upon emotional factors, even though organic changes of non-psychogenic origin are present. This second group is even more important than the first from the standpoint of diagnosis and treatment. These psychosomatic problems often are very complicated, and because serious organic disease may be present, the psychic factor is capable of doing more damage than in the first group. This phase of the subject is especially well illustrated by many instances of organic heart disease. For while a neurotic with a normal heart may suffer a great deal subjectively and may even have a disturbance of cardiac function marked by various forms of arrhythmia, the heart, certainly in the majority of such patients, remains structurally healthy. But the neurotic patient, who has organic heart disease, may add a real burden to the work of his heart either through constant tension of psychic origin or more especially by means of acute episodes of emotional origin. This may hasten a cardiac breakdown which might be postponed indefinitely, if there were no psychic stress. Thus the psychic factors may be even more important than the physical in producing incapacity.

(3) Psychosomatic medicine is much interested in disorders generally considered wholly within the realm of "physical disease", which have to do with the vegetative nervous system, such as migraine, asthma, peptic ulcer and essential hypertension. It is believed that psychic factors may be of great importance in their etiology and even more importantly in their management.

(4) Here we touch upon a fourth problem, related to 2 and 3, in which studies are just beginning to be made, that is, the possible relationship of psychological disturbances to structural alteration. The viewpoint of disease bequeathed to us from the nineteenth century could be indicated in the following formula:

Cellular disease → Structural alteration → Physiological (or functional) disturbance.

In the twentieth century this formula underwent alteration in some situations. For example, in essential hypertension and vascular disease the formula was altered to read:

Functional disturbance → Cellular disease → Structural alteration.

We are still in the dark as to what may precede the functional disturbance as in the example just cited of essential hypertension and the resulting vascular disease. It seems possible that future investigations will permit us to say that it is possible for a psychological disturbance to antedate the functional alteration. Then the formula would read:

Psychological disturbances → Functional impairment → Cellular disease → Structural alteration.

With the last problem, however, this discussion is not greatly concerned. It is restricted for the most part to known psychosomatic relationships, in other words, a discussion of clinical problems for which there are immediate practical applications.

The Present Management of Psychosomatic Problems

The Illness Is "Functional"

How does modern medicine handle these patients? When we review our present management, we find that the patients in group (1) are commonly told that no organic disease is present and that the whole thing is "functional". They are dismissed often without further care, only to land eventually in the hands of some irregular practitioner or quack healer. Certainly in dealing with many of these patients it is necessary to do more than assure the patient of the absence of physical disease. Nor does it do to dismiss a patient with the statement that his illness is "functional". To the physician this term usually means "psychogenic", although he does not always admit it, even to himself. All kinds of twists and turns are taken to avoid the use of the hated term, psychogenic. Often "neurogenic" replaces it, and thus the physician is permitted to hold on to the notion that somehow there is a physical answer to the problem. This point will be discussed shortly.

Hamman[1] has written with a great deal of understanding on this subject: "When I was a student, the course in psychiatry consisted of lectures upon insanity and the demonstration of patients with gross disorders of thought and conduct. I had no interest in the topics and the patients distressed and disturbed me. I was greatly relieved when the course was over and never dreamed that I should find any occasion upon which to apply what I had heard and seen. I fully determined to have nothing further to do with psychiatry and unfortunately I held very obstinately to this determination. As a matter of fact, I still hold to it as regards what I then considered to be the province of psychiatry. I say that this determination was unfortunate because it prevented me from understanding what is the true domain of psychiatry, and so blinded me that it was many years before I could see the fruitful application of psychiatry to the daily problems of practice. In a word, the practicing physician is not at all interested in what he scornfully regards as the medicine of the madhouse and the asylum; but he is vitally interested in what we may call every day psychiatry. At least he becomes interested in it when his interest is properly aroused by the demonstration of the importance and value of the application of psychiatry to his daily work. He must know a little about gross disorders of the mind, but only enough to see clearly that these extreme alterations are merely exaggerations of trends and reactions that he may observe in himself, in his friends, in his patients. If a physician is once persuaded to look within himself and to learn to identify unaccountable variations in mood and energy as the analogue of a manic-depressive cycle, the habit of ascribing failure and disappointment to ill luck or persecution as the promptings of paranoia, day dreams (in which satisfaction is secured for the rubs and indignities of life and retributive disaster showered upon enemies) as the harmless whisperings of schizophrenia, certain exaggerated reactions as the masks for defeats and inadequacies, various somatic symptoms as excuses for retreat from difficult or unpleasant situations, he will forever have an enduring interest in psychiatry."

Suspicion of Physical Disease

Sometimes the patient is told that the physician does not think that anything is the matter, but suspicion is cast upon some organ or system which needs watching and care. For example, the patient with symptoms referred to the heart region is told that his heart is all right. Nevertheless he is cautioned to rest, medicine is given, and each time that he visits the physician his heart is examined again, or his blood pressure is taken. It is impossible to eradicate the suspicion of organic disease under such circumstances. This point will be considered later, but here it may be emphasized that in dealing with the majority of "functional" problems we must examine thoroughly, satisfy ourselves as to the absence of physical changes and then stop examining with the firm statement, "You have no evidence of organic disease".

Pathological Curiosities

Very frequently following "thorough study" by means of the usual medical history physical examination and laboratory investigation, some "pathologic curiosity"* is discovered, which really has nothing to do with the illness, but the patient then is treated from the standpoint of disease and is subjected to unnecessary medical or surgical treatment, which in many instances intensifies the neurotic condition. For example, a common cause of fatigue is not infection but emotional conflict which uses up so much energy that little is left for other purposes. A patient with chronic fatigue may be studied from every possible physical standpoint and finally, especially in the presence of long continued, low fever, suspicion rests upon minimal and obsolete tuberculosis of the lungs.

* By "pathologic curiosity" is meant some congenital or acquired lesion that has no significance from the standpoint of the present illness.

Long periods of rest in bed or sanitarium may follow. The error in the study of such cases is the fixation on physical factors and the absence of attention to emotional factors so that the physician himself becomes a "pathogenic agent" in helping to "fix the neurosis".

In other words the attitude of modern medicine is not so very different toward these patients from that described in 1884 by Clifford Allbutt,[2] the great English clinician, who said in speaking of the visceral neuroses: "A neuralgic woman seems thus to be peculiarly unfortunate. However bitter and repeated may be her visceral neuralgias, she is told either that she is hysterical or that it is all uterus. In the first place she is comparatively fortunate, for she is only slighted; in the second case she is entangled in the net of the gynecologist, who finds her uterus, like her nose, is a little on one side, or again, like that organ, is running a little, or it is as flabby as her biceps, so that the unhappy viscus is impaled upon a stem, or perched upon a prop, or is painted with carbolic acid every week in the year except during the long vacation when the gynecologist is grouse-shooting, or salmon-catching, or leading the fashion in the Upper Engadine. Her mind thus fastened to a more or less nasty mystery becomes newly apprehensive and physically introspective and the morbid chains are riveted more strongly than ever. Arraign the uterus, and you fix in the woman the arrow of hypochrondia, it may be for life."

The Organic Tradition in Medicine

As a consequence of this structural and physiological tradition in medicine a large number of physicians pride themselves upon their unwillingness to concede the absence of physical disease when dealing with an obscure illness. In discussing such a patient they are apt to say "but there must be something the matter", meaning that there must be a physical basis for the illness. And they furthermore believe that future researches along the lines of physical medicine will eventually uncover the hidden causes, infectious, allergic, endocrine or metabolic, responsible for such obscure illnesses.

Still another group of physicians are willing to believe that psychic factors have something to do with illness, but they have only a vague notion of the part that such factors play. These physicians recognize that there is a "neurogenic factor" or a "large nervous element" present, but they look upon this feature as a secondary one and probably a consequence of the physical disorder. While freely acknowledging the relation of psychic causes to such physiological phenómena as blushing, weeping, gooseflesh, vomiting and diarrhea, nevertheless they find it difficult to believe that more prolonged, chronic disturbances of a physiological nature possibly can be psychic in origin.

They are the physicians, who often remark about a patient, "but he does not look neurotic", perhaps imagining that such a patient should by his general apprehension or by evidences of physical nervousness betray the fact that neurosis is present. Their approach to the emotional problem is apt to consist of the question, "Are you worried about anything?" Unfortunately most neurotics do not betray their neurosis in their appearance, nor is the approach to their emotional problem so simple that the direct question, "Are you worried about anything?", will produce material of importance.

Diagnostic Problems in Psychosomatic Medicine

More specifically then, what are some of the diagnostic and therapeutic problems of psychosomatic medicine and how are they to be approached?

First, there is the failure to recognize neurosis and treatment of the patient as "organically" diseased. This happens most frequently, as already suggested, because modern clinical medicine attempts to establish the diagnosis of "functional" disease by ruling out "organic" disease through medical history, physical examination and laboratory investigation. The point that I particularly wish to make is that the diagnosis of "functional" illness must be established not simply by exclusion of "organic" disease but on its own characteristics as well. In other words neurosis has its own distinctive features to be discovered by psychosomatic study, for only in this way can serious errors in diagnosis and treatment be avoided. If the above statements are admitted to be correct, it must follow that personality study is just as important in the problems of illness as laboratory investigation.

This kind of approach will do a great deal to relieve the fear of the physician that he is missing something organic, because it will supply him with additional information to confirm his diagnosis of functional disease. It is perfectly true, of course, that structural alterations can be overlooked and the patient treated only as a functional case, which is the reverse of the situation above mentioned. Physicians are constantly harassed by this fear of overlooking "organic" disease. They are of the opinion, when dealing with this class of patients, that the structural disease is hidden and will come to light with the passage of time. Again this may be true but in the majority of instances is not.

A recent study from the Mayo Clinic is illuminating in this regard. Macy and Allen[3] studied the records of 235 patients approximately six years after the diagnosis of chronic nervous exhaustion had been made with the idea that, if the clinical picture at the first examination was due to unrecognized "organic" disease, such "organic" disease should be detected by subsequent examinations over a period of years. The accuracy of the diagnosis proved to be 94 per cent., which seems to indicate that this kind of "functional" illness, at any rate, is not due to "organic" disease. It is interesting to note in passing that 289 separate operations had been performed on 200 patients of the group that they studied.

The "Either-Or" Concept

When emotional factors are associated with actual "organic" changes, too little attention is paid to the emotional factors. The feeling exists and the statement is made that "the physical findings are sufficient to account for the illness". In this connection let me again emphasize that just as we cannot limit ourselves simply to the exclusion of "organic" disease in dealing with the purely "functional" group, so even more importantly in the second group is there the necessity for not resting content with the finding of an "organic" lesion. The day is near at hand for the final outmoding of the "either-or" concept, either functional or organic, in diagnosis and to place in its stead the idea of how much of one and how much of the other, that is, how much of the problem is emotional and how much is physical and what is the relationship between them. This is truly the psychosomatic concept of medicine.

In a well written and remarkably lucid consideration of the "cause" of illness Halliday[4] indicated the approach to this complicated problem with a simple illustration.

Let us take, says Halliday, a fragment of conversation, which may be overheard when a toddler begins to howl in the street.

> Onlooker to mother: "Why is he crying?"
> Mother: "Oh, he cries at anything; he is just a baby".
> Small brother: "He saw a cat and it frightened him".
> Onlooker: "Well, he has got a fine pair of lungs anyway".

"These remarks provide an explanation of the child's mode of behavior in terms of the three fields of etiological discourse. In the field of the *individual* the cause is announced to be the characteristic of 'being a baby': in the field of *environment* the encounter with a cat: in the field of *mechanism* the lungs in their instrumental perfection. It will be noted that, if any mode of behavior is to take place, 'cause' must operate in all three fields at a particular point in time. In the example quoted, we may assume that the behaviour called crying would not have appeared in the absence of (a) the characteristic of being a baby, or (b) the environment factor of the cat, or (c) the mechanism integrity of the respiratory organs."

Halliday then explains that, when the findings as to cause in each of the three fields of "etiological discourse" can be related to one another, we may say that the illness is explained. Thus, in diphtheria "the cause in the first field is the characteristic summarized by the phrase 'being Schick-positive'; cause in the second field is an encounter with the diphtheria bacillus; cause in the third field is the toxin produced on the fauces . . ."

When we think in terms of the psychosomatic point of view, we must employ the same approach. Thus in peptic ulcer we must think (1) of the individual, "what kind of person is he?" (predisposition, physical and psychological); (2) of the environment, "what has he met?" (tobacco and food, social and psychological problems), and (3) of mechanism, "what happened?" (vascular supply, hyperacidity, hypermotility, etc.)

Here the psychic element is an integral part of the study, one of many and diverse etiological factors, emerging at various levels of the personality development.

At this point it may not be amiss to quote further from Halliday in regard to that long confused subject "functional" versus "organic" disease.

Functional and Organic

"Another source of obscurity is to confuse the technique of approach with the object of study. A common example is the mysterious phrase 'mind and body'. This seems to indicate that an individual is composed of two distinct and contrasted entities, a mind entity and a body entity. If the phrase has any meaning, it is this; the individual may be studied by a psychological approach, and the individual may be studied by a structural or physical approach. It is our techniques or methods of investigation which are diverse and multiple, not the individual, who is a unity."

"The words functional and organic suggest that illness may be divided into two distinct kinds, and much has been written on this faulty premise. For example, it has been stated that, if an unorthodox healer cures a patient, the illness must have been functional and presumably not the concern of the scientific medical man, who deals only in true or organic illness. Again, it has been stated that the word "functional" is applicable to a morbid process which is "reversible". But what of lobar pneumonia, warts and on occasion even lipoma? A little consideration shows that the words organic and functional are merely examples of technical slang, which express in convenient form the following: In certain illnesses or in certain stages of these illnesses a structural technique or approach, e.g. anatomical, histological, provides a positive finding; in slang terms the illness is organic. In other illnesses the application of the structural approach provides a negative finding, whereas the application of other techniques of approach provides a positive finding; in slang terms the illness is functional. Many writers, failing to appreciate the only meaning which can be given to these terms, seem to have imagined that by using them a fundamental etiological basis for the division of illness has been achieved."

The following diagrams are used frequently in illustrating this topic. Fig. 1 illustrates the usual approach in the study of illness which presumably will lead to a diagnosis. It consists of the bare facts of the medical history, the physical examination and the various laboratory investigations. It is diagnosis by exclusion and fails in so many instances simply because the life situation of the patient, in other words, a study of the emotional life, which may provide the key to the solution of the problem, is neglected completely or at most investigated inadequately. The proper psychosomatic approach is shown in Fig. 2 where the personality study occurs at the same time as the physical and laboratory study.

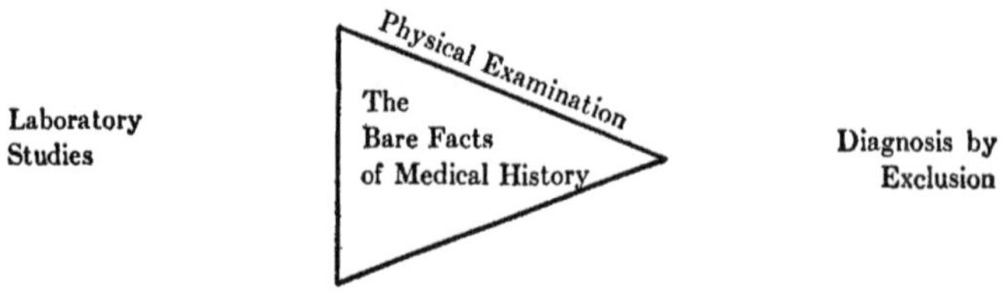

FIG. 1*

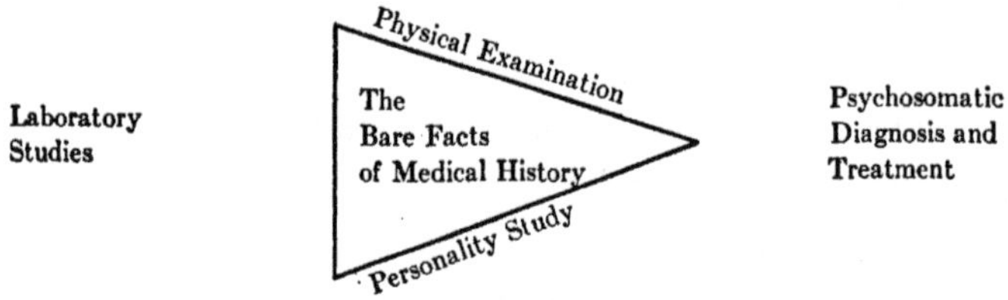

FIG. 2

THE NATURE OF EMOTIONAL PROBLEMS

We know that these patients have been badly handled. Can we do any better? What is the matter with them and how should they be treated? First of all let us say that these patients are suffering from disturbances in their emotional lives; that is, the illness is wholly or in part of psychological origin and can be studied satisfactorily and treated only if this factor is dealt with adequately. The ill health arises in a predisposed individual usually from long standing dissatisfactions in the business, social or home life, and this failure of adjustment to environment is manifested by a disturbance in some part of the personality either as bodily symptoms of various kinds capable of mimicking almost any disease or as affections of the spirit resulting in attacks of anxiety, obsessions, phobias, depression and other disturbances of mood. What is not so generally realized is that the mere discovery of the so-called dissatisfactions or unpleasant occurrences in the life situation of the individual is not a sufficient explanation nor even an adequate indication of the psychic background of the illness. In

* From Weiss, E., and English, O. S.: Psychosomatic Medicine, p. 7.[10]

other words, besides excluding physical disease in the one case and correctly evaluating the part it plays in another, it is of the greatest importance to know the patient's ability to adjust to certain life situations, his pattern of reacting to them, the degree of anxiety in his make-up and the nature and seriousness of his conflicts. Psychosomatic study is necessary, if we are to establish a specific relationship of the psychic situation to the personality of the individual. Just as the typhoid bacillus, specific for typhoid fever, depends upon the susceptibility of the individual, so does specificity of the psychic event depend upon personality structure of the person. To make such studies one must have some training in psychopathology. When psychopathology is given an equal place with tissue pathology in our medical curriculum and is as well taught, we will finally realize that psychotherapy is an integral part of our medical discipline.

Psychopathology

It would seem that we are rapidly approaching such an understanding. The great impetus given to this subject by military medicine surely will result in the proper emphasis in medical teaching. It can be truly said that World War I established psychiatry on a firm scientific basis, and World War II is seeing its final integration into general medicine, in other words, psychosomatic medicine. When this integration has been satisfactorily accomplished, there will no longer be need for the term, psychosomatic; both parts of the term will be implicit in the word medicine.

It is impossible in a short discussion to cover the subject of psychopathology. Only a few principles can be mentioned. There is no sharp line between normal and neurotic. Anyone may "break under pressure", in other words, become neurotic. Witness the combat neuroses of World War II; robust men with previously healthy personalities succumbed to "combat fatigue", when enough pressure was put upon them. The same thing is true in civil life, although not so common. Generally speaking persons, who develop severe psychosomatic disorders or pronounced neurotic disturbances, are people who have been predisposed by psychopathology established early in life. In other words an adult neurosis depends to a great extent upon a childhood neurosis.

Influence of Childhood Environment. — A point of view which I have tried to stress is that for the most part psychotherapy is necessary because our educational processes are confined to the intellect. In other words our children receive scientific management from an intellectual standpoint, but for a variety of reasons, mainly constitutional and family influences, the emotional growth is stunted. It is the retarded emotional development which is fundamentally responsible for psychosomatic illness. In other words, if the intellectual age and the emotional age differ sharply, the background for illness of psychological origin exists. One might go further to say that man has four ages, first, his *chronological age*, second, his *physical age*, third, his *intellectual age* and fourth, his *emotional age.* For example, one easily can think of an adult, who is chronologically forty, physically fifty, intellectually twelve and emotionally only five. And it might be said that, if these various ages are in harmony, he is apt to be well, and if they are in disharmony, he is apt to be ill. Such persons, and the world is full of them, furnish the soil for the development of psychosomatic illness. Psychotherapy is a process which aims to bring about reëducation of the emotions and the psychosomatic approach takes cognizance of all factors, physical, intellectual and emotional.

It is not unusual for physicians to recommend pregnancy and parenthood as a cure for neurotic illness, instability in the husband or threatened divorce or separation. This prescription is rarely, if ever, of value. It is a pretty safe rule that the unstable person will not be helped by becoming a parent but usually will be made worse as a result of the added responsibility. How often upon taking the history of neurotic persons, and especially women, do we hear, "I was perfectly well until my first child was born; I haven't had a well day since." It is true that some neurotic women will feel better during pregnancy, but they pay dearly for their short period of improvement. Nor should the cost to the child be forgotten. Not only does parenthood not cure neurosis, but it prepares the way for another spoiled life, because this is surely one of the ways in which neurosis is perpetuated. The atmosphere of the home, in which there is serious emotional maladjustment, creates the culture medium for the development of further emotional problems. This is the real "social disease". The advice to an incompatible couple, "What you need is a child — then you will have a common interest", is as unenlightened as it is dangerous. While it may succeed in holding the marriage together, who can say how many children thus are sacrificed on the altar of incompatibility.

Pregnancy, like marriage, is an excellent institution and undoubtedly will persist, but it is not to be recommended for therapeutic reasons. My feeling is that we must reverse the process of recommending parenthood for emotional maladjustment and instead advise birth control until there is adequate emotional development for rearing a child.

What has just been said suggests that there is such a thing as "psychological infection" and that the atmosphere of the home is the source of contagion.

The Rôle of Anxiety. — The central problem of disturbances of emotional origin is anxiety. One cannot be well oriented in the field of psychiatry or psychosomatic medicine without considerable knowledge of the rôle of anxiety in the development of illness of emotional origin. It lies at the root of all psychopathology and for that matter plays an important part in normal behavior. The human being from birth onward has a need for optimum conditions of comfort as the growth processes advance. During the first months of life the body needs food and warmth not only because of their importance for physical growth but also for emotional satisfaction. The world of the infant is small, and what would seem to be of little consequence in the life of the adult may be of primary importance in his life.

The Feeding Process. — The sensual pleasure derived from the feeding process is an example. The total nutritional process will leave a pleasant memory impression upon the mind, if the good will and esteem of those who take care of the child are added to the feeding process. A sufficiency of food of the right kind, given at regular intervals and administered by one who loves the child, does much to lay the groundwork for a relaxed personality which feels the world to be a friendly place. Thus the nutritional process, a feeling of security and the capacity to love are blended harmoniously.

If, on the other hand, there is insufficient food or a sudden change in the type of food or method of feeding, or if there is impatience or hostility on the part of the one who feeds the child, then the distress of hunger or of cold or the lack of emotional warmth produce anxiety. There seems to be a blind sense, which we may be permitted to call instinct, that, if such conditions continue long enough, death will ensue. In the beginning this apprehension that something threatens the integrity of the self is a reflex pattern, and as a matter of fact much of it remains reflex throughout life. An important part of the therapeutic educational process is the effort to help the individual to understand the source of his anxiety and to teach him what he must do to relieve it. It is fundamental to our understanding of personality development to realize how much basic insecurity and resulting anxiety may occur through deprivation of food, warmth or love or through misunderstanding of the physiological rhythms during the early weeks and months of life, and that such difficult situations in the life of a child will produce anxiety through a definite physiological mechanism.

The Components of Anxiety. — Anxiety has two elements, a psychic and a somatic or physiological component. The psychic component of anxiety is the sensory cortical registration of displeasure and apprehension, the instinctual awareness that something is wrong, and the somatic component is the motor response of rapid heart action, rapid or embarrassed respiration, flushing, perspiration and even a disturbance in the function of the gastrointestinal tract. Anxiety can make its effects felt in every tissue of the body, although in many cases it seems to limit its expression predominantly to those organs and tissues supplied by the autonomic nervous system.

The Unconscious. — Parents, unaware of the serious effects of trauma and deprivation in the life of the child, may permit much psychopathology in the form of anxiety to develop in the first year of life. Unwanted children are neglected often and fed carelessly as to rhythm or improperly as to the type of food, or they are weaned forcibly and without regard for the limited adaptive powers of the infant to a new experience. Depending upon the constitution of the infant, such treatment is apt to cause anxiety. Memory impressions are made, and psychological reflexes are built up. These patterns are "forgotten" with the passing of time, but if numerous or highly charged with anxiety, they may form the nucleus of illness later on. Very little of what happens to us is truly forgotten. Each event is registered on the brain as a memory with varying degrees of clearness, and what cannot be recalled is referred to as unconscious. That part of the mental mechanism, which holds these memories and their accompanying charges of emotion, is called the *unconscious*, commonly referred to as the *unconscious mind*. The more pain, shame, disgust or other painful affect that occurs during development, the more likely that repression will occur, and the more difficult it will be to recall the traumatic event in later life. The emotions combined with the memories and ideas accumulated during growth make the unconscious a dynamic center of psychic energy rather than a static storehouse of innocuous impressions.

Anxiety and the Gastrointestinal Tract.— The digestive processes form the most important phase of the child's life during the first year. If this function has been exposed to, and associated with, too much strife, deprivation or ill will, they become associated in the mind of the infant. One is "conditioned" to the other. The memories of unpleasant experiences associated with the gastrointestinal function exist in that part of the mind we call the unconscious. As the child grows older, life conditions often improve, but a revival of the same situation of deprivation at the hands of fate or ill will from classmates, business associates or spouse may reactivate anxiety. Now, if this anxiety and its cause are recognized and can be dealt with through escape, compromise or sharing with some stronger person the experiences and their effects, thus gaining reassurance and new strength, a solution is found. If the anxiety is not recognized and is not adequately discharged, it finds no release and must exert its force upon the body itself. Then some organ or organ system is very apt to bear the brunt of this potent force and will function badly as a result. If during the years, when the swallowing and digestive processes are of paramount importance in the life of the child, there were anxiety-producing experiences, then similar experiences later in life are likely to reproduce symptoms of the upper gastrointestinal tract.

Organ Neurosis.— With regard to other related factors one may say that the earlier in life and the more profound the psychological traumatic experience, the more serious the resulting psychosomatic affection may prove to be. The term organ neurosis is used frequently to designate the disturbance in the working of a bodily organ resulting from psychic forces. But there are various degrees of organ neurosis. Perhaps the most simple expression of psychological conflict is the so-called conversion hysteria in which the symptom is the symbolic expression of the psychological conflict. Thus nervous vomiting may have disgust as one of its meanings. A more severe degree of organ neurosis, or what is sometimes referred to as a vegetative neurosis, is a disorder in which actual physical changes take place as a result of a profound psychological disturbance. Cardiospasm is an example. Just as psychosis probably represents in the mental sphere earlier and more serious emotional traumatic experience than neurosis, so does vegetative neurosis represent earlier and more profound psychological disturbance than conversion hysteria so far as psychosomatic medicine is concerned.

Relation of Symptoms to Life Situation. — There are certain epochs in life when psychosomatic affections are apt to make their appearance. These are outlined in Table I.

TABLE I *

CORRELATION OF LIFE SITUATION AND SYMPTOM FORMATION

Oral Stage (first year of life)	
Food and love are being given to the child with no responsibilities exacted in return.	Refusal to nurse; fretfulness when nursing is over, or contentment? Protest to weaning (crying or vomiting)?
Anal Period (1–3 years)	
Responsibility of cleanliness and neatness has to be taken over in toilet habits and in other activities. This is not easy, and the child needs much friendliness, understanding and patience to accomplish it without anxiety or detriment to personality development.	Is toilet training accepted, or is child stubbornly resistive, wetting and soiling beyond usual age of established cleanliness? Is there constipation, temper tantrum, stubbornness, resentment, destructiveness?
Genital Period (3–6 years)	
Period of increasing general and sexual curiosity. Period of beginning tender attachment to parent of opposite sex.	Excessive masturbation, fretfulness, disobedience, aggression, cruelty, eneuresis, poor adjustment to other children.
Latent Period (6–12 years)	
Period of primary education, identification with ideals and authority.	How is social adjustment? Does he do well in studies? Does he mix well in classroom and playground? Is there sexual delinquency, truancy, aggressiveness, cruelty, poor sportsmanship, seclusiveness?
Puberty (12–15 years)	
Period of maturity and beginning activity of sex glands. Extra impetus given to entire emotional life, especially emotional patterns pertaining to love and sexuality.	Are there anxiety attacks; fears of disease, of death, of harming others; nightmares, irritability, social anxiety, seclusiveness, loss of appetite, vomiting, diarrhea, cardiac palpitation?

* From Weiss, E., and English, O. S.: Psychosomatic Medicine, p. 541[10].

TALE I—(*Continued*)

Adolescence (15–21 years) Period of secondary and college education. Often the need to leave. the home and live among strangers. Beginning of love relationships. Planning for life work, career, home, marriage. The fields of competition widen. Conflicts over religion or ideals and current behavior.	Are there symptoms occurring on leaving home, on beginning or ending a love affair, because of inability to compete? Are there seclusiveness and anxiety? A period in which the incidence of somatic symptoms is high!
Early Adult Life (21–40 years) Decisions must be made about love, marriage, work, parenthood. Parental support drops away after 21, if not before. Responsibilities of adulthood are thrust upon one. They catch up with one whether he is prepared for them or not. May be stress of military service.	Symptoms may appear in relation to engagement, marriage, pregnancy, childbirth, loss of job, failure to adjust in marriage, or new environment. "War neuroses".
Middle Adult Life (40–60 years) Period when anticipated ambitions are lost or realized. Children begin to leave home. Women go through menopause. Both sexes have to adjust to changing values.	Women have to cope with the menopause and loss of companionship of the children. May not be resourceful enough, become depressed and anxious. For men it is the age of business success and failure. Of divorce. Reactions to physical disease. Cancerophobia, depression and suicide.
Late Adult Life and Old Age Period (60 years plus) Period of retirement for men, forced or voluntary. Dependency on children for support in both sexes. Problems of physical disease (geriatrics) and the need for care by others.	Symptoms of anxiety often appear after retirement, and many symptoms are due to the frictions incident to living with children and in-laws. Arteriosclerosis and senile dementia usually make social adjustment more difficult.

In the beginning of this discussion I suggested that there was no sharp line between normal and neurosis. Nevertheless there are certain distinguishing features, and indeed one of the first problems that presents itself to the physician in dealing with a patient is to try to determine whether one is dealing with a normal, a neurotic or a psychotic personality. Glover[5] has defined the normal personality as being (1) free of symptoms, (2) unhampered by mental conflict, (3) having a satisfactory working capacity and (4) being able to love someone other than oneself. Neurosis and psychosis show pronounced deviations in each of these spheres as shown in Table II.

TABLE II *

NORMAL PERSONALITY		NEUROSES	PSYCHOSES
EMOTIONAL FEATURES			
Unhampered by mental conflict	Ability to reach a decision without too much stress or delay	Hampering mental conflicts Mild mood disturbances Capacity for decision impaired	Mental conflicts Severe mood disturbances Capacity for decision impaired
Satisfactory work capacity	Enjoys work No undue fatigue No need for frequent change Maintains optimum efficiency	Work not enjoyed Fatigue a frequent and pronounced symptom Impairment work efficiency	Severe disturbances in efficiency; concentration upon or participation in work may be totally impossible
Ability to love someone other than self	Takes pleasure in social relationships, marital relationships, parental relationships. Can understand the emotional needs and point of view of others and make appropriate response	Disturbances in ability to enjoy social relations, *i.e.*, inability to relate themselves to others in such a way as to gain security and emotional response. Limited capacity to give emotionally, yet some conventional relation to others is maintained even though imperfect and at the cost of anxiety	Severe disturbances in ability to relate themselves to others, in fact, they tend to renounce their relations to others more or less completely
PHYSICAL STATUS Absence of symptoms (of neurotic origin)		Conversion of emotional stress (anxiety) into somatic symptoms in one or many parts of body	Somatic symptom formation during onset of illness, but eventually symptoms are in sphere or control of emotion, thought, speech, action Varying amount of loss in control of well integrated thought, emotion and speech, and regressions to childish levels—and/or solution of anxiety through false beliefs or false sensory perception

* From Weiss, E., and English, O. S.: Psychosomatic Medicine, p. 42[10].

Psychosomatic Study in Illness

In a general way it may be stated that in addition to the physical study the psychosomatic approach consists in getting to know the patient as a human being rather than as a mere medical case. Too often, as already stated, the patient is looked upon as only a physiological mechanism and is studied by means of medical history and physical examination aided by "instruments of precision" and chemical tests. Tape measure and test tubes carry the erroneous notion of exactness and thoroughness, erroneous because the emotional life of the individual, which may hold the key to the solution of the problem, is not investigated or at best, inadequately so.

While the subject cannot be discussed in detail, usually the best procedure in dealing with these patients is as follows.

(1) To satisfy ourselves and establish their confidence, a thorough medical history should be taken; this must contain more information regarding the family and social background of the patient than most of our present histories do. Many years ago Kilgore[6] criticized the standardization of hospital clinical records. His criticism, part of which follows, still stands. "The amazing epidemic of standardization that has been visited upon American institutions in this century has not permitted our clinical records to escape. In practically all hospitals with any pretensions one finds the clinical records usually in trim aluminum covers with some variation in charts and laboratory sheets but with the clinical history proper invariably displayed under a stereotyped system of paragraphs with or without the guidance of printed forms. The histories thereby are given an orderliness, which is pleasing to the eye, and which makes a tacit claim to the admirable quality of thoroughness.

"And yet these standardized histories are open to a very serious criticism. My criticism may be interpreted from the following illustration: In a medical ward of a class A teaching hospital I recently saw a Jewess, aged forty-five years. Five minutes' conversation brought out the facts that she had always been in reasonably good health until after the death of her husband a year ago, that she then looked hopefully for support from her eldest son, but that about three months ago she gradually experienced the final and crushing conviction that his talents were limited to the selling of newspapers, which yielded a profit of less than a dollar a day. She, therefore, in addition to caring for her home and the younger children, took employment in a restaurant, standing eight hours a day washing dishes. Then came backache, sleepless nights of worry, anorexia, loss of 20 pounds, nervousness, utter exhaustion, hospitalization. Cursory examination revealed only the ordinary effects of such a life including possibly some thyroid disturbance.

"Now I ask of you sticklers for form and order, what do you suppose that woman's folder contained? Five and one-half closely written pages of matter comprised under twenty-eight captions, all neatly underlined with red ink and ruler! Figure out the time that probably took, and then ask yourselves how much time and energy remained to devote to the clinical problem of that woman. We toil through those five and one-half pages in search of useful bits of information. Here and there we find a few, fragmentary and uncorrelated. In the place for 'social condition' it is stated that she is a widow; under 'occupation' that she is a housewife; under 'marital history' that she has four children, but not a word about that fiasco of the eldest son. The paragraph on 'habits' speaks of weight loss but gives no hint of the possible cause. Breathlessly we work down to the captions 'complaint', 'onset of present illness' and 'course of present illness' and find only some sketchy references to pains in the back, palpitation, breathlessness on effort, gas in the stomach and so on, but never a word of the restaurant or the thoughts in the poor woman's head. Then comes the sacred array of paragraphs on the various systems with reiteration of shortness of breath under 'cardiorespiratory system' of stomach gas under 'gastrointestinal', etc., etc.

"The writer of this history was evidently painstaking and industrious, and yet what a mess he made of it! There is not the slightest doubt that if, before he ever set foot in the medical school, he had been confronted with this patient and had been asked to write down what he could find out about her condition, he would have done incomparably better. And as a commentary on the teaching of clinical history-taking is not that the height of irony? The reason for this enormity is obvious. The writer of the history has been so occupied in constructing and polishing the frame in order to meet the standard specifications that he has been unable to paint the picture; indeed, he has scarcely seen the patient and her experiences at all.

"This case, to be sure, is worse than many of our hospital clinical histories, but it is none the less a good illustration of a valid general criticism of unrestrained standardization, namely, stereotypism, perfunctoriness, mediocrity."

(2) After a medical history, which takes account of personal factors as well as "medical facts", we should make a complete physical examination and such laboratory tests as are necessary to exclude physical disease or to establish the precise nature of the organic problem and the amount of disability which it in itself is capable of causing.

(3) Having assured the patient that no physical disease is present in the first instance, or that it is present to a certain extent in the second group, but that the disability is out of proportion to the disease, it is usually easy by examples of psychic causes for such physiological disturbances as blushing, gooseflesh, palpitation and diarrhea to make the patient understand that a disturbance in his emotional life may be responsible for the symptoms.

(4) Then important clues for this disturbance usually can be found by en-

couraging a discussion of problems centering around vocational, religious, marital and parent-child relationships. Usually this is best accomplished indirectly rather than by direct questions. The more one can persuade such a patient to talk about "his other troubles" the sooner do we come to an understanding of the "present troubles". The greater our success in switching the conversation from symptoms to personal affairs, the sooner do we come into possession of the real problem disturbing the patient. We are all familiar with the patient, who is preoccupied with his bowel function and wants to talk about nothing else, whose whole life really seems to surround his daily bowel movement. It is the physician's duty tactfully to switch him from a discussion of his symptoms to a discussion of his personal life. Encourage him to talk about himself as a person rather than as a medical case. In adults domestic problems and professional and business relationships play a large part in functional illness. In young, unmarried people, family relationships, choice of a career and often religious and sexual problems are important topics for discussion.

Usually one or more of three special fears are uppermost in the minds of such patients. One of the most common is fear of cancer, cancerphobia. A great many patients think they have cancer, and indeed most women who consult physicians will have the idea at some time. They do not always express it; in fact, they rarely directly express their cancer fears. They often disguise it by a complaint about a lump, a swelling or a curious sensation in the abdomen or breast, and when they are assured at the end of a complete physical examination that they are free from organic disease, they heave a sigh of relief and say, "Oh, I am so glad because I thought I might have a cancer". With all of the propaganda for the early detection of cancer these fears are exaggerated, and I presume it is the price that we must pay for instructing people about cancer. I am not, of course, advising against such instruction; it is only that we must realize that we add to the apprehension of many patients by our emphasis upon the early detection of cancer.

Another common fear, as already suggested, is the fear of heart disease. When pain in the precordial region as well as rapid beating of the heart, breathlessness and fatigue occur, suspicion of heart disease often arises. If we remember that the pain of cardiac neurosis bears no definite relationship to effort, is frequently described as sticking, needle-like or soreness, that often it is associated with inframammary tenderness and hyperalgesia, so that the pressure of the stethoscope sometimes elicits it, and that it may be accompanied by a sense of choking as well as sighing respirations, we will have no difficulty in the differential diagnosis, particularly when we associate these symptoms with the whole picture and life situation of the individual with cardiac neurosis.

(5) The inability to concentrate often gives rise to the fear of "losing the mind". Along with this fear frequently there are ideas of suicide. Both are

very distressing to the patient and usually are not volunteered. When the patient is assured that it is his feelings which are involved and not his "mind", and that the reason his "memory fails him" is because he is so preoccupied with concern over his problems, then he may confess his fear that he was "losing his mind" or his ideas of doing away with himself.

Once these ideas are brought to the surface and ventilated, and the patient receives sufficient reassurance, then often much improvement occurs. Indeed the intensity of the fear and the amount of reassurance necessary to abolish it serve as a crude index to the depth of the neurosis.

The Anxiety Attack

Quite frequently the first pronounced evidence of neurosis may be an anxiety attack, and again and again in studying the histories of patients with chronic invalidism of emotional origin we find that the first outspoken manifestation of illness was the sudden onset of anxiety with apprehension and dread. There is a feeling of weakness, sweating and a sensation that something terrible is about to happen. There is dyspnea, palpitation and sometimes, nausea. The attacks usually last only a few minutes and subside rather quickly but may last for an hour or more.. Weakness and fatigue follow. The emotional as well as the physical distress is so marked as to cause the patient to conclude that some very serious physical disability is present. Almost never does he conclude that his difficulty is emotional. Most people prefer to think that physical distress means physical disease, and unfortunately physicians too frequently have assisted them in this belief. When a patient with an acute anxiety attack is first examined, the physician notes the rapid pulse and listens to the pounding heart and all too often permits the patient to believe that the heart is diseased, that hyperthyroidism is present or covers his unwillingness to make a diagnosis of a psychological disorder by using some such term as neurocirculatory asthenia or autonomic imbalance. This is immediately reassuring but ultimately harmful. Sedatives are of very little help; if the anxiety is acute, sedation does not occur until the attack has spent itself anyhow. To be consistent one gives no treatment other than personal reassurance. To give drugs and do nothing about fear is to mislead the patient into feeling that his distress is due to altered physical pathology rather than to psychopathology.

In treating the personality for the factors which produce anxiety we must realize that the patient is apt to be an elusive, disinterested individual who, once over the first attack, does not want anyone to probe his feelings. When he begins to have frequent attacks and is afraid to go where the attack may occur, street, subway, stores, etc., he has regressed to a position in relation to his family which unconsciously he wishes to maintain. Hence the cooperation of the family is necessary to make him come to his physician where he can be apprised of his real troubles and learn to correct them.

Organ Language

A method of helping patients to understand their symptoms, which I find useful, is based upon the symbolism of symptoms. Patients are told that if they cannot find an outlet for tension of emotional origin by word or action, the body will find a means of expressing this tension through a kind of "organ language". The psychopathology responsible for "organ language" cannot be discussed in detail, but many clinical instances can be cited.

For example, if a patient cannot swallow satisfactorily, and no organic cause can be found, it may mean there is something in the life situation of the patient that he "cannot swallow". Nausea in the absence of organic disease sometimes means that the patient "cannot stomach" this or that environmental factor. Frequently a feeling of oppression in the chest accompanied by sighing respirations, again in the absence of organic findings, indicates that the patient has a "load on his chest" that he would like to get rid of by talking about his problems. The patient, who has lost his appetite and as a consequence has become severely undernourished, so-called "anorexia-nervosa", which in its minor manifestations is such a common problem, is very often emotionally starved before he becomes physically starved. When he learns to taste life, he will begin to taste food. The common symptom, fatigue, very often is due to emotional conflict, which uses up so much energy that little is left for other purposes. Again emotional tension of unconscious origin frequently expresses itself as muscle tension giving rise to aches and pains, and sometimes these are represented by sharp pains such as atypical neuralgia. Thus, we suggest that atypical neuralgia of the arm or face may be due to focal conflict as well as focal infection. An ache in the arm, instead of representing the response to a focus of infection, may mean that the patient would like to strike someone but is prevented from doing so by the affection or respect that is mingled with his hostility. Itching, for which no physical cause is found, very often represents dissatisfaction with the environment which the individual takes out upon himself; martyr-like he scratches himself instead of someone else. "All-gone" feelings in the epigastrium, "shaky legs" and even vertigo are common physical expressions of anxiety, and the anxiety attack, so frequently called a heart attack, a gall-bladder disturbance, hyperthyroidism, neurocirculatory asthenia, hyperinsulinism, etc., is still far from being understood in general clinical medicine in spite of the fact that Freud[7] described it more than forty years ago.

Many more examples could be given but are unnecessary. Only one more point remains before concluding this part of the discussion, and that is that the gastrointestinal tract is, above all other systems, the pathway through which emotions are often expressed in behavior. Why this is so becomes apparent in the study of psychopathology.

This whole approach can be summed up in the following fashion: Understanding illness and treating sick people consist of something more than a knowledge of disease; they necessitate looking upon illness as an aspect of behavior. It means that the nature of bodily disorders can be appreciated only when emotional factors are investigated in addition to physical factors. Such an approach can be applied to a wide variety of ailments and can be utilized very generally in talking with patients. Nor does it require a very high degree of intelligence on the part of the patient to follow this simple explanation. Patients in the clinic as well as those in private care can be dealt with in this fashion; they are just as susceptible to these psychosomatic disorders.

Sexual Factors

This again is a subject that cannot be treated in detail, but one point of importance does deserve consideration at this juncture, and that is the relation of sexuality to neuroses.

Ever since the introduction of the epoch-making studies of Freud to the problems of neurosis, medicine has misunderstood his conception of sexuality. He has been quoted often to the effect that disturbances in genital activity are the sole causes of the neuroses. This is very far from the truth. It is rather that difficulty in the sexual sphere appears as a revealing index to a neurotic personality and can be looked upon in that light. In other words, in much the same manner that urea retention serves as an index to an impending uremia, so do disturbances in the sexual life of the individual, such as varying degrees of frigidity in the female and varying degrees of impotence in the male, serve as a reliable index to the kind of personality that is very apt to develop a neurosis. Sexual difficulties are rarely in themselves the cause of the kind of the illness under consideration; when they are important and the patient has a satisfactory relationship to the physician, sufficient confidence will be gained eventually to permit discussion of these intimate matters. In women questions regarding menstruation and child-bearing often will lead naturally to such a discussion.

In this connection let me suggest a cautious attitude in regard to marital maladjustments, which are often in the background of obscure illnesses. The better these problems are understood from the standpoint of personality study, the clearer it becomes that serious emotional maladjustment is behind the marital problem. Consequently, casually to give advice regarding marriage and child-bearing, divorce and extramarital relationships as short cuts to involved emotional problems is to assume knowledge beyond present human understanding.

Psychotherapy

And now to come to a question frequently raised regarding these matters; "Suppose you do find something of importance in the emotional life of a patient, some conflict that is causing illness; What good does it do the patient to know? What can you do about it?"

First of all, it is often a great help to the patient to know that the ailment is not organic but is due to a disturbance in his emotional life. When a neurotic symptom is divorced from a fear of organic disease, cancer, for example, it loses its force, whereupon the slogan "carry on in spite of symptoms" often helps the patient a great deal. This is especially true, if the psychological approach, which we have discussed, is a part of the study, and the emotional background of the illness is made clear to the patient.

What Is Psychotherapy?

What, indeed, is psychotherapy? Too often it is assumed to be something vaguely referred to as "the application of the art of medicine". This defies analysis but seems to represent a combination of the experience and common sense of the seasoned practitioner, an intuitive knowledge of people, the cultivation of a charming bedside manner, such trifles as serving food in attractive dishes and the generous use of reassurance. The psychological approach in medicine, essential for psychotherapy, consists of something more. It is a medical discipline to an equal degree with internal medicine itself. It is an effort to understand the personality structure of patients, the mental mechanisms which are at work and the specific relationships of psychological situations in the precipitation of the illness.

Reassurance, in the majority of instances, unless combined with an analysis of the illness from the standpoint of the behavior, gives only temporary help and depending upon the degree of anxiety has to be repeated constantly, like a dose of digitalis in a failing heart. Closely allied to reassurance is another superficial treatment that rarely results in more than temporary help, i.e., environmental manipulation, without any attempt to give the patient insight into his conflicts.

Real psychotherapy, which is directly the opposite of simple reassurance, tries to make the patient understand the meaning of his symptoms and the nature of his conflicts. It is a process of reëducation and, when properly done, leads to sufficient emotional development so that the necessity for symptom formation is abolished. The best example of this kind of psychotherapy is psychoanalysis, but for various reasons this method cannot be applied directly to the majority of patients. Nevertheless, psychoanalytic insight and guidance prove adequate to handle the emotional factor in the majority of psychosomatic disturbances.

Between simple reassurance at one end of the scale and adequate psychoanalysis at the other there are all degrees of psychotherapy, which can be applied depending upon the degree of illness and the circumstances of the patient.

It is my hope that every physician will be trained in psychological medicine so that he may be able to understand and manage the many emotional problems that are presented to him daily. It is possible that some internists will wish to perfect themselves in psychosomatic medicine in the same way that others interest themselves chiefly in cardiology, gastroenterology and other fields. Certainly better training facilities should be developed for residents in medicine to acquire the psychosomatic approach to medical problems. At the same time an opportunity for residents in psychiatry to have more medical training would do a great deal to break down the false alignment between psychiatry and medicine. It would provide us with capable teachers, who could cooperate in giving medical students the psychosomatic point of view. Therein lies our hope for an important development in medicine. As a part of this process and essential for its development general hospitals must establish divisions for the observation and treatment of psychoneurotic and psychosomatic problems. The time has passed for psychiatry to lead an isolated existence. Until it is brought into physical proximity with general medicine it cannot achieve final integration into the body of medical knowledge.

Major and Minor Psychotherapy

A considerable number of the patients, whom we have been considering, cannot be sent to psychiatrists, nor is it necessary. Not that there is anything reprehensible about consulting a psychiatrist, this too is a problem of education, but there are not enough psychiatrists to take care of the thousands of patients, and moreover, as I have tried to show, a great part of this work lies in the field of general medicine. Another way of stating the problem is to say that there is a major and a minor psychotherapy just as there is a major and a minor surgery. Many physicians, who practice general medicine, feel themselves capable of doing minor surgery, but only a few have the skill to attempt major surgery. They would not permit themselves to attempt something for which they are not prepared. This is just as true in regard to psychotherapy. The general physician must be able to treat the minor ailments, but he must be able also to recognize when the problem is beyond him, and then refer the patient elsewhere for major psychotherapy. Such knowledge and such an approach frequently will save the patient from unnecessary troublesome and expensive medical or surgical treatment with a resulting further degree of invalidism. So much for some of the more obvious benefits to be achieved by the psychosomatic approach. But as a part of what is intended as a practical introduction to psychosomatic medicine a word must be said about the cost of psychotherapy.

Cost of Psychotherapy

What about the question of time, effort and the expense of psychotherapy? True it is that all of this takes time and effort and must be paid for, yet when we look into the time, effort and expense that have been expended by many patients or by institutions taking care of these patients in the usual medical approach, we realize that an hour or two well spent in a discussion of the life situation of such patients would obviate a great deal of this expense. It is amazing what the total expense of a great many of these unnecessary studies amounts to so far as the institution is concerned, and of course the same thing is true in the case of private patients. The day is close at hand, when we will regard some of these thick-chart patients, this polyphysical approach, with the same amusement and disdain with which we now regard the polypharmacy of a bygone age in medicine. Hospitals are beginning to understand that it is not only intelligent but economical to utilize the service of a psychiatrist in the general medical division, and this same idea could be applied with great benefit to the much discussed medical insurance plans. To quote Dunbar[8] on this subject; "Although the psychic factor is more regularly overlooked in the case of severe somatic damage . . ., and in the handling of convalescence and chronic illness, it is no less important in our failures — patients who wander from physician to physician and clinic to clinic. If a patient has received treatment from a dozen or two private physicians and half a dozen clinics and has submitted to elaborate and expensive laboratory procedures in each place, one may be justified in suspecting that his physicians have in some way failed to find out what was the matter. Usually when this happens it is because a prominent psychic factor is present. Such patients are a real drain on hospital and clinic time and funds. They can be effectively treated only if equal attention is given to the psychic and somatic aspects of their illness.

"There is need of an adequate basis for the inclusion of attention to the psychic component in illness in our public health program. Its inclusion is exigent, both because of the facts just stated and in view of the problems of health insurance and socialized medicine with which we are confronted. A major weakness of such systems as are in operation results from a lack of knowledge concerning emotions and physiological changes. . . . It is chronic illness as well as those illnesses which have the greatest tendency to become chronic in which the psychic component is of the greatest significance to therapy."

Summary

The main point of this discussion can be stated briefly; the study and treatment of illness constitutes much more than the investigation and eradication of disease. Yet there is nothing new or startling in this viewpoint. We have heard a great deal in recent years about the study of the organism-as-a-whole, but for most part we have been paying only lip service to this concept. We have been led to believe that the art of the physician, having to do with his common sense or intuition, as opposed to his science, is sufficient to grasp the problems that we have been considering. It is not enough. A real understanding of psychopathology is necessary in order to study the emotional life in relation to ill health. In other words, the physician must be able to define the specific mental factors producing the illness, rather than to be satisfied with vague generalizations about "neurogenic background". Just as we would criticize the physician of today, who would call all fevers malaria, so we must criticize the physician of tomorrow, who hints vaguely at nervous factors in the background of an illness and makes no effort really to understand the psychic situation.

In his "History of Medicine" Garrison states that the fundamental error of medieval medical science, as originally pointed out by Guy de Chauliac and elucidated by Allbutt, was in the divorce of medicine from surgery. He might have added that the fundamental error of modern medical science has been in the divorce of both from psychiatry.

BIBLIOGRAPHY

1. HAMMAN, L.: Relationship of psychiatry to internal medicine, Ment. Hyg., 1939, XXIII, 177.
2. ALLBUTT, T. C.: Visceral Neuroses, p. 17, P. Blakiston's Son and Co., Philadelphia, 1884.
3. MACY, J. W. and ALLEN, E. V.: Justification of diagnosis of chronic nervous exhaustion, Ann. Int. Med., 1934, VII, 861.
4. HALLIDAY, J. L.: Principles of etiology, Brit. Jour. Med. Psych., 1943, XIX, 367.
5. GLOVER, E.: Medico-psychological aspects of normality, Brit. Jour. Psychol., 1932, XXIII, 152.
6. KILGORE, E. S.: Clinical records; criticism of present vogue, Jour. Am. Med. Assoc., 1931, XCVII, 93.
7. FREUD, S.: Collected Papers, Vol. I, p. 76, Internat. Psychoanalyt. Press, New York, 1924.
8. DUNBAR, F.: Psychosomatic Diagnosis, pp. 696–697, Paul B. Hoeber, Inc., New York, 1943.
9. DUNBAR, F.: Emotions and Bodily Changes, Columbia University Press, New York, 1938.
10. WEISS, E. and ENGLISH, O. S.: Psychosomatic Medicine, W. B. Saunders Co., Philadelphia, 1943.

April 1, 1945.

CHAPTER XXI

PHYSICAL MEDICINE

By FRANK H. KRUSEN

Table of Contents

LOCAL APPLICATION OF HEAT

The application of heat locally is one of the most common procedures in the practice of medicine. Heat may be applied by conduction, convection or conversion. The application of conductive heat by direct application of water is discussed later in the section on *Hydrotherapy*. The procedures for applying conversive heat locally are described in the section on *Electrotherapy*. The majority of the methods of applying conductive heat and the procedure for application of convective heat are considered here.

Conductive heating can be accomplished by the direct application of a warm object to a bodily surface. Conductive heating devices can be heated by means of (1) warm air, (2) warm water, (3) chemicals or (4) electrical resistance coils. Previously heated solids or semisolids also can be employed for conductive heating.

Convective heating usually is accomplished by reflection of infra-red or luminous radiant energy on some region of the body.

Methods of Applying Heat Locally

Conductive Heat

Warm Air Devices. — Hot air chambers, blowers or applicators heated from within by means of hot air have been used medically. Hot air chambers (Fig. 1), constructed of wood or metal and lined with asbestos, were developed by August Bier[1] and described by Willy Meyer[2] more than forty years ago. Although such chambers have been abandoned to a large extent in this country, they still are employed enthusiastically by South American and Italian physicians. The chambers have an opening at one end to permit the insertion of an arm or leg. Usually they are heated by an alcohol lamp or by a can of solidified alcohol. The air within the chamber usually is extremely hot, attaining a temperature of 250° to 260° F. (121° to 125° C.).

Recently the Council on Physical Therapy of the American Medical Association approved a device which circulates warm air within a sleeve fastened to an extremity. An apparatus which circulates hot air within a distensible rubber bag also is being recommended currently. The bag is inserted into the vagina for treatment of pelvic inflammatory disease. The pressure usually is 1 to 1½ pounds (0.5 to 0.7 kg.) and the temperature not more than 130° F. (54.4° C.)[3].

Warm Water Devices. — The time-honored hot water bottle falls in this category as does the so-called Elliott treatment regulator. The hot water bottle is sufficiently well known to preclude the necessity of careful

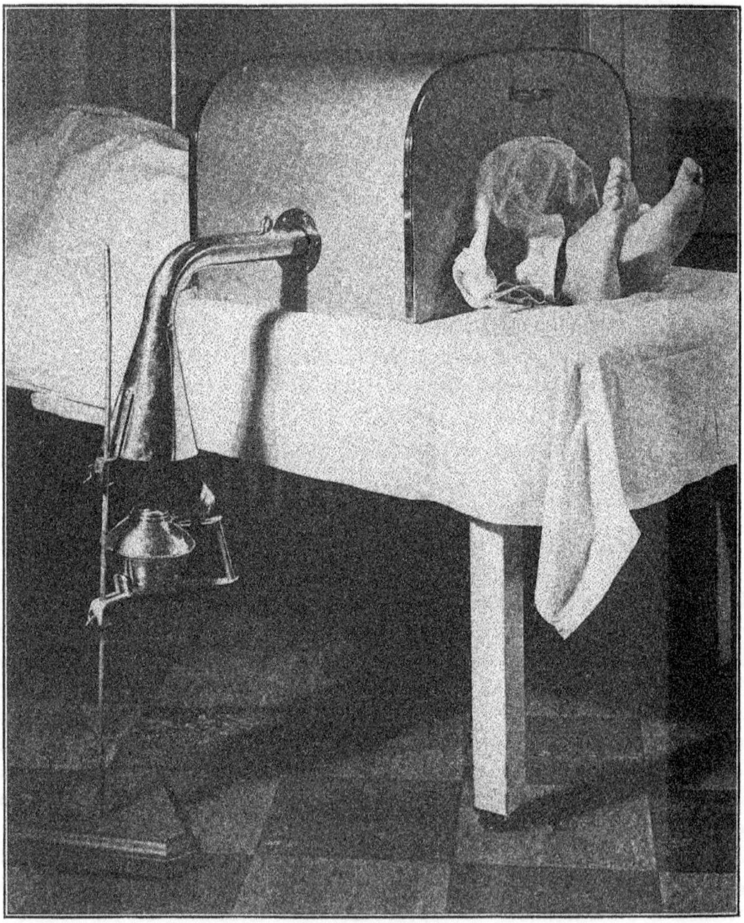

FIG. 1. A hot air chamber for local application of heat. Although still employed enthusiastically in some parts of the world, in the United States this device now has become almost obsolete.

description. Recently an electrical immersion heater has been developed which can be inserted in the standard hot water bottle in place of the usual cap. Its purpose is to maintain the temperature of the water within the bag at a constant level.

The Elliott apparatus heats and circulates water which is passed under pressure through thin rubber applicators. These applicators are constructed for insertion into various bodily orifices.

Chemical Devices. — Pads which make use of the latent heat of crystallization to produce prolonged heating effects have been employed therapeutically. These pads have been constructed for application to the eye[4], to the frontal region[5] or to other regions of the body[6]. One type[4, 5] of chemical heating pad contains sodium acetate 90.5 per cent., glycerin 3 per cent., sodium sulfate crystals 2 per cent. and anhydrous sodium sulfate 4.5 per cent. These chemicals are sealed inside the rubber applicator which is boiled for ten minutes before use. The pad then will remain at a temperature of about 108° to 114° F. (42.2° to 45.5° C.) for approximately an hour. It has a lifetime of about 600 hours of service.

The other type of chemical heating pad[6] depends on the chemical reaction which occurs when water is added to a mixture of finely divided iron 84 per cent., sodium chloride 6 per cent. and manganese dioxide 10 per cent. The chemicals are placed in a canvas bag enclosed in flexible rubber. If 2 drachms (7.5 c.c.) of water are placed inside the container, heat will be liberated. After use, if the cover is removed, it will cool rapidly. It has a useful life of 80 to 125 hours.

Devices Containing Electrical Resistance Coils. — Pads containing electrical resistance coils with a flexible insulated covering are used commonly today. In fact, they have become household utility devices. Such pads are not satisfactory for therapy. They tend to become too hot; temperature control is inadequate, and the fact that they produce burns or shocks occasionally is reported.

Electrical pads which can be controlled more accurately than the household heating pad have been constructed for therapeutic use. One such device[7] consists of a flat coil contained in a waterproof cover. A thermostat of considerable accuracy permits minute adjustments of temperature. A mercury thermometer, inserted in a pocket in the cover, allows close observation of the temperature. The pad is intended to be used for the purpose of keeping hot moist dressings at a constant temperature.

Parts of an electrically heated suit, similar to those worn by deep sea divers and stratosphere fliers, have been employed therapeutically for local application of heat to a certain region of the body. Brown and Allen[8] used cuffs or sleeves of this sort in treatment of peripheral vascular diseases. Recently I have had constructed a device of this type for application of conductive heat to the shoulder and upper part of the arm (Fig. 2). It has the advantage of providing uniform heating of all the surfaces of the shoulder and arm surrounded by it. All or any part of an electrically heated suit thus can be constructed so that regulated conductive heat can be applied to all sides of various regions of the body.

Recently an ingenious electric blanket (Fig. 3) has been developed; this was intended primarily for household employment but may be found extremely useful in medical practice[9]. A transformer within the control

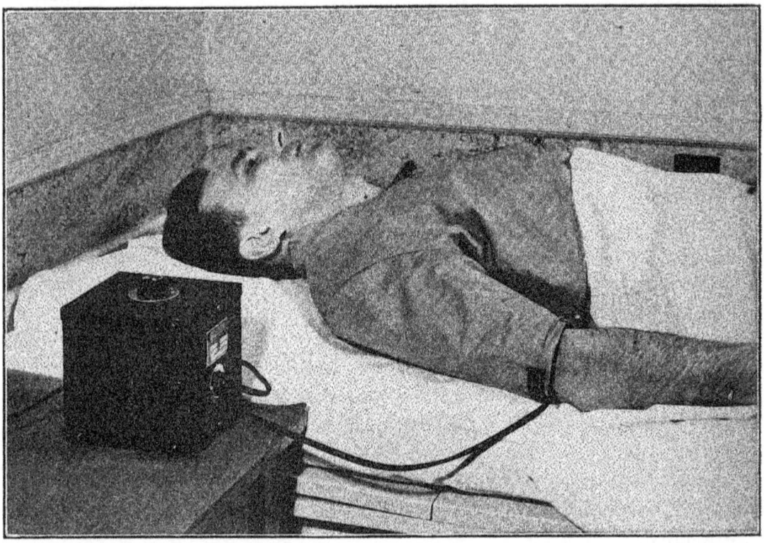

FIG. 2. A new type of electrically heated shoulder and arm pad with an accurate thermostatic control. It has the advantage of providing uniform heating of all surfaces.

box reduces the usual 115 volt current to 18 volts at the blanket. This practically eliminates the danger of electrical shock. A thermostat in the control box can be adjusted manually to the desired level of temperature. It then will maintain this level despite changes in the temperature of the room. If the environmental temperature rises, the blanket will cool, and conversely, if the room becomes cool, the blanket will warm up until the predetermined level is reached.

This type of blanket should prove valuable for maintenance of a constant, optimal bodily temperature in certain cases of peripheral vascular disease. It might prove valuable also for keeping tuberculous patients at a constant comfortable warmth while sleeping in well ventilated rooms during cold weather. Likewise, it should be valuable in providing a safe type of warm bed to combat postoperative surgical shock. There would not be the danger, which has been observed so often in the past, of burning semiconscious patients with hot water bottles.

Previously Heated Solids and Semisolids. — The ancient household custom of applying hot irons, hot bricks, hot salt bags or hot sand bags to various regions of the body for relief of pain or of muscular spasm has declined recently. This is largely because of the fact that the temperature

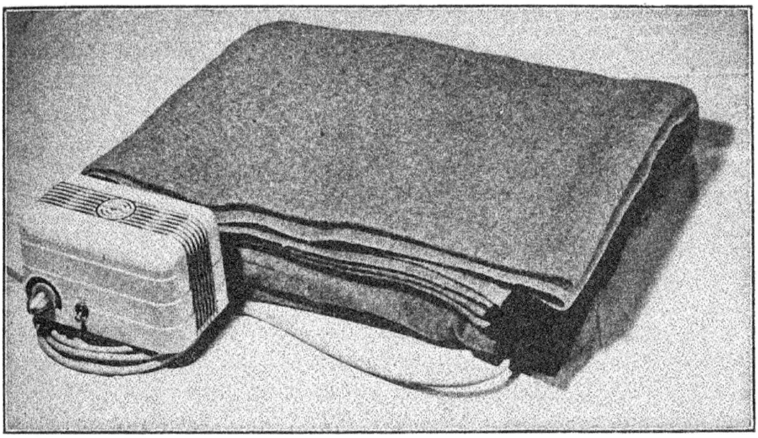

FIG. 3. An automatic electric blanket, the temperature of which can be adjusted to the desired level. This temperature is maintained by means of a thermostat despite changes in environmental temperature (From Krusen, F. H.: Physical Medicine, Saunders, Philadelphia, 1941).

of the simple devices of a similar nature, which are now readily available, can be controlled more accurately.

The employment of hot mud packs has been popularized commercially by certain European spas. The claims for alleged specific effects of various types of "therapeutic" muds have been vague and completely unconvincing. Typical examples of this kind of supposedly therapeutic mud are the "piestany" mud and the "fango" mud. There is no convincing evidence that such muds contain constituents which enhance their effectiveness when they are applied to the surface of the body.

Working in my department, R. L. Bennett checked the action on photographic paper of the allegedly radioactive "fango" mud. He found that there was insufficient radioactivity to fog the paper, even after exposure for twenty-four hours. It was concluded that the supposed radioactivity would have a negligible therapeutic effect. In addition, comparative clinical tests were performed which revealed no essential differences between the thermal effects of "fango" mud, ordinary garden mud and Mississippi valley clay. It would seem that "therapeutic" muds have no particular advantage over simpler and cleaner methods of applying heat.

Hot paraffin can be applied easily to local regions and is clean and effective. All the materials which are necessary are "jelly wax" or ordinary commercial paraffin, a kitchen stove and a double boiler, such as can be found in any kitchen. I frequently recommend that paraffin be employed for local application of heat when the patient lives in a house which is not equipped with electricity to operate a homemade baker or a simple heat lamp. But even in well-supplied institutions paraffin frequently is employed in preference to other local heating measures. The paraffin is placed in the inner pan of the double boiler, and water is poured into the outer pan. The boiler then is placed on the stove and heated until all the paraffin has melted. It is permitted then to cool until a thin film of solidifying paraffin has formed on the surface. At this time the paraffin will be at its low melting point which is approximately 167° to 176° F. (75° to 80° C.).

The paraffin then is painted over the region which is to be treated. About a dozen coats are applied in rapid succession. The layers of paraffin solidify almost instantly to form a thick warm covering of the surface. This covering is left in place for at least thirty minutes. Variations include dipping of a part, usually a hand or foot, in the paraffin about six times to form a similar warm paraffin pack, applying alternate layers of bandage and paraffin to a joint to provide a warm firm supporting dressing, or leaving the part immersed in a special large paraffin bath for thirty minutes or longer.

I have placed thermocouples beneath paraffin packs or dressings and have found that the temperature is kept above normal levels for more than an hour.

Convective Heat

Convective heating is accomplished by irradiation of the surface of the body with rays from the visible and infra-red regions of the electromagnetic spectrum. A beam of visible light can be split by means of a triangular prism into the various colors of the rainbow. Above the violet end of this rainbow are situated the invisible ultraviolet rays; below the red end lie the invisible infra-red or heat rays.

A variety of infra-red generators has been marketed for therapeutic use. The units commonly employed at present consist of a spiral coil of resistant metal wire wound around a cone made of steatite or porcelain, or plates, rods or disks of resistant metal such as carborundum. These units usually are placed in a cup-shaped reflector which will cause the rays to converge on the part which is to be treated (Fig. 4). The infra-red lamp

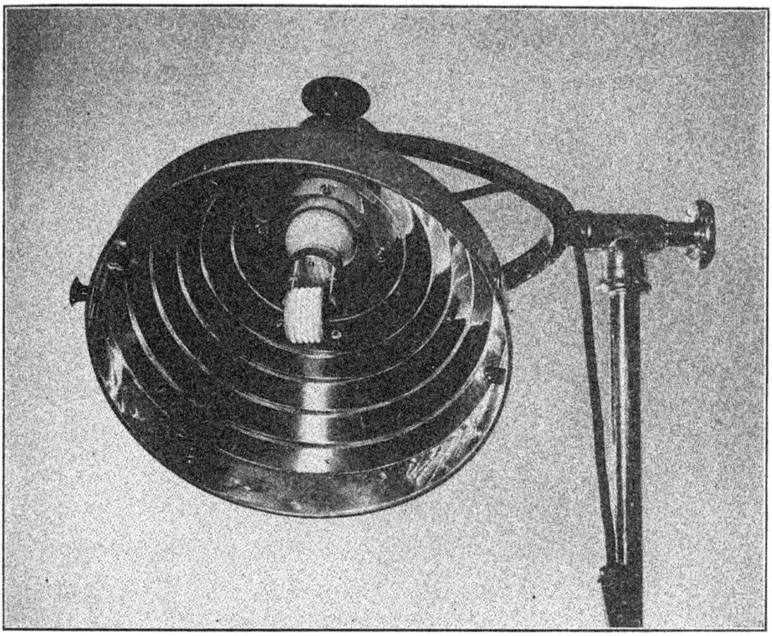

FIG. 4. An infra-red unit, nonluminous variety, in the usual type of cup-shaped reflector which causes the radiation to converge to a focal point.

employed by the physician differs little from the familiar household electric heater (Fig. 5). The chief difference is in the shape of the reflector. The household heater has a flatter, platelike reflector, which diffuses the heat rays through the room, while the infra-red lamp has a more concave, cup-shaped reflector, which concentrates the rays on a small local region. The heating units themselves can be used interchangeably because the radiation from one is practically identical with that from the other.

It is obvious, therefore, that infra-red rays are not mysterious or unusual. However, even though infra-red rays simply are heat rays, they are, nevertheless, of considerable usefulness in therapy. For many years illumination engineers have known that radiation from luminous sources, such as tungsten or carbon filament bulbs, penetrates human tissues to a greater depth than that from nonluminous sources such as the infra-red coils or plates. Oddly enough, physicians have not been familiar, as a rule, with this fact. Somehow, many physicians have entertained the erroneous idea that the radiation from infra-red coils penetrates to great depths. Actually, the rays from the far portion of the infra-red spectrum, which are produced by these nonluminous or "black body" radiators, penetrate in appreciable amounts to a depth of less than 1 mm.

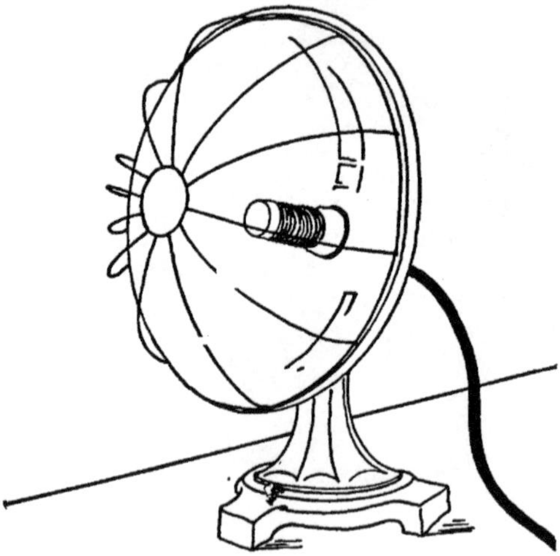

FIG. 5. An ordinary household electrical heater. The heating unit produces radiation similar to that emitted by the therapeutic infra-red unit, but the flatter reflector tends to diffuse the radiation (From Krusen, F. H.: Light Therapy, Ed. 2, Hoeber, New York, 1937).

The greatest amount of penetration of convective heat can be obtained from luminous sources, which produce considerable amounts of radiation in the near portion of the infra-red spectrum, such as carbon filament or tungsten filament lamps (Fig. 6*a* and *b*). These infra-red luminous bulbs can be placed in the same cup-shaped reflectors which are employed for the nonluminous infra-red coils. The penetration through human tissues of radiation from the luminous bulbs has been estimated variously up to depths of 1.5 cm. Recently, however, Hardy and Muschenheim[10] reported careful investigations, which indicated that the transmission through skin of even these most penetrating infra-red rays

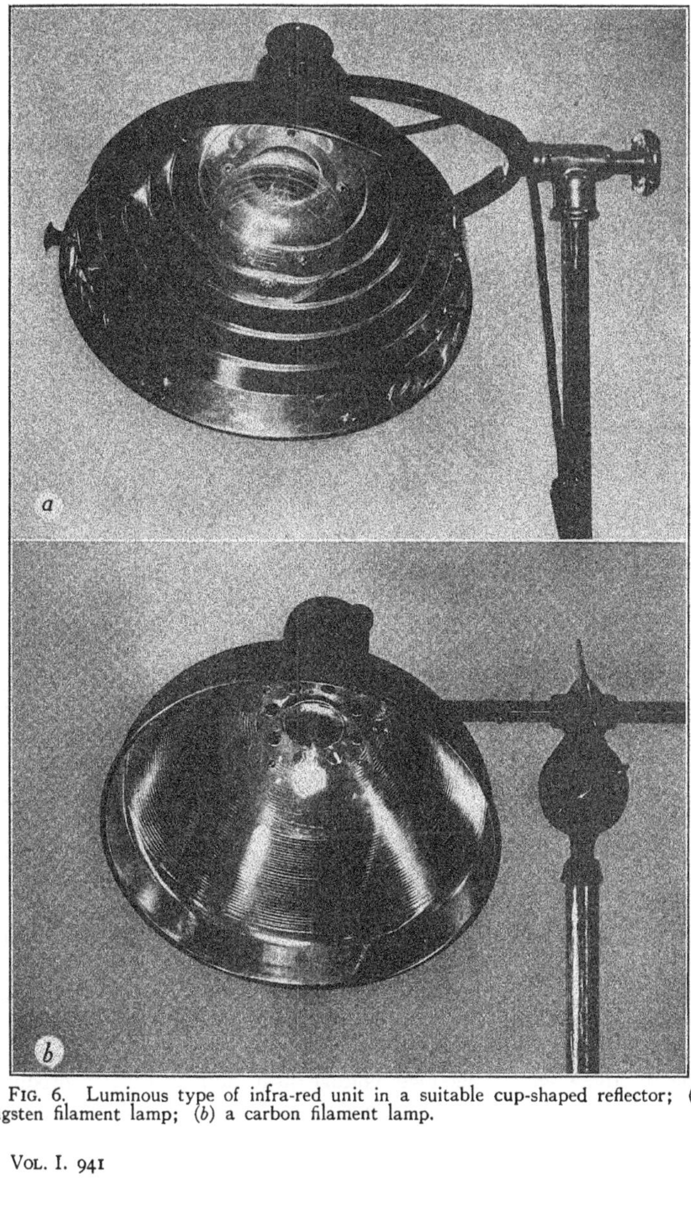

FIG. 6. Luminous type of infra-red unit in a suitable cup-shaped reflector; (*a*) a tungsten filament lamp; (*b*) a carbon filament lamp.

is slight. They found that about 95 per cent. of the rays were absorbed within 2 mm. of the surface and 99 per cent. within 3 mm.

For most therapeutic applications it will be advisable to employ a source of radiation which is rich in the more penetrating near infra-red rays. Therefore, convective heat treatments usually should be administered with a device which converges the rays from a luminous source on

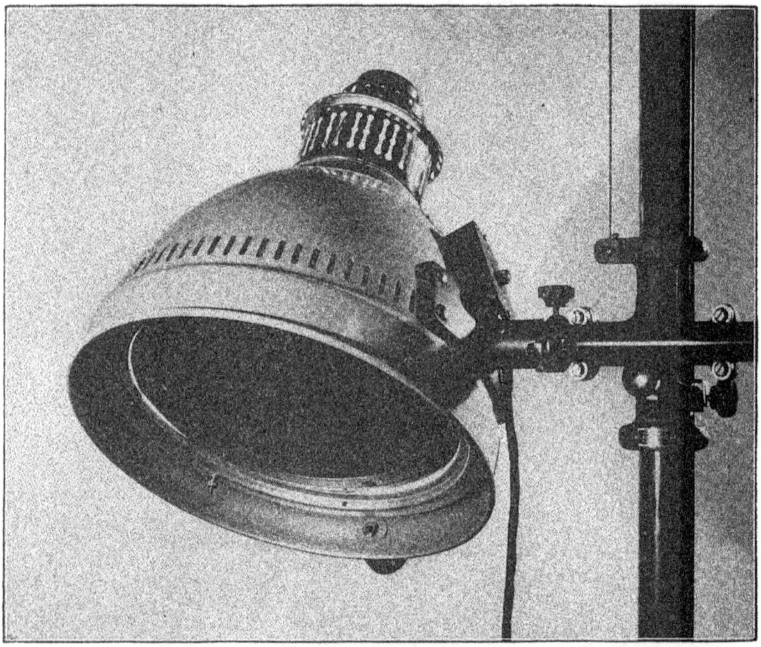

FIG. 7. A radiant heat lamp, luminous type of infra-red bulb, with a special black glass filter, which eliminates glare but does transmit most of the more penetrating near infra-red rays (From Krusen, F. H.: A new type of filter for efficient infra-red radiation, Proc. Staff Meet., Mayo Clin., 1941, XIV, 22).

the part to be treated. For example, one type of luminous therapeutic heat bulb, which is known as the "Mazda CX" bulb, is particularly rich in the slightly more penetrating near infra-red rays. Thirty per cent. of the radiation from this type of bulb is within the most penetrating range with wavelengths between 770 and 1,200 millimicrons.

One disadvantage of the high voltage heat bulb is that it produces considerable glare. I recently have described[11] a new type of infra-red lamp with a special black glass filter which transmits most of the penetrating near infra-red rays but cuts off practically all of the visible rays and thus eliminates glare (Fig. 7). This lamp seems to be especially valuable

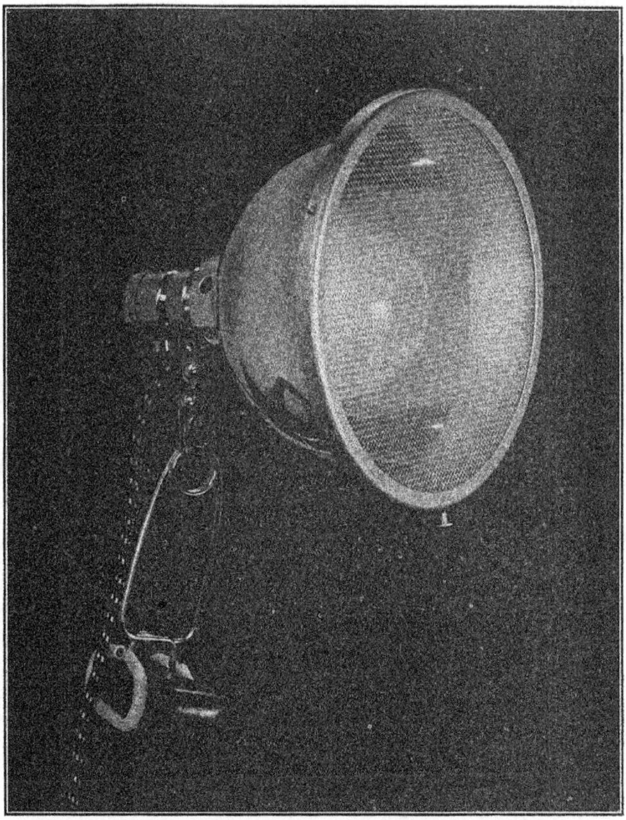

FIG. 8. An inexpensive "clamp lamp" which can be employed at home for prolonged local heating of various regions of the body (From Krusen, F. H.: Physical therapy in arthritis, with special reference to home treatment, Jour. Am. Med. Assoc., 1940, CXV, 605).

for application of heat to the face and to the upper anterior part of the body because the patient is not annoyed by glare.

A strange phenomenon has been the development in this country of small inexpensive heat lamps consisting of a bulb on a small reflector attached to a handle. It is undoubtedly of great usefulness to have inexpensive heat lamps readily available, but the catch is that almost nobody wishes to hold such a lamp steadily in his hand long enough for it to produce any marked therapeutic effect. It usually requires at least thirty minutes of local application of heat to produce an effective increase in temperature of the tissues. It is extremely tiresome, even if the hands are shifted, to hold a lamp steadily in one position for thirty minutes.

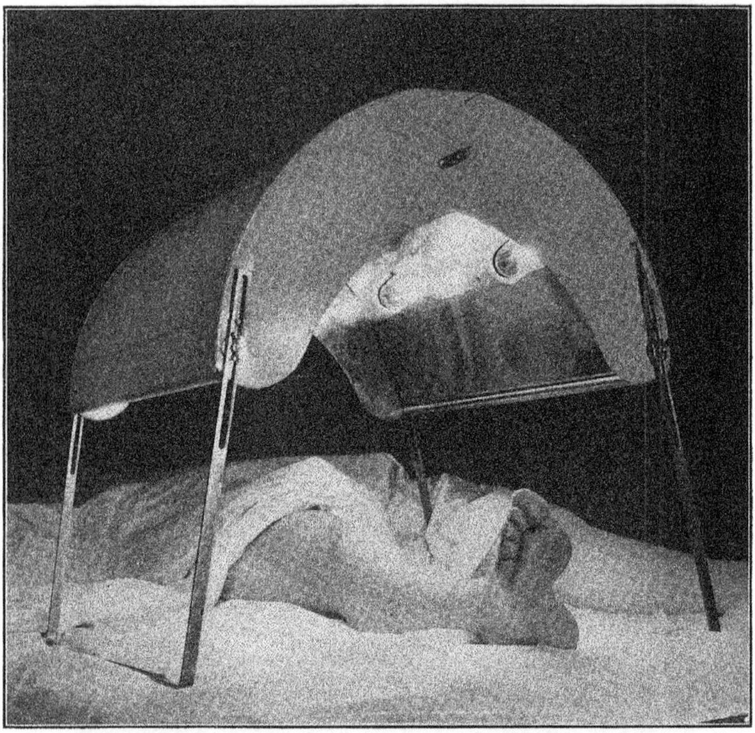

FIG. 9. Institutional type of baker. This is a luminous heat device containing usually four to twelve light bulbs.

To obviate this difficulty, I have had constructed an inexpensive "clamp lamp" which was described a few years ago[12]. This lamp has a cup-shaped reflector containing a luminous heat bulb. Instead of a handle a clamp similar to that employed for "photo-flash" lamps is provided. This inexpensive clamp lamp can be attached to the side of a bed or to the back of a chair. A ball and socket joint permits adjustment of the reflector at any angle. The lamp can be employed easily for prolonged heating of various local regions of the body (Fig. 8).

Still extremely serviceable is the old style "baker" which consists of a slightly curved rooflike reflector supported by adjustable legs. Beneath this reflector are several small electric light bulbs. This tunnel-like heating device can be placed over a leg, an arm or the back (Fig. 9). A

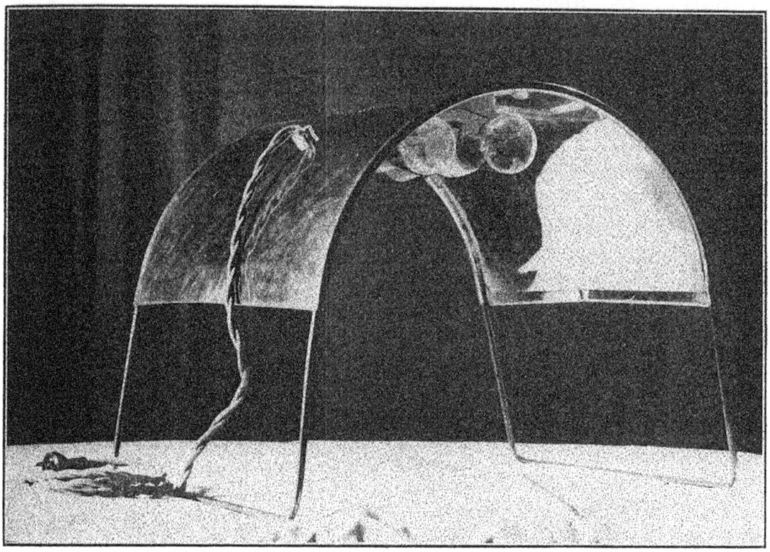

FIG. 10. Inexpensive homemade baker. Four bulbs are covered by a reflector of sheet tin on framework of iron rods.

similar, less elaborate baker for home use can be constructed of four light bulbs covered by a piece of polished sheet tin supported on a light framework of iron rods (Fig. 10).

PHYSICAL PRINCIPLES CONCERNED IN THE LOCAL APPLICATION OF HEAT

Since heat is a form of irregular molecular motion, thermal energy can be transmitted from one body to another by continuation of this molecular motion. Interchanges of this sort are taking place continually between the human body and its environment. As previously mentioned, such transmission of molecular motion can take place by conduction, convection or conversion.

All of the conductive methods, which have been described, require direct application of the hot applicator to some surface of the body.

Luminous and infra-red rays result from electromagnetic disturbances of the ether. According to Huygen's wave theory there is a propagation of energy in the form of waves. Wavelength is the distance between the crests of adjoining ether waves.

Because the frequency of vibration of a given source of heat energy is uniform, and the velocity of the radiation is constant, the distance between any two adjacent waves will be identical with the distance between any other two waves derived from the same source.

The electromagnetic spectrum can be defined as a graphic representation of the various waves of energy in ascending order of length (Fig. 11). Starting with the shortest known rays, the cosmic rays, it will be seen that the next shortest in ascending order are the gamma rays of radium. Forming a continuous spectrum in succession of increasing wavelengths from these are the roentgen rays, ultraviolet rays, visible light, infra-red rays, hertzian waves including the short and long radio waves and alternating current waves.

Those portions of the spectrum which contain radiations employed for convective heating are the visible and infra-red regions. The wavelengths of the rays from this portion of the spectrum vary between 290 and 15,000 millimicrons.

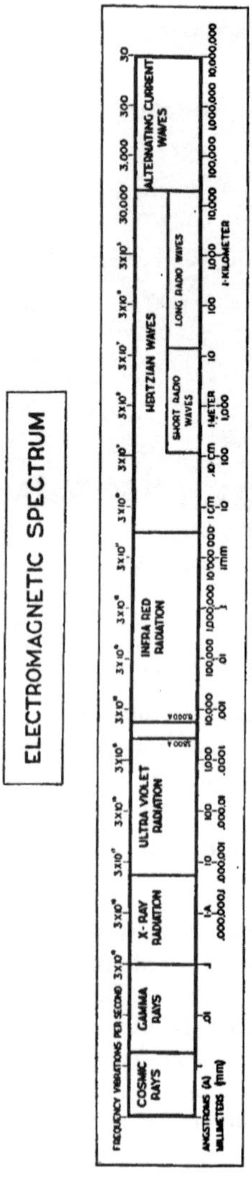

FIG. 11. Graphic representation of the electromagnetic spectrum (Courtesy of the Council on Physical Therapy of the American Medical Association).

Action and Uses of Local Heating Devices

The action of conductive or conversive heating is superficial because the penetration of heat is always slight. Normally the temperature of the blood in various peripheral regions of the body is lower than the central temperature of approximately 98.6° F. (37° C.). The temperature of the skin, fat and muscle in peripheral regions varies and usually is considerably lower than the rectal temperature.

Local applications of heat will tend to raise the temperature in peripheral regions.

It is probable that bodily tissues cannot tolerate a *prolonged* increase of external temperature to more than 113° F. (45° C.) without being damaged. For *short periods* of time they can tolerate changes of external temperature exceeding 36° F. (20° C.) without evidence of injury. Local application of heat produces dilatation of blood vessels and an increase in the rate of flow of the blood. The tendency toward rapid dissemination of the heat finally may result in an increase in the systemic temperature. There is evidence that the heat causes increase of phagocytic and local metabolic activity. Heating of the blood increases carbon dioxide tension and acidity. It has been suggested[13] that these changes may be of some value in modifying the reactions of tissues to infection.

A point worth keeping in mind is that local exposure to infra-red radiation will produce a rise of temperature of a considerable volume of blood as it circulates through the cutaneous capillaries. The temperature of the blood will reach a level exceeding that of the average systemic fever without any appreciable rise in the systemic temperature. Local applications of heat possibly may stimulate intracellular oxidation. Likewise sweating and muscular relaxation are produced by local heating.

Daily treatments for thirty minutes in the hot air chambers and blowers have been recommended particularly as an adjunct in the management of various forms of arthritis. The vaginal applicator, which is heated by circulating hot air, usually is employed for sessions of one hour daily in treatment for specific and nonspecific inflammatory disease of the pelvis.

Like the hot air device, the Elliott apparatus, which circulates hot water through a distensible rubber bag within the vagina, is employed chiefly for pelvic inflammatory disease. The water pressure meter should register 2 or 3 pounds (0.9 or 1.4 kg.). Hourly treatments usually are given once or twice a day. Randall and I[14] found that complete clinical remissions were obtained in 55 per cent. of our 45 cases of chronic gonorrheal inflammatory disease of the pelvis in which treatment with the Elliott device was employed; in an additional 22 per cent. negative cultures developed, but there was evidence of residual salpingo-oöphoritis; in 11 per cent. improvement did not occur, and in 11 per cent. insufficient treatment was received. Of our group of 173 patients suffering from nonspecific pelvic inflammatory disease 30 per cent. were greatly improved after Elliott treatment; 27.7 per cent. were moderately improved; 9.8 per cent. were slightly improved, and 5.7 per cent. were unimproved. Surgical treatment was required in 26.5 per cent. of the cases. Pelvic heating with the Elliott device was employed successfully to promote absorption of exudates following pelvic operation.

The Elliott treatment has been applied through a rectal applicator for chronic prostatitis, specific and nonspecific, and a urethral applicator was employed by Emmett in treatment for nonspecific urethritis among females. Welch and I have administered Elliott treatments through a colonic stoma to lessen edema of the spur and to permit earlier application of clamps for the second stage of the Mikulicz operation.

The chemical heating pads have been employed chiefly for chronic inflammation of the eye or nasal accessory sinuses. The larger chemical heating pad has been used as a substitute for the hot water bottle and has the advantage that it will remain hot for a longer period.

Ordinary electrical heating pads should not be used unless more suitable methods of heating are not available. The compress with accurate thermostatic control can be employed to maintain the warmth of wet dressings at proper level for infections, acute inflammations, cutaneous diseases and surgical conditions. The electrically heated sleeves, cuffs and pads, which have accurate control, can be employed for peripheral vascular diseases, arthritis and traumatic lesions.

Applications of hot paraffin have been recommended chiefly for contractures, arthritis, fibrositis, post-traumatic stiff joints and lacerations.

The application of infra-red radiation has been advocated for numerous conditions. It tends to promote absorption of exudates because heat produces not a passive congestion but an active hyperemia with an increase in the volume of blood flowing through the region rather than engorgement and stagnation.

Local treatment with infra-red radiation has been recommended[15, 16] for various types of neuritis, myositis, fibrositis and arthritis, for circulatory diseases, for certain types of paralysis and also for traumatic lesions such as sprains, contusions, dislocations and fractures. It always should be remembered that various conductive methods of applying heat often can be substituted for infra-red radiation or vice versa. The therapeutic effects are essentially the same. The choice of the superficial heating agent will be largely a matter of convenience.

Following trauma heat should not be applied until the danger of capillary oozing with extravasation and ecchymosis has ceased. This usually will require twenty-four to forty-eight hours. During this time tight dressings, immobilization and applications of cold are in order. As soon as this danger disappears, applications of heat for periods of thirty minutes or longer, once or twice a day, should be begun. After the applications of heat, massage sometimes can be administered. The heat and massage will tend to promote absorption and to prevent the formation of organized hematomas.

Traumatic synovitis, tenosynovitis, bursitis, spastic muscles and strained muscles often can be benefited by local applications of conductive or convective heat.

Contraindications to the Local Application of Heat

The great danger in applying any form of therapeutic heating is that burns may be caused. Patients have been known to permit themselves to be burned thinking that they were supposed to tolerate the pain. It is not sufficient to give the patient a bell and to tell him to ring it if the part becomes too hot. I recall one patient who, although he had been so instructed, promptly permitted himself to be burned and then explained that he did not know how much "too hot" was. Therefore, the patient must be told that he should feel only comfortable warmth; that the minute he feels the slightest discomfort, he should ring. He should be warned that excessive heat will do more harm than good.

Heat always must be applied with extreme caution to extremities in which the circulation is impaired. In the presence of peripheral vascular disease heat will be disseminated poorly by the impaired circulation; therefore, burns are more likely to occur. Furthermore, if a burn does result, slowly healing lesions or even gangrene may occur in the devitalized tissue. It should be remembered in dealing with peripheral vascular diseases that the local application of heat to an unaffected region may produce vasodilatation in the affected part. Local heating of an uninvolved region may be just as effective as direct heating, and it is much safer. If heat is to be applied locally to the affected extremity, prolonged applications at fairly low temperatures, 91.4° to 95° F. (33° to 35° C.), are safer than short exposures at high temperature.

Heat always must be applied with great caution over old scars which are comparatively avascular and will blister readily. It often is wise to cover small scars in a region which is to be heated. Likewise heat must be applied with extreme caution over anesthetic regions. Because there is no sensation, the patient may be burned without realizing it.

Knapp[17] recently has expressed the opinion that in most instances just sufficient heat should be applied to produce a faint pink blush on the skin. He concluded that, if there was a mottled erythema of the skin, the heat was too intense. It seems obvious that the mottling, so commonly observed during intense heating of the skin, indicates unequal distribution of the hyperemia in the region under treatment. Certainly it is safer to avoid the mottling when possible.

Local exposures to heat may aggravate certain cutaneous rashes. As a rule, local heat should not be applied in febrile conditions. Occasionally sensitivity to heat, attributable usually to derangement of the heat regulating mechanism, may be encountered. In such instances local heating must be applied with great caution.

When Elliott treatments are administered to the vagina, incorrect placing or improper distention of the applicator may produce excessive localization of heat in a small region, and severe burns may ensue. Large sloughs of the anterior vaginal wall have been reported after incorrect employment of the procedure.

If hot paraffin is used for local heating, in rare instances a mild paraffin rash may be produced.

Summary of Data on Local Heat

There are numerous, readily available sources of heat which can be employed in local treatment for various diseases. Devices heated by warm air, warm water, chemicals, electrical coils, previously heated solids and semisolids and several sources of infra-red radiation can be used.

These devices are employed chiefly to increase local temperature and circulation, to increase local metabolism, to promote absorption and to relieve muscular spasm. Local applications of heat are indicated especially in the management of acute and chronic inflammations, impairment of circulation and various traumatic lesions. Heat should be applied with great caution in the presence of peripheral vascular disease, scars or anesthesia of the skin.

BIBLIOGRAPHY OF LOCAL HEAT APPLICATIONS

1. BIER, AUGUST: Hyperemia as a Therapeutic Agent, (translated by G. M. Blech), Frank S. Betz Co., Hammond, Indiana, 1913.
2. MEYER, W. and SCHMIEDEN, V.: Bier's Hyperemic Treatment in Surgery, Medicine and the Specialities; a Manual of its Practical Application, Saunders, Philadelphia, 1908.
3. NEWMAN, L. B.: An improved method for applying pelvic heat using air, Am. Jour. Obst. and Gynec., 1939, XXXVIII, 725.
4. COUNCIL ON PHYSICAL THERAPY: Altherm eye pad acceptable, Jour. Am. Med. Assoc., 1934, CIII, 563.
5. COUNCIL ON PHYSICAL THERAPY: Altherm sinus pad acceptable, Jour. Am. Med. Assoc., 1936, CVI, 921.

6. COUNCIL ON PHYSICAL THERAPY: Thermat self-heating heat pad acceptable, Jour. Am. Med. Assoc., 1935, CV, 118.
7. COUNCIL ON PHYSICAL THERAPY: Cooley compress acceptable, Jour. Am. Med. Assoc., 1939, CXIII, 1139.
8. BROWN, G. E., Jr. and ALLEN, E. V.: Personal communication to the author.
9. KRUSEN, F. H.: Physical Medicine, Saunders, Philadelphia, 1941.
10. HARDY, J. D. and MUSCHENHEIM, C.: Radiation of heat from the human body. V. The transmission of infra-red radiation through skin, Jour. Clin. Invest., 1936, XV, 1.
11. KRUSEN, F. H.: A new type of filter for efficient infra-red radiation, Proc. Staff Meet., Mayo Clin., 1941, XVI, 22.
12. KRUSEN, F. H.: A simple inexpensive heat lamp, Jour. Am. Med. Assoc., 1936, CVII, 780.
13. BAZETT, H. C.: The physiological basis for the use of heat. In Principles and Practice of Physical Therapy, Vol. I, pp. 1–29, Prior, Hagerstown, Maryland, 1934.
14. RANDALL, L. M. and KRUSEN, F. H.: A consideration of the Elliott treatment of pelvic inflammatory disease of women, Arch. Phys. Therapy, 1937, XVIII, 283.
15. TROUP, W. A.: Therapeutic Uses of Infra-red Rays, Actinic Press, London, 1930.
16. TROUP, W. A.: Infra-red and U-V irradiation of injuries in sport, Brit. Jour. Phys. Med., 1935, IX, 172.
17. KNAPP, M. E.: Personal communication to the author.

Sept. 1, 1941.

GENERAL APPLICATION OF HEAT

The general or systemic heating of the human body for therapeutic purposes now is spoken of commonly as "fever therapy". There are several methods of obtaining increases in bodily temperature by physical means, and recently much interest has developed in the employment of these devices for the production of artificial fevers.

A few decades ago fever was considered by physicians to be a manifestation of disease which should be combated. Therefore, much of the internal medication, chiefly with the derivatives of coal tar, was directed toward abolishing fevers. At present it is believed that spontaneous fever often is an indication of the benign efforts of nature to overcome disease. Today in certain types of disease, in which spontaneous fever does not occur, the physician makes a therapeutic effort to produce a fever by physical or other means.

Recently much fundamental and clinical research has been done in this field. Fever therapy, at least when high temperatures are used, now is considered a major procedure, which should be employed only in well-equipped institutions possessing skilled personnel. The procedure seems logical and appears to have far-reaching possibilities.

Methods of Producing General Heating of the Body (Fever Therapy)

Rises in systemic temperature can be produced physically by the use of (1) cabinets within which circulates hot humid air, (2) cabinets heated by luminous heat bulbs or nonluminous heating coils, (3) diathermy, (4) hot tub or spray baths or (5) conductive heating by means of heated blankets or sleeping bags.

Hot Humid Air Cabinets. — The device for inducing fever by physical means which is employed most commonly in this country is the hot humid air cabinet. A plan of one of the earlier models, known as the Kettering hypertherm, is illustrated in Fig. 12. One of the newer models of the "hypertherm" is illustrated in Fig. 13*a* and *b*. This type of apparatus was developed by Simpson and Kendell[1, 2] at the Kettering Institute for Medical Research in Dayton, Ohio. I have employed it extensively and have found it satisfactory for the production and maintenance of prolonged high fevers.

Warm humid air is circulated slowly through the cabinet. The air temperature varies between 110° and 130° F. (43.3° and 54.4° C.), and the humidity usually is kept above 80 per cent. Temperature and humidity

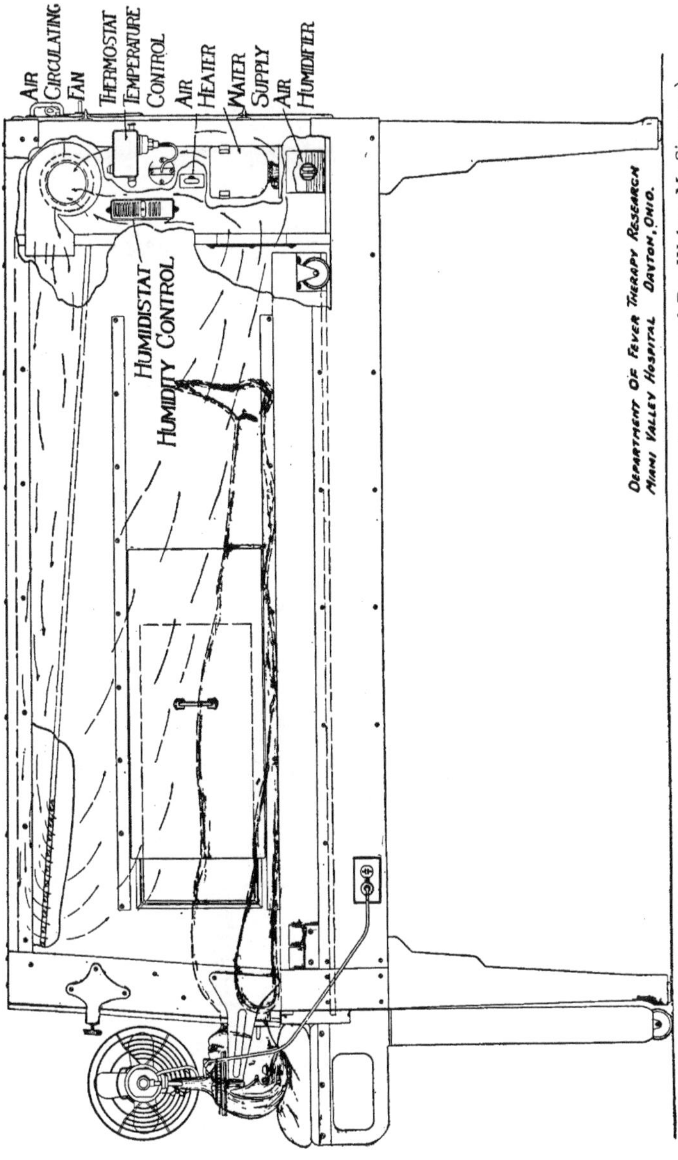

FIG. 12. Plan of the hot, humid air, fever cabinet (Kettering hypertherm) (Courtesy of Dr. Walter M. Simpson).

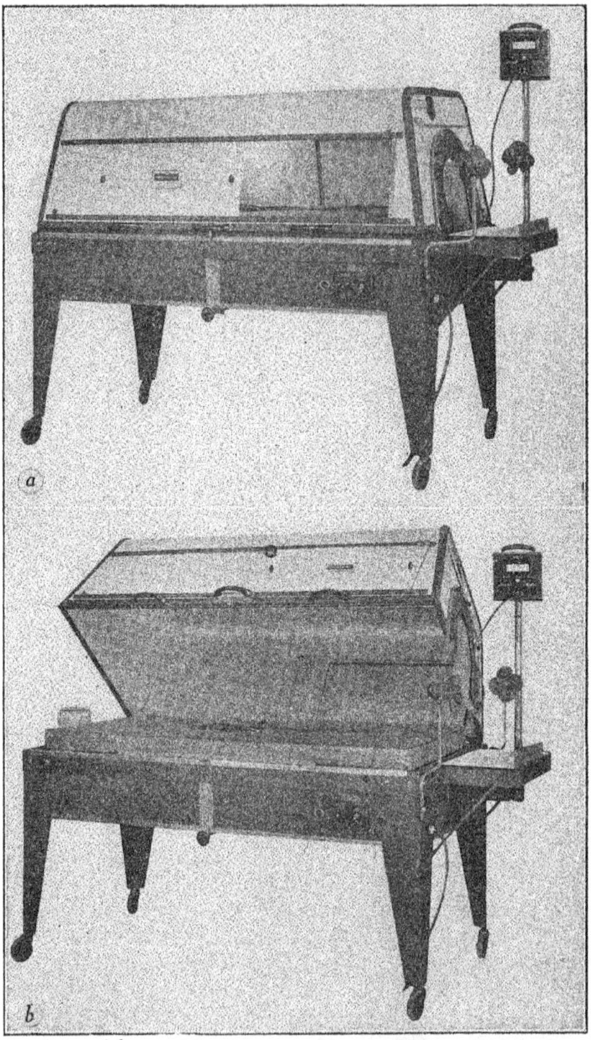

FIG. 13. A metal fever cabinet known as the hypertherm, which has been developed on the same principles as the original Kettering hypertherm; (*a*) cabinet closed; (*b*) cabinet open.

are modified readily, as desired, so that the procedure is excellent, because it permits such accurate control of bodily temperature.

Cabinets Heated by Luminous Bulbs or Nonluminous Heat Coils. — A fever cabinet heated by luminous bulbs can be constructed for about \$150[3]. Another one has been described[4], which can be built for considerably less than \$100. The plan of such a cabinet, which was developed by Sheard, is illustrated in Fig. 14. Sheard's cabinet differs from the other

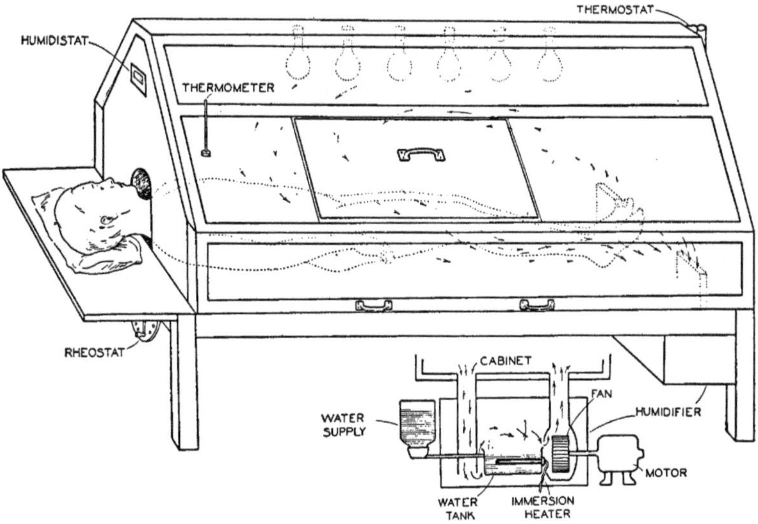

FIG. 14. Plan of the Sheard luminous heat fever cabinet (From Krusen, F. H.: Physical Medicine, Philadelphia, Saunders, 1941).

luminous heat cabinets in having a humidifying mechanism attached and in being more heavily insulated. The other luminous cabinets mentioned depend on moisture from the perspiration of the patient to humidify the still air of the cabinet. This latter plan is feasible because, if the cabinet is kept closed, the air soon becomes saturated with moisture as the patient's temperature rises and he begins to perspire.

Various types of fever cabinets, which have been heated by nonluminous heating elements, have been marketed also. This type of cabinet has not been employed so extensively as have other kinds of fever producing machines.

Diathermy. — A method of heating the entire body by means of conventional diathermy formerly was employed for the production of artificial fevers, but this procedure now has become obsolete. At present the newer short wave diathermy machines frequently are used for induction of artificial fevers. A common procedure is to introduce a long induction cable from a short-wave diathermy machine into one of the humid air cabinets (Fig. 15). The diathermy is used to induce the fever which then is maintained by means of the insulated cabinet. I have obtained equally satisfactory results by induction of fever with the hot humid air alone and prefer this simpler method, although there is no great objection to inducing the fever with diathermy.

Halphen and Auclair[5] employed a powerful short-wave diathermy ma-

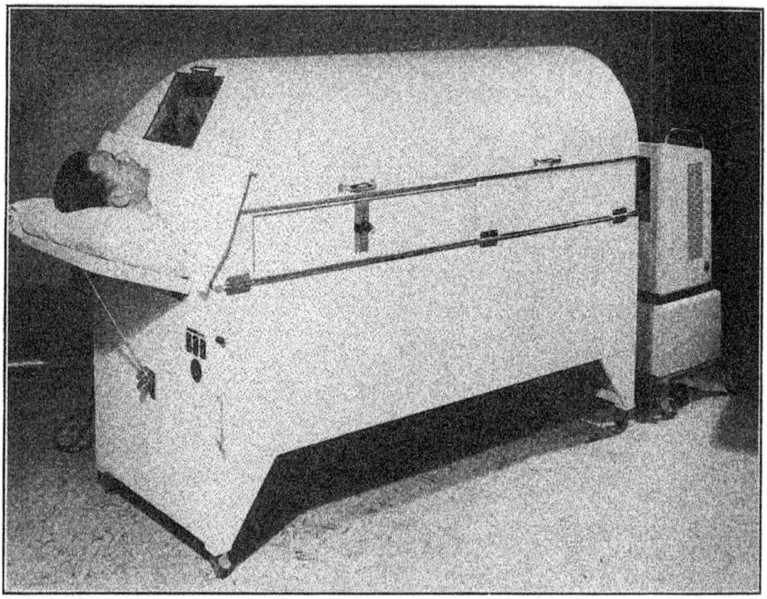

FIG. 15. A fever cabinet into which extends a short wave diathermy induction coil. Diathermy is employed to induce the fever which is maintained by the insulated cabinet (From Krusen, F. H.: Physical Medicine, Philadelphia, Saunders, 1941).

chine and a nonmetallic treatment bed. The patient, dressed in a bathrobe, lay on the bed and was covered with blankets. Two large flat diathermy electrodes were placed on the same plane beneath the bed at a distance of approximately 10 cm. from the patient's back. The patient's body thus was within the high frequency electrical field adjacent to the electrodes, conversive heat within his body caused his systemic temperature to rise, and loss of heat was prevented by the blankets. The great objection to the use of blankets for insulation is that as the temperature rises, the patient becomes uncomfortable under the heavy coverings.

Hot Tub or Spray Baths. — Tub baths can be employed to advantage for the induction of short low fevers. Prolonged hot tub baths are depressing and may be dangerous. Deaths from prolonged hot baths have been reported. I frequently employ the short hot baths for therapeutic effects, but these baths never are permitted to last more than an hour and usually do not last more than thirty minutes.

The method consists of immersing the patient to the neck in water which is at a temperature of 105° to 110° F. (40.5° to 43.5° C.). He remains in the tub until his systemic temperature is within 1.5° F. (0.83° C.) of the desired level. Then the water is cooled to the temperature of the patient, or he is removed from the tub and placed in a blanket, sleeping bag or insulated cabinet. Usually his temperature will continue to rise until it reaches the desired level and will tend to remain there as long as he remains covered. The method is comparatively safe and simple, if it is not desired to increase the systemic temperature to more than 103° to 104° F. (39.4° to 40° C.).

Hot spray cabinets have been manufactured, which resemble somewhat the other types of fever cabinets. The patient's head protrudes from one end of the cabinet, and his nude body is sprayed with a mist of nebulized hot water. This form of fever apparatus has been used successfully in some institutions.

Conductive Heating. — Electrical blankets, hot water bottles and blankets, and fever bags, all, have been employed to heat and to insulate the body of the patient in order to produce artificial fever. Unless some means of keeping the heavy coverings off the patient's body is employed, all such methods are extremely uncomfortable. Like hot baths they should not be used to raise the systemic temperature to more than 103° to 104° F. (39.4° to 40° C.).

Physical Principles Concerned in the General Application of Heat

The production of artificial fevers by physical means depends on two factors; increased input and decreased output of heat energy. Practically all of the methods for physical induction of fever employ both factors. Some method of increasing temperature is used in conjunction with some method of insulating the body to limit loss of heat. The input of heat generally is achieved by increasing the environmental temperature of the patient or by the application of high frequency currents, and the egress of heat usually is lessened by placing the patient in an insulating medium of some sort.

From a physical standpoint the regulation or prevention of loss of heat is more important than the application of heat in producing artificial fevers. This is owing to the fact that the heat eliminating mechanism of human beings, when performing in a normal manner, can rid the body of an excess of heat at a rate which is twelve times as great as the basal rate of heat production.

Action and Uses of Devices for the General Application of Heat (Fever Therapy)

High physically induced fevers increase the pulse and circulatory rates. The velocity of the blood may be increased as much as 400 per cent. During induction of fever the cardiac filling time is shortened temporarily so that partial decompensation may occur. When fever therapy is accompanied by profuse sweating, the reduction in blood plasma may be so great that peripheral vascular collapse ensues. During fever therapy the visible capillaries of the nail beds are increased in size and number. Physically induced fevers produce leukocytosis. An initial decrease in the number of leukocytes is followed immediately by a tidelike increase; the new cells are added in waves for several hours after completion of the febrile session. The number of leukocytes then gradually diminishes and attains prefebrile levels in about twenty-four hours. Leukocytosis is greater several hours after the end of the fever session than at its close. At the peak there may be more than 40,000 leukocytes per cubic millimeter of blood. There is a relative increase in neutrophils and a relative decrease in lymphocytes following fever therapy. Excessive perspiration accompanying fever therapy may cause a marked decrease in the chlorides of the blood serum.

At the beginning of a session of fever the content of oxygen and the oxygen combining power of the venous blood are increased. Despite this increase of oxygen, the increased metabolic activity and the increased demand for oxygen in the tissues may result finally in anoxia of the tissues, particularly if the circulation begins to fail because of circulatory collapse. The danger of anoxia and likewise the danger of circulatory collapse owing to loss of bodily fluids from excessive perspiration always are present during prolonged sessions of artificial fever.

The growth of certain organisms is destroyed or attenuated at temperatures induced by artificial fever. The *Neisseria gonorrhœæ* generally is destroyed at a temperature of 106° to 107° F. (41.1° to 41.6° C.) in 6 to 34 hours, the mean number of hours being 16.1. The thermal death time of the *Treponema pallidum* at 102.2° F. (39.0° C.) is five hours and at 106.8° F. (41.5° C.) is one hour. Nearly all strains of *meningococci* are attenuated greatly or destroyed at temperatures of 104° to 107.6° F. (40° to 42° C.) applied for five hours.

Arthritis. — Fever therapy has been employed in treatment for acute and chronic atrophic arthritis. It seems of benefit in a certain percentage of the acute cases. Short sessions of thirty minutes, given every day or so, seem to assist in controlling exacerbations of chronic atrophic arthritis.

Bronchial Asthma. — For bronchial asthma, which has failed to respond to the usual therapeutic procedures, fever therapy has been used. Although this treatment has not been too successful, nevertheless in some instances it has caused remission of symptoms for a year. Usually the remission, if it occurs at all, lasts only for a few weeks.

Sydenham's Chorea. — Fever therapy now is considered by some authorities[6] "the method of choice in chorea". Of 76 collected cases of Sydenham's chorea in which fever treatment was given, I found that in more than 72 per cent. recovery occurred, and in an additional 21 per cent. marked improvement was noted. Neymann's[7] previous analysis of 69 cases indicated recovery in 77 per cent. and improvement in 17 per cent.

Endocarditis Lenta. — The use of fever therapy in treatment for endocarditis lenta, subacute bacterial endocarditis, is particularly interesting. In 1933 Bierman[8] employed fever therapy without additional chemotherapy for subacute bacterial endocarditis. He reported that in this case "showers of numerous emboli caused an exitus". In 1936 I[9] reported that I had tried artificial fever therapy in endocarditis lenta and had abandoned it because of the apparently increased danger of embolism. In 1937 Dry and Willius[10] treated four patients, who had subacute bacterial endocarditis, with fever therapy and came to the conclusion that, despite the fact that fever therapy enhanced cellular reactions and bodily defense processes, *Streptococcus viridans* seemed to be able to resist the highest temperatures which were humanly tolerable.

In 1941 Bierman and Baehr[11] reported two cases of subacute bacterial endocarditis in which treatment with a combination of sulfanilamide and fever proved successful. Their first patient was treated in 1938. In 1940 Bennett and I[12], following up Baehr and Biérman's successful 1938 case, reported six cases of subacute bacterial endocarditis in which treatment with combined fever and sulfanilamide was unsuccessful. The combined therapy in our opinion appeared to have a definite though transient influence on the disease, for, despite the ultimate failure, culture of the blood following treatment revealed either a definite decrease in the number or a temporary complete disappearance, of bacterial colonies.

In 1941 Lichtman and Bierman[8] reported that of 200 cases of subacute bacterial endocarditis caused by nonhemolytic *Streptococcus viridans*, in which the sulfonamide drugs were administered, recovery occurred in 12 (6 per cent.). Recovery occurred in 5 (11.6 per cent.) of 43 cases in which combined chemotherapy and heparin were used and in 9 (20 per cent.) of 45 cases in which combined chemotherapy and fever therapy (either physically induced or induced by typhoid-paratyphoid vaccine) were employed. They concluded: "The combined methods of therapy seem to promise a greater incidence of recovery than may be anticipated in the natural course of the disease or after treatment with sulfonamide drugs alone."

The series of cases reported to date is too small to have any great statistical significance; it is possible that the 6 failures, reported by Bennett and myself, happened to be drawn from the large group of patients who failed to respond. In the light of present evidence, therefore, it seems logical to consider the use of combined fever and chemotherapy in this nearly hopeless group of cases. Additional experience may modify this opinion. At present there seems to be nothing better to offer. Bierman and Baehr[11] concluded that their experience indicated "that physically induced pyrexia enhances the value of chemotherapy in the treatment of subacute bacterial endocarditis". Their clinical results supported "the in vitro observations of White[13] that the effectiveness of the sulfonamide drugs is materially enhanced at sustained higher elevations of temperature".

Gonorrhea. — I have been interested especially in the treatment of gonorrhea by means of fever therapy and more recently in treatment by means of a combination of fever therapy and the sulfonamide drugs for gonorrhea which is resistant to chemotherapy alone. In a series of 415 cases of proved gonorrhea in which adequate fever therapy was administered, after an average of four fever sessions per patient, Randall, Stubler and I found that there were apparent, complete, clinical remissions in 94.1 per cent[14]. Follow-up studies revealed that the disease recurred in not more than 3 to 5 per cent.[15]. Of 1,157 collected cases of acute and chronic gonorrhea treated by artificial fever I[16] found that apparent cures were reported in 87.4 per cent. and failures in 12.6 per cent.

Despite these excellent results with fever therapy alone with the advent of the sulfonamide drugs it became apparent that they would have a curative effect in a high percentage of cases of gonorrhea. The administration of these drugs under proper control is certainly a much less rigorous procedure than is fever therapy. Therefore, it is recommended at present that chemotherapy be tried first before fever therapy is administered for gonorrhea.

Chemotherapy has failed to cure gonorrhea in 32 per cent. of the cases reported by Dees and Young[17] in their recent review of the literature. It is in this group of highly resistant cases, chemotherapy failures, that the combination of fever and chemotherapy seems to be particularly valuable. For such cases I now administer a single 10 hour fever at 106.8° F. (41.5° C.) at a time when there is a high hemal concentration of the sulfonamide drug. This is strictly an institutional procedure and should be attempted only by a well-organized group of fever therapists.

I[16] found that in a group of 43 patients suffering from resistant gonorrhea, all of whom had failed to respond to unfortified sulfonamide therapy, an average of 1.2 treatments with combined chemotherapy and artificial fever for 10 hours effected apparent, complete, clinical remissions for 95.4 per cent. Thus it seems that the combined procedure is by far the most potent means of treating gonorrhea; this method always is to be considered, when unfortified chemotherapy fails.

Kendell, Rose and Simpson[18] agree with me because recently they reported: "All of 31 unselected consecutive patients treated with sulfanilamide or promin for eighteen hours before a single 10 hour fever session at a rectal temperature of 106.6° F. were cured." They studied 83 patients suffering from complications of gonorrhea, resistant or intolerant to chemotherapy. "Of those refractory patients, receiving fever therapy alone, only 12.5 per cent. were cured following a single 8 hour treatment at 106.6° F.; 62.5 per cent. were cured following a single 10 hour treatment at 106.6° F."

I have been using the 10 hour sessions of fever at approximately 106.8° F. (41.5° C.) routinely for resistant gonorrhea since January 1937, because previously I had come to the conclusion that this was the most satisfactory way of treating resistant gonorrhea. The observations of Kendell and his associates confirm these views.

With the introduction of chemotherapy this procedure was combined with the 10 hour sessions of fever with even better results. Kendell and his associates observed that "a 10 day period of intensive sulfanilamide therapy prior to fever therapy is without value in sulfanilamide-resistant patients, provided none of the drug is present in the body fluids at the time of the fever treatment." This confirms my previous contention that there must be a high hemal concentration of the drug at the time of the fever treatment.

Kendell and his associates came to a conclusion with which I agree; namely, that: "The combination of a single 10 hour session of artificial fever therapy combined with the administration of adequate sulfanilamide or promin for eighteen hours prior to the fever treatment appears to be the procedure of choice in the treatment of chemotherapy-resistant gonococcic infections."

Gonorrheal Arthritis. — Fever therapy is the most effective means of treatment for gonorrheal arthritis. In the "Fifth Rheumatism Review"[6] there was a summary of fifteen reports in which results of fever therapy in approximately 380 cases of gonorrheal arthritis were presented. About 90 per cent. of these 380 patients, who had acute or chronic gonorrheal arthritis, became free of symptoms. Fever therapy was spoken of variously as "specific", "the procedure of choice", "the best treatment now available" and "the treatment of choice to be used at the earliest available opportunity" in cases of gonorrheal arthritis.

Recent advances in chemotherapy undoubtedly have lessened the incidence of this later manifestation of gonorrhea. But whenever chemotherapy fails to prevent the development of a gonorrheal arthritis, the combined fever-chemotherapy regimen should be attempted at once. It is unwise to delay the combined procedure too long, because the earlier the combined treatment is given, the less is the likelihood of permanent damage to the involved joint or joints.

Gonococcal Septicemia. — There have been several reports[19, 20, 21, 22] of cases of gonococcal septicemia in which cure followed fever therapy. In two instances[19, 22], even though there was an associated gonococcal endocarditis, recovery occurred. In Elkins' and my[23] case of gonococcal endocarditis, in which fever therapy was used, recovery did not occur. In the light of present knowledge the combination of fever and chemotherapy always should be considered when gonococcal septicemia is encountered.

Meningococcal Septicemia. — For this condition combined fever and chemotherapy may be curative. Elkins and I[23] reported successful employment of this procedure in one such case. Four cases of meningococcal septicemia, in which unfortified fever therapy has produced cures, have been reported[24, 25]. The combined procedure seems worthy of trial in selected cases of meningococcal infection.

Multiple Sclerosis. — Fever therapy, although often recommended, seems to be of limited, if of any, value for multiple sclerosis. After treating 10 patients with discouraging results, I abandoned the procedure. A review of the conclusions of five other investigators[7, 26–29] led to the conclusion that the results of fever therapy for multiple sclerosis for the most part have been unfavorable[16]. Recently Bennett and Lewis[30] checked 51 cases of multiple sclerosis for an average of thirty-one months after artificial fever therapy. Although they expressed the opinion that the procedure still should be tried early, when the patients were "ambulatory without assistance", they concluded that "on the whole, except in the early group of cases and those having signs which suggest infection, there is little evidence that fever therapy has any markedly beneficial results in multiple sclerosis". Furthermore they stated that in "the bedridden group", fever therapy "does no good and may do harm".

Mycosis Fungoides, Neuritis and Radicular Pain. — Fever therapy has been employed in treatment of mycosis fungoides with transitory improvement. Of 10 cases reported in the literature[31, 32] moderate and temporary improvement was noted in 8. I have seen temporary but distinct improvement in 2 cases. Fever therapy may retard the disease sufficiently to warrant its employment.

For neuritis and radicular pain artificial fever of low temperature has been recommended[33] as a safe and efficient means of treatment.

Rheumatic Fever. — Treatment for rheumatic fever by means of physical fevers, especially when combined with chemotherapy, sometimes may be justifiable. In one series of cases[34] there often was relief from pain and from swelling of joints as well as a final reduction in the number of leukocytes and in the sedimentation rate of the erythrocytes. In two-thirds of this small series of 9 cases inactivity occurred in an average of 24 days after an average of 5 fever treatments.

Syphilis. — Investigations[35] of the treatment for early syphilis by physically induced fevers revealed that artificial fevers combined with antisyphilitic chemotherapy afford better results than can be obtained from the use of either one alone. In an experimental study[2] of the combined procedure for treatment of early syphilis it was found that artificial fever fortifies and intensifies the curative action of chemotherapeutic agents and that the time required for treatment can be reduced greatly by the combined treatment method. In its present stage of development fever therapy cannot possibly be made available to the average patient, who has a primary syphilitic lesion, but it is possible that it may be employed routinely for primary syphilis at some future time. A final evaluation of the procedure will not be possible for many years.

For dementia paralytica physically induced fevers frequently can be used to great advantage. There still is much controversy concerning the comparative value of physical fever and malarial fever in treatment for paresis. Enthusiasts about malarial fever have been slow to recognize the undoubted effectiveness of physically induced fever for dementia paralytica.

Probably the most authoritative comparative study of the relative merits of the two procedures is that recently published by physicians from a group of co-operating clinics working in conjunction with the United States Public Health Service[36]. This group, whose chairman was O'Leary, carefully studied 1,100 patients, who were treated with malaria as compared with 320 patients, who received physically induced fevers. The number of cases was large enough to be of some statistical significance, and there was much evidence to indicate the slight superiority of physical fevers over malarial fevers.

The Committee studied patients "under treatment-observation" for three or more years. Of the patients, who had mild paresis, 52.4 per cent. of those treated with malarial fever and 59.3 per cent. of those receiving physical fever obtained remissions. Of those who had intermediate paresis 27.3 per cent. of the patients, who were treated with malaria, and 28.1 per cent. of those treated by physical fevers obtained remissions. For severe paresis an even more striking difference was found: only 0.8 per cent. of the malaria treated group as compared with 12.0 per cent. of those treated by physical fevers had remissions. Furthermore the "crude death rate" in the malaria treated group was 13.4 as compared with only 8.1 in the cases treated with physically induced fever.

In only one respect did the statistical evidence seem to reveal a superiority of the malarial therapy over the artificial fever therapy. "In patients treated with fever plus chemotherapy the annual rates of spinal fluid as well as blood reversal were consistently higher with malaria than with artificial fever." But even here there was an explanation because "this difference was assumed to be due to the greater amount of chemotherapy, 17 per cent. more, administered to the malaria patients".

More studies, of course, will be necessary, but as evidence piles up, it becomes increasingly evident that physical fevers are equally as effective, if not more effective, than malarial fevers in the treatment of dementia paralytica. In addition any procedure, which will lessen the mortality by more than 5 per cent., should be given careful consideration.

For tabes dorsalis fever therapy sometimes has been recommended. In a report[1] of the results of this treatment of 15 patients, 8 were said to be greatly improved, 6 moderately improved and 1 was unimproved. One of the most constant results has been relief of gastric crises and tabetic pains. Another investigator[7] reported that two-thirds of 114 tabetic patients exhibited definite improvement following fever therapy.

Fever therapy has been reported also as being of much value in the treatment of ocular syphilis. Culler[37] found the combination of fever and chemotherapy useful for syphilitic interstitial keratitis, exudative uveitis and choroiditis.

Tetanus. — An interesting case in which fever therapy was employed in my department as an adjunct in treatment for tetanus was reported recently by Heersema[38]. In this case fever therapy was administered in conjunction with the use of antitoxin. Despite the fact that he had failed previously to respond to large doses of antitoxin, when fever therapy was inaugurated, the patient began to improve, and he finally recovered. Heersema commented that; "it is not impossible to postulate a more effective interrelationship of the toxin and antitoxin facilitated by the hyperthermia. For the present, however, the symptomatic relief obtained is sufficient to warrant further trial of this method. There was no doubt of this patient's improvement by the third day of treatment, whereas the clinical course before initiation of hyperthermia was definitely downward."

Malignant Tumors. — Warren[39] of Rochester, New York, has employed a combination of roentgen therapy and physical fever in treatment of malignant tumors. He stated that the growth of tumors is inhibited more completely by the combined procedure than by roentgen therapy alone. Jares[40], also working at Rochester, New York, studied the thermal death time of animal tumor cells in vitro. He came to the conclusion that the combined effects of fever and roentgen rays are superior to the effect of either alone. The most destructive combination was simple, fractional doses of roentgen rays, about 300 r. daily, plus fever treatment immediately afterward.

In a recent report[41] on the studies at Rochester, New York, on the combined effects of high voltage roentgen therapy and artificial fever on carcinoma the author stated; "The summative effects of the two radiations, x-rays and heat, appear to be more destructive to the carcinoma and normal structures than either alone. Since the dosage values are not well understood the experiments have been restricted to hopeless cases. The delayed effects (telangiectases, edema, cutaneous degeneration and the like) seem to be more marked, probably because of the summative effect.

"The following dosage has been used with safety, though it should not be attempted by any one not well versed in both irradiation technic and fever treatment technic: Daily for six days 250 roentgens is given in the usual manner for any one port. On the third day in this schedule a five hour fever bout at 41.5° C. (106.7° F.), rectal temperature is administered and at the end of the fever, while the body temperature is up, that day's x-ray treatment is given. A second fever bout of one hour (or more if the patient is not too much intoxicated by the tumor destruction) is given on the fifth day with the x-ray treatment again administered at its end. Several portals may be treated simultaneously except that great caution must be exercised not to overtreat (i.e. not over 1,800 roentgens given to any one skin area) within a given course. Courses have been repeated in six months without catastrophe, although the damage to the skin was considerable.

"At present this method is purely experimental and is not advocated for general use until its merits are more clearly defined."

At this time, there is no indication for the clinical employment of fever therapy as a therapeutic measure for malignant tumors.

Undulant Fever (Brucellosis). — Fever therapy has proved to be of distinct value in treatment for undulant fever. Prickman, Bennett and I[42] reviewed the results obtained in 21 cases of brucellosis following treatment by means of physically induced fever and found that in approximately 80 per cent. apparently complete clinical remissions occurred. Recently Moor[43] reported on 15 cases of brucellosis treated by fever therapy. Nine patients, 60 per cent., obtained "unqualified recovery"; one was "much improved"; one was "improved", and the other four were only "temporarily improved". Zeiter[44] at the Cleveland Clinic and several others[16] also have reported successful treatment of brucellosis by means of fever therapy. Results have been most encouraging throughout; although the series still is small, there is increasing evidence of the value of fever therapy in this disease.

Contraindications to the General Application of Heat (Fever Therapy)

Serious complications of fever therapy are heat stroke, heat exhaustion and circulatory collapse, which are followed by anoxia and finally hemorrhagic changes and damage to nerve tissues. Minor complications include tetany, heat cramps, delirium, mild dehydration with resultant nausea and vomiting, superficial burns and herpes labialis. Skillful treatment will prevent or minimize many of these complications. Important factors in management include the administration of sufficient amounts of fluid either orally or intravenously to prevent circulatory collapse, the employment of inhalations of oxygen throughout the treatment in order to prevent anoxia and proper cooling of the patient in case the temperature becomes too high.

Apparently several deaths have occurred because of incorrect attempts at lowering bodily temperature during excessive hyperpyrexia. In several instances patients have been placed in ice packs in an attempt to lower rapidly their high systemic temperatures. Actually this procedure constricts the peripheral capillaries, lessens the amount of radiation of heat, drives the hot blood from the surface into the splanchnic regions and often causes a slight additional rise of the rectal temperature. The correct method of lowering the bodily temperature, if it becomes too high, consists of removing the patient from the fever producing device, sponging his nude body with tepid water and turning a fan so that it blows across the surface of the body. Bodily heat thus will be dissipated rapidly by evaporation, and the high temperature will tend to fall rapidly to normal.

A treatment as heroic as fever therapy is not without a definite element of danger. According to the most accurate compilation I have been able to make the mortality rate per patient from fever therapy now is less than 0.2 per cent. This compares favorably with the mortality from simple appendectomy. In one average hospital, 685 appendectomies were performed and there were 8 deaths, a percentage mortality rate per patient of 1.16.

Fever therapy is contraindicated in about the same conditions as is a major operation. It should not be administered to patients who have severe cardiovascular-renal disease, evidences of damage to the liver or sensitivity to heat. Its employment is contraindicated at the extremes of age. The very young and the very old do not tolerate fever therapy well. It always should be used with caution for patients who are asthenic or dehydrated. A careful general physical examination and accurate laboratory studies should be performed before administration of fever therapy.

Summary of Data on Fever Therapy

There are numerous effective methods for the general application of heat to the human body. The procedure usually is called "fever therapy". Elevations of systemic temperature can be accomplished by means of heated cabinets, diathermy, hot baths or by heated blankets or packs. The hot humid air cabinet seems to be the most satisfactory device for producing artificial fever by physical means.

High artificial fevers produce profound physiological changes which have been investigated rather extensively in the past few years. Fever therapy has become a therapeutic agent of considerable usefulness, and it gives promise of being still more valuable as more information is ascertained concerning it.

Fever therapy often is of value in treatment for resistant gonorrhea and its complications and for syphilis and its various forms. The value of fever therapy for syphilis of the nervous system is becoming recognized. It has been employed also, to more or less advantage, in the management of atrophic arthritis, intractable bronchial asthma, Sydenham's chorea, endocarditis lenta, meningococcal septicemia, mycosis fungoides, neuritis, rheumatic fever, tetanus and undulant fever. The combined application of fever and chemotherapy apparently is going to be extremely useful in a number of diseases. Fever therapy requires a trained personnel and proper equipment. In unskilled hands the procedure is potentially extremely dangerous. The development of fever therapy is a distinctly valuable contribution to the advance of modern therapeutics.

BIBLIOGRAPHY OF FEVER THERAPY

1. SIMPSON, W. M. and KENDELL, H. W.: Artificial fever therapy, Colorado Med., 1937, XXXIV, 782.
2. SIMPSON, W. M. and KENDELL, H. W.: Experimental treatment of early syphilis with artificial fever combined with chemotherapy, pp. 143–145, in Fever Therapy; abstracts and discussions of papers presented at the First International Conference on Fever Therapy, Hoeber, New York, 1937.
3. BISHOP, F. W., LEHMAN, E. and WARREN, S. L.: A comparison of three electrical methods of producing artificial hyperthermia, Jour. Am. Med. Assoc., 1935, CIV, 910.
4. ATSATT, R. F. and PATTERSON, L. E.: Fever therapy apparatus, Arch. Phys. Therapy, 1936, XVII, 108.
5. HALPHEN, A. and AUCLAIR, J.: Short waves; a perfect pyretogenic agent, pp. 21–23, in Fever Therapy; abstracts and discussions of papers presented at the First International Conference on Fever Therapy, Hoeber, New York, 1937.
6. HENCH, P. S., BAUER, W., DAWSON, M. H., HALL, F., HOLBROOK, W. P. and KEY, J. A.: The problem of rheumatism and arthritis; review of American and English literature for 1937 (fifth rheumatism review), Ann. Int. Med., 1939, XII, 1005, 1295.
7. NEYMANN, C. A.: Artificial Fever Produced by Physical Means; its Development and Application, Thomas, Springfield, Illinois, 1938.
8. LICHTMAN, S. S. and BIERMAN, W.: The treatment of subacute bacterial endocarditis, Jour. Am. Med. Assoc., 1941, CXVI, 286.
9. KRUSEN, F. H.: The present status of fever therapy produced by physical means, Jour. Am. Med. Assoc., 1936, CVII, 1215.
10. DRY, T. J. and WILLIUS, F. A.: Fever therapy for subacute bacterial endocarditis, Proc. Staff Meet., Mayo Clin., 1937, XII, 321.
11. BIERMAN, W., and BAEHR, G.: The use of physically induced pyrexia and chemotherapy, Jour. Am. Med. Assoc., 1941, CXVI, 292.
12. KRUSEN, F. H. and BENNETT, R. L.: Unsuccessful treatment of subacute bacterial endocarditis with combined fever and sulfanilamide therapy, Proc. Staff Meet., Mayo Clin., 1940, XV, 328.
13. WHITE, H. J.: The relationship between temperature and the streptococcidal activity of sulfanilamide and sulfapyridine in vitro, Jour. Bact., 1939, XXXVIII, 549.
14. KRUSEN, F. H., RANDALL, L. M. and STUHLER, L.: Fever therapy plus

additional local heating in the treatment of gonococcic infections, pp. 168–170, in Fever Therapy; abstracts and discussions of papers presented at the First International Conference on Fever Therapy, Hoeber, New York, 1937.

15. KRUSEN, F. H.: Summary of results of fever therapy for gonorrhea with follow-up reports, Proc. Staff Meet., Mayo Clin., 1938, XIII, 297.
16. KRUSEN, F. H.: Physical Medicine, Saunders, Philadelphia, 1941.
17. DEES, J. E. and YOUNG, H. H.: Present status of sulfanilamide therapy in gonorrhea, Ven. Dis. Inform., 1939, XX, 33.
18. KENDELL, H. W., ROSE, D. L. and SIMPSON, W. M.: Combined artificial fever-chemotherapy in gonococcic infections resistant to chemotherapy, Jour. Am. Med. Assoc., 1941, CXVI, 357.
19. FREUND, H. A. and ANDERSON, W. L.: Recovery in a case of gonococcic endocarditis treated by artificial hyperpyrexia, pp. 178–180, in Fever Therapy; abstracts and discussions of papers presented at the First International Conference on Fever Therapy, Hoeber, New York, 1937.
20. HAZEL, O. G. and SNOW, W. B.: Gonococcic septicemia with purpura and arthritis successfully treated by hyperthermia, Jour. Am. Med. Assoc., 1937, CIX, 1275.
21. WARREN, S. L.: Personal communication to the author.
22. WILLIAMS, R. H.: Gonococcal endocarditis treated with artificial fever (Kettering hypertherm), Ann. Int. Med., 1937, X, 1766.
23. KRUSEN, F. H. and ELKINS, E. C.: Fever therapy for gonococcemia and meningococcemia with associated endocarditis; report of two cases, Proc. Staff Meet., Mayo Clin., 1937, XII, 324.
24. BENNETT, A. E., PERSON, J. P. and SIMMONS, E. E.: Treatment of chronic meningococcic infections by artificial fever, Arch. Phys. Therapy, 1936, XVII, 743.
25. PLATOU, E. S., McELMEEL, E. and STOESSER, A.: Artificial fever in the treatment of meningococcus infection, Minnesota Med., 1936, XIX, 781.
26. WALTHARD, K. M. and HERTENSTEIN, H.: Some remarks on short wave fever therapy, pp. 118–119, in Fever Therapy; abstracts and discussions of papers presented at the First International Conference on Fever Therapy, Hoeber, New York, 1937.
27. DESJARDINS, A. U. and POPP, W. C.: Our experience with fever therapy, pp. 7–8, In Abstracts of Papers and Discussions, Fifth Annual Fever Conference, May 2 and 3, 1935.
28. BENNETT, A. E. and AUSTIN, B.: Preliminary report of the University of Nebraska fever research project, pp. 23–24, in Abstracts of Papers and Discussions, Fifth Annual Fever Conference, May 2 and 3, 1935.
29. HEFKE, H. W.: Report on the first year of fever therapy at the Milwaukee hospital, pp. 29–30, in Abstracts of Papers and Discussions, Fifth Annual Fever Conference, May 2 and 3, 1935.
30. BENNETT, A. E. and LEWIS, M. D.: Artificial fever therapy in multiple sclerosis; a study of fifty-one cases, Jour. Nerv. and Ment. Dis., 1940, XCII, 202.

31. KLAUDER, J. V.: Fever therapy in mycosis fungoides, Jour. Am. Med. Assoc., 1936, CVI, 201.
32. PEYRI, J.: Quelques commentaires à notre casuistique de mycosis fungoides, Ann. de Dermat. et Syph., 1935, VI, 481.
33. BENNETT, A. E. and CASH, P. T.: The relief of neuritic pain by artificial fever therapy; results obtained in 40 cases, pp. 91–92, in Fever Therapy; abstracts and discussions of papers presented at the First International Conference on Fever Therapy, Hoeber, New York, 1937.
34. SIMMONS, E. E.: Value of fever therapy in the arthritides, Am. Jour. Med. Sci., 1937, CXCIV, 170.
35. NEYMANN, C. A., LAWLESS, T. K. and OSBORNE, S. L.: The treatment of early syphilis with electropyrexia, Jour. Am. Med. Assoc., 1936, CVII, 194.
36. O'LEARY, P. A., BRUETSCH, W. L., EBAUGH, F. G., SIMPSON, W. M., SOLOMON, H. C., WARREN, S L., VONDERLEHR, R. A., USILTON, L. J. and SOLLINS, I. V.: Malaria and artificial fever in the treatment of paresis, Jour. Am. Med. Assoc., 1940, CXV, 677.
37. CULLER, A. M.: Artificial fever therapy of ocular syphilis, pp. 105–106, in Abstracts of Papers and Discussions, Fifth Annual Fever Conference, May 2 and 3, 1935.
38. HEERSEMA, P. H.: Management of tetanus with report of use of hyperthermia in one case, Minnesota Med., 1940, XXIII, 636.
39. WARREN, S. L.: Preliminary study of the effect of artificial fever upon hopeless tumor cases, Am. Jour. Roentgenol., 1935, XXXIII, 75.
40. JARES, J. J., JR.: The in vitro thermal death time of animal tumor cells, pp. 114–115, in Fever Therapy; Abstracts and Discussions of Papers Presented at the First International Conference on Fever Therapy, Hoeber, New York, 1937.
41. QUERIES AND MINOR NOTES: Combined fever and roentgen therapy for cancer, Jour. Am. Med. Assoc., 1940, CXV, 2106.
42. PRICKMAN, L. E., BENNETT, R. L. and KRUSEN, F. H.: Treatment of brucellosis by physically induced hyperpyrexia, Proc. Staff Meet., Mayo Clin., 1938, XIII, 321.
43. MOOR, F. B.: Personal communication to the author.
44. ZEITER, W. J.: Treatment of undulant fever by artificial fever therapy, Cleveland Clinic Quart., 1937, IV, 309.

Sept. 1, 1941.

LOCAL AND GENERAL APPLICATIONS OF COLD

Applications of cold both locally and generally have been employed for therapeutic purposes. There has been considerably less investigation of hypothermy than of hyperthermy. The therapeutic administration of cold has been called "cryotherapy" or "crymotherapy", and prolonged systemic applications of cold have been spoken of as "hibernation" or "refrigeration therapy".

Recently considerable unfortunate publicity has been given to the possibilities of benefiting carcinoma by such general applications of cold. As yet there is no convincing evidence that any such possibility does exist. While studies in a few cases have indicated that prolonged general applications of cold effect apparent modifications in malignant cells, the number of cases studied is so meager as to preclude serious consideration at this time.

Although local applications of cold long have been used in therapy, the general application of cold has not been established as yet as a rational therapeutic procedure.

Methods of Applying Cold

Cold water or ice can be applied directly or indirectly to a small or large area of the human body to produce local or systemic effects. In some instances ordinary refrigerating units, similar to those employed in the household, electrical iceboxes, are connected with metallic coils or blankets, which are applied to the entire body of the patient in order to effect lowering of the systemic temperature.

In other instances an air cooling unit, similar to that employed for air conditioning of rooms in the summer, is employed to cool a small room, in which the nude patient lies on a bed, in order that his systemic temperature may be lowered. Another arrangement, which I have seen, consisted of a cold air blower connected to the top of a tent which was placed over the bed of the patient. The cold air blew down over the patient and cooled him effectively. In still another arrangement the patient is placed in a large bag containing within its walls serpentine coils, through which is circulated a cooling fluid derived from a regular refrigeration unit, which is placed at the foot of the patient's bed.

For local application of cold the time-honored ice bag, the cold compress and the ice pack still are extremely useful. A refinement of technic consists of the construction of sets of metallic applicators, which can be connected to a refrigeration unit and through which the refrigerating mixture is circulated (Fig. 16). These small applicators can be applied to various regions or orifices of the body in order to administer intense cold. Little is known, as yet, concerning the value of, or indications for, the use of these applicators, which were constructed primarily for use in conjunction with "hibernation therapy" for malignant lesions. The thought

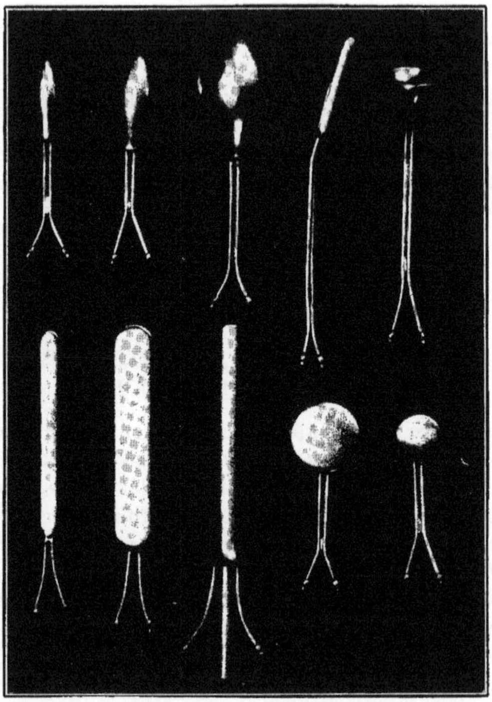

FIG. 16. Applicators through which a cooling mixture can be circulated from a refrigeration unit to permit local applications of intense cold.

was that these applicators could be applied directly over the growth to produce additional local cooling during the period when the bodily temperature was lowered.

I have had no personal experience with the methods for treatment of malignant lesions by means of general and local applications of cold and sincerely doubt that the procedures ever will be of much, if of any, value. Nevertheless it seems worth while to consider the whole subject of cold therapy, because there have been so many recent inquiries concerning it, and because its distinct limitations should be stated.

Physical Principles Concerned in the Application of Cold

There is an extreme dearth of information concerning the physics of cold. Textbooks on physics neglect this subject in an amazing fashion. From a therapeutic standpoint, however, it is necessary merely to know that, in order to apply cold to all, or to a part, of the human body, it must be placed in a cold environment or in contact with a cold substance.

Action and Uses of Cooling Procedures

Cooling of the surface of the body without compensation produces definite systemic changes. Constriction of the peripheral vessels occurs with associated peripheral stasis and anoxemia. There is a lowered leukocytic response, and the phagocytic capability of the fixed tissue cells is impaired. These changes are the reverse of those observed on applications of heat. Processes of immunity unquestionably are delayed in local regions which are cooled. Locally the volume of blood will be diminished, and local metabolic activity will decrease. Application of cold to the abdomen tends to cause a temporary increase in peristalsis, which is followed later by a decrease.

Placing the forearm in cold water lessens the rate of circulation so greatly that eventually even comparatively deep tissues may have a temperature little higher than that of the bath. Local application of cold to any region of the body will tend to cause generalized vasoconstriction. Drinking of cold water likewise causes vasoconstriction.

Hypersensitivity to cold occasionally is observed. Horton and his associates[1] studied 22 hypersensitive persons and noted that locally there was cutaneous pallor during exposure; redness, swelling and increased local temperature appeared on removal from the cold environment. After a latent period of three to six minutes the systemic reaction developed; this consisted of flushing of the face, a sharp drop in blood pressure, a rise in pulse rate, a tendency toward syncope and then transitory recovery in five or ten minutes. These studies suggested that a chemical substance, which causes a histamine-like reaction, is produced in the skin following exposure to cold.

Although in most instances applications of cold impair circulation, occasionally applications of mild cold, which will cause slight vascular constriction and moderate reduction of capillary pressure, actually may cause a more rapid flow of blood than would application of heat.

Reactions to thermal changes are very complex. They are, in general, vasodilatation on heating and vasoconstriction on cooling. If the cold is intense, it may cause vasodilatation. Arterioles, capillaries, arteriovenous aneurysms and veins are involved. There may be considerable local increase or decrease in the flow of blood. These changes are caused partly through nervous reflexes. Application of cold to an extremity may cause vasoconstriction in a distant region such as an opposite limb which is not primarily affected by the change in temperature.

Peripheral vasoconstriction caused by local application of cold is balanced by opposite changes in the remaining vessels, particularly the splanchnic or other deep vessels. Bazett[2] has shown that the vasodilatation caused by extreme cold occurs only when the temperature of the skin is less than 64.4° F. (18° C.). The reflex that produces such dilatation probably is akin to a mild inflammatory reaction. This reaction may protect the peripheral region from injury.

Brooks and Duncan[3] recently have conducted interesting studies on the effects of temperature on the survival of anemic tissue. These experiments demonstrated conclusively "that temperature is a powerful factor in determining the length of time tissues rendered completely anemic remain viable". Although usually it has been contended that in the presence of threatened gangrene the part should be kept in a warm environment to maintain viability and to promote normal circulation, these investigators found that completely anemic tissues became gangrenous much sooner at high temperatures than at low ones. Brooks in discussion stated that the experiments have convinced him of "the inadvisability of applying unregulated heat to an anemic extremity and have, at least, raised the question of the possible benefits of the employment of a method for maintaining temperature of anemic tissue below that which it would assume under ordinary clinical conditions". Here, possibly, is a new indication for the employment of local applications of cold.

General applications of cold cause distinct changes in the circulation time. These have been investigated carefully by Oppenheimer and McCravey[4]. They observed the circulation time of human beings subjected to "refrigeration" and found that it was increased from an average of 17.2 seconds at normal bodily temperature to 23.5 seconds in the same individuals during "hibernation". They observed an "apparent correlation" between prolongation of circulation time and reduction in rectal temperature; the circulation time increased approximately 5 per cent.

for each degree Fahrenheit the temperature decreased. The bleeding time has been shown[5] to be reduced in partially frozen animals.

If the systemic temperature of rabbits is decreased to less than 75.2° F. (24° C.), frostbites will occur. Shivering ceases at this temperature level, and the lethal general temperature for rabbits is approximately 60.8° F. (16° C.). Oppenheimer has informed me that human beings cease to shiver as the body is cooled, and shivering does not return as the body is gradually warmed again. Large amounts of heat are required to restore the normal temperature of animals or human beings after cooling. Troedsson[7] found that, when the temperature of rabbits was lowered to 73.4° F. (23° C.), the number of leukocytes decreased from 10,300 to 5,200 per cubic millimeter; the relative number of polymorphonuclear leukocytes increased, and the lymphocytes decreased.

Experimental studies by Meader and Marshall[8] revealed that mice were able to survive an internal temperature of 47.3° F. (8.5° C.). Cooling produces an initial acceleration of the respiratory rate which is followed by a reduction of rate. The respiratory rate diminishes approximately 10 excursions per minute per degree centigrade of loss of heat, until an internal temperature of 53.6° to 60.8° F. (12° to 16° C.) is reached. Thereafter it diminishes approximately 20 excursions per minute per degree centigrade.

Rapid freezing of aqueous suspensions of bacteria leads to death of a constant proportion of cells, varying from about 80 per cent. of the most sensitive organisms, *Pseudomonas aeruginosa* (*Bacillus pyocyaneus*), to a slight percentage or no destruction of the least sensitive structures, spores[9].

A significant study, which suggests the futility of employing cold as a curative agent for malignant disease, is that of Breedis and his associates[10]. They found that although the transmitting agent of leukemia in mice, presumably malignant leukocytes, is inactivated by rapid freezing to −22° F. (−30° C.), it nevertheless remains viable even at −94° F. (−70° C.) when frozen slowly. These investigators found also that sarcomatous tissue of mice can be frozen to at least −94° F. (−70° C.) without being inactivated, and that this tissue can be preserved at this temperature with little or no subsequent deterioration during at least 56 days. In the light of these facts it seems that it is utterly useless to attempt to destroy or to inhibit the growth of malignant cells in the living human being by gradual reduction of the systemic temperature to levels between +88° and 90° F. (+31.1° and 32.2° C.) for periods of five or six days.

Local Applications of Cold. — These have been employed therapeutically for conditions in which peripheral vàsoconstriction is desirable. Contusions, sprains or other superficial traumatic lesions, in which there is danger of extravasation of blood and lymph into the perivascular tissues, often can be treated best during the first forty-eight hours by local applications of cold.

Cold often is applied locally for acute inflammation or congestion of superficial regions in order to produce vasoconstriction and to relieve pain, but cold cannot be used to allay inflammations within the abdomen, because now it is believed generally that local application of cold to the abdomen produces little, if any, change in the temperature of the underlying viscera. Intense cold can be used to destroy superficial cutaneous lesions. Usually a carbon dioxide pencil is employed for this purpose.

Occasionally when a local rise of temperature in an extremity is desirable, and a rise of systemic temperature is contraindicated, the general rise can be avoided by placing another extremity in moderately cold water while the affected extremity is being heated. This is known as the Lovén reflex.

Patients, who are hypersensitive to cold, can be desensitized by the simple expedient of immersing one hand in cold water at a temperature of 50° F. (10° C.), for one or two minutes twice a day for three or four weeks[1].

Systemic Applications of Cold. — These have been tried clinically for patients who have advanced malignant disease. In some instances local applications of cold have been used in conjunction with the general cooling. Theorizing that increased temperature alone is required to bring into existence activation of the rapid embryological cellular division in hen's eggs, that in plant life darkness and sustained abnormally high temperatures give rise to overgrowth and delayed maturity, and that intense sunlight and sustained low temperatures tend toward a slow and stunted maturity, Fay and Henny[11] advocated trials of "refrigeration" in cases of carcinoma. They reported five cases in which "responses" were noted. They claimed "definite relief of local pain" and "apparent gross retardation in growth as well as diminution in the size of the carcinomatous lesions".

Later Smith and Fay[12], expanding on the hypothesis that carcinomatous metastatic lesions are most common in bodily segments in which the temperature is highest, again advocated "refrigeration" therapy. They reported that local application of cold at approximately 36° F. (2.2° C.) to the pelvis of a patient, who had a massive pelvic extension of a carcinoma of the cervix, caused relief from pain in 48 hours, that within 5 days there was devascularization of the carcinomatous region with shrinkage, and within 3 weeks there was evidence of repair with fibrous tissue.

Prolonged intense cold applied to normal tissues could be expected to produce much the same effects, and in the light of the studies of Breedis and his associates[10], previously mentioned, the temperatures employed could have little effect on the malignant cells. In normal tissues cold always will tend to produce devascularization, shrinkage and tissue damage which, of course, will be followed by repair with fibrous tissue.

Therefore, the hypotheses, which have been set forth by Fay and his associates as bases for suggesting this form of therapy in cases of carcinoma, are debatable. The number of cases reported to date is so limited that the whole problem remains in the realm of pure conjecture. I would not give the question so much attention here, were it not for the fact that much publicity regarding this work has swamped me with numerous inquiries concerning it.

Until definite proof is forthcoming, it seems evident that no clinician is justified in employing the procedure as a therapeutic measure in carcinoma, unless he desires to do so from an experimental angle in an institution properly equipped for such investigative work.

Systemic applications of cold have been suggested in treatment for lymphatic leukemia, but again the studies of Breedis and his associates[10] suggest the futility of the method, and there is no clinical proof of its effectiveness. Troedsson[7] stated that mild generalized "hypothermy" might be found useful in reducing a temporarily high fever, a high metabolic rate or rapid cardiac action "to give the heart a rest". At present none of these procedures has been investigated sufficiently to warrant its general use. Currently local applications of cold can be said to be of clinical value, but systemic applications of cold have not been developed to a point at which they can be employed in clinical practice.

Contraindications to Applications of Cold

Cold should not be employed for patients who have a definite hypersensitivity to it, nor should it be applied to the skin in the presence of cutaneous atrophy, radiodermatitis or melanotic nevus. It has been suggested[13] that prolonged cold therapy for inflammations may lessen vitality and hinder repair.

The danger signs noted during systemic application of cold include slowing of pulse and respiration and lowering of blood pressure. Although general applications of cold have not been employed sufficiently for one to define the contraindications clearly, it seems obvious that the procedure should not be employed in asthenic individuals or in the presence of any marked circulatory or renal disturbance. Respiratory infections also would seem to contraindicate its employment. Acute pancreatitis has occurred following "refrigeration therapy".

Summary of Data on Cold Applications

Local or general applications of cold will cause profound physiological changes. There are numerous methods of applying cold therapeutically. There are several indications for the local applications of cold. Chief among them are traumatic lesions, inflammations and congestions. General application of cold is still in the experimental stage of development, and there are, at present, no indications for its clinical employment.

BIBLIOGRAPHY OF COLD APPLICATIONS

1. HORTON, B. T., BROWN, G. E. and ROTH, G. M.: Hypersensitiveness to cold with local and systemic manifestations of a histamine-like character; its amenability to treatment, Jour. Am. Med. Assoc., 1936, CVII, 1263.
2. BAZETT, H. C.: The physiological basis for the use of heat, Vol. I, pp. 1–29, in Principles and Practice of Physical Therapy, Prior, Hagerstown, Maryland, 1934, Chapt. I.
3. BROOKS, B. and DUNCAN, G. W.: The effects of temperature on the survival of anemic tissue; an experimental study, Ann. Surg., 1940, CXII, 130.
4. OPPENHEIMER, M. J. and McCRAVEY, A.: Circulation time in man at low temperatures, Am. Jour. Physiol., 1940, CXXIX, 434.
5. HARKINS, H. N. and HARMON, P. H.: Experimental freezing; bleeding volume, general and local temperature changes, Proc. Soc. Exper. Biol. and Med., 1935, XXXII, 1142.
6. OPPENHEIMER, M. J.: Personal communication to the author.
7. TROEDSSON, B. S.: Experimental lowering of body temperature of rabbits and its possible application in man, Arch. Phys. Therapy, 1939, XX, 501.
8. MEADER, R. G. and MARSHALL, C.: Studies on the electrical potentials of living organisms: II. Effects of low temperatures on normal unanesthetized mice, Yale Jour. Biol. and Med., 1938, X, 365.
9. HAINES, R. B.: The effect of freezing on bacteria, Proc. Roy. Soc., London, s. B., 1938, CXXIV, 451.
10. BREEDIS, C., BARNES, W. A. and FURTH, J.: Effect of rate of freezing on the transmitting agent of neoplasms of mice, Proc. Soc. Exper. Biol. and Med., 1937, XXXVI, 220.
11. FAY, T. and HENNY, G. C.: Correlation of body segmental temperature and its relation to the location of carcinomatous metastasis; clinical observations and response to methods of refrigeration, Surg., Gynec. and Obst., 1938, LXVI, 512.
12. SMITH, L. W. and FAY, T.: Temperature factors in cancer and embryonal cell growth, Jour. Am. Med. Assoc., 1939, CXIII, 653.
13. BUNCH, G. H.: Ischemic necrosis from ice bag "burn", Am. Jour. Surg., 1936, XXXII, 519.

ULTRAVIOLET RADIANT ENERGY

Ultraviolet therapy consists of treatment by means of radiation from the ultraviolet portion of the electromagnetic spectrum (Fig. 11). Sunlight, particularly during the summer months, is a more or less satisfactory source of ultraviolet radiation. The wavelengths of ultraviolet rays vary between 13.6 and 390 millimicrons.

Ultraviolet rays with wavelengths between 13.6 and 290 millimicrons are spoken of as "far ultraviolet rays", those with wavelengths between 290 and 390 millimicrons as "near ultraviolet rays". Properly employed ultraviolet radiation has a considerable field of usefulness in medicine.

Methods of Applying Ultraviolet Radiant Energy

There are several sources of ultraviolet energy which can be employed for therapeutic purposes. These include the sun, various types of quartz mercury vapor arcs and carbon arcs. To select a source of ultraviolet radiation, it is necessary to know which rays the source produces, their quantity and their physiological effects. Different ultraviolet lamps produce different amounts of radiation from various regions of the spectrum. Because of these variations, different types of ultraviolet lamps may produce distinctly different physiological effects.

It is apparent that the user of such a lamp must know the rays produced and their effects. Practically all sources of ultraviolet radiation commonly employed produce not only ultraviolet rays but also visible and infra-red rays.

The Sun. — Radiation from the sun has its spectral limits at about 290 millimicrons in the ultraviolet portion of the electromagnetic spectrum and 4,000 millimicrons in the infra-red portion. The greatest intensity is at about 490 millimicrons. The sun emits very little ultraviolet radiation of wavelengths shorter than 350 millimicrons. The intensity of the rays of wavelengths of less than 350 millimicrons is slight; the intensity then increases rapidly to 490 millimicrons and above that decreases gradually to 4,000 millimicrons in the infra-red region. Sunlight contains approximately 1 to 5 per cent. ultraviolet radiation, 41 to 45 per cent. visible or luminous radiation and 52 to 60 per cent. infra-red radiation.

The sun is an unreliable source of ultraviolet radiation because it emits an appreciable amount of such rays, especially during winter, only for about three or four hours in the middle of the day. The intensity of ultraviolet radiation is much greater at high altitudes than at sea level.

Much of the radiation is absorbed by water vapor at the lower atmospheric levels.

The Quartz Mercury Vapor Arc. — Radiation from the quartz mercury arc lamp consists of a series of intense spectral lines, namely, at 257, 265, 280, 297, 302, 313, 334 and 365 millimicrons, superimposed on a faint continuous spectrum extending throughout the visible and into the infra-red region. The radiation from such a lamp is composed of approx-

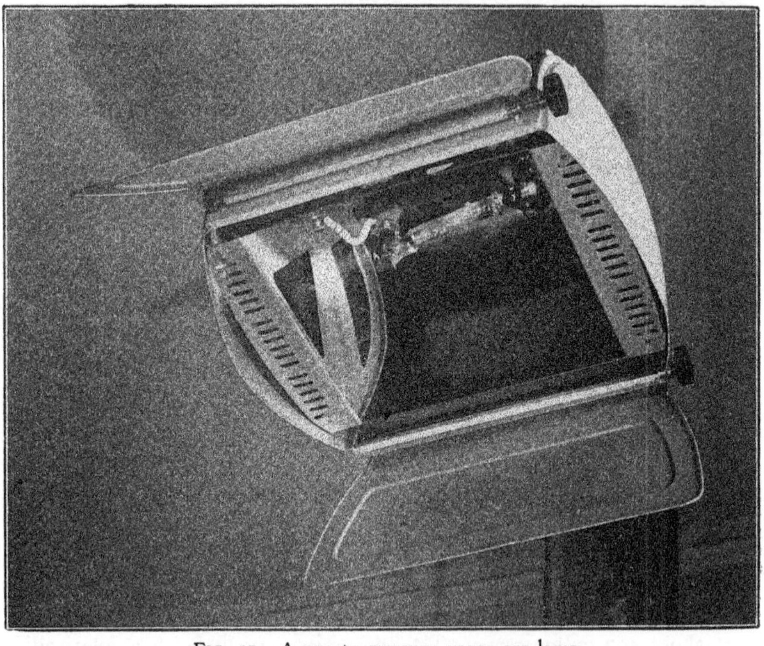

FIG. 17. A quartz mercury vapor arc lamp.

imately 6 per cent. far ultraviolet rays, which have a high germicidal action, and which are completely absent in sunlight, 28 per cent. total ultraviolet rays, 20 per cent. luminous rays and 52 per cent. infra-red rays.

Quartz tubes containing a mercury vapor arc usually are enclosed in an adjustable reflector and applied over large regions of the body for purposes of general irradiation (Fig. 17). Smaller quartz tubes containing a mercury arc sometimes are enclosed in a water jacket to cool the burner so that it can be brought close to the skin. These water-cooled quartz lamps often are called "Kromayer" lamps.

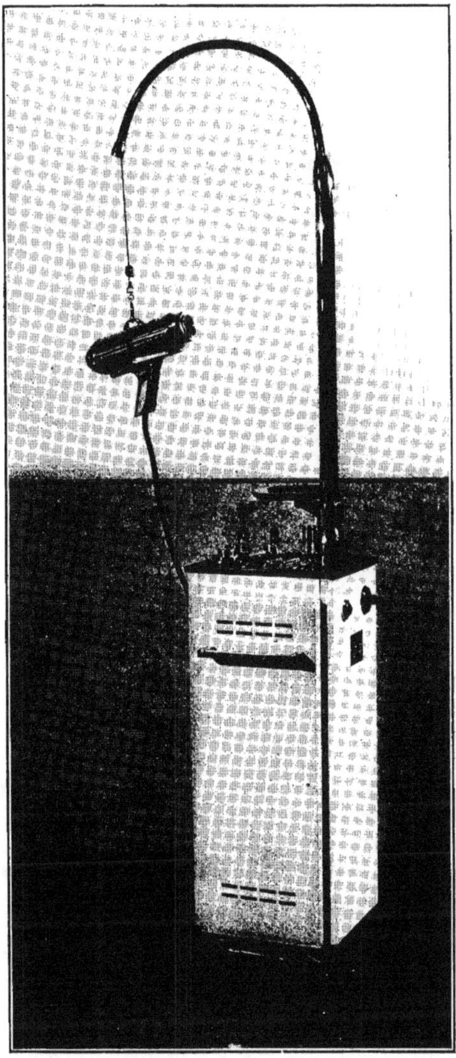

FIG. 18. A new type of air-cooled Kromayer lamp.

Recently an air-cooled Kromayer lamp (Fig. 18) has been developed for local irradiation; this is rather similar to the old water-cooled units with the exception that the small burner is cooled by means of an air blower and not by circulating cold water. Quartz rods and disks can be placed over the window of this lamp for the purpose of conducting the radiation to the surface or to the orifice which is to be exposed (Fig. 19).

The Carbon Arc. — Radiation from a carbon arc lamp varies according to the kind of "carbon pencils" employed. Electrodes of pure carbon are not employed therapeutically. The pencil-like carbon electrodes contain a core composed usually of metallic salts. By varying the constituents of these cores the arc can be altered and its radiation modified.

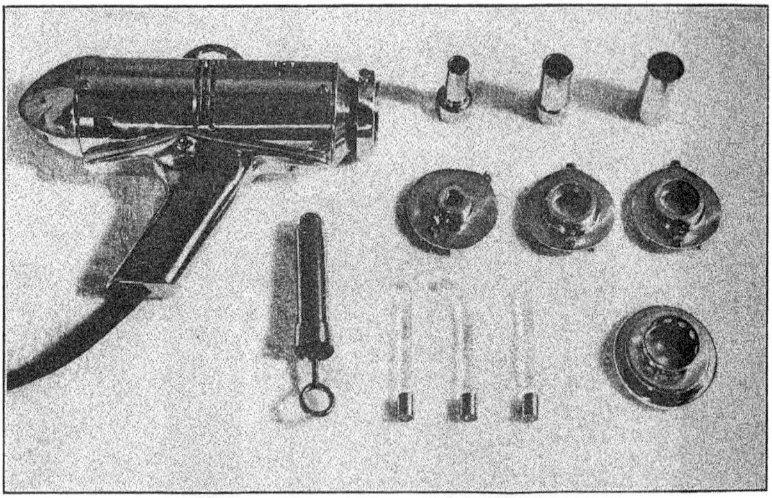

FIG. 19. Quartz disks and rods, which are employed with the Kromayer lamp to conduct the radiation into bodily orifices or to small local regions of the body.

Carbons which contain such metallic cores are spoken of as "impregnated carbons".

The "A" or "sunshine" carbon. The type of carbon most commonly used in therapeutic lamps is known as an "A" or "sunshine" carbon. It is impregnated with "rare earth" oxides, and its arc produces radiation which has a spectral range from 220 millimicrons in the ultraviolet region to more than 4,000 millimicrons in the infra-red region. The spectrum, which it produces, approaches that of sunlight but still is far from being an exact match. Radiation from this source contains 5 per cent. ultraviolet rays, 50 per cent. luminous rays and 45 per cent. infra-red rays.

The "B" carbon. The "B" carbon is similar, but it is impregnated with iron oxide, and its spectrum more nearly resembles that of the mercury arc. This carbon is particularly rich in radiation of wavelengths shorter than 310 millimicrons.

The "C" carbon. The "C" carbon is impregnated with calcium oxide and is particularly rich in radiation in the region between 290 and 320 millimicrons. Its arc emits 9 per cent. ultraviolet rays, 24 per cent. luminous rays and 67 per cent. infra-red rays.

The "E" carbon. The other type of carbon, which commonly is employed therapeutically, is known as the "E" carbon. The radiation, which is emitted by its arc, is similar to that produced by a tungsten filament lamp; it is, therefore, a good source of near infra-red rays. The radiation is particularly rich in rays from the spectral region between 550 and 750 millimicrons in the orange and red portions of the visible spectrum. It emits much radiation in the near infra-red region.

Usually therapeutic carbon arc lamps consist of two carbons arranged end to end in a suitable reflector (Fig. 20). The carbons are connected to a source of electricity. When they are brought together momentarily, the electrical circuit is completed, and then when they are separated slightly, an intense electrical arc forms between the tips of the carbon electrodes. The carbon electrodes are consumed gradually and must be replaced from time to time.

The chief advantage of the carbon arc lamp is that the carbons can be changed to vary the radiation produced. Thus different therapeutic effects can be achieved with the same lamp.

The "Cold Quartz" Lamp. — In the past few years an ultraviolet lamp, which is practically devoid of heat, has been marketed. It, therefore, has been called a "cold quartz" lamp. It consists of quartz tubing containing neon and mercury vapor through which is passed an electric charge of high voltage. The appearance of the tubing is similar to that of the familiar neon signs commonly used in advertising. This tubing usually is shaped into a serpentine grid which is placed over the face of a reflector.

The radiation from this lamp consists of one very intense spectral line at 254 millimicrons and a series of a few much less intense lines. The lines at 297 and 313 millimicrons are fairly intense, but 95 per cent. "of the total radiation of wavelengths less than, and including, 313 millimicrons is contained in the resonance emission line at 254 millimicrons". Because of its limited range of radiation this type of lamp has a limited field of usefulness.

Sun Lamps. — In the past few years several kinds of sun lamps have been constructed for home use. Typical of this group of lamps is the

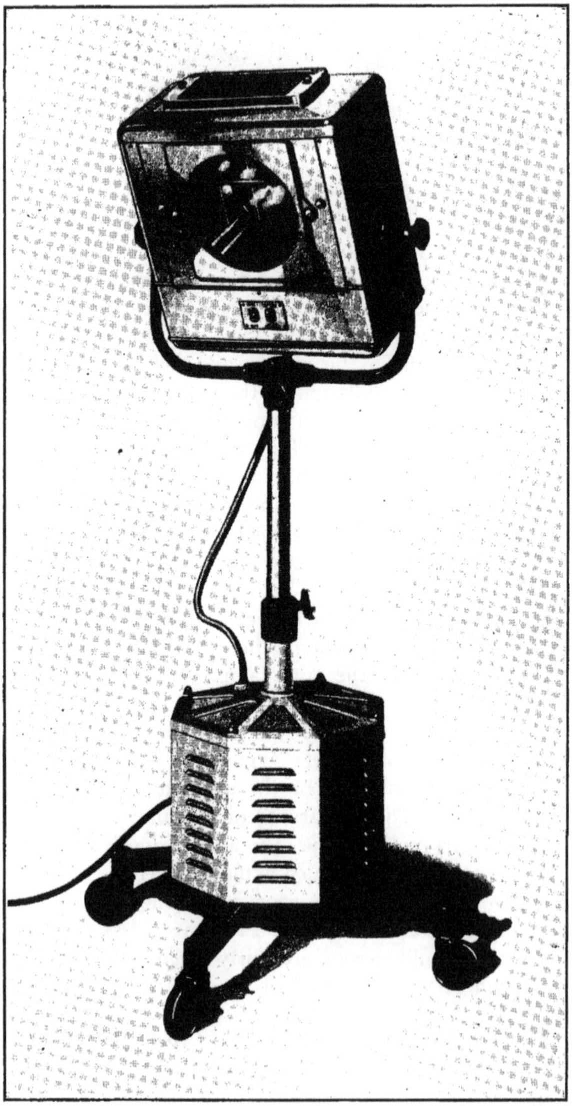

FIG. 20. A carbon arc lamp of the type commonly employed in a physician's office.

"S-1" lamp. It consists of a tungsten filament, two tungsten electrodes and a drop of mercury enclosed in a bulb of ultraviolet transmitting glass. When it is turned on, the filament becomes hot, and the mercury vaporizes and forms a mercury vapor arc between the electrodes. This arc emits ultraviolet rays (Fig. 21). The radiation is not unlike that of the other

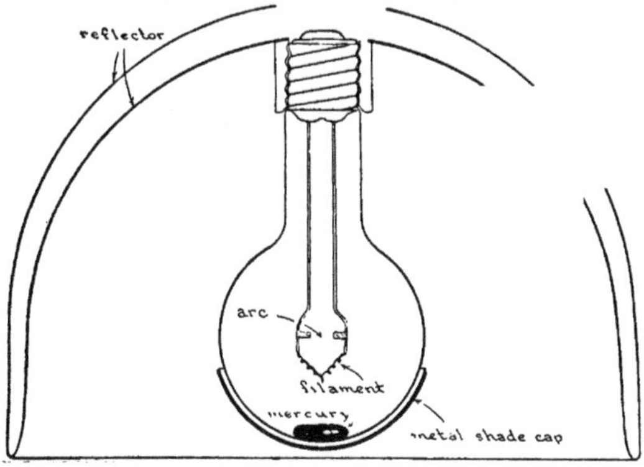

FIG. 21. An S-1 lamp, which is a suitable source of ultraviolet radiation for use in the home (From Krusen, F. H.: Physical Medicine, Saunders, Philadelphia, 1941).

hot mercury quartz lamps. It emits 5 per cent. ultraviolet rays, 78 per cent. luminous rays and 17 per cent. infra-red rays. At a distance of 2 feet, 60 cm., its output of ultraviolet rays is about equivalent to that of noontime sunlight in June.

Other similar sun lamps, which recently have been approved as suitable devices by the Council on Physical Therapy of the American Medical Association, are the "S-4" lamp and the "L. M.-4" lamp. Still another suitable sun lamp, which produces radiation similar to that of the "S-1" lamp, is the "type G mercury glow lamp". These lamps will not be described in detail.

PHYSICAL PRINCIPLES CONCERNED IN THE APPLICATION OF ULTRAVIOLET RADIANT ENERGY

The electromagnetic spectrum already has been mentioned briefly. The physician, who uses ultraviolet radiation therapeutically, must be familiar with the properties and the effects of the rays derived from various portions of this spectrum, if he is to use his lamp intelligently.

The unit of measurement of wavelength of radiation, which is employed commonly by the United States Bureau of Standards, is the millimicron, usually abbreviated mμ. The other unit of measurement of wavelength, which sometimes is employed, is the Angström unit, usually abbreviated A. U. or A.°. An Angström unit is 0.1 millimicron (Table I). The electromagnetic spectrum is represented in graphic form in Fig. 11 and in tabular form in Table II.

The ultraviolet rays with wavelengths ranging between 13.6 and 390 millimicrons possess varying physical properties and produce a variety of effects which are chiefly of a chemical nature. For example, there is a band of ultraviolet rays between 290 and 315 millimicrons, sometimes called the "vital ultraviolet band", which possesses antirachitic properties, and which converts more than 60 per cent. of the provitamin, ergosterol or 7-dehydrocholesterol, into vitamin D. On the other hand the group of ultraviolet rays, the wavelength of which is shorter than 280 millimicrons, are chiefly bactericidal and abiotic, capable of destroying tissue cells, and tend to destroy vitamin D.

It is apparent that, to obtain the maximal antirachitic effect from a source of ultraviolet radiation, the lamp used should produce little or none of the rays of wavelength shorter than 290 millimicrons and should be rich in radiation from the "vital ultraviolet band". Similarly, if a maximal bactericidal effect is desired, a source rich in the ultraviolet rays of shorter wavelength should be employed.

Penetration of ultraviolet rays through the skin or through mucous membranes never exceeds a depth of 2 mm. Various substances not only absorb such radiation but also reflect some of the rays. The most absorbent substance will reflect some of the rays, and conversely the most efficient reflector will absorb some of the radiation. The amount of absorption by human tissues depends largely on the wavelength of the radiation and the output of energy from the source.

Action and Uses of Ultraviolet Radiant Energy

Exposure to ultraviolet rays produces[1] photochemical effects with activation of certain substances in the skin and also possibly in the blood. Also certain biological effects have been observed such as stimulation of metabolism and growth and increase of circulation and cellular activity.

Ultraviolet rays of wavelengths between 290 and 315 millimicrons have the specific property of preventing and curing rickets. Radiation from this same "vital" region possesses the ability to impart an antirachitic potency to fats, milk, ergosterol, 7-dehydrocholesterol (the sterol, found in human skin, which can be activated), oils and vegetables. If pregnant or

TABLE I

UNITS OF MEASUREMENT OF WAVELENGTHS

One angstrom unit (A. U. or A.°)	One-tenth millimicron or one-ten-millionth millimeter
One-millimicron (mμ)	Ten angstrom units or one-millionth millimeter
One micron (μ)	One-thousandth millimeter
One millimeter (mm.)	One-tenth centimeter or one-thousandth meter

TABLE II

ELECTROMAGNETIC SPECTRUM

Rays		Extent of wavelengths
Gamma rays		0.001 to 0.14 mμ
Roentgen rays		0.14 to 13.6 mμ
Ultraviolet rays	far	13.6 to 290. mμ
	near	290. to 390. mμ
Visible rays	violet	390. to 450. mμ
	blue	450. to 490. mμ
	green	490. to 550. mμ
	yellow	550. to 590. mμ
	orange	590. to 630. mμ
	red	630. to 770. mμ
Infra-red rays	near	770. to 1,400. mμ
	far	1,400. to 15,000. mμ
Hertzian waves		15,000. mμ to several kilometers

nursing mothers or cows are exposed to these rays, their milk will develop an antirachitic potency.

Ultraviolet rays will cause a delayed or latent erythema in the skin of human beings. Repeated exposures to erythemal doses lead to the production of diffuse pigmentation of the skin of the white man. Such pigmentation probably assists in the absorption of radiant energy which is transformed into heat.

There is evidence to indicate that ultraviolet irradiation of the human being causes improvement of the tone, color and elasticity of the skin and presumably also increases the secretory and protective powers of the skin. Exposures of large portions of the cutaneous surface to ultraviolet radiation produces activation of a constituent of the cutaneous cholesterol, 7-dehydrocholesterol, to form vitamin D, which in turn stimulates absorption of calcium and phosphorus from the intestinal tract and increases metabolic efficiency. Phytosterol of plants is activated similarly.

It has been reported that ultraviolet irradiation causes an increase of the active oxygen content of the lipids of the skin and consequently an increase in their bactericidal action. It is possible also that exposure to ultraviolet rays leads to the formation of hormones in the skin and accomplishes the activation of useful cutaneous reflexes.

On general exposure to ultraviolet radiation the number of erythrocytes, leukocytes, blood platelets and hemoglobin of the circulating blood may increase slightly, and the hydrogen ion concentration, coagulation time and eventually the volume of blood may decrease. In general darkness produces a reverse effect with the exception that the blood volume seems to be diminished. Exposure to ultraviolet rays produces an increase in serum globulin. Ultraviolet irradiation is believed to cause a possible increase in bodily resistance by increasing the bactericidal power of the blood which depends largely on the leukocytic reaction. Such radiation probably does not influence specific immunity.

In moderate doses ultraviolet radiation causes an increase in carbon dioxide tension and a relative alkalosis, while in heavy doses it produces a decreased carbon dioxide tension and acidosis. It has been demonstrated that ultraviolet irradiation causes a lessening of the toxicity of the serum of the patient who has pernicious anemia.

General ultraviolet irradiation produces a transient lowering of blood pressure. The factors, which probably are responsible for the reduction of blood pressure, are the production of cutaneous hyperemia, the decrease in the viscosity of the blood, the development of cutaneous depressor substances and the production of sympathetic hypotonia. Activation of the circulation has been attributed to the vasodilating effect of the ultraviolet erythema and its continuous tonic action on the nerve endings. It has been shown also that these rays cause increased permeability of cell membranes and capillaries.

In general ultraviolet rays of wavelengths longer than 290 millimicrons produce presumably stimulative effects on the human body, but if the rays are of wavelengths shorter than 290 millimicrons and in large quantities, they will have a lethal effect on the cells of the human body. In smaller quantities the rays of shorter wavelength may have a stimulative action on the cells. These effects are due, perhaps, to the production of a toxic photo-product, which in large quantities is lethal and in small quantities acts as a stimulant to cell division.

Other general effects of ultraviolet irradiation have been noted; these include improvement of muscular tone, increase in protein and mineral metabolism, possible lowering of sympathetic tone, possible stimulation of intracellular oxidation and possible increase in the rate of bodily growth.

The application of ultraviolet rays does not act as a substitute for dietary deficiencies but produces an increase in the ability of the organism to utilize more effectively materials which are present but are not otherwise available. It is said that general exposure to ultraviolet rays causes a decrease in the rate, but an increase in the depth, of respiration.

Finally ultraviolet radiation has a definite bactericidal action. The line at 266 millimicrons is the most highly bactericidal; it is followed in order of effectiveness by the lines at 254, 280, 248 and 270 millimicrons. It has been demonstrated recently that the very short rays with wavelengths of less than 240 millimicrons have some germicidal action. Stimulation of bacterial growth has not been observed to result from exposure to ultraviolet rays.

The use of ultraviolet radiation in the treatment of disease has been most extensive, but much of the literature on the subject has been written poorly and is of an unconvincing nature. It is essential, therefore, that physicians make a careful analysis of the writings on this subject and accept only those which seem to have proved their claims by properly controlled studies[2].

Diseases of the Alimentary Tract. — There is now sufficient evidence to indicate that ultraviolet irradiation may be of distinct value in the treatment of *tuberculous peritonitis and enteritis*. Since intestinal tuberculosis is one of the most frequent complications of pulmonary tuberculosis, occurring as it does in from 50 to 80 per cent. of all fatal cases, any measure that will be of benefit is of the utmost importance. Ultraviolet irradiation is one of the most important factors in the arrest and treatment of intestinal tuberculosis. In a survey of the records of 8,087 routine postmortem examinations evidence of pulmonary tuberculosis was found in 886 cases and of intestinal tuberculosis in 233 cases. The ratio of pulmonary to intestinal tuberculosis was, therefore, approximately

4:1. Of 180 patients, who had intestinal tuberculosis and had received treatment at Saranac Lake, 65 per cent. of those treated with ultraviolet light were alive, whereas of those not so treated only 17 per cent. were alive at the time of the report. At the Trudeau Sanatorium of a series of 106 patients, who had intestinal tuberculosis, 88 per cent. of those treated by ultraviolet light survived, whereas only 25 per cent. of those not so treated survived.

Following the use of the mercury quartz lamp in the treatment of intestinal tuberculosis, tubercle bacilli often disappear from the stools; pain, nausea and vomiting are relieved, but the diarrhea and intestinal disturbances tend to resist the longest. In the treatment of tuberculous peritonitis the best results are obtained in the ascitic type. In abdominal tuberculous adenitis it may be unwise to temporize with light therapy, since in more than three-fourths of the cases it is possible to excise the affected glands.

Ultraviolet irradiation has been recommended in the treatment of *pylorospasm*. It is possible that, when this condition, as seems often the case, is associated with calcium deficiency, ultraviolet irradiation may be of value.

Diseases of the Blood and Circulatory System. — In the treatment of *secondary anemia* it has been suggested that one of the important factors in an ideal program consists of adequate exposure to ultraviolet radiation. There is considerable similarity between anemia and rickets, a disease cured and prevented by ultraviolet irradiation, when there is an adequate intake of calcium and phosphorus. In both diseases there is lowered gastrointestinal acidity, pH, which interferes with the absorption of calcium and with the absorption of iron, with a resultant decrease in the amount of iron available for regeneration of blood. In both diseases changes in the bone marrow and modifications in the types of cells may be seen. Ultraviolet irradiation may be beneficial in the treatment of either disease.

In a study conducted for a period of more than eight years in an artificial light clinic for school children it was found that after twelve or more exposures to irradiation from a carbon arc lamp the amount of hemoglobin of anemic children increased by approximately 10 per cent. Another controlled study of the use of ultraviolet irradiation in 54 cases of secondary anemia indicated greater increases in hemoglobin and in the number of erythrocytes and leukocytes in the treated than in the control group. It has been suggested that further studies of patients, who have secondary anemia, may indicate a possible influence of ultraviolet irradiation on the chemical constituents of the blood. Although various studies indicate that ultraviolet radiation may be a useful adjunct in the treatment of secondary anemia, there are still insufficient data to indicate the exact value of this therapeutic measure.

Various observers have shown that ultraviolet irradiation does produce transient *reduction in blood pressure.* The work of Laurens[3] and his coworkers in this field has been most convincing. As a therapeutic measure, however, it is doubtful whether ultraviolet irradiation can be considered more than a slight adjunct to the treatment of hypertension.

Ultraviolet irradiation has been employed for *carbon monoxide poisoning* because Haldane and Hartridge showed that the dissociation of carbon monoxide and hemoglobin was increased markedly under the influence of ultraviolet light. Such treatment has been found to be beneficial.

Diseases of the Respiratory System. — Many articles have been prepared, pro and con, with regard to the use of general ultraviolet irradiation in the prevention and treatment of the *common cold.* At Cornell University[4] small groups of male students were irradiated with minimal erythema doses of ultraviolet rays once weekly during the winter months. There was an apparent reduction in the incidence of colds ranging from 27.9 to 55.5 per cent. At Vanderbilt University[5] an investigation on the management of common colds revealed decided improvement in cases in which ultraviolet irradiation was used.

At the Cook County Hospital[6] ultraviolet irradiation was recommended in the treatment of *chronic coughs.* It was said to have a stimulating effect on general metabolism and on resistance to infection, provided the optimal dose was not exceeded and the patient was free from fever.

On the other hand some investigators have been of a contrary opinion; thus it has been concluded that, although the mercury quartz lamp has been used extensively to enhance individual resistance to colds, well-controlled studies on both infants and adults nevertheless have failed to corroborate claims for its value. Hill and Clark[7] found little to support the view that ultraviolet irradiation was capable of increasing a person's natural resistance. Other investigators have performed experiments similar to those conducted at Cornell with results, which were for the most part negative, although they did find that in certain tests the resistance of the irradiated group was greater than that of the control group. Still other investigators observed 363 adults for thirty-five weeks; during the first thirty-one weeks approximately half the group were given frequent ultraviolet irradiations, a single minimal erythema dose being applied either to the chest or to the back at each treatment. The incidence of colds during the period of study was slightly higher in the irradiated group than in the control group. However, it should be pointed out that failure to benefit from treatment may have been due to inadequate dosage. Only a quarter of the body was treated at any session, and the dose was not increased at subsequent sessions. It is agreed generally that to produce beneficial systemic effects a series of irradiations to the entire body should be given and that the dose should be increased gradually.

Further investigations will be necessary before final conclusions can be drawn concerning the value of ultraviolet irradiation in treating common colds.

In the treatment of *pulmonary tuberculosis* there likewise has been much controversy concerning the use of ultraviolet irradiation. Although ultraviolet light frequently is used in Europe for the treatment of pulmonary tuberculosis, in this country it often has been thought to be dangerous. It has been stressed especially that there is danger of producing pulmonary hemorrhage. My own controlled studies[8] on 60 patients, who were receiving routine sanatorium care, indicated that hemoptysis did not contraindicate the judicious employment of heliotherapy, and a number of other investigators have reached similar conclusions following controlled studies. It has been said that treatment, which brings about improvement in the general health of the patient, is the best means of combating pulmonary, as well as surgical, tuberculosis.

Observations on 115 patients treated by carbon arc irradiation led to the conclusion that minimal, moderately advanced or even far advanced pulmonary tuberculosis may be benefited by graduated irradiation, if the patient's temperature does not rise above 37.5° C. (99.5° F.) and his general physical condition is satisfactory. In Denmark treatment of pulmonary tuberculosis with light now is almost universal, and in Britain detailed results in a series of 123 cases led to the conclusion that, if patients are selected carefully, chronic pulmonary tuberculosis may be treated not only with safety but with good results.

Recently a number of writers in the United States have expressed a similar opinion. It has been reported that clinical experience will convince one of the value of the mercury quartz vapor lamp in the treatment of pulmonary tuberculosis of children. Tuberculous infants, who have excessive pulmonary infiltration, even with cavity formation, may recover.

Although I believe that, judiciously employed in conjunction with routine institutional care, light therapy may be of value as an adjunct in the treatment of pulmonary tuberculosis, its indiscriminate use is fraught with danger. Of 71 competent observers 47 obtained favorable and 24 either poor or no results following the use of ultraviolet irradiation in the treatment of pulmonary tuberculosis. This indicates an almost 2:1 preponderance in favor of the judicious application of ultraviolet radiation. For far advanced toxic or advancing active, exudative pulmonary tuberculosis light therapy should not be employed, but incipient pulmonary tuberculosis, especially of children, and nontoxic lesions, which have reached the stage of chronicity, may be benefited by the careful administration of small doses of general ultraviolet radiation. Abundant rest, an increased intake of food and proper hygienic measures are more important in the treatment of tuberculosis than is ultraviolet therapy, which is merely an adjunct to these other measures.

Diseases of the Bones and Joints. — In a study of 22 children, who had *tuberculosis of the bones or joints* and were treated throughout the winter and spring with radiations from a carbon arc light of high intensity, it was found that the majority showed a rise in the blood count, a tendency to gain weight and likewise, a marked improvement in the local tuberculous lesions.

An extensive study on the nonoperative treatment of *tuberculous joints* of the lower extremities revealed that, over a period of years, 65 per cent. of the adult patients under treatment for all extrapulmonary tuberculous lesions had definite, though usually inactive, pulmonary tuberculosis. Conservative treatment by heliotherapy in conjunction with routine care was used in this large series of cases. Of 437 patients with tuberculosis of the bones and joints and 72 with nontuberculous osteomyelitis, who remained on an institutional regimen for three months or longer, the following conditions were revealed on dismissal: 53.8 per cent. apparently had recovered; the tuberculosis of 23.1 per cent. was arrested; 10.7 per cent. were improved; 7.8 per cent. were unimproved, and 4.5 per cent. had died. A follow-up of these patients revealed that between 80 and 87 per cent. were working, an additional 8 to 10 per cent. were ambulant but unable to work, and between 3 and 5 per cent. were confined to bed. It was concluded that such conservative treatment usually resulted in healing with useful motion. Operative interference should not be attempted until after prolonged heliotherapy has been tried.

Bernhard[9], as a result of twenty-five years' experience, was of the opinion that in the treatment of *surgical tuberculosis* heliotherapy was the method of choice. In his first 1,000 cases of surgical tuberculosis in which heliotherapy was employed, 858 patients were cured, 120 were improved, 14 were unimproved and 8 had died, a mortality rate of only 0.8 per cent. Six of the patients, who were unimproved, died later, raising the final mortality to 14 or 1.4 per cent. The effect of heliotherapy in one case is shown in Fig. 22.

Osteomalacia, fragilitas osseum and *delayed union of fractures* are conditions which may be due to faulty calcium metabolism, and ultraviolet irradiation may be of value. In a study of experimental fractures of the fibula in 25 normal dogs and 80 normal rats measured amounts of carbon arc radiation were administered during the period of healing. During

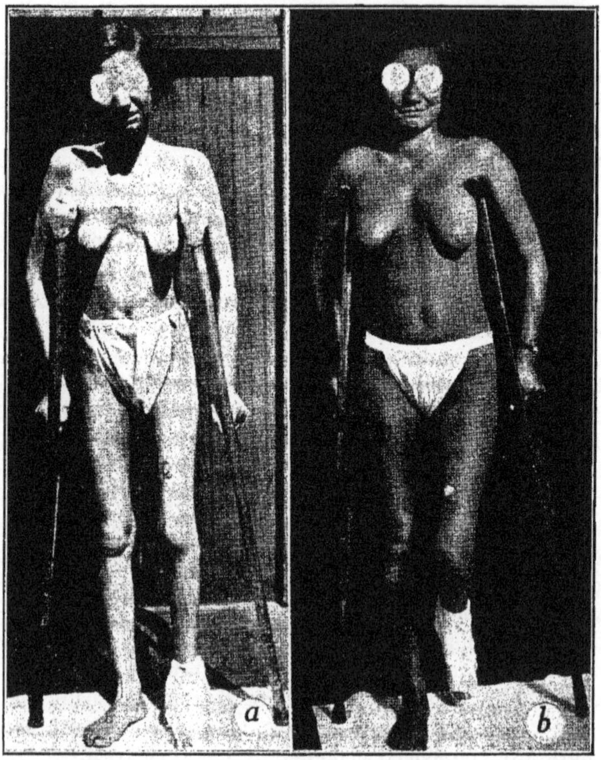

FIG. 22. Patient with extrapulmonary tuberculosis; (*a*) before heliotherapy, in April, 1927; (*b*) after heliotherapy, in December, 1927 (Courtesy of Dr. Richard T. Ellison; from Krusen, F. H.: Light Therapy, Ed. 2, Hoeber, New York, 1937).

this period 73.9 per cent. of the fibulas of animals irradiated with "sunshine" carbons, 26.9 per cent. of those irradiated with "C" carbons and 41.3 per cent. of those of the controls healed. The average healing time for fractures was 3.7 days shorter when the animals were irradiated than when they were not. In fractures of the long bones it has been reported that among patients, who were given irradiated ergosterol, the density and the amount of callus increased as compared with a control group of patients. These changes were greatest in children and in the aged, and they began to appear about three weeks following injury. On the other hand, in rabbits and rats, given respectively 3 and 1.25 gm. of irradiated ergosterol by mouth, the rate of healing or amount of callus in fractures of the tibia and fibula did not increase.

In rats, on which parathyroidectomy has been performed with consequent parathyroid deficiency, calcification does not occur regularly in the callus following fracture, if calcium is lacking also in the diet; under such conditions administration of irradiated ergosterol promotes calcification of callus.

It seems logical to presume that ultraviolet irradiation has little influence on healthy individuals, whose calcium metabolism is normal, but it would seem that it might be of value for patients with faulty calcium metabolism, who sustained fractures.

A number of authors have recommended the use of ultraviolet radiation for both *atrophic* and *hypertrophic arthritis*. Although there is no specific effect, it is believed by many clinicians that ultraviolet irradiation is of value, particularly when there is an associated secondary anemia, or when the patient has been confined to bed for a long period.

It has been claimed that ultraviolet irradiation tends to counteract the decalcifying process in the bones and to have an accessory nutritional influence in managing the anemia, debility and allied conditions so frequently found in chronic infectious arthritis. It has been pointed out, however, that chronic infectious arthritis can continue as a progressive crippling disease even in the Arizona desert unless therapeutic measures other than sunlight and climate are utilized.

It has been recommended that for chronic infectious arthritis of children reasonable exposure to sunlight or to quartz lights be utilized during the winter months. Ultraviolet irradiation has been recommended especially in the treatment of *psoriatic arthritis*. A combination of crude, coal tar ointment and ultraviolet irradiations is applied to the psoriatic lesions, and heat, massage and exercise are applied locally to the involved joints (see also treatment of psoriasis in the latter part of this section under the subheading, *Diseases of the Skin*).

Diseases of the Genito-urinary System. — In a series of 26 cases following nephrectomy for *renal tuberculosis* ultraviolet irradiation proved to be a most helpful therapeutic measure for the cure of the tuberculous sinuses and visceral ulceration incident to the disease. It has been said likewise that in tuberculosis of the genito-urinary tract surgical treatment frequently offers prompt relief if combined with postoperative heliotherapy.

Direct irradiation of the bladder for the treatment of *tuberculous ulceration* or *cystitis* has been recommended by a number of observers.

Diseases of the Eye. — Following a study of eighteen years' duration, ultraviolet irradiation was reported to have proved its worth in the treatment of diseases of the eye. Such treatments, for example, had reduced the proportion of losses in *ulcus serpens* from 30 to 6 per cent. Ultraviolet irradiations likewise had produced favorable results in other *diseases of the cornea, conjunctiva* and *sclera.* Excellent results have been reported in the treatment of corneal ulcers by accurately localized ultraviolet irradiation.

Ultraviolet radiation often is of benefit in the treatment of *tuberculous lesions of the eye.* A study of the combined use of local and general ultraviolet irradiation for the treatment of tuberculous lesions of the eye in 100 children revealed some improvement in every case.

Diseases of the Ear. — It has been claimed that irradiation by means of a "Kromayer" lamp with a small quartz rod in many instances will abort *furunculosis of the external auditory canal.* Combined local and general ultraviolet irradiations have been reported to be of definite value in the treatment of *tuberculosis of the middle ear.*

There is little evidence that ultraviolet radiation is of value in the treatment of *chronic otorrhea,* for which it occasionally has been recommended; it has been pointed out that even a thin layer of mucus or pus will filter out the ultraviolet rays and prevent any favorable action.

Diseases of the Nose. — Ultraviolet irradiation has been recommended as an adjunct to the surgical removal of *tuberculous lesions of the nose.* It likewise has been said that ultraviolet irradiation is of value in the treatment of *infected wounds* and of certain *nasal dermatoses,* and its use has been suggested for *ulcerations of the nose,* especially septal ulcers. Ultraviolet rays likewise have been said to be of value in the treatment of *lupus* of the nasal mucosa.

Diseases of the Throat. — Combined general and local ultraviolet irradiation has been recommended in the treatment of *tuberculous laryngitis.* Strandberg[10] reported a series of 203 cases of tuberculous laryngitis in which treatment with general ultraviolet irradiation was followed by cauterization. One hundred and thirteen patients were reported as cured of the disease of the larynx, and the majority of the others were said to have improved. Thomson[11] challenged these results and said that 32 patients, who had pulmonary tuberculosis, had been treated according to the Finsen plan without any striking evidence of benefit. In only two or three of these cases could some improvement be claimed.

Stevenson[12] observed 320 cases of tuberculous laryngitis. Thirty-eight of the patients obtained clinical cure, 101 were improved, 81 were unimproved, 59 were worse, and 41 had died. All of Stevenson's patients received routine sanatorium care, vocal rest and various local applications to the throat as well as ultraviolet irradiation. It is impossible, therefore, to say which was the most important factor in treatment.

In a study of 452 cases of pulmonary tuberculosis tuberculous laryngitis was present in 19.2 per cent. of the cases. It was felt that reflected sunlight was of value occasionally in supervised cases, particularly during the early stages. It would seem that in tuberculous laryngitis general and local ultraviolet irradiation in conjunction with routine care may be of some value in selected cases and certainly is worthy of trial. Several observers have felt that the local applications of ultraviolet light were a valuable adjunct.

Diseases of the Skin. — In no phase of ultraviolet therapy have there been more irrational and hyperenthusiastic claims than in that dealing with treatment for cutaneous diseases. In a bewildering mass of hastily written literature concerning ultraviolet therapy claims are made that this physical agent will cure almost any cutaneous disease "from acne to zoster[13]".

It has been stated[14] that among the diseases of the skin ultraviolet irradiation acts specifically only on *lupus vulgaris* and this only, when treatment is strictly on the Finsen principle. Likewise ultraviolet irradiation may have a favorable action in other dermatoses, *scrofuloderma, erythema induratum, psoriasis, pustular folliculitis, indolent ulcer, furunculosis, acne vulgaris, angioma serpiginosum, parapsoriasis* and *pityriasis rosea.*

Ultraviolet irradiation has been recommended for various forms of *acne, acne conglobata, acne cachecticorum, acne varioliformis* and particularly, *acne vulgaris.* In treatment for acne vulgaris it generally is considered best to produce a second degree erythema of the entire region covered by the lesions; this will be followed by desquamation. The most satisfactory results are obtained in the early stages of the disease when slight, acute inflammation and only a few comedones are present. Response to treatment often is slow. Proper dietetic management and medication should be used in conjunction with ultraviolet irradiation. Patients always should be told to expect severe reddening of the skin from the second degree erythemal dose which is to be administered. They frequently object to heavy doses of ultraviolet radiation on the face which is a common site of the lesions. In persistent cases of acne vulgaris, it is said, irradiation with a "cold quartz" lamp often frees the patient from the lesions and lessens the degree of scarring. In local treatment for acne vulgaris, particularly of the juvenile type, ultraviolet irradiation in erythemal doses, which produces exfoliation, may be used to advantage in conjunction with other measures. It is indicated especially for patients ten to fourteen years of age before complete development of adolescence, at which time roentgen therapy is contraindicated. It has been said that, although roentgen rays undoubtedly are best in local treatment for acne vulgaris, their improper use often is followed by disastrous results. Ultraviolet light applied locally in combination with astringent lotions is helpful in certain cases.

In treatment of *adenoma sebaceum* the use of blistering doses of ultraviolet irradiation has been recommended, and it has been said to be useful occasionally for this purpose. Erythema of second or third degree must be produced which will be followed by marked desquamation.

It has been reported that local applications of moderate doses of ultraviolet radiation may improve the lesions of *angioma serpiginosum.* Satisfactory results have been reported in treatment by means of ultraviolet irradiation for *infected granulating regions* following extensive burns, in preparation for Thiersch grafts. It was said that the effect of such rays on these wounds might be attributed to the following factors; (1) a bactericidal effect on the organisms on the surface, (2) production of active hyperemia which increased nutrition and resistance of tissues locally and (3) perhaps a stimulation of cell growth.

In regard to treatment for *cicatrices* heavy doses of ultraviolet radiation may be found serviceable in the removal of small pitted scars, particularly the type encountered following acne.

Many authors have reported favorable effects from treatment for *erysipelas* by means of ultraviolet irradiation. Excellent results were reported by one investigator, who said that each of 91 patients, who had erysipelas, was given a single, simple, ultraviolet treatment, which was inexpensive and without danger. The results were believed to be as satisfactory as those to be obtained from the use of antitoxin, roentgen rays or any other accepted method of treatment. It is necessary usually to obtain only one heavy dose of erythema of second degree or even third degree over the entire lesion, including 2 inches (5 cm.) of normal skin in every direction around the borders of the lesion. The common error in treatment is to give insufficient exposure. Fifteen to twenty times the minimal erythemal dose often should be administered. Even with smaller doses results may be good. Thus one author reported that exposures of only fifteen to sixty seconds at a distance of 20 to 30 inches (51 to 76 cm.) to a mercury quartz lamp in 10 cases produced results that were better than those of any other treatment which had been given. It was stressed that treatment should be begun at the earliest possible moment, especially before the lesion has had time to extend into the hair or to the external auditory meatus.

In a report on 340 cases of erysipelas of all types, in which treatment with ultraviolet radiation was employed, double the erythemal dose with the hot quartz lamp at a distance of only 8 inches (20 cm.) from the lesion or twenty times the erythemal dose with a "cold quartz" lamp were used. Twenty-seven patients, 7.94 per cent., died of erysipelas, and 313 recovered. The average time between treatment and restoration of normal temperature was 3.9 days. The average duration from the time of treatment to the time of dismissal was 8.67 days. The average duration from onset to dismissal was 11.34 days. It was concluded that ultraviolet irradiation was an effective treatment for erysipelas, for consistently good results were obtained in this study which covered a period of seventeen years.

The following technic for local application of ultraviolet rays for erysipelas has been suggested. The region of involvement and the normal adjacent skin, at least 2 inches (5 cm.) beyond the border of the lesion, should be exposed to ultraviolet radiation. A mercury quartz burner may be used. The lamp is permitted to run for ten minutes before treatment is begun in order that the lamp may reach its maximal efficiency. The rays must strike the diseased region and the adjacent skin at right angles to its surface for ten minutes at a distance of 12 inches (30 cm.) provided the erythemal dose of the lamp is approximately one minute at that distance. For infants and very young children the time of exposure may be reduced to five minutes and occasionally, to three minutes. If the lesion of erysipelas shows evidence of spreading, a second treatment will be required. Usually one intense treatment suffices.

It has been said that ultraviolet irradiation may be beneficial in treatment for *erythema induratum.* Local irradiation also may improve the lesions of *pustular folliculitis.* Although it has been said that ultraviolet radiations are of questionable value for *furunculosis*, other authorities have believed that such lesions sometimes may be improved by judicious irradiation.

Concentrated ultraviolet irradiation undoubtedly is the best local treatment for *lupus vulgaris.* The carbon arc light of the Finsen type is said to be more satisfactory than the "Kromayer" lamp. It has been reported that cure was obtained in only 29 per cent. of cases when a "Kromayer" lamp was used and in 90 per cent. of cases when a carbon arc lamp was used. At the Finsen Institute during a period of ten years treatment was given in 957 cases of lupus vulgaris. In 735 of these cure apparently resulted; in 75 treatment was still being carried out, and in

147 adequate treatment had failed, for one reason or another, to be accomplished. If this latter group is omitted, there are 810 cases, in which adequate treatment was received, and in 735 of these, 90.7 per cent., the lesions apparently were cured. Further study revealed that of the 735 patients, who received adequate treatment and apparently were cured, 44 showed signs of recurrence later. Nevertheless the results were excellent. It is felt that ultraviolet irradiation still may be considered the standard form of treatment for lupus vulgaris.

The interesting and valuable observation has been made that in cases of lupus vulgaris the tuberculous skin is more pervious to luminous and to ultraviolet radiation than is normal skin. The energy penetration becomes relatively greater as the wavelengths grow shorter, until at 313 millimicrons the tuberculous skin may be three to six times as pervious as normal skin. Thus, greater action of the radiant energy on the diseased skin is to be presumed.

In cases of *nevus flammeus*, port wine mark, ultraviolet irradiations may be very useful; excellent results may be obtained with the use of an air-cooled ultraviolet lamp and thorough-going blanching may be produced readily. *Parapsoriasis* and *pernio* also may be improved by ultraviolet irradiations.

In cases of *pityriasis rosea* in conjunction with the use of soothing lotions such as calamine lotion or mild protective ointments such as boric acid, zinc oxide or 2 per cent. sulfur ointment ultraviolet irradiation may be used routinely. However, ointments and oily applications sometimes may aggravate the condition, and calamine lotion without phenol is said to be by great odds the best local application. It has been suggested also that erythemal doses of ultraviolet radiation from either "cold quartz" or hot quartz lamps are too irritating and are unnecessary. However, divided suberythemal doses are recommended, and they usually quiet the itching and promote exfoliation of the lesions within two or three weeks. Although previously I have recommended the production of a second degree erythema in order to obtain desquamation, I now feel that the suberythemal doses are more satisfactory. As I pointed out previously, after the use of a second degree erythema the itching, fawn-colored lesions on the trunk are replaced by generalized sunburn. Because the disease is self-limited and because the discomfort from the sunburn is considerable, it might be preferable to use other palliative measures and permit the disease to run its course. By using suberythemal doses recovery may be hastened without producing any discomfort to the patient; this procedure is advocated as an adjunct to other forms of treatment.

Although it has been reported that ultraviolet irradiation may cause improvement or may be injurious in cases of *psoriasis*, nevertheless, with judicious applications, ultraviolet radiation may be very beneficial. If the affected skin is covered with a thin film of crude coal tar ointment and then irradiated with ultraviolet light, better results can be obtained than by the use of either one of these agents alone. The ointment should consist of gr. 30 (2 gm.) each of crude coal tar and pulverized zinc oxide, mixed with 2 ounces (56.7 gm.) each of corn starch and petrolatum.

The ointment is applied to the patches for twenty-four hours and then is removed with olive oil. Vigorous efforts at cleansing are postponed until after the lesions have been exposed to a mercury quartz ultraviolet lamp. Thus a thin film of the ointment remains on the lesion during irradiation. Only after ultraviolet irradiation may the patient take a bath with soap and water or oatmeal and soda which by aiding in the removal of the remaining débris enhances the effect of the tar and light. The light usually is applied at a distance of 30 inches (75 cm.) for one minute, the time being increased one minute daily for three or four days. If the patient then shows no signs of reaction, the time of irradiation is increased rapidly, and the distance between the lamp and the lesion is decreased.

An effort is made to avoid any marked cutaneous reaction, but an attempt is made to produce tanning as soon as possible. If the therapist is acquainted thoroughly with the effectiveness of his lamp, and if he handles it deftly, "it should be possible to remove all patches of psoriasis in practically all cases in from three to four weeks".

Patients who have psoriasis are likely to experience the development of arthritis. In a series of 936 cases of psoriasis studied at the Mayo Clinic arthritis was associated with 133, 14 per cent., of them. In 40 of these 133 cases systematic treatment with tar and ultraviolet irradiation was given. The eruption responded as readily in these cases as in those in which arthritis was not present. It was a striking fact that in about half of these cases the active symptoms of the arthritis entirely disappeared without any other treatment.

Employed judiciously a combination of local and general ultraviolet irradiation may be of benefit to *scrofuloderma*. There is sufficient evidence to justify the statement that ultraviolet irradiation is of value for certain types of cutaneous tuberculosis, scrofuloderma.

Indolent ulcers occasionally may be caused to heal more rapidly by the use of erythemal doses of ultraviolet radiation or by daily exposures to graduated doses of solar radiation. In regard to wounds, particularly *indolent wounds*, the use of unaltered sunlight has been recommended highly. I have been able to obtain what I consider to be comparable results by exposing the indolent wound first to a radiant heat lamp and then to a mercury quartz lamp.

There is a difference of opinion regarding the value of ultraviolet irradiation for about thirty additional dermatoses.

Miscellaneous Diseases. — In *rickets* it is believed that ultraviolet irradiation furthers the absorption from the intestine of either phosphorus or calcium or both. It is probable that the hydrogen ion concentration is the limiting factor in such action. A number of investigators have shown that, to produce beneficial effects in the treatment of rickets, it is necessary to administer only comparatively small doses of effective ultraviolet radiation.

For example, a single weekly exposure to one erythemal dose of ultraviolet rays was sufficient to produce healing of rachitic lesions of infants. Irradiations from a mercury quartz lamp, front and back, for four to five minutes once weekly, until approximately 100 minutes of exposure had been given, was sufficient to effect cure in a series of 43 rachitic nurslings so treated.

Heavy doses of ultraviolet light did not prevent rickets in rats, which had been placed on a rickets-producing diet, provided they were prevented from licking their fur or eating their excretions. If, however, the rats were shaved, the skin sterol then was activated by irradiation, absorbed and exerted antirachitic effects.

It has been shown that the provitamins D exhibit pronounced ultraviolet absorption. Of the eight to ten provitamins D, which are said to exist, only two, ergosterol and 7-dehydrocholesterol, appear to be very common. When irradiated, these provitamins become extremely active, and 5 mgm. of either is equivalent in potency to 1 liter of good cod liver oil. Direct irradiation of the skin by ultraviolet rays may be specific in the treatment of rickets.

Results comparable to those obtained in the treatment of rickets may be obtained also by the use of ultraviolet irradiation in cases of *tetany* and *spasmophilia.*

Among the *unusual uses of ultraviolet irradiation* may be mentioned its employment for diagnostic purposes, for the identification marking of newborn infants, for the purpose of producing hardening of the nipples prenatally and for the sterilization of air in operating rooms. It has been pointed out that prenatal irradiation and the irradiation of the nursing mother are efficacious in the prevention of rickets in the child, and that direct irradiation of cows will impart an antirachitic potency to their milk.

Contraindications to the Application of Ultraviolet Radiant Energy

Ultraviolet irradiation is contraindicated in the presence of cardiac insufficiency, valvular heart disease, advanced myocarditis, arteriosclerosis, nephritis, advanced bilateral renal tuberculosis with impending uremia and pulmonary tuberculosis of the advancing exudative type.

It sometimes is contended that previous exposure to roentgen rays contraindicates subsequent exposure to ultraviolet radiation. The idea probably arises from the fear of a possible cumulative action produced by the latent erythema from the roentgen rays added to the erythema from the ultraviolet rays. With this exception there is no apparent contraindication to combining the two procedures. Recently Ellis and Kirby-Smith[15] studied 11 patients who had been given from 10 to 16 one-third erythemal doses of roentgen rays and from 4 to 20 erythemal doses of ultraviolet rays. None showed any evidence of roentgen ray dermatitis. They concluded that roentgen therapy has simply an additional action separate from the effect of the ultraviolet radiation on the skin. For example, if R represents the permanent or late effect of the roentgen rays and A the permanent actinic cutaneous change, then the total late changes will equal R plus A. When roentgen (R) and ultraviolet irradiations (A) are given simultaneously, alternately or later, neither exerts a beneficial or deleterious effect on the other, but there is only a summation of the effect of one plus that of the other.

Ultraviolet irradiation may cause an exacerbation, provoke an attack or produce other injurious effects in such cutaneous lesions as eczema, lupus erythematosus, herpes simplex, erythema solare perstans, xeroderma pigmentosum, freckles, atrophy, keratoses and permaturely senile skin.

Exposures to ultraviolet radiation should not be employed for tuberculosis of the suprarenal glands or for certain types of tracheobronchial adenitis. Such exposures are contraindicated also in the presence of hyperthyroidism and diabetes, because pruritus and heightened irritability may result. Still other contraindications to the use of ultraviolet irradiation are advanced cachexia, inanition, extreme age and acute forms of generalized dermatitis.

Summary of Data on Radiant Energy

Ultraviolet irradiation has been used extensively but indiscriminately in the practice of medicine. However, in a rather large number of conditions the evidence indicates that ultraviolet irradiation is, or gives promise of being, valuable. Among these conditions may be mentioned tuberculous peritonitis and enteritis, calcium deficiency diseases, secondary anemia, carbon monoxide poisoning, pulmonary tuberculosis, tuberculosis of bones and joints, atrophic and hypertrophic arthritis, tuberculosis of the genito-urinary tract, ulcus serpens, corneal ulcer, tuberculous lesions of the eye, ear or nose, nasal ulcerations, tuberculous laryngitis, certain cutaneous diseases, rickets, tetany and spasmophilia.

BIBLIOGRAPHY OF RADIANT ENERGY

1. KRUSEN, F. H.: Light Therapy, Ed. 2, Hoeber, New York, 1937.
2. KRUSEN, F. H.: Medical application of ultraviolet radiant energy, Ann. Int. Med., 1940, XIV, 641.
3. LAURENS, H.: The Physiological Effects of Radiant Energy, The Chemical Catalog Co., New York, 1933.
4. MAUGHAN, G. H. and SMILEY, D. F.: Irradiations from a quartz-mercury-vapor lamp as a factor in the control of common colds, Am. Jour. Hyg., 1929, IX, 466.
5. ZERFOSS, T. B.: The management of colds, Journal-Lancet, 1935, LV, 792.
6. FANTUS, B.: The therapy of the Cook County Hospital, Jour. Am. Med. Assoc., 1936, CVI, 375.
7. HILL, C. M. and CLARK, J. H.: The effect of ultraviolet radiation on resistance to infection, Am. Jour. Hyg., 1927, VII, 448.
8. KRUSEN, F. H.: Heliotherapy in the treatment of pulmonary tuberculosis, Am. Rev. Tuberc., 1927, XVI, 180.
9. BERNHARD, O.: Quoted by Laurens, H.[3].
10. STRANDBERG, O.: Traitement photothérapique de la tuberculose du larynx. Traitement spécial par bains de lumière chimiques artificiels, combiné avec un traitement chirurgical intralaryngé, Ann. d. Mal. de l'Oreille, du Larynx, 1927, XLVI, 653.
11. THOMSON, St. C.: Quoted by Stevenson, R. S.[12].
12. STEVENSON, R. S.: The treatment of tuberculosis of the larynx, Brit. Med. Jour., 1933, II, 960.
13. WILLIAMS, H. B.: The need of research in physical therapy, In Vol. I, pp. 1–3, Principles and Practice of Physical Therapy, Prior, Hagerstown, Maryland, 1934.
14. COUNCIL ON PHYSICAL THERAPY: Regulations to govern advertising of ultraviolet generators to the medical profession only, Jour. Am. Med. Assoc., 1932, XCVIII, 400.
15. ELLIS, F. A. and KIRBY-SMITH, H.: Effect of ultraviolet radiation on roentgen rays: do ultraviolet rays have deleterious effect on roentgen rays when applied to the skin? Arch. Dermat. and Syph., 1940, XLII, 466.

Sept. 1, 1941.

HYDROTHERAPY

Although it is one of the oldest forms of therapy and one which often can be employed to advantage, hydrotherapy has been neglected recently. Interest in the employment of water for therapeutic purposes has waxed and waned throughout the centuries but never has ceased entirely. Baruch[1] said: "Of all remedial agents in use since the dawn of medicine, water is the only one that has survived all the vicissitudes of doctrinal changes because its rise or fall was always contemporaneous with the rise and fall of intelligence among medical men". If this is true, we modern physicians should look to our laurels and inquire into the present state of our collective intelligence. The current medical literature is woefully lacking in careful, scientific evaluations of the various phases of hydrotherapy.

It has been said: "Hydrotherapy includes the application of water in any form from the solid and fluid to vapor, from ice to steam, internally and externally". Water can be applied either locally or generally.

Methods of Applying Hydrotherapy

Local Application. — Among the methods of applying water locally for therapeutic purposes can be mentioned local baths, sitz baths, contrast baths, whirlpool baths, local douches, irrigations and compresses.

Local Baths. The arm, hand, leg, foot or other local region of the body can be immersed in water at different temperatures to cause local effects which uusally are of a thermal or mechanical nature. Baths for the extremities usually are administered in specially shaped containers which conform to the shape of the limb. A large oval dishpan can be used for the arm and a large bucket or tub for the leg. In the so-called half bath only the pelvis, hips and lower extremities are immersed in water contained in an ordinary bath tub.

In the *sitz* (*hip*) *bath* the patient sits in water with only the hips, pelvis and external genitalia immersed. In institutions special tubs are employed for administration of these baths, but in the home a wash tub can be substituted.

Alternate applications of hot and cold water, *contrast baths*, to the extremities are very useful in treatment for hypertrophic arthritis and for certain circulatory diseases. The usual plan of alternately immersing the part in hot and then in cold water for intervals of one minute is not so satisfactory as are immersions for longer periods of time. Woodmansey and his associates[2] in England found the best circulatory responses when the hot water was applied for six minutes and the cold water for four minutes. Our American patients, possibly because they are accustomed to warmer houses, dislike the more prolonged periods of cold.

Checking the work of Woodmansey I found that patients in this country responded best to a routine which employed either five minutes of heat and two minutes of cold or four minutes of heat and one minute of cold. To obtain the best vascular response the patient always should start and end with the hot water. The cold water should be kept at a temperature of 50° to 65° F. (10° to 18.3° C.) and the hot water at 100° to 110° F. (37.8° to 43.3° C.) If the first routine is employed, the treatment should last for either 19 or 26 minutes, thus 5–2–5–2–5 or 5–2–5–2–5–2–5. If the latter procedure is employed, treatments will require 19 or 24 minutes, thus 4–1–4–1–4–1–4 or 4–1–4–1–4–1–4–1–4.

Baths of whirling aerated water, *whirlpool baths*, at a temperature of 110° F. (43.3° C.) have been employed extensively in civilian hospitals for increasing the peripheral circulation of the extremities. These baths, which were developed during the World War of 1914–1918, still are considered to be extremely useful, especially in the management of fractures of the extremities. Specifications for the construction of a simple, "homemade", whirlpool bath are illustrated in Fig. 23. For institutional work specially shaped whirlpool baths are available for immersion of the leg; there is another type which is raised on a pedestal for immersion of the arm. Portable whirlpool baths also are available. These contain an immersion heater and a mechanical electrically operated device for agitating and aerating the water.

Various *sprays* and *douches* can be employed therapeutically. The ordinary bath spray, sometimes called a "rose spray", can be used to shower a local region with hot or cold water, or it can be employed to administer contrast baths to regions, such as a shoulder, which cannot be immersed readily in a tub.

The *jet douche* is a stream of water projected from an ordinary hose nozzle. If the water from such a nozzle is spread in the shape of a fan by placing a finger over the opening, it is called a "*fan douche*". If the circular aperture in the nozzle is extremely small so that a very fine, forceful stream of water is projected on the body, it is spoken of as a "*filiform douche*". Such a stream may be sufficiently forceful to destroy surface epithelium and even to cause bleeding.

Irrigations are used chiefly for flushing of various bodily cavities, that is, the colon, vagina, ear, nose, throat, urinary bladder or stomach. In the few instances in which irrigation of the colon is necessary, the physician can employ an ordinary bed, a plain glass irrigation jar on a stand, a rectal tube (no. 34, French), a Y tube with two clamps and a large closed jar to receive the return flow. This simple equipment is equally as effectual as the elaborate colonic irrigation tables covered with chrome metal and fancy gadgets which so frequently are marketed for this purpose.

For irrigation of the vagina the usual irrigation can or fountain syringe

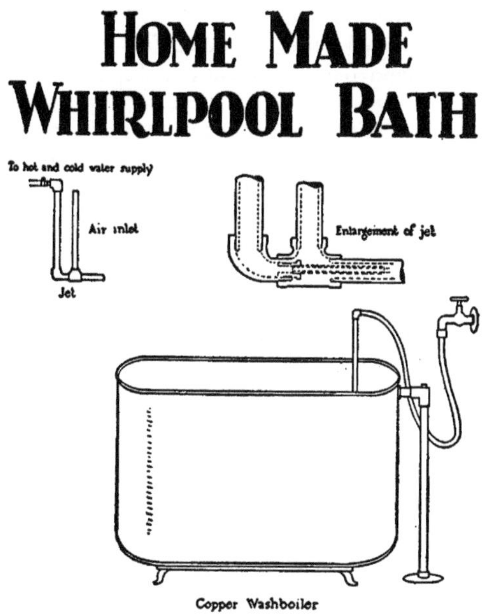

FIG. 23. Specifications for the construction of a homemade whirlpool bath (Courtesy of the Council on Physical Therapy of the American Medical Association).

with a hard rubber tip, which is sufficiently large to prevent its passage into the cervical canal, can be employed.

For irrigation of the ear, nose or throat the usual irrigation can or rubber bag and tubing can be employed. A very satisfactory irrigation tip can be made by inserting the glass portion of an ordinary eye dropper into the end of the tubing. Irrigation of the bladder is performed by connecting the fountain syringe to an ordinary urethral catheter.

Finally irrigation of the stomach can be accomplished by the employment of one of several types of tubes. The large rubber stomach tube, which varies in caliber from no. 12 to no. 30, French, can be used. Or a large, no. 30, French, Boas tube, a nasal catheter with a soft rubber tip or a small caliber Rehfuss tube with a metal tip can be employed. Fluids can be introduced through a funnel or by means of a syringe and can be removed by siphonage or by means of the syringe.

Cloths partially wrung out after dipping in hot or cold water can be applied to some region of the body to produce a local circulatory reaction. These are spoken of as "*compresses*" or "*packs*".

General Application. — Among the methods for the general application of water can be mentioned baths, including full baths, brine baths, effervescent baths and bland baths, Hubbard tanks, pools, showers, douches and packs.

A cold plunge in a *full bath* at a temperature of 50° F. (10° C.) occasionally is employed as a powerful excitant. The tepid full bath at temperatures between 80° and 92° F. (26.7° and 33.3° C.) sometimes is used therapeutically. A neutral bath is one which is kept at a temperature of from 92° to 97° F. (33.3° to 36.1° C.) while the hot bath is applied at temperatures between 98° and 108° F. (36.7° and 42.2° C.) *Continuous full baths* sometimes are employed. They are kept at neutral temperature, and the patient lies on a canvas hammock which is beneath the water in a large tub.

The chief advantage of the *brine bath* is its buoyancy. It usually contains from 5 to 30 pounds, 2.3 to 13.6 kg., of sodium chloride to 40 gallons, 160 liters, of water. Little salt is absorbed through the skin. It is employed usually for administration of certain types of underwater exercise.

Baths containing carbonated water, *effervescent baths*, commonly known as carbon dioxide or "Nauheim" baths, occasionally are employed in treatment of certain types of cardiac disease. Usually ½ pound, 0.2 kg., of sodium bicarbonate is placed in a tubful of salt water. Then six or eight large tablets of specially prepared acid sodium sulfate are arranged along the floor of the tub. A chemical reaction follows which causes the liberation in the water of large quantities of carbon dioxide. The patient then is immersed in this bath.

Sometimes oxygen is bubbled into a tub of water through rattan reeds to provide an "oxygen bath". This type of effervescent bath was recommended by Nylin[3].

Sometimes, soothing or *bland baths* are used in treatment of certain acute inflammations of the skin. They usually are kept at neutral temperature, and soothing medication is added to the water. A suitable bland bath can be prepared by adding to the full, neutral temperature bath a decoction consisting of 5 pounds (2.3 kg.) of starch in 1 gallon

(4 liters) of water or 3 pounds (1.4 kg.) of wheat bran in the same amount of water.

In order that underwater exercises can be administered easily a special butterfly-shaped tank has been constructed. This kind of tank, usually called a "*Hubbard tank*", now is employed extensively in the various hospitals of the United States. A simple type can be constructed for home use; specifications are obtainable from the Council on Physical Therapy of the American Medical Association.

Therapeutic pools have been developed to a high degree of efficiency. They are employed extensively for underwater exercises and can be found in many large hospitals, schools for crippled children and orthopedic institutions.

The overhead *shower bath*, often called a "*rain douche*", and the *needle shower* sometimes are employed therapeutically. The latter is composed of semicircles of shower heads which spray many fine, forceful streams of water onto the surface of the body. The pressure of the water causes the needle-like streamlets to sting the skin; hence the designation "needle shower".

If the surface of the body is sprayed alternately by forceful jets of hot and cold water, the procedure is called a "*Scotch douche*". This treatment, when properly applied by a skillful individual, has a distinctly invigorating and refreshing effect.

The *full wet pack*, the *blanket pack* and the *towel pack* all have been employed therapeutically. In each the patient is wrapped in cold or hot moist coverings. Usually the patient is wrapped in a cold, wet covering and then quickly enveloped in warm coverings. A reactive hyperemia occurs, and he soon feels warm and begins to perspire. As the patient remains in the pack, it finally begins to produce a distinctly sedative effect.

Physical Principles Concerned in the Employment of Hydrotherapy

Water solidifies at 32° F. (0° C.); as ice it can be applied locally. Water occasionally is applied locally through a jet in its gaseous form, steam. However, in most instances water is applied in its liquid form when local effects are desired. Because of this flexibility of application water often is applied generally in solid, liquid or gaseous form. A general application of the solid form is the ice pack, of the liquid form the full bath and of the gaseous form the steam bath.

Water is an excellent medium for producing, by conduction, changes in the temperature of the bodily tissues. It is said that it imparts its temperature to bodily tissue more readily than does air at the same temperature. A sensation of chilliness will be observed much more rapidly by anyone lying quietly in a tub of still water at 80° F. (26.7° C.) than by anyone lying in still air at the same temperature. Also water has a high specific heat, that is, a large amount of heat is required to raise its temperature. Conversely, when it cools, it liberates a large amount of heat to substances with which it is in contact. Therefore, water is a very satisfactory means of applying conductive heat.

Hydrotherapeutic procedures can cause mechanical as well as thermal effects. The impact of water applied under pressure to the skin will tend to have a stimulating effect on the sensory nerve endings. A shower bath generally is considered to be more stimulating and refreshing than a tub bath.

Action and Uses of Hydrotherapy

With regard to the local effects of hydrotherapy one of the most interesting of the recent observations is that of Blair[4]. His studies on the physiological effects of alternate increase and decrease of the blood supply may aid in explaining the value of contrast baths in the treatment of fractures. Furthermore Blair's observations may explain in part the reason for the varied opinions concerning the effect of hyperemia on calcification of bone. He concluded that it was the alternate increase and decrease in the volume of blood, which promoted calcification of bone, whereas prolonged hyperemia produced decalcification of bone, and prolonged ischemia caused calcium deposition and ossification.

Normally the volume of blood reaching the bones of the extremities is varied by the alternate contraction and relaxation of muscles which take place during the usual activity of the part. Following a fracture prolonged immobilization prevents this activity. Blair concluded that contrast baths which have been used for years "to hasten healing of fractures" probably caused "an alternation of blood supply to the part" and were advantageous because "alternating ischemia and hyperemia maintain normal calcification of bone". If Blair's observations are correct, then contrast baths followed by massage and muscle setting exercises, alternate static contraction and relaxation of muscles, should be particularly effective in promoting healing and calcification of fractures.

It has been pointed out by McClellan[5] that hydrotherapeutic procedures cause chiefly thermal and mechanical stimulation. This stimulation acts as an irritant to the sensory nerve endings and may produce a response locally by reflex action. The local reaction to cold water is contraction of elastic and muscular fibers in the cutaneous and subcutaneous regions, which results in ischemia. When the application of cold ceases, the fibers relax with the result that hyperemia occurs. Hot applications tend to result in an atonic reaction and cold applications in a tonic reaction.

The chief effect of generalized application of water is thermal. The bodily temperature will tend to rise or fall according to the temperature of the bath. The physiological effects of general exposure to heat or to cold already have been discussed in the sections dealing with applications of heat and cold.

Most writers on hydrotherapy stress the importance of obtaining a good "reaction". The "action" caused by brief applications of cold water consists of peripheral vasoconstriction, pallor, chilliness, shivering and increases in respiratory and pulse rates. The "reaction", which starts immediately and lasts for about twenty minutes, consists of peripheral vasodilatation, redness of the skin, warmth, relaxation and slowing of the respiratory and pulse rates. Likewise a "reaction" may be noted following a brief application of hot water. This reaction has been said[6] to consist of muscular relaxation, lowered arterial tension and increase in the pulse rate with shallow respirations. In order to produce a marked hyperemia, alternate applications of hot and cold water often are recommended.

Cold baths increase the general metabolic rate and the amount of oxygen inspired. Hot baths also will increase the metabolic rate, if they are administered for a period which is sufficiently long to raise the systemic temperature, but the amount of oxygen which is inspired will be decreased.

Local Application. — Warm or hot *local baths* are applied to the upper or to the lower extremity in treatment of arthritis, burns, cellulitis, circulatory diseases, contusions, sprains and infected wounds. Cold foot baths have been recommended in treatment of bromidrosis and for persistent coldness of the feet. Cold sitz baths have been recommended in treatment of such conditions as amenorrhea, prostatorrhea, atony of the bladder, atonic constipation and sexual impotence. The hot sitz baths have been suggested in treatment of dysmenorrhea, amenorrhea, prostatitis, tenesmus, ureteral colic, pelvic inflammation and gluteal fibrositis.

Contrast baths are especially useful in treatment of hypertrophic arthritis of the hands and feet and in the management of fractures, sprains and contusions. Such baths have been employed also for peripheral vascular disease.

In the auxiliary treatment of fractures of the extremities after removal of dressings whirlpool baths often are valuable. This type of bath improves circulation, relaxes muscles and seems to have a sedative effect, thus preparing the part for subsequent massage and exercise. Indications for use of whirlpool baths are much the same as those for the contrast baths. Whirlpool baths, too, are used in treatment of traumatic lesions, such as sprains, contusions, dislocations and of arthritis, peripheral vascular diseases and infected wounds of the extremities.

Warm or hot *irrigations* of the ear, nose or throat are employed to relieve inflammation and to remove exudate in the presence of such conditions as otitis media, furunculosis of the external auditory canal, chronic rhinitis, acute nasopharyngitis or peritonsillar abscess.

Irrigations of the stomach are used for relief of gastric retention in association with pyloric stenosis or carcinoma. They have been employed also to remove recently ingested poisons. Vaginal irrigations often are indicated in the management of leucorrhea, vaginitis, endocervicitis, endometritis and pelvic inflammatory disease.

There are very few indications for the use of *colonic irrigations.* It is possible that they may be useful occasionally for removal of masses of impacted feces from the lower part of the bowel. Such irrigations should not be employed routinely. Even occasional irrigations rarely are indicated.

Hot *compresses* are employed, at times, in treatment of muscular spasm or of acute inflammatory processes. Cold compresses sometimes are applied over the precordium in treatment of tachycardia and cardiac neurosis.

General Application. — The *cold full bath* has been recommended to improve functional activity, to stimulate general metabolism and to combat the debility associated with sedentary living. It was recommended by Brand in treatment of typhoid fever. The *tepid bath* has been employed chiefly as a sedative or to combat excessive febrile reactions. *Neutral baths* are used occasionally to treat insomnia or to allay nervous excitability. *Warm baths* have been used for convulsions of infancy, to diminish the cerebral manifestations of certain acute febrile disorders and to treat such conditions as acute sciatica, dysmenorrhea, amenorrhea and insomnia. *Hot baths* often may be employed to advantage in controlling acute exacerbations of chronic atrophic arthritis as well as for fibrositis, myositis, neuritis, muscular spasm and abdominal cramps. *Continuous baths* are used particularly in the control of acute manias. They have been employed also in treatment of extensive burns, indolent ulcers, cutaneous diseases, suppurating wounds and large abscesses. *Brine baths* have been used especially for arthritis, fractures, dislocations, fibrositis, myositis and osteomyelitis.

Effervescent baths have been used for cardiac disease, especially for valvular or myocardial lesions. The oxygen bath has been recommended for hypertension and cardiac neurosis and as a mild sedative for advanced cardiac disease. *Bland baths* are used to relieve generalized pruritus and dermatitis.

Underwater exercises in tanks or pools are employed chiefly for poliomyelitis, spastic paralysis and certain orthopedic and neurological conditions. *Douches* and *showers* are employed to improve peripheral circulation and to act as general stimulants. Neurasthenics and debilitated individuals often are benefited by the Scotch douche. *Packs* can be used to advantage in home treatment of arthritis, fibrositis or myositis as well as for control of delirium, psychosis, hyperexcitability and insomnia.

Contraindications to the Employment of Hydrotherapy

Very hot or very cold sitz baths should not be administered during pregnancy or the menstrual period. Cold local baths or extremely hot baths at a temperature higher than 105° F. (40.6° C.) are not to be used in the presence of advanced peripheral vascular disease. The former aggravate the condition, and the latter may cause burns, which would heal slowly, if at all.

In irrigation of the nose the force of the stream must not be too great, or else infected material may be carried into the eustachian tube or the nasal accessory sinuses. In irrigating the throat, if the stream of fluid is directed on the soft palate or uvula, it may cause gagging. Irrigation of the stomach should not be employed to remove corrosive poisons because the pressure of the fluid may cause perforation of the eroded wall of the stomach.

Routine daily irrigations of the vagina are potentially harmful because they may remove the normally germicidal, vaginal secretions. Colonic irrigations may increase rectal discharges, irritate the anus, disturb a chronic ulcer of the bowel, produce nausea or cause fatal intussusception or volvulus. It has been reported that they may cause also rectal bleeding, from hemorrhoids, a fissure or an ulcer, or cause a torn rectal valve. In one instance perforation by the rectal tube of a diverticulum of the sigmoid has been reported.

Cold compresses should not be used in the presence of impaired circulation, sensitivity to cold or asthenia. Hot compresses should be employed with caution for peripheral vascular disease because of the danger of burns with their disastrous consequences.

General cold baths should not be used, if there is hypersensitivity to cold, because collapse may occur. Urticaria also may be produced by cold baths. The cold bath should not be employed in the presence of arteriosclerosis, nephritis, spastic paralysis, nervous irritability or cardiac weakness. Neutral baths are contraindicated, if the patient has hypotension or a subnormal bodily temperature. Hot baths are not to be employed in the presence of marked hypertension, advanced debility, functional neurosis or conditions in which hemorrhage impends.

Among the dangers of continuous baths have been mentioned heat prostration, chilling, scalding, convulsions and drowning. Continuous baths should not be employed in the presence of cardiac disease, hypotension or asthenia. Carbon dioxide baths should not be used for patients who have marked cardiac decompensation, congestive heart failure or advanced syphilitic heart disease.

Underwater exercises are contraindicated for acute infections or febrile diseases, acute inflammations of joints, acute neuritis, tuberculosis of joints and during the acute painful stage of early poliomyelitis. General packs should not be employed when there is severe circulatory disturbance, advanced cardiac disease or extreme exhaustion, or when it is evident that a "reaction" may not occur.

Summary of Data on Hydrotherapy

Many local and general hydrotherapeutic procedures are simple of application and can be employed with ease in the patient's home. Physicians often have neglected to use these effective procedures, probably because they are not taught properly in our medical schools.

There is little room to doubt the efficacy of contrast baths, whirlpool baths, irrigations, hot tub baths, underwater exercises and packs in the management of certain pathological conditions. These procedures should be employed more extensively in general practice.

BIBLIOGRAPHY OF HYDROTHERAPY

1. BARUCH, S.: An Epitome of Hydrotherapy for Physicians, Architects and Nurses, Saunders, Philadelphia, 1920.
2. WOODMANSEY, A., COLLINS, D. H. and ERNST, M. M.: Vascular reactions to the contrast bath in health and in rheumatoid arthritis, Lancet, 1938, II, 1350.
3. NYLIN, J. B.: Hydrotherapy, in MOCK, H. E., PEMBERTON, R. and

COULTER, J. S., Principles and Practice of Physical Therapy, Vol. III, Chapt. XX, Prior, Hagerstown, Maryland, 1934.

4. BLAIR, H. C.: The alternation of blood supply as a cause for normal calcification of bone, Surg., Gynec. and Obst., 1938, LXVII, 413.

5. McCLELLAN, W. S.: Hydrotherapy and balneotherapy. In BARR, D. P., Modern Medical Therapy in General Practice, Vol. I, pp. 711–750, Williams and Wilkins, Baltimore, 1940.

6. WRIGHT, R.: Hydrotherapy in Hospitals for Mental Diseases, Tudor Press, Boston, 1932.

Sept. 1, 1941.

ELECTROTHERAPY

The types of electrical current commonly employed in modern medical practice are the constant current, the faradic current, the various sinusoidal currents and the high frequency or diathermy currents.

THE CONSTANT CURRENT

The constant or galvanic current is a unidirectional current of low voltage (tension) and amperage (volume). The current possesses polarity, there being a positive and a negative pole. The current is capable of producing migration of ions; it can be used in medicine to deposit ions of certain salts on or in the superficial layers of the skin or mucous membranes. If these ions are concentrated in a small region, destructive chemical effects of a caustic nature can be obtained.

The constant current is employed therapeutically chiefly for electrolysis, particularly for epilation, and for common ion transfer, iontophoresis, of a few medicinal ions. The Council on Physical Therapy of the American Medical Association[1] has said that the interrupted low frequency current and the constant electric current "are widely used in medical practice and are unquestionably of value in the treatment of a limited number of conditions".

Methods of Applying the Constant Current

The constant current can be derived from a battery of electrical cells, which usually are connected in series or from the main supply current, if this is of the direct (D. C.) rather than of the alternating (A. C.) variety. If the latter is used, a "shunt resistance" is placed in the patient's circuit to reduce the amount of current.

In the United States the house current usually is of the alternating (A. C.) variety; this can be employed as an indirect source of the therapeutic constant current only by the introduction of a motor generator, a rectifier or a "B-battery eliminator" between the house outlet and the patient.

The chief advantages of a therapeutic device, which derives its constant current from a battery of dry cells, are that it is portable and that it is not dependent on any outside electrical circuit. The specifications for construction of a simple, low cost, constant current generator have been prepared by the Council on Physical Therapy of the American Medical Association (Fig. 24).

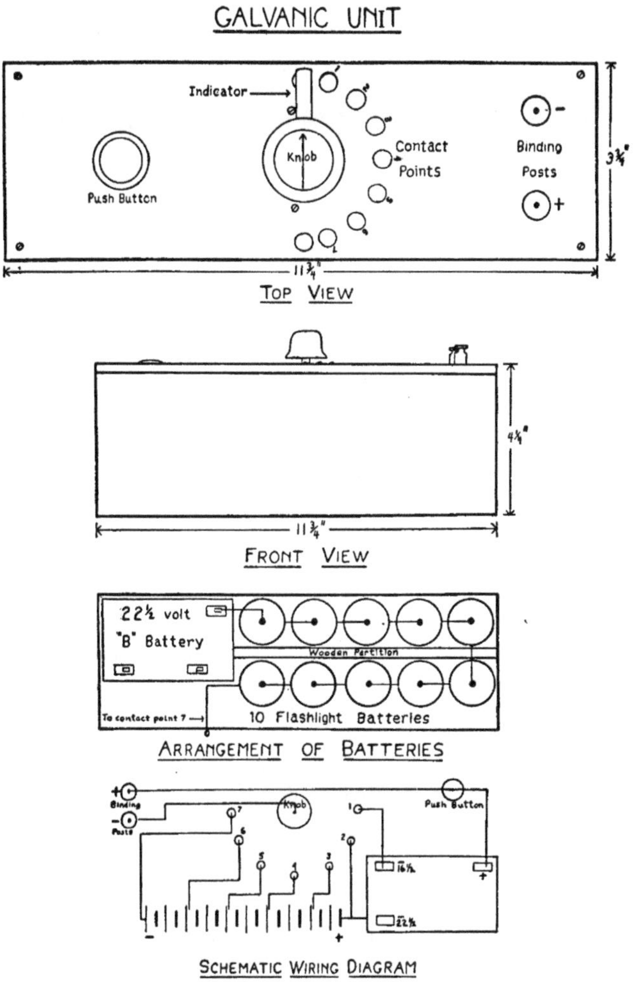

FIG. 24. Specifications for the construction of a constant, galvanic, current generator of low cost (Courtesy of the Council on Physical Therapy of the American Medical Association).

Physical Principles Concerned in the Therapeutic Application of the Constant Current

Certain substances, when dissolved in water, form a solution that possesses an osmotic pressure greater than that of water. Such a solution will conduct a constant current. The molecules are decomposed by the current, and their components collect at either the positive or the negative pole of the current. Acids, bases and salts are included among the substances which act in this manner. They are called "electrolytes" and the smaller particles into which they are decomposed are called "ions".

When the constant current is passed through an aqueous solution of sodium chloride, a migration of ions will occur. Some will collect at the positive and others at the negative pole. Similarly, if the constant current is passed through the bodily tissues, a migration and a concentration of their ions will occur beneath the electrodes connected to the two poles of the source of the current. The therapeutic effectiveness of the constant current depends on this ability to cause migration of ions.

Action and Uses of the Constant Current

When applied diffusely to the skin, the constant current, because of its stimulating effect on sensory nerve endings, will produce reflex vasodilatation. However, there are other simpler methods of obtaining this effect.

When concentrated at the tip of a needle, the constant current will cause chemical changes, owing to the collection of ions, which are so intense that caustic effects are obtained. Caustic destruction of the tissues ensues.

The ions of certain metals such as copper or zinc and of certain other substances such as histamine hydrochloride and mecholyl, acetyl-beta-methylcholine chloride, have been introduced into the superficial layers of the skin or mucous membranes by means of the constant current for therapeutic purposes.

The positive pole repels metals and alkaloids into the tissues; the negative pole repels acids, acid radicals and halogens. This should be remembered, when attempts are made to introduce these substances into the tissues, in order that the correct pole will be employed.

When *iontophoresis* is employed, the penetration of ions never will be greater than a fraction of a millimeter; nevertheless certain valuable superficial effects can be obtained. The low velocity of the ions and the low potential, at which they are introduced, preclude deep penetration, but the ions can be absorbed into the circulation from the superficial layers of the skin and thus produce distinct local and even systemic effects.

Electrolysis achieved by sharp localization of caustic products at the tip of a needle is a suitable method for obtaining destruction of certain lesions of the skin and mucous membranes. The indications for electrolysis are comparatively few. In many instances the newer and more readily controlled high frequency currents are used for destruction of small superficial lesions. There are, however, several conditions for which electrolysis still is considered the method of choice. Both MacKee[2] and Cipollaro[3] recommended electrolysis for destruction of certain cutaneous lesions, such as adenoma sebaceum, dilated capillaries, benign cystic epitheliomas, hemangiomas, hydrocystomas, hypertrichosis, keratosis, pigmented hairy moles, spider nevi and syringocystadenomas. By far the most common and important indication for electrolysis is hypertrichosis. As Cipollaro[3] stated: "It is the only method for permanent and safe removal of unwanted hairs."

For selected cases of chronic otorrhea Friel[4] has recommended the employment of *zinc iontophoresis*. Lierle and Sage[5] were not impressed so favorably with the procedure, and Hollender[6] concluded that, although the method may be useful in selected cases, the evidence presented to date is insufficient to place the procedure on a firm scientific basis. Recently zinc iontophoresis has been recommended in treatment of hay fever and rhinitis. The method may cause fibrosis of the nasal submucosa without damage to the superficial epithelium. Local application of phenol can produce a similar effect. At best the procedure is palliative and not curative. It has seemed to be more effective in non-allergic rhinitis than in seasonal hay fever. Its value and dangers as yet have not been determined fully.

Kovács[7] has recommended the employment of *iontophoresis of mecholyl*, acetyl-beta-methylcholine chloride, in treatment of varicose ulcers. *Zinc* or *copper iontophoresis* has been employed in the past for indolent ulcers.

Kling[8] advocated the use of *histamine iontophoresis* in treatment of peripheral circulatory diseases. He was of the opinion that the procedure was more effective than were inunctions of histamine. Neither procedure is particularly effective in peripheral vascular diseases. I have tried histamine iontophoresis and could see no advantage over other simpler methods of producing hyperemia.

Several authors[8, 9, 10, 11] have urged strongly the use of iontophoresis of histamine or of mecholyl (acetyl-beta-methylcholine chloride) in treatment of atrophic, hypertrophic or traumatic arthritis. It was thought that the procedure caused local vasodilatation within the joint over which it was applied. It has been commented that this can be "little more than pure conjecture". I have found little to recommend the procedure and prefer simpler methods of producing vasodilatation in treatment for arthritis.

Copper iontophoresis has been employed for many years in treatment for endocervicitis, but no one seems to have compared it carefully with other methods of treatment. Tovey[12], for example, recommended the procedure enthusiastically but presented no statistical or comparative studies to support his views.

Contraindications to the Employment of the Constant Current

Following iontophoresis of either histamine or mecholyl (acetyl-beta-methylcholine chloride) untoward systemic reactions may occur which must be guarded against. When electrolysis is performed, care should be taken to avoid application of the current from the positive pole through a steel needle, or else a tattoo may result. Incorrect technic in electrolysis may cause painful, disfiguring or even dangerous lesions. Infections, keloids or regions of depigmentation may occur. Incomplete destruction of a benign melanoma may cause it to become malignant.

Use of excessive amounts of current in copper iontophoresis of the cervix may produce sloughing and subsequent stenosis of the cervical canal. Improper employment of zinc iontophoresis in the nose may result in impairment of the sense of smell.

Summary of Data on the Constant Current

The constant current is useful chiefly for electrolysis and for iontophoresis. Electrolysis is indispensable for safe epilation and can be employed to advantage also for destruction of a few cutaneous lesions.

Iontophoresis of certain medicinal ions may be employed occasionally for therapeutic purposes. The constant current has a distinct but limited field of usefulness in medicine.

The Faradic Current

The therapeutic use of the faradic current followed the discovery by Michael Faraday in 1831 of electromagnetic induction. Guillaume Duchenne is believed to have been the first to employ the faradic current in medicine. He thought that faradic stimulation aided in the recovery of weakened muscles by increasing their circulation. He was sufficiently observant to realize, however, that the procedure was not so effective in strengthening weakened muscles as was voluntary contraction.

The faradic current, which is employed for therapeutic purposes, is an intermittent, asymmetrical, alternating current obtained from the secondary winding of an induction coil. Like the constant current its field of usefulness is distinctly limited. At present it is employed chiefly for stimulation of weak or atrophied muscles, which have a normal nerve supply, for testing for the reaction of degeneration and as a means of suggestion for treatment of hysteria.

Methods of Applying the Faradic Current

Small faradic units long have been marketed for medical use. Any electrician can build one at small cost by following the directions which have been prepared by the Council on Physical Therapy of the American Medical Association (Fig. 25).

This device employs a sliding iron core which permits the current in the secondary coil to be varied smoothly in a surging manner. This surging of the current by sliding the core in and out permits the operator to produce rhythmic graduated contractions of muscles through which the current is passed.

More elaborate types of the faradic unit dispense with the manual production of variation in the current and employ motor driven cams or other mechanisms to vary its intensity. A suitable portable faradic coil, which has been employed extensively in England, has been developed by Sir Morton Smart[13, 14].

Physical Principles Concerned in the Therapeutic Application of the Faradic Current

The device for production of a faradic current consists of a constant current source such as a battery of electrical cells, an induction coil and a current interrupter. The primary coil of the apparatus consists of a few turns of copper which encircle a core made of a bundle of soft iron wires. The secondary coil consists of many turns of fine copper wire which encircle a hollow fiber cylinder. This cylinder is made to ensheathe the primary coil. Either this cylinder or the iron core is arranged so that it can be slid in or out to vary the amount of induced current in the secondary coil.

The asymmetrical current, which flows from the secondary coil, will

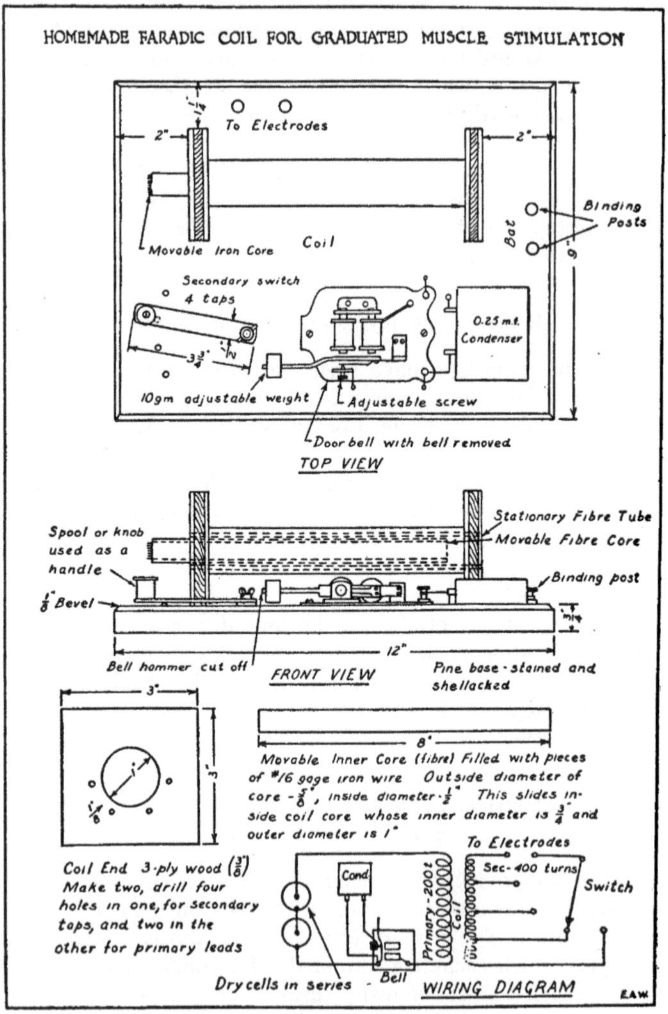

FIG. 25. Specifications for the construction of a simple faradic coil (Courtesy of the Council on Physical Therapy of the American Medical Association).

stimulate contractions of normal muscles but will not cause muscles, which have lost their nerve supply, to contract.

Action and Uses of the Faradic Current

The physiological effect of faradic stimulation of muscles is similar to that of other forms of electrical stimulation. However, the method of accomplishing the muscular contraction differs from that of other currents.

The effective phase of the secondary faradic current occurs at the "break". These "break" phases occur at a rate of 50 to 100 times per second. These "break" stimuli follow one another so rapidly that the muscle, which possesses a normal nerve supply, will have no time to relax between stimuli, and a smooth even tetanus will result. The very short "break" stimuli, lasting 0.001 second, although very suitable for stimulating the normal muscle, which has a chronaxia of 0.0015 second, will not produce any effect on a paralyzed muscle which, because of its lack of innervation, has a chronaxia of 0.01 to 0.1 second.

These facts form the basis for the employment of the faradic current in testing for reaction of degeneration. A muscle with an intact normal nerve supply will respond to faradic stimulation, whereas if the nerve supply is damaged or degenerated, the muscle will not respond. The details of the test for reaction of degeneration will not be described here but can be found in other books[15, 16].

As has been mentioned, the faradic current is employed chiefly for performing this test or for stimulation of muscles which have poor tone but possess a normal nerve supply. It is particularly useful in stimulating muscles which have lost tone and have become atrophied following prolonged disuse. The current also can be applied by means of a special brush electrode to cause strong, painful, muscular contractions as a means of inducing suggestion in cases of hysteria. Another valuable application of the faradic current is for the purpose of teaching a patient to contract one muscle independently. Muscle setting exercises often are valuable, but it may be difficult to train a patient to contract the correct muscle or muscles. Faradic stimulation of the muscles in question immediately will demonstrate to the patient which muscles are to be contracted. Once he feels these muscles contract, he may be able to continue the contractions voluntarily. The electrical stimulation may save several hours of explanation and practice.

Faradic stimulation occasionally can be employed to produce rhythmic contractions of muscles which the patient cannot or will not contract of his own volition. Smart[13, 14] recommended its employment for many conditions including such as strains, muscular atrophy, fibrositis, tenosynovitis, sprains, dislocations, fractures, arthritis and certain forms of paralysis.

Contraindications to the Use of the Faradic Current

Faradic stimulation is contraindicated in treatment during the acute stage of sprains in which the muscular contractions, which it produces, might cause further extravasation of blood and lymph into the tissue spaces and might interfere with normal repair. Stimulation of muscles by the faradic current should be used with caution in recent fractures because of the danger of disturbing the alignment of the fragments. It should be remembered that voluntary exercises are to be preferred to faradic stimulation of the muscles.

Summary of Data on the Faradic Current

As with other low voltage therapeutic currents the faradic current has a small but definite field of usefulness. The current is derived from a fairly simple apparatus and is easy to apply. It is indispensable for use in performance of the test for reaction of degeneration and is valuable for stimulating weak and atrophied muscles.

The Interrupted Galvanic and Sinusoidal Currents

The interrupted or waved currents of this group are of low voltage and amperage. The group includes the interrupted galvanic current, the slow sinusoidal current and the rapid sinusoidal current. There are numerous modifications of these basic forms of current, for which a uniform nomenclature has not been determined.

The interrupted galvanic current is a unidirectional current which is made and broken, turned on and off, sharply. When passed through normal muscles, it will produce quick, brief, muscular contractions at each make and break of the current. The slow sinusoidal current is an alternating current, the volume of which can be represented as traveling in the course of a sinusoid. In other words a graph of the current volume looks like a series of symmetrical waves. The potential rises slowly from zero to maximum, then gradually returns to zero; it then reverses and repeats this action. The rate of alternation usually is 5 to 30 per minute. Smooth muscles and skeletal muscles, which are in a state of flaccid paralysis, usually will respond to this current.

The rapid sinusoidal current is similar to the slow sinusoidal current with the exception that its rate of oscillation is much greater, the rate being 120 alternations, 60 cycles, or more per second. The rapid, sinusoidal current alternates so rapidly that, although it will cause smooth tetanization of normal skeletal muscles, no single stimulus is long enough to produce a contraction in a paralyzed muscle.

Modifications of these basic interrupted or waved currents include various types of surging, such as the types known as the surging sinusoidal current and the surging sinusoidal current with a sustained peak.

When employed for stimulation of muscles, the sinusoidal currents are somewhat less unpleasant than is the faradic current because their alternations are perfectly smooth. The indications for their use are practically the same as those for the faradic current.

Methods of Applying the Interrupted Galvanic and Sinusoidal Currents

The interrupted galvanic current is produced by the apparatus for generation of the constant, galvanic current with the exception that some method must be provided for making and breaking the electrical circuit. A make and break key or button can be used to permit manual interruption of the current, or some mechanical interrupter such as a metronome, rotating cam or automatic switch can be employed.

To obtain the slow sinusoidal current a source of galvanic current can be employed in conjunction with a variable resistance and current reverser which will wave the current in the form of a sinusoid. The rapid sinusoidal current usually is derived from an alternating current main and is modified and protected suitably. Elaborate machines, which produce the three basic currents variously modified, have been marketed.

Physical Principles Concerned in the Application of the Interrupted Galvanic and Sinusoidal Currents

The physics of the interrupted galvanic current is the same as that of the constant current. The ordinary house current usually is a rapid sinusoidal current of 60 cycles and of such high voltage and amperage that, unmodified, it cannot be employed for therapeutic purposes. If the voltage and amperage are reduced to tolerable volumes, then the current can be employed for stimulation of muscles possessing a normal nerve supply.

No rate of oscillation ever has been agreed on as the dividing line between rapid and slow sinusoidal currents. It has been suggested that, if no single wave before reversal of flow lasts longer than 1/50 (0.02) of a second, such a sinusoidal current should be called "rapid"; that if the length of time for the completion of one wave is greater than 1/50 (0.02) of a second, then the current can be considered to be a slow sinusoidal current.

Usually with the rapid sinusoidal current the duration of the period of flow before reversal will be from 1/50 (0.02) to 1/200 (0.005) of a second. With the current of 60 cycles the duration would be 1/120 (0.008) of a second because there are 120 alternations to 60 cycles.

Action and Uses of the Interrupted Galvanic and Sinusoidal Currents

When these interrupted or waved currents are passed through human tissues, the electrochemical changes, which are produced, may stimulate nerves or cause muscles to contract. The action has been attributed to concentration of hydrogen or hydroxyl ions.

The contractions caused by the interrupted galvanic current are separate and brief; hence, they do not resemble normal muscular contractions. Voluntary muscular contractions are more prolonged and result from a series of nerve stimuli, which are said to occur at the rate of more than twenty per second. Therefore, the interrupted galvanic current is not the most suitable current for therapeutic use, and it is employed only for stimulation of weak, paralyzed muscles, which will not respond to the waved currents. There has been a great deal of controversy concerning the rôle of electrical stimulation in treatment for various types of lesions of the lower motor neurons with resultant paralysis. .Some physicians[17, 18] contend that electrical stimulation will maintain contractility, irritability, tone and nutrition until such time as regeneration of the nerve takes place, if it takes place at all. Others[19, 20] are equally positive that electrical stimulation has no place whatever in the treatment of paralysis and may do much harm.

Because of this controversy the comparatively recent studies of Fischer[21] are significant. He noted that in spite of this prolonged clinical dispute concerning the value of electrotherapy in treating paralyzed muscles, almost no experimental data could be found to support the contention of either group. He performed tests on laboratory animals with either a tetanizing faradic current from an induction coil or an interrupted galvanic current from dry cells. After extensive study and experimentation he reached a number of interesting conclusions. Among these were the following: If a denervated muscle has been left untreated for about two weeks or more, faradic stimulation no longer produces an appreciable contraction. In such instances galvanic stimulation will provoke contractions, and repeated daily treatments will delay the lengthening of chronaxia to some extent but not nearly so markedly as will early treatment by faradic current. The fact that electrical treatment of muscles decreases the rate, previously increased by denervation, at which weight and water content are lost and also increases "the quantitatively raised, but qualitatively impaired, metabolism" seems to afford a clue for the explanation of the beneficial effect of the treatment. This effect is identical with the training effect on normal muscle produced by electrical stimulation. In normal muscles, also, the weight increases, and the metabolism is raised and increased in efficiency by strong electrical stimulation. A treated muscle five weeks after denervation has about the same weight as an untreated muscle about one week after denervation. The power of a muscle treated for five weeks is appreciably greater than that of its untreated partner. It is noted especially that the treated muscle is less fatigable. Despite remarkable retardation of loss of weight and diminished loss of dry substance, the treatment has failed to improve the contractile mechanism. But after reinnervation it seems reasonable to assume that a treated muscle with its higher excitability, its greater weight, its lower content of water and its increased metabolism could be restored more easily to normal function than an untreated muscle. These studies seem significant and would seem definitely to refute the claims of those who say that electrical stimulation plays no part in the treatment of paralyzed muscles.

The uses of the interrupted galvanic current in medicine are few. It, of course, is employed routinely in conjunction with the faradic current in performance of the test for reaction of degeneration. It is used occasionally also for stimulation of extremely weak, paralyzed muscles which will not respond to the slow sinusoidal or to other waved galvanic currents.

The slow sinusoidal current is used for stimulation of unstriped muscles and sometimes can be used to produce contractions of paralyzed skeletal muscles. The rapid sinusoidal current is employed for stimulation of weak or atrophied muscles which have a normal nerve supply. For this purpose it is somewhat less unpleasant than the faradic current.

Not only have the interrupted galvanic and slow sinusoidal currents been employed in treatment for lesions of the lower motor neurons, but their use has been suggested[1] also for lesions of the upper motor neurons such as hemiplegia or myelitis. Electrical stimulation has been employed for prevention of atrophy of the quadriceps or deltoid muscle following injury to the knee or shoulder, to improve muscular tone in cardiovascular disorders and to initiate respiration in asphyxia of the newborn.

The rapid sinusoidal current can be used interchangeably with the faradic current. Therefore, the indications listed under Action and Uses of the Faradic Current can be consulted for further information concerning possible uses of the rapid sinusoidal current.

Contraindications to the Application of the Interrupted Galvanic and Sinusoidal Currents

Electrical stimulation is contraindicated in cerebrospastic paralysis, combined sclerosis of the spinal cord, progressive muscular atrophy and myasthenia gravis. In stimulation of paralyzed muscles excessive treatment may produce fatigue and do more harm than good. Such stimulation always should be applied within limits of fatigue. If there is slowing of muscular response, which is the first sign of fatigue, treatment should be stopped at once.

It has been said that, if alternating or sinusoidal currents are applied to the cardiac region, they may cause cardiac fibrillation. It must be stressed once more that electrical stimulation always is less valuable than is voluntary exercise.

Summary of Data on the Interrupted Galvanic and Sinusoidal Currents

A few simple modifications of the three basic currents, which have been discussed, are all that is necessary for satisfactory electrical stimulation of muscles. Elaborate apparatus is not required for this purpose. The simpler devices are entirely satisfactory for production of muscular contractions. There are several uses for such apparatus.

Diathermy

By far the most valuable form of electrical current for use in medicine and surgery is the high frequency, or diathermy, current. It has been found that, if an electrical current is made to oscillate at an extremely rapid rate, it can be passed through the tissues of the human body without producing any neuromuscular response; hence no electrical "shock" is produced. Under such circumstances both the voltage and the amperage of the current can be increased so that an increase in temperature will develop in the tissues traversed by the current.

In this manner a means of producing deep local heating of bodily tissues is obtained without any other effects on these tissues. To employ a crude analogy, just as the filament of an ordinary electric light bulb glows to white heat owing to the resistance it offers to the flow of a 60 cycle current of relatively high voltage, so to a lesser degree will the bodily tissues become heated owing to the resistance which they offer to the flow of this current of relatively high voltage and very high frequency. The patient would receive a severe electrical shock from a 60

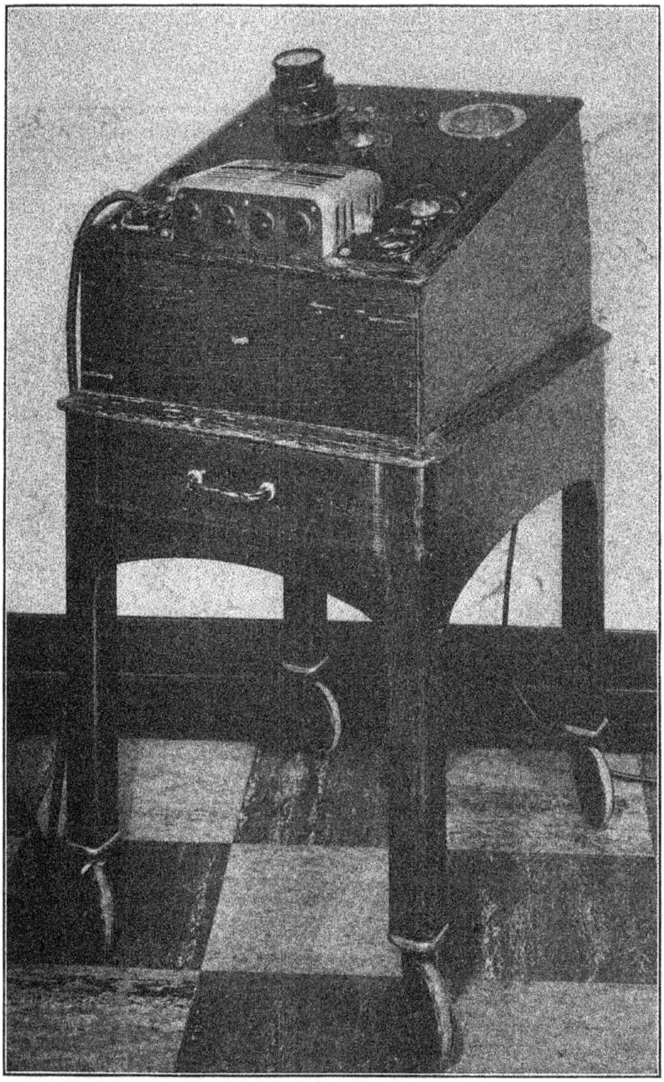

FIG. 26. A conventional diathermy machine (From Krusen, F. H.: Physical Medicine, Saunders, Philadelphia, 1941).

cycle current of sufficient voltage and amperage to heat the tissues, but he receives no such shock from the current of high frequency.

Because of the heating of the tissues which are traversed by the current, the procedure has been called "diathermy". This designation has become well established as the proper term for the description of the application of high frequency currents of relatively long wavelengths, 500,000 to 3,000,000 cycles per second.

Following the development of the triode principle of electronic oscillations, radio engineers were able to construct excellent vacuum tube oscillators which would produce currents of much higher frequencies, and shorter wavelengths, than previously had been employed. The newer machines, which employed vacuum tubes, were able to produce an oscillating current of extremely high frequency, from 10,000,000 cycles per second and a 30 meter wavelength to 100,000,000 cycles per second and a 3 meter wavelength.

With the development of these new machines it has become the custom in the United States to call longer wavelength machines "conventional diathermy" apparatus and the new shorter wavelength devices "short wave diathermy" machines. In Europe the much less explicit and less descriptive designation "short wave therapy" still is employed frequently.

Methods of Applying Diathermy

A typical apparatus for producing conventional diathermy consists of (1) a source of alternating, 60 cycle, current, (2) a switch, (3) a choke coil, current intensity regulator, (4) a step-up transformer, (5) spark gaps, (6) condensers, (7) a solenoid and (8) an inductor (Fig. 26). Such an arrangement delivers a moderately high frequency current to a patient. Wires leading from the machine to metal plates on the surface of the patient's body will provide a conductive type of high frequency current for passage through the body. With the development of the newer short wave diathermy machine the older conventional diathermy apparatus largely has been discarded. Nevertheless it still is useful and sometimes can be employed to better advantage than the newer machine for localizing heat in a small region.

The most common type of apparatus for production of short wave diathermy current consists of a simple two tube, "push-pull" circuit (Fig. 27). The circuit consists of three essential parts; (1) the power supply, (2) the oscillating circuit and (3) the output circuit. For further details, the reader can consult an article by Hemingway and Stenstrom[22] in which the circuits are well described. The appliance for the production of short wave diathermy resembles in construction a short wave radio transmitter with the exception that the electrical energy, instead of being dispersed from antennas as in broadcasting, is confined mostly between

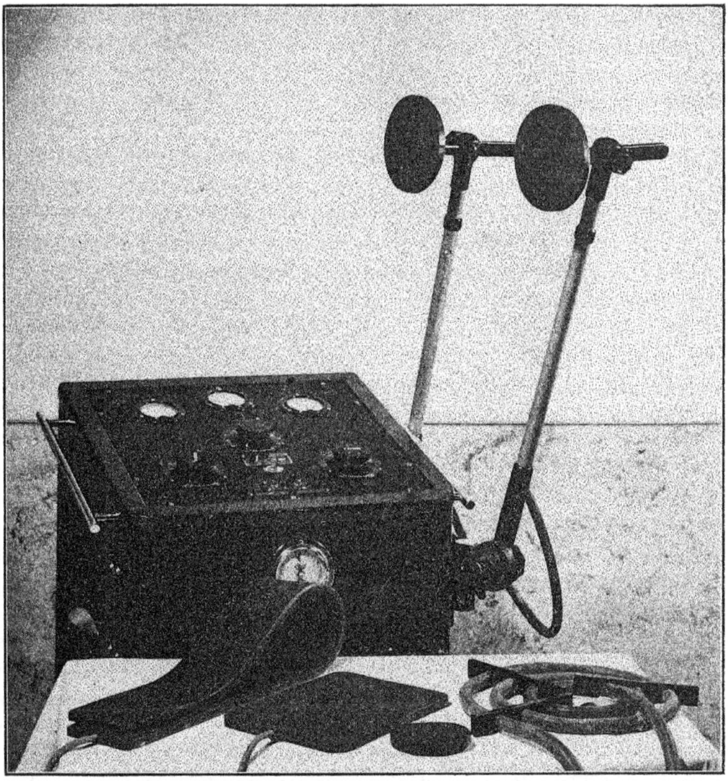

FIG. 27. A short wave diathermy machine (From Krusen, F. H.: Physical Medicine, Saunders, Philadelphia, 1941).

condenser plates to produce an electrical field or is confined within a coil to produce an electromagnetic field.

Human tissues, acting partly as conductors and partly as dielectrics, when placed within these fields, presumably are heated by the production of ionic oscillations and molecular friction. Power losses occur, and heating of the deep tissues is produced.

Physical Principles Concerned in the Application of Diathermy

With regard to the position of electrodes with conventional diathermy it is necessary to have the electrodes in direct contact with the skin or the mucous membranes. This may be unsatisfactory, especially if a large electrode is to be used over an irregular surface. However, if short wave diathermy is to be employed, an insulating pad or layer of air can be interposed between the electrode and the surface of the body. Thus, by applying short wave diathermy electrodes at a distance from the surface, it is possible to heat a deeper region of the body without undue heating of the skin.

Selective Heating. — It has been claimed that the newer short wave diathermy currents will produce "selective heating" of various bodily tissues; that is, because different tissues have different dielectric constants, they will be heated to a greater or lesser degree. Basing their claims on this therapeutic conception, a number of enthusiasts have concluded that it would be possible, therefore, to heat one organ of the body to a greater degree than another. Although it is true that short wave diathermy will produce selective heating of inorganic substances and of dead tissues, it now has been demonstrated repeatedly that in the living animal, owing to dissipation of heat by the circulation, no such selective heating of tissues can be expected.

Thermopenetration. — For various physical reasons it is evident that short wave diathermy should produce more uniform and deeper penetration of heat than does conventional diathermy. As yet, despite a number of investigations of the problem, there is no conclusive proof of this. Further observations eventually may indicate the comparative thermopenetration of these two forms of diathermy.

Dosage. — At present there is no means for accurate determination of the dosage of short wave diathermy. Watt meters are being developed which may help to give some indication of proper dosage; however, these are not entirely accurate. At present the physician, who applies short wave diathermy, must rely on his careful observation of the sensation of heat felt by the patient and from this must govern the dosage as accurately as possible. Because of this need for careful observation of the sensations of the patient by a skilled physician or technician no patient ever should be permitted to control the dials of the apparatus himself.

Wavelength. — It has been claimed by various investigators that different wavelengths produce different effects on the bodily tissues; however, as more and more experimental evidence is amassed, it becomes evident that the only effect of short wave diathermy on the bodily tissue is a thermal one, and that within the range between 3 and 30 meters one wavelength has no particular advantage over another.

Action and Uses of Diathermy

It has been demonstrated that appreciable rises in temperature of more than 5° F. or of 2.75° C. can be obtained at a depth in comparatively avascular tissues. If the tissues are highly vascular, little increase in temperature, not more than 0.9° F. or 0.5° C., will be found. It frequently has been claimed by enthusiasts that short wave diathermy will produce certain physiological effects other than those attributable to heating, but a large amount of experimental data now has been amassed, which seems definitely to indicate that no specific physiological effects other than those attributable to heating exist.

The numerous scientific investigations of the effect of diathermy on bacteria now permit the conclusion that neither in vitro nor in vivo are there specific bactericidal effects other than those attributable to heat.

Whereas high frequency currents may be employed to great advantage for electrosurgery, fulguration, desiccation, coagulation and electric cutting, such applications are outside the realm of this chapter. The surgeon, who desires additional information on this subject, should refer to other sources[23, 24, 25] for details concerning their employment. Short wave diathermy currents are not suitable for fulguration, desiccation or coagulation but are excellent for purposes of cutting. A conventional diathermy, spark gap, apparatus should be employed for fulguration, desiccation or coagulation.

For medical purposes, that is to heat the bodily tissues within physiological limits, short wave diathermy is most effective. For such local heating of tissues there are three general types of electrodes; condenser plates or pads may be placed on each side of the part to be treated, cuffs may encircle an extremity above and below the region to be treated, or an induction coil may be wrapped around an extremity or formed in the shape of a flat pancake and placed over a certain region. The electrodes always should be spaced away from the bodily surface for a distance of about 2 inches (5 cm.) by means of felt pads or folded turkish towels. The apparatus then is adjusted to provide comfortable warmth in the region which is exposed to the current.

Despite frequent claims that short exposures of not more than ten minutes are sufficient to produce proper heating of the tissues, repeated studies in my own department[26] have indicated that it requires at least thirty minutes of exposure to short wave diathermy to obtain an optimal increase in temperature, and the usual exposure time should be thirty to forty-five minutes. For further details concerning the technic of application of short wave diathermy other more complete publications should be consulted[16, 27].

Short wave diathermy has been recommended especially in the treatment of suppurative processes, diseases of the bones and joints such as sprains, dislocations, arthritis, osteomyelitis and periostitis. There still is considerable argument concerning the usefulness of short wave diathermy in the management of fractures. Some investigators have expressed the belief that hyperemia caused by diathermy produces demineralization of bones, whereas others have felt that the increased circulation accelerates the formation of new bone.

Some have stated that the heat produced by diathermy is valuable in the treatment of fractures because of its favorable influence on the associated injuries to soft tissue. When so employed, it often should be administered in conjunction with massage and exercise. Diathermy also has been recommended in the treatment of various types of endarteritis to promote circulation. However, in such cases there is always danger of producing burns and subsequent gangrene, if too intense diathermy is applied directly to the involved extremity. Its employment has been recommended also in treatment for varicose ulcers.

In the field of cutaneous diseases continental workers have recommended particularly that diathermy be applied for furuncles, carbuncles, cellulitis and paronychia. To date there is no conclusive evidence that diathermy is more effective in such localized infections than are other forms of mild local heating. For certain gastrointestinal diseases such as diverticulitis, acute enteritis and spastic colitis diathermy has seemed to be of value as a palliative measure. A number of good investigators have stressed the value of local applications of intrapelvic diathermy in the treatment of chronic inflammation in the pelvic region as well as for nonspecific prostatitis, epididymitis and cystitis. Among the diseases of muscles, tendons and bursæ, for which diathermy has been recommended, may be mentioned contusions, muscular strains, myositis, fibrositis, tenosynovitis and bursitis. Among the diseases of the nervous system, in which local heating by diathermy sometimes is useful, may be mentioned neuritis, particularly ischemic neuritis and such conditions as brachial neuritis, intercostal neuritis, sciatica and trifacial neuralgia. Short wave diathermy has been recommended to promote healing and to allay pain in otitis media and in the treatment of furunculosis of the external auditory canal.

Among diseases of the respiratory system, for which short wave diathermy has been recommended, may be mentioned sinusitis. Although after adequate drainage has been established local applications of heat may be of slight value in the presence of inflammation of the accessory nasal sinuses, the procedure is merely palliative, and there is no conclusive evidence that the procedure, as often has been claimed, ever is a specific in this condition. Diathermy has been recommended also as an adjunct in the management of various pulmonary lesions such as bronchitis, bronchial asthma and both bronchial and lobar pneumonia. In such conditions it must be considered simply as another means of applying heat, and it should be employed only as an auxiliary measure in conjunction with other forms of treatment.

Contraindications to the Employment of Diathermy

Diathermy should not be employed in the treatment of any condition in which there is danger of hemorrhage. Because of the danger of burns the application of diathermy is contraindicated also over regions in which sensation is impaired. It should not be administered to the abdomen, lower portion of the back or pelvis during pregnancy or during the menstrual period. Also it should not be applied over regions in which there may be a malignant growth or tuberculous lesion. Some authors believe that diathermy should not be applied in the presence of phlebitis because of the danger of embolism.

Summary of Data on Diathermy

It is wise to employ only such diathermy apparatus as has been accepted by the Council on Physical Therapy of the American Medical Association. The various diathermy machines which have been considered acceptable, information about their degree of efficiency and the approved technics for their use are listed in a booklet entitled "Apparatus Accepted by the Council on Physical Therapy of the American Medical Association"[1]. Every effort should be made to avoid the use of diathermy except when it definitely is indicated. Certainly there are enough rational indications for its employment to warrant its frequent use. It should not be forgotten, however, that simpler methods of applying heat may be equally effective for the treatment of superficial lesions. Short wave diathermy finds its greatest usefulness for treatment of deeper lesions. It unquestionably is the most valuable form of electrotherapy available today. When employed in a rational manner, it may be used for a multitude of purposes both in medicine and in surgery.

BIBLIOGRAPHY OF ELECTROTHERAPY

1. COUNCIL ON PHYSICAL THERAPY: The interrupted low frequency and the constant electric current in medicine, in Handbook of Physical Therapy, Ed. 3, pp. 205–213, American Medical Association Press, Chicago, 1939.
2. MACKEE, G. M.: The treatment of skin diseases by physical therapeutic methods, Jour. Am. Med. Assoc., 1932, XCVIII, 1646.
3. CIPOLLARO, A. C.: Electrolysis; a discussion of equipment, method of operation, indications, contraindications, and warning concerning its use, in Handbook of Physical Therapy, Ed. 3, pp. 268–279, American Medical Association Press, Chicago, 1939.
4. FRIEL, A. R.: Electric Ionization; a Practical Introduction to its Use in Medicine and Surgery, Wood, New York, 1922.
5. LIERLE, D. M. and SAGE, R. A.: Underlying factors in the zinc ionization treatment of middle ear infections, Ann. Otol., Rhin. and Laryng., 1932, XLI, 359.
6. HOLLENDER, A. R.: Physical Therapeutic Methods in Otolaryngology, Mosby, St. Louis, 1937.
7. KOVÁCS, J.: Iontophoresis of varicose ulcers, Arch. Phys. Therapy, 1937, XVIII, 103.
8. KLING, D. H.: Histamine iontophoresis in rheumatic and peripheral circulatory disturbances, Arch. Phys. Therapy, 1935, XVI, 466.
9. KOTKIS, A. J. and MELCHIONNA, R. H.: Physiologic effects of acetyl-beta-methylcholine chloride by iontophoresis; preliminary report, Arch. Phys. Therapy, 1935, XVI, 528.
10. KOVÁCS, J.: The iontophoresis of acetyl-beta-methyl-choline chloride in the treatment of chronic arthritis and peripheral vascular disease, Am. Jour. Med. Sci., 1934, CLXXXVIII, 32.
11. KOVÁCS, R. and KOVÁCS, J.: Newer aspects of iontophoresis for arthritis and circulatory disturbances, Arch. Phys. Therapy, 1934, XV, 593.
12. TOVEY, D. W.: Copper ionization treatment of cervicitis, (Spec. Sect.), Am. Med., 1932, XXXVIII, 2.
13. SMART, M.: The Principles of Treatment of Muscles and Joints by Graduated Muscular Contractions, Oxford University Press, London, 1933.
14. SMART, M.: Graduated Muscular Contractions; a Short Description of Principles and Technique, Oxford University Press, London, 1936.
15. CUMBERBATCH, E. P.: Essentials of Medical Electricity, Ed. 6, Mosby, St. Louis, 1929.
16. KRUSEN, F. H.: Physical Medicine, Saunders, Philadelphia, 1941.
17. KOVÁCS, R.: Electrotherapy and Light Therapy, Ed. 3, Lea and Febiger, Philadelphia, 1938.
18. CUMBERBATCH, E. P.: Essentials of Medical Electricity, Ed. 8, The Sherwood Press, Cleveland, 1939.
19. CHOR, H., CLEVELAND, D., DAVENPORT, H. A., DOLKART, R. E.

and BEARD, G.: Atrophy and regeneration of the gastrocnemius-soleus muscles; effects of physical therapy in the monkey following section and suture of sciatic nerve, Physiotherapy Rev., 1939, XIX, 340.

20. OBER, F. R.: Physical therapy in infantile paralysis, Jour. Am. Med. Assoc., 1938, CX, 45.

21. FISCHER, E.: The effect of a faradic and galvanic stimulation upon the course of atrophy in denervated skeletal muscles, Am. Jour. Physiol., 1939, CXXVII, 605.

22. HEMINGWAY, A. and STENSTROM, K. W.: Physical characteristics of short wave diathermy, in Handbook of Physical Therapy, Ed. 3, American Medical Association Press, Chicago, 1939.

23. MOCK, H. E.: Electrosurgery in thyroidectomy, Jour. Am. Med. Assoc., 1930, XCIV, 1365.

24. KRUSEN, F. H. and ELKINS, E. C.: Electrosurgery, South. Surgeon, 1938, VII, 61.

25. KRUSEN, F. H. and SCHULHOF, M. G.: Electrosurgery, in The Cyclopedia of Medicine, Surgery and Specialties, pp. 454-469, Davis, Philadelphia, 1939.

26. KRUSEN, F. H.: Short-wave diathermy, Military Surgeon, 1940, LXXXVII, 158.

27. BIERMAN, WILLIAM: The Medical Applications of the Short Wave Current, Wood, Baltimore, 1938.

Sept. 1, 1941.

MASSAGE

"Massage" is a term used to describe a group of systematic and scientific manipulations of the tissues of the body which are performed best with the hands for the purpose of affecting the general circulation and the nervous and muscular systems.

A better understanding by physicians of the subject of massage undoubtedly would lead to its more extensive use and to methods of application which would be more suitable for the individual patient. Too frequently the physician requests a technician to give a patient "some massage" without specifying the type, duration or other details concerning the method of massage to be followed. Although on the European continent it frequently is the custom for the physician himself to apply massage, among American and British physicians it usually is customary to delegate this work to technicians. Because of the fact that in the United States there are skillful registered physical therapy technicians and in Britain well trained members of the Chartered Society of Massage and Medical Gymnastics, who are well instructed in anatomy and kinesiology, the custom usually is acceptable. Nevertheless even the most skillful technician is untrained in diagnosis and has only a limited knowledge of morbid physiology and pathology, so that the physician always should assume direct supervision of the massage, even though the technician does the actual work.

Mennell[1] said pertinently: "When a medical man orders massage he should not try to hand over his responsibility to the masseur. He should consider the prescription of massage treatment in the same light as he would consider that of a potent drug and watch its effects no less closely, varying the dose and the nature of the dose from time to time according to indications."

Methods of Applying Massage

The massage movements in the order of their importance are as follows; (1) effleurage (stroking), (2) pétrissage (kneading), (3) friction (a circular rolling movement), (4) tapotement (percussion) and (5) vibration (a tremulous or vibratory movement).

Stroking, kneading and friction are the only movements which are employed routinely for therapeutic purposes. Vibratory and percussion movements usually are applied to the healthy individual and rarely are applied to the sick person.

Effleurage or Stroking. — Stroking is the most common form of massage. The hand is moved slowly, gently and rhythmically in long, stroking movements. Light, superficial stroking produces reflex effects, and deep stroking will produce actual mechanical emptying of the veins and lymphatic vessels.

Pétrissage or Kneading. — Kneading is a wringing or compression movement in which the muscles are picked up and rolled, squeezed or wrung.

Friction. — Friction is not, as the name might suggest, a rapid rubbing of the technician's hand over the skin to produce a frictional effect. On the contrary, it is a circular, rolling movement, in which the patient's skin is moved over the subcutaneous structures in small circles. The fingers of the masseur remain at one point on the patient's skin and move it around. This type of massage tends to loosen superficial scars and adhesions. Friction usually is preceded and followed by stroking.

Tapotement or Percussion. — There are various types of percussion. If the surface of the patient's body is struck lightly and alternately first with the ulnar surface of one hand and then with the ulnar surface of the other hand, the procedure is called "hacking". If the part is struck lightly and rapidly with alternate slightly cupped palms of the hands, the procedure is called "cupping". If the tips of the fingers are employed for percussion, the method is spoken of as "tapping". When the flattened palms are employed for percussion, the procedure is termed "slapping". Finally, if the relaxed half-clenched fists are used for percussion, the designation "beating" is employed. Percussion movements will produce stimulating effects and induce peripheral hyperemia.

Vibration. — Vibration is a continuous trembling movement which is applied to the surface of the patient's body through the tips of the technician's fingers or through his whole hand. The vibratory movement is initiated by the muscles of the technician's shoulder and forearm. It is an extremely difficult movement and soon tires the masseur. For this reason in the few instances, in which vibration is required, a mechanical device may be attached to the back of the technician's hand to produce the vibratory movement.

In most instances the numerous mechanical devices, which have been marketed in profusion for pushing, pulling, twisting, turning and otherwise manipulating the human contours, are utterly useless. For example about ten years ago the public was swept with a wave of enthusiasm for machines which allegedly supplied massage and exercise by means of a strong vibrator attached to a wide belt. These so-called health exercisers were much in vogue for a short time, but because they were, like most such devices, almost useless as a means of applying either massage or exercise, they soon fell into disrepute.

In 1930 Pemberton, Coulter and Mock[2] commented concerning these "health exercisers" as follows: "Doctor Gustaf Zander of Stockholm, about 1857, was the first to use mechanical means for massage and exercise. His machines will do anything that any of the highly advertised mechanical vibrators will do. These machines were given a trial in this country, and several large hospitals completely equipped Zander rooms. These forms of apparatus have fallen into disuse, as will the present widely advertised mechanical exercisers." The prediction of these physicians was correct; the "health exerciser" no longer is heard of, and such has been the case with all similar mechanical massaging devices.

Physical Principles Concerned in the Application of Massage

Massage is an entirely mechanical procedure. Usually the hands of a skilled masseur or masseuse serve as the therapeutic agents. Mechanical apparatus of various types has not proved suitable for massage because the movements are too complex to be produced satisfactorily by a machine.

Mennell[1] said that only two possible effects were obtainable from massage, a mechanical effect and a reflex effect. It generally is believed that superficial stroking will produce reflex diminution of muscular spasm. Physicians usually are more familiar with reflexes, such as the cremasteric or the plantar reflexes, which are produced by irritation of the skin and cause muscular contraction, and often they have not realized that the soothing effect of light stroking of the skin may produce reflex muscular relaxation. It is easy to demonstrate such reflex muscular relaxation by applying superficial rhythmic stroking in the presence of a recent fracture with associated muscular spasm. The gentle stroking often produces sufficient relaxation to permit easier reduction of the fracture.

Action and Uses of Massage

Pemberton[3] said aptly: "There is probably no other measure of equal known value in the entire armamentarium of medicine which is so inadequately understood and utilized by the profession as a whole." Mennell[4], Coulter[5] and Pemberton[3] all have made definite contributions to our modern knowledge of the action of massage. Massage can be employed for its direct action on the surface of the skin to remove detritus and excessive secretions and to cleanse the openings of sweat and sebaceous glands. This procedure is particularly useful at the time of removal of splints or casts following fracture. Rosenthal[6] found that massage of the skin could cause an increase of local temperature of 3.6° to 5.4° F. (2° to 3° C.). He attributed these increases of temperature not only to direct mechanical action but also to indirect vasomotor effects.

The mistaken general impression still exists that massage will remove deposits of fat from local regions of the body. Careful clinical investigations do not support this impression. In experimental studies of this problem Rosenthal[6] found that vigorous massage of the abdominal wall of animals produced no destructive effect on the adipose tissue. Following the heavy massage histological sections of the adipose tissue exhibited no destruction of the fat, although the pressure of the massage had been sufficiently heavy to produce multiple hemorrhages.

It is believed[3] that massage of muscles may improve the supply of blood and tend to remove the excess of lactic acid which develops following exercise. Massage can be employed as a mechanical means of stretching or breaking adhesions of intramuscular connective tissue. Although it often is thought that massage of muscles may increase their strength, this is not the case. Muscular strength can be improved only by active exercise.

Centripetal stroking will improve circulation by aiding mechanically the return of venous blood and lymph toward the heart. It may produce also reflex contraction of the unstriped muscles of the walls of the vessels, thus assisting in the maintenance or restoration of the tone of these muscular fibers. The lightest stroking will empty the superficial veins and lymphatic vessels of an extremity, and the pressure in the deeper veins rarely exceeds that of 5 or 10 mm. of mercury. In order to obtain mechanical assistance to circulation in the deeper vessels, the muscles must be well relaxed.

Best and Taylor[7] pointed out that light stroking causes the "white reaction", which attains its maximal intensity in thirty to sixty seconds and then gradually fades in about three to five minutes. They concluded that this reaction did not have a nervous basis but was due to direct stimulation of the walls of the capillaries. They thought that heavy stroking would produce more enduring dilatation.

Massage often is valuable as an adjunct to elevation in the relief of edema of an extremity. Massage will assist gravity and also aid in restoring vasomotor tone.

Observations[3] through a permanent window of the capillary circulation of the ear of a rabbit have revealed that following massage there is an increase in the rate of flow of blood and a change in the walls of the capillaries which is evidenced by sticking and emigration of leukocytes. It was concluded that the massage produced an increased interchange of substances between the blood stream and tissue cells with an altered and presumably improved metabolism of tissues.

For necessarily inactive patients and especially for patients with cardiac decompensation massage can be employed to compensate for the lack of contraction of the muscles of locomotion which normally contributes to the return of venous blood to the heart. I agree with Pemberton[3] that this form of massage "is not utilized clinically to the extent that it should be".

It is said that the influence of massage in increasing the amount of hemoglobin and the number of erythrocytes of the circulating blood "is beyond question". Massage does not increase the lactic acid content of the blood, and the change in the hydrogen ion concentration is not comparable to that observed following exercise. Massage produces no change in the percentage of oxygen saturation, but it does cause a slight rise in the oxygen capacity of the blood.

If massage is applied skillfully, it can be employed to produce either a sedative or a stimulating effect on the central nervous system. Massage does not have any immediate effect or great influence on general metabolism. There is no immediate or delayed effect on the basal consumption of oxygen, the pulse rate or blood pressure of normal persons.

Arthritis. — Massage is of considerable value in preventing or delaying the muscular atrophy which often is associated with arthritis. Properly applied, it can be employed also in arthritis to improve local metabolism, increase circulation and lessen edema. In most cases of arthritis massage is preceded by applications of heat and followed by exercise. For atrophic arthritis massage alone is useless. Usually massage is applied to the muscles above and below the joint rather than directly to the arthritic joint. In the management of atrophic arthritis general massage often can be employed advantageously in conjunction with local massage. In hypertrophic arthritis especial care must be exercised to avoid heavy massage over, or too close to, the articular structures. Massage never should add to the trauma which already has been inflicted on such joints.

A leading specialist[8] on arthritis said that "few, if any, advanced cases of arthritis of either the atrophic or the hypertrophic type . . . can be expected to recover without recourse to the principles of physical therapy, intelligently ordered rest and massage in particular".

Fibrositis. — Many English writers have urged the employment of a special type of extremely firm massage in treatment for fibrositis of either the intramuscular or the periarticular type. All these authors[9, 10, 11, 12, 13] agreed that in conjunction with fibrositis, fibrous nodules will be found which can be "massaged away".

Despite the fact that this condition commonly is unrecognized in the United States, it seems safe to conclude that the numerous English observers are correct in their conclusions. They contended that there is a form of muscular rheumatism, commonly called "fibrositis", which is characterized by the formation of fibrous nodules, bands or indurated regions, which are acutely tender at first and are associated with muscular spasm, and that, if the condition becomes chronic, the tenderness and muscular spasm tend to disappear.

Furthermore English physicians have claimed repeatedly that such indurations can be broken up and made to disappear by means of a special type of heavy stroking and kneading which should be applied directly to the indurations. The heavy massage, if continued for a sufficiently long period, tends to relieve pain, tenderness and muscular spasm. Apparently fibrositis frequently is overlooked, and the value of heavy massage in treatment often has been unrecognized. The procedure is palliative rather than curative, and recurrences are frequent, so that often it will be necessary to employ other methods of treatment in conjunction with renewed applications of firm massage.

Diseases of the Muscles. — In muscular spasm of the occupational type, such as "writer's cramp", a small localized region of tenderness often is present. Friction and deep stroking frequently relieve such tenderness. Continued deep stroking and kneading may prove to be a valuable adjunct in treatment.

Brisk general massage in conjunction with stroking and kneading of the affected regions has been employed in treatment for pseudohypertrophic muscular dystrophy. The massage usually is administered in conjunction with the passive exercise of joints to prevent contractures. These procedures, of course, are merely palliative.

For muscular contusions gentle stroking and later kneading may be valuable in relieving pain and stiffness and in promoting absorption of exudate. The massage should not be begun until forty-eight hours after the injury was sustained.

Obesity. — It has been mentioned that massage is incapable of removing local deposits of adipose tissue, but general massage employed in conjunction with exercise and reduction of caloric intake may be of slight usefulness in the management of obesity. The massage sometimes can be employed as an adjunct in the early treatment of weak, obese individuals; later it can be replaced by carefully graduated mild exercises.

Circulatory Diseases. — When there is cardiac decompensation, skillful massage may aid in restoring compensation by improving the peripheral circulation. Curiously enough, although massage has an obvious field of usefulness in improving circulation, and although it frequently is employed for this purpose on the European continent, it rarely is put to this use by American physicians. Every clinician determines the presence of edema by making pressure with a finger to displace fluids. It is obvious that massage could perform the same function on a larger scale and free an extremity of some of the edema. This fact, however, seems "to have escaped large recognition in this country[8]".

Furthermore in cases of circulatory failure, when the patient must remain at absolute rest, massage can be employed as a substitute for the normal muscular contractions which usually assist circulation. Moderately deep stroking sometimes can be employed in conjunction with other therapeutic measures in treatment of peripheral vascular diseases.

Neurological Diseases. — Massage sometimes is employed to combat the fatigue, depression and irritability often associated with neurasthenia. Massage sometimes can be employed to advantage in the management of hysteria, but the technician must be familiar with psychotherapeutic methods and must employ massage only as it may be needed. For most neuroses massage should not be used indiscriminately. Coulter[5] has said that in most cases of traumatic neurosis "more symptoms have been rubbed in with massage than have been rubbed out".

Massage has been employed as a palliative measure in the management of such neurological conditions as Parkinson's syndrome, syringomyelia and Sydenham's chorea. Light sedative massage occasionally is used in treatment of peripheral neuritis. In certain forms of paralysis, such as "crutch paralysis" and "Bell's palsy", massage can be very useful in maintaining tone and nutrition of the muscles until volitional control returns.

Orthopedic Conditions. — Massage has been employed for sprains, strains, dislocations and fractures to promote circulation, relieve muscular spasm, overcome adhesions and restore function. It is valuable also in conjunction with exercise in the management of postural backache, sacroiliac or lumbosacral strain and coccygodynia. In the latter condition both external and internal massage are employed occasionally. In some instances coccygodynia seems to be due to spasm of the piriformis, coccygeus and levator ani muscles, and such spasm sometimes can be relieved by internal massage through the rectum.

Following amputation massage often is useful in the preparation of the stump to receive the prosthesis.

Obstetrical Conditions. — Massage frequently is valuable during and following the puerperium. Certain conditions which contribute to the discomforts of pregnancy can be benefited distinctly by correct application of massage. These include nervous headaches, cramps of the legs, backache resulting from muscular strain and mild edema of the legs resulting from simple venous obstruction. During labor massage of the uterus often is employed by the obstetrician. Following delivery massage of the fundus of the uterus is practiced in order to hasten involution. On the third day after delivery massage of the legs can be started.

Contraindications to the Application of Massage

Massage should not be employed in the presence of malignant growths, acute inflammatory processes, certain cutaneous affections such as eczema and acne, tuberculous lesions, acute systemic diseases which are accompanied by fever, acute phlebitis, thrombosis or lymphangitis. Other conditions, which contraindicate the employment of massage, are undrained osteomyelitis, gastric or duodenal ulcer, hernia, debilitating diseases, advanced arteriosclerosis, abscesses, aneurysm, advanced nephritis and acute communicable diseases. Heavy massage should not be applied to the abdomen during the later months of pregnancy.

Summary of Data on Massage

There is a distinct need for a better understanding on the part of physicians of the action and uses of massage. Its limitations also should be known. Massage can be employed satisfactorily only if each step in its application is directed properly by a physician, who is familiar with its effects, and who knows how to modify them to suit the indications. The numerous contraindications to the use of massage always should be kept in mind.

BIBLIOGRAPHY OF MASSAGE

1. MENNELL, J. B.: Massage; its Principles and Practice, Ed. 2, Blakiston, Philadelphia, 1920.
2. PEMBERTON, R., COULTER, J. S. and MOCK, H. E.: Massage, Jour. Am. Med. Assoc., 1930, XCIV, 1989.
3. PEMBERTON, R.: Physiology of massage, in Handbook of Physical Therapy, pp. 78–87, Ed. 3, American Medical Association Press, Chicago, 1939.
4. MENNELL, J. B.: Physical Treatment by Movement, Manipulation and Massage, Blakiston, Philadelphia, 1934.

5. COULTER, J. S.: Massage, in PIERSOL, G. M.: The Cyclopedia of Medicine, Vol. VIII, pp. 598–617, Davis, Philadelphia, 1933.
6. ROSENTHAL, C.: Quoted by Pemberton, R.[8].
7. BEST, C. H. and TAYLOR, N. B.: The Physiological Basis of Medical Practice; a University of Toronto Text in Applied Physiology, Ed. 2, Williams and Wilkins, Baltimore, 1939.
8. PEMBERTON, R.: Massage in internal medicine, in Handbook of Physical Therapy, Ed. 3, pp. 105–114, American Medical Association Press, Chicago, 1939.
9. STOCKMAN, R.: Rheumatism and Arthritis, Green and Son, Edinburgh, 1920.
10. COPEMAN, W. S. C.: The Treatment of Rheumatism in General Practice, Wood, Baltimore, 1933.
11. POYNTON, F. J. and SCHLESINGER, B.: Recent Advances in the Study of Rheumatism, Blakiston, Philadelphia, 1931.
12. THOMSON, F. G. and GORDON, R. G.: Chronic Rheumatic Diseases; their Diagnosis and Treatment, Oxford University Press, Edinburgh, 1926.
13. CYRIAX, E.: On fibrositis of the neck, Brit. Jour. Phys. Med., 1935, X, 49.

Sept. 1, 1941.

CORRECTIVE OR THERAPEUTIC EXERCISE

The methods of exercise employed in modern therapy have sprung from three systems of exercise; (1) the Swedish system introduced by Ling and Spiess, (2) the Turnverein system founded in Germany by Jahn and (3) the Delsarte system developed by the French.

The modern American technician, as a rule, does not follow any one of these systems but has adopted that which is best from all of them and has introduced much in addition. The Swedish system for some reason has caught the popular fancy in this country, and many physicians as well as laymen have the erroneous fancy that anyone who is a native of Sweden is endowed with great skill in massage and gymnastics. As a matter of fact the American physician, who is familiar with modern corrective exercise, immediately becomes suspicious of the individual who claims to be an expert in Swedish exercises, because he knows that the modern American technician should be familiar with the best methods of exercise derived from all the ancient systems and should not confine himself to one system only.

Today the old systems and the Zander equipment no longer are employed in the hospitals. Corrective or therapeutic exercises now are administered, usually as free exercises without the aid of apparatus, by skilled technicians who are well trained in anatomy and kinesiology. Working under direct medical supervision, such technicians are capable of providing an infinite variety of corrective exercises which can be modified from day to day to fit the needs of the individual patient.

The scope of therapeutic exercise is much broader than most physicians realize. It is apparent that every physician should be familiar with the various forms of corrective exercise, and that the supervision of the therapeutic exercises should be entirely in his hands. As is the case with regard to massage, or for that matter, any form of treatment, the responsibility should not be delegated to a layman.

Corrective or therapeutic exercise can be defined as "the scientific application of bodily movement designed specifically to maintain or to restore normal function to diseased or injured tissues". Exercise can be employed to rehabilitate patients suffering from a wide variety of diseases.

Methods of Applying Therapeutic Exercise

Exercises can be performed either actively or passively. In passive exercise the motion of a segment of the body is imparted by some outside force. The outside force usually is derived from the hands of the technician but can be obtained also from voluntary effort of another segment of the patient's own body or from a machine. Active exercise is accomplished by volitional movement by the patient of the involved segment or segments of the body.

Therapeutic exercise is classified best under four headings; (1) passive exercise or relaxed movement, (2) active assistive exercise, in which the patient makes a voluntary movement and is assisted in making it by the technician or by some other force, (3) active or free exercise and (4) active resistive exercise, in which the patient makes a voluntary effort to move the part and is resisted in such movement by the technician, by some other outside force or by his own physiologically antagonistic muscles.

Passive exercise may vary from the gentlest of slow rhythmic movements, such as are employed in the early stages of post-fracture mobilization, to the extremely forceful movements, sometimes used to overcome fibrous ankylosis of joints, which are so rigorous that they must be administered only when the patient is anesthetized. Practically all forms of manipulative surgical procedures can be classified under the heading of passive exercise. Between the two extremes of passive exercise lie various gradations of passive movement which must be understood thoroughly by the technician.

Although *active exercises* usually result in movement of joints, there is one form which frequently is employed for therapeutic purposes, in which movement of the joints does not occur. This form of active exercise is called *static exercise* or *muscle setting.* In muscle setting the patient simply contracts and relaxes a muscle or a group of muscles without moving a joint. The procedure has been likened to a "muscle dance" and has the advantage of maintaining circulation and muscular tone and of preventing atrophy without disturbing the position of bones and joints. It often is employed to exercise the muscles of an extremity during a period of enforced immobilization.

Correct use of *resistive exercise* often is the only way to make one group of muscles work alone and to exclude its antagonists.

Physical Principles Concerned in the Application of Therapeutic Exercise

As with any mechanical device in the mechanical acts of the human body movement is obtained by the action of a force on a lever. Each of the 434 skeletal muscles is a simple independent force capable of producing motion. These muscles act on the three orders of levers commonly encountered in the skeletal mechanism.

With a lever of the first order the joint, which serves as the fulcrum, lies between the weight and the insertion of the muscle which serves as the power. With a lever of the second order the weight lies between the point of application of power and the joint. With a lever of the third order, the type most commonly found in the human body, the power is applied at a point between the weight and the fulcrum.

The great importance of the normal functioning of these mechanisms in preserving health is stressed by Mackenzie[1], who thought that in most instances health depended on "a correlation of all the bodily systems to the erect posture", and ill health depended on "a failure of one or more systems to correlate to it".

No matter which order of lever is encountered in the human body, practically all of them are arranged so that the distance between the fulcrum and the point of application of power is short. For this reason even a slight pathological, muscular contracture may cause a relatively marked angulation of a joint. Also with this type of lever a muscle must be strong in order to mobilize the joint.

Action and Uses of Therapeutic Exercise

Whereas an ordinary locomotive may be only 4 per cent. efficient, the human body is much more efficient; it varies in efficiency from about 20 to 40 per cent.[2]. When a muscle is subjected to stress, it will respond by increase in tension. This is known as the "stretch reflex". A muscle, which is held in a shortened position, tends to become tonically shortened; one, which is kept in an elongated position, tends to become permanently stretched.

Passive movements at first produce little change in the rate of the pulse, but as the part becomes fatigued, there may be a slow rise in the rate of the pulse. On voluntary contraction of muscles the rate of the pulse increases more rapidly. The extent of the increase in cardiac rate depends to a great extent on the physical condition of the subject. Although the pulse rate of an untrained individual may increase 25 to 40 beats per minute from moderate volitional exercise, this can be considered a normal response to moderate exercise. The trained athlete's cardiac rate will increase very little, because his heart responds to increased effort by increase in the stroke volume of the heart rather than by increase in the rate of contraction. It has not been proved, however, that this increase in the stroke volume is any easier on the heart itself than is an increase in rate.

The cardiac rate of the normal individual should return to normal levels within a half hour following moderate exercise. If the exercise has been exhausting, the rate of the pulse may remain accelerated for several hours. Because of these facts it becomes obvious that measurements of the rate of the pulse and the length of time that the pulse remains accelerated are good indexes of the amount of exercise which a patient can tolerate.

Best and Taylor[3] have estimated that the flow of blood through active muscles may be twenty or more times as great as the flow during rest. During exercise a much greater portion of the capillary bed is supplied with blood. Both arterial and venous blood pressures are increased during exercise. The part, which active exercise takes in assisting circulation, is appreciated insufficiently by many physicians, and the deleterious effects of prolonged rest often are overlooked.

Exercise tends to increase general metabolic activity. Even very slight exercises, such as writing, may increase the metabolic rate 25 to 50 per cent. above the basal level. Vigorous exercise may increase the metabolic rate to ten to twenty times the basal level.

It is impossible within the limits of this chapter to describe in detail the exercises which should be employed for various diseases. Therefore, when possible, I shall refer the reader, who wishes detailed exercises, to suitable sources of information.

Corrective exercises may be extremely useful in the management of postural deformities. The physician, who is interested in this subject, should refer to the report of the Subcommittee on Orthopedics and Body Mechanics of the White House Conference on Child Health and Protection[4] and to the textbooks by Goldthwait and his associates[5] and by Phelps and Kiphuth[6] which deal fully with this important problem. Elsewhere[7] I have described the exercises employed at the Mayo Clinic for treatment of weakness and pronation of the feet as well as exercises for postural backache, lumbar lordosis and scoliosis. Kleinberg[8] has written an excellent monograph on scoliosis.

One of the most interesting recent developments in the field of therapeutic exercise concerns its employment for the control of some of the symptoms of bronchial asthma. The Asthma Research Council of King's College, London[9], has published an excellent small booklet, which is well illustrated and inexpensive, and which can be employed by the patient as an instruction manual while learning the exercises. Livingstone and Gillespie[10] and Bray[11] have reported favorably concerning the efficacy of these exercises in relieving some of the distress of the asthmatic attacks and even in aborting the attacks. These exercises for asthma are directed especially toward teaching the patient to make a prolonged voluntary expiratory effort and to develop ability in abdominal breathing.

Exercises play an extremely important part in the management of the residual effects of poliomyelitis. The physician desiring detailed information concerning such exercises should consult the excellent small and inexpensive booklets on this subject by the Kendalls[12] and by Greteman and Jackson[13] as well as the free booklet by Stevenson[14]. Other valuable communications on this subject include those of Hansson[15], Legg and Merrill[16] and Lovett[17].

Another group of patients, who have been neglected much, and who receive great benefit from prolonged training in corrective exercise, is the throng of children suffering from cerebral palsy. Because of the limited facilities which are available for proper training of these unfortunate youngsters, and it has been estimated that there are 108 treatable cases of cerebral palsy for each 200,000 population, it often becomes necessary for a parent to carry on the training of the child at home. I have found that Girard's excellent monograph[18] is a valuable guide for such parents. Other books to which these parents can refer include the ones by Fischel[19], Rogers and Thomas[20] and Abele and Greteman[21]. In addition every patient with cerebral palsy can get a great deal of inspiration by reading the semibiographical book by Earl R. Carlson[22], himself a sufferer from cerebral palsy, who has devoted his career as a physician to the treatment of "the severely birth-injured".

Coulter[23] has described a set of modified Frenkel co-ordination exercises which can be employed to advantage in the treatment of combined sclerosis and tabes dorsalis. He has given also an excellent description of the proper methods of employing exercise in cardiac diseases and in the management of hemiplegia. Sever[24] has presented detailed information concerning the employment of corrective exercises for obstetrical paralysis. Elsewhere I[7] have given a description of exercises of individual joints following trauma.

Occupational therapy is a form of therapeutic exercise and anyone interested in this extensive field of therapy should refer to the writings of Davis and Dunton[25], Dunton[26], Mock[27] and Mock and Abbey[28].

To summarize concerning the uses of therapeutic exercise, one may say that general postural exercises are required in the management of such conditions as scoliosis, kyphosis and lordosis. Postural exercises may benefit or may prevent orthostatic albuminuria, postural backache, chronic postural strain, exhaustion states or functional decompensation of the muscles of the back. Foot postural exercises may be useful in treatment of pronation of the feet or in treatment of breaking down of the longitudinal or transverse arches of the feet. Exercises may be valuable in overcoming muscular, tendinous or fascial contractures.

Among the medical conditions, which often can be benefited by exercises of certain types, can be mentioned asthma, arthritis, cardiac disease, cerebral palsy, combined sclerosis, hemiplegia, poliomyelitis and tabes dorsalis. Among the surgical lesions, which can be helped by various types of exercise, can be mentioned contusions, sprains, strains, dislocations, fractures, amputations, peripheral nerve lesions and obstetrical paralysis. Exercises of the legs may prevent postoperative thrombosis, and abdominal exercises can be employed to strengthen the muscles following pregnancy or prior to herniorrhaphy.

Contraindications to the Employment of Therapeutic Exercise

There are few contraindications to the use of exercise because activity is a normal state. In some instances, however, exercises are overdone or are performed incorrectly. Following injury to certain joints, particularly the elbow, if exercise is started too early, or if passive movement is applied too vigorously, further trauma and eventually ankylosis may result.

Patients, who have neurocirculatory asthenia, or "effort syndrome", tolerate exercise poorly. In the presence of cardiac disease exercise, although not usually contraindicated, should be employed only with great caution and after proper testing of the tolerance of the patient to exercise.

If employed injudiciously, exercise may precipitate hemorrhage, loosen emboli or cause similar disastrous results.

Summary of Data on Therapeutic Exercise

Corrective or therapeutic exercise now is applied or directed usually by skilled technicians working under direct medical supervision. Exercise, if at all strenuous, should be prescribed only after a careful examination of the cardiovascular system. Such exercise is useful in many diseases and is an indispensable part of modern therapy.

BIBLIOGRAPHY OF THERAPEUTIC EXERCISE

1. MACKENZIE, C.: The Action of Muscles Including Muscle Rest and Muscle Re-education, Ed. 2, Hoeber, New York, 1930.
2. SCHNEIDER, E. C.: Physiology of Muscular Activity, Saunders, Philadelphia, 1933.
3. BEST, C. H. and TAYLOR, N. B.: The Physiological Basis of Medical Prac-

tice; a University of Toronto Text in Applied Physiology, Ed. 2, Williams and Wilkins, Baltimore, 1939.

4. REPORT OF SUBCOMMITTEE ON ORTHOPEDICS AND BODY MECHANICS: Body Mechanics; Education and Practice, White House Conference on Child Health and Protection, The Century Company, New York, 1932.
5. GOLDTHWAIT, J. E., BROWN, L. T., SWAIM, L. T. and KUHNS, J. G.: Body Mechanics in the Study and Treatment of Disease, Lippincott, Philadelphia, 1934.
6. PHELPS, W. M. and KIPHUTH, R. J. H.: The Diagnosis and Treatment of Postural Defects, Charles C. Thomas, Springfield, Illinois, 1932.
7. KRUSEN, F. H.: Physical Medicine, Saunders, Philadelphia, 1941.
8. KLEINBERG, S.: Scoliosis; Rotary Lateral Curvature of the Spine, Hoeber, New York, 1926.
9. ASTHMA RESEARCH COUNCIL, KING'S COLLEGE, LONDON: Physical Exercises for Asthma, Ed. 3, Chicago Medical Book Company, Chicago, 1939.
10. LIVINGSTONE, J. L. and GILLESPIE, M.: The value of breathing exercises in asthma, Lancet, 1935, II, 705.
11. BRAY, G. W.: Recent Advances in Allergy (Asthma, Hay-fever, Eczema, Migraine, etc.), Ed. 2, Blakiston, Philadelphia, 1934.
12. KENDALL, H. O and KENDALL, F. P.: Care during the recovery period in paralytic poliomyelitis, Public Health Bulletin 242, United States Treasury Department, Public Health Service, 1938.
13. GRETEMAN, T. J. and JACKSON, R. B.: Care of Infantile Paralysis in the Home; a Handbook for Parents, John S. Swift Co., Inc., St. Louis, 1938.
14. STEVENSON, J. L.: The Nursing Care of Patients with Infantile Paralysis, The National Foundation for Infantile Paralysis, New York, 1940.
15. HANSSON, K. G.: After-treatment of poliomyelitis, Jour. Am. Med. Assoc., 1939, CXIII, 32.
16. LEGG, A. T. and MERRILL, J. B.: Physical therapy in infantile paralysis, Reprinted from Principles and Practice of Physical Therapy, Prior, Hagerstown, Maryland, 1932.
17. LOVETT, R. W.: The Treatment of Infantile Paralysis, Ed. 2, Blakiston, Philadelphia, 1917.
18. GIRARD, P. M.: The Home Treatment of Spastic Paralysis Written in a Simple, Practical Way with Many Detailed Drawings, Lippincott, Philadelphia, 1937.
19. FISCHEL, M. K.: The Spastic Child; a Record of Successfully Achieved Muscle Control in Little's Disease, Mosby, St. Louis, 1934.
20. ROGERS, G. G. and THOMAS, L. C.: New Pathways for Children with Cerebral Palsy, Macmillan, New York, 1935.
21. ABELE, J. F. and GRETEMAN, T. J.: Care of the Spastic Paralytic Child in the Home; a Handbook for Parents, Children's Hospital, Iowa City, Iowa, 1938.

22. CARLSON, E. R.: Born That Way, John Day Company, New York, 1941.
23. COULTER, J. S.: The use of therapeutic exercise in internal medicine and in neurology, in Principles and Practice of Physical Therapy, Vol. III, pp. 1–68, Prior, Hagerstown, Maryland, 1934.
24. SEVER, J. W.: The physical therapy of obstetrical paralysis, in Principles and Practice of Physical Therapy, Vol. II, pp. 1–26, Prior, Hagerstown, Maryland, 1934.
25. DAVIS, J. E. and DUNTON, W. R., JR.: Principles and Practice of Recreational Therapy for the Mentally Ill, A. S. Barnes and Company, New York, 1936.
26. DUNTON, W. R., JR.: Occupational therapy, in Principles and Practice of Physical Therapy, Vol. I, pp. 1–48, Prior, Hagerstown, Maryland, 1934.
27. MOCK, H. E.: Reconstructive surgery and functional recreation, in Principles and Practice of Physical Therapy, Vol. II, pp. 1–12, Prior, Hagerstown, Maryland, 1934.
28. MOCK H. E. and ABBEY, M. L.: Occupational therapy, in Handbook of Physical Therapy, Ed. 3, pp. 165–178, American Medical Association Press, Chicago, 1939.

Sept. 1, 1941.

CHAPTER XXII

THE PHARMACOLOGICAL BASIS OF MEDICINE

By L. G. ROWNTREE

Table of Contents

Introduction

To the thinking physician treatment does not consist merely in applying measures of relief. The essence of treatment consists: in recognizing the pathological process; in understanding its nature, its cause, the mechanism involved in its production and in the development of its clinical manifestations; in knowing the character, extent, and probable outcome of the resulting functional and morphological changes; in valuing correctly the significance of clinical and laboratory findings; in ascertaining the indication for, in knowing the mode of action of, and the most effective methods of applying measures for its prevention, abortion, amelioration, or cure.

A correct diagnosis is the first essential to treatment. Direct and specific therapy begins with diagnosis, failing which, general or palliative measures only are possible. It is to be recognized that, with or without diagnosis, cures result at times, the work of nature, not of medicine.

Doctrines control therapy. Treatment is good or bad according to whether doctrines are true or false. These are subject to evolution. Verified and established they constitute the science of medicine. Their relation to treatment is twofold. They concern the nature and mechanism of pathological processes on the one hand, and on the other, the mode of action of measures of relief.

In treatment there are two fundamentally different points of view of disease; viz., the morphological and the functional. Both are important. The former as pathology has dominated the field of medicine. The latter, pathological physiology, is more difficult to acquire, but is essential to therapy, since, generally speaking, drugs affect function rather than form. Not until the physician sees a deranged function as well as a lesion will he become a master of treatment. Recognition of derangement of function presupposes a knowledge of normal function. Physiology, therefore, becomes the basis or starting-point of therapy, the diagnosis incorporating a physio-pathological conception of disease.

Pharmacology deals with the action of drugs. Though it be youthful, it is already a vigorous science. It brings with it to the bedside the tools of science; investigation, experimentation, standards, exactness in measurement, observation, and analysis. It necessitates and hence develops critical judgment. It reveals facts concerning changes in bodily function wrought by the action of drugs, the mechanism whereby these changes are effected, and not infrequently uncovers physiological processes previously unrecognized. It yields quantitative results. One of the great weaknesses of drug therapy today is the lack of quantitative determination of results. Many drugs are threshold bodies, that is, they must reach certain levels in the body before they exercise beneficial effects. On the other hand, the majority of them, in the event of overdosage, lead to untoward effects resulting in the nullifying of therapeutic action, to exacerbations of the original symptoms, or in the appearance of other untoward clinical manifestations.

In practice the end may be attained by various measures acting in different ways. In order to obtain maximum results familiarity with the mode of action of the remedy is essential, and a treatment must be employed which combats the pathological process as near its source as possible, preferably by one which eradicates the cause.

Health is the normal balance in physiological functions. In the organism factors of safety are large. Nature has provided many defenses against disease and is ingenious in meeting difficulties and dangers. Vicarious activity and sharing of function is resorted to repeatedly. Successively or simultaneously several lines of defense may be called into play and must be overcome before a vital function is actually endangered. Where the cause is beyond attack, treatment may so affect this balance that, despite an irremovable cause and an all but exhausted reserve, function is maintained and life goes on without disabling symptoms and perhaps without serious restrictions.

The requisites of treatment are: (1) correct diagnosis; (2) a true conception of the cause and nature of the derangement; (3) familiarity with the manner in which the derangement can be corrected; and (4) knowledge concerning the means whereby this may be effected.

These appear simple matters, withal, but they are the revelations of succeeding ages—the handiwork of evolving science. Now, as in the days of Hippocrates, "Experience is fallacious and judgment difficult."

Oliver Wendell Holmes says, "The débris of broken systems and exploded dogmas form a great mound, a Monte Testaccio of the shards and remnants of old vessels which once held human beliefs. If you take the trouble to climb on top of it, you will widen your horizon, and in these days of special knowledge your horizon is not likely to be any too wide." We can, with profit, consider the evolution of medical doctrines underlying the treatment of the past, study the methods and beliefs of our forefathers, observe their mistakes and successes, and the causes of each, and compare in these respects the medicine of the past with that of to-day.

The Historical Evolution of Medical Doctrines

Primitive man found himself confronted with functional disabilities. He suffered, not from disease, but from symptoms; headache, jaundice, chills, blindness, or weakness. The cause, nature, or the significance of the symptoms, the underlying disease, the nature of the derangement, prognosis, and the treatment were all unknown. Doctors, textbooks, and medicine were not in existence. Biology, anatomy, physics, chemistry, physiology, pathology, pharmacology, and therapeutics were still undreamed of. Education, mental training, observation, logic and experimentation, drugs and instruments were all lacking. When sick he had recourse merely to his fellowmen, to the animal world about him, and to himself. He could observe, listen, imitate, speculate, imagine, and obey. He already believed in a supernatural being who was responsible for all he could not understand. Surrounded by ignorance and superstition, he was the recipient of kind-hearted, well-meaning advice or treatment, born of actual experience in some instances, more often of pretense of knowledge assumed for gain or prestige. He desired relief from sufferings and restitution to health. He followed his instincts or natural inclinations, usually adopting the expectant principle of treatment, lying at rest awaiting recovery. This failing, he consulted with his fellowman and adopted his advice or appealed to the supreme being for relief. In the event of recovery, he sang the praises of the treatment and its author or lifted his voice in thanks to the Almighty.

The savage's conception of disease is essentially spiritualistic. Supernatural agencies are of various kinds: (1) independent devil-born demons of disease; (2) departed spirits, ghosts, or spirits of the dead; (3) spirits of slain animals; (4) human enemies who act through their own supernatural powers by casting spells or indirectly through one or other of the types of spirits already mentioned; and (5) spirits acting through the direction of the Almighty to aid in the administration of punishment or the wreaking of vengeance on man for his manifold shortcomings and sins. The latter group is the most important, since in them belief still exists to some extent even among civilized nations, and they were responsible to a large extent for the sacerdotal trend of early medicine.

According to Withington ([1]) three methods of procedure have been found effective by the savage medicine man in combating supernatural agencies of disease: (1) rendering the body an unpleasant abode for the intruding spirit through squeezing, beating, starving, or fumigating it, or through the use of nauseating drugs which result in vomiting; (2) offering the spirit a more pleasant abode, for instance, the demon of jaundice can be enticed into a yellow canary, and that of ague into a cold, clammy frog; (3) the intervention of other spiritual forces.* The first, or what may be considered as expulsion by violence, is represented by emetics and massage; the second, or wily seduction, finds expression in the "signatures" of the middle ages and perhaps in the "similia similibus curantur" of our day; and the third, or the intervention of other spiritual forces, is largely responsible for the rôle played by the priesthood in the history of medicine.

Our knowledge of the medicine of uncivilized or early civilized man is derived largely through ancient writings or their translations, through folklore, through the tracing back of peculiar customs, and through investigations of recent date of peoples still uncivilized (Madagascar, Tahiti, Indians of North and South America).

* This idea also resulted in the belief in witchcraft, wherein the same power was used for purposes other than good.

Egyptian Medicine

This is revealed through the study of tombs, pyramids, and ancient writings. From the tombs we learn of Sekhet'-enanch, the first physician known to history, who lived about 3000 or possibly 3500 B.C., and of the existence in his day of the lancet and of a cupping instrument. But our chief knowledge of Egyptian medicine is derived through the Ebers Papyrus, which was written about 1550 B.C. This is mainly a collection of receipts, and from it we learn something of the therapy of early Egypt, thus " Sçhepen " (probably the poppy) is useful to soothe crying babies. "Against all kinds of witchcraft, a large beetle, cut off his head and wings, boil him, put him in oil and apply to the part. Then cook his head and wings, put them in serpent's fat, warm it, let the patient drink it." "To make the skin of the face smooth, soak meal in spring water. Let her wash her face daily and then apply the meal." "To keep away mice, smear everything possible with cat's fur." Pills, potions, inunctions, inhalations, and plasters were all used in these days.

It also contains some remarkable passages relating to diagnosis. One reference to the circulatory system is particularly interesting: "The vessels are said to run in pairs . . . and to contain not only blood, but air, water, milk, and other fluids." In the doctrine of the heart as the center of the vascular system, and in the importance attributed to the pulse, the Egyptians were in advance of Hippocrates. "If the physician place his fingers on the head, neck, hands, arms, feet, or body, everywhere he will find the heart (i.e. the pulse), for the vessels go to all parts." *

The Berlin Papyrus, which is of somewhat later date, contains many prescriptions and abounds in incantations. More than the Ebers Papyrus it emphasizes the supernatural origin of disease.

Egyptian medicine, just as Egypt itself, marked time for nearly 3,000 years. In fact, judging from the relative popularity and success of Egyptian and Greek physicians at the time of Hippocrates, and also later, the Egyptian physicians appeared to be hopelessly outclassed.

Hindu Medicine

Our knowledge of Hindu medicine is revealed through the Vedas or "Works of Wisdom." The 4th or Atharva Veda, written about 700 B.C., and later supplementary Vedas, are the most important from the standpoint of medicine. From them we learn of the medical work of

* From Withington's (1) "Medical History from the Earliest Times." To Withington the author is indebted for most of the historical sketch here presented. Garrison (1) and Baass (1) have also been freely consulted.

Charaka and Susruta, which indicate that the Hindu medicine of 300 B.C. to 750 A.D. (the period of Buddhist predominance) compares favorably with the contemporary Hellenic medicine. The Hindu medicine contributed much to surgery, and to organized medical effort such as medical teaching, army sanitation, hospitals, and asylums for the blind and lame.

Surgery was favored rather than medicine, thus by Susruta new noses were created from cheek and forehead flaps, supraorbital nerves were sectioned in neuralgia, even laparotomies were suggested. In writing of his calling, he says, " Surgery is the first and highest division of the healing art, least liable to fallacy, pure in itself, perpetual in its application, the worthy product of heaven, the source of fame on earth."

Early Greek Medicine

Hippocrates was the founder of Greek medicine and of medicine in general. However, prior to his time medicine had made considerable progress. Homer's account of medicine relates mostly to surgery, but he introduces us to drugs " pharmakon," which in the " Iliad " refers to remedies externally applied and in the " Odyssey " to either poisons or charms. He also intimates that knowledge of drugs constitutes a criterion for judging the ability of a physician. In his time medicine and surgery were definitely distinguished, the distinction having been made primarily by Æsculapius; for Machaon, one son, was endowed with skilled hands to draw out darts and make incisions, while to Podalirius, the other, was given all cunning to find out things invisible and to " cure that which healed not." In Homer's day " incubation " flourished before the altars of the Asclepieia or temples of Æsculapius. The patient, after priestly preparation, lay down to sleep before the altar, whereupon was revealed to him by dreams or through the priests those things necessary for recovery. In this way many miracles were wrought.

Empedocles, B.C. 490-430, is also worthy of mention because he laid the foundation for the humeral pathology of Hippocrates, and introduced the four elements into medical philosophy. Withington (1) presents a fragment of one of his poems " On Nature."

> "Listen first, while I sing the fourfold root of creation,
> Fire, and water, and earth, and the boundless height of the ether,
> For thereupon is begotten what is, what was, and what shall be."

Hippocrates adopted this idea of " fire, water, earth, and air," but enlarged upon it. He considered heat, cold, dryness, and moisture as four corresponding qualities, and blood, phlegm, yellow bile, and black bile as the four corresponding bodily juices or humors. Each humor had its own seat: thus for the blood, the heart; for phlegm, the brain; for yellow bile, the liver; and for black bile, the spleen. Health was unimpaired so long as each humor remained in its own place and in its proper proportion relatively, but disease resulted from disproportionate amounts and from an element out of its proper sphere. In this conception quantities and interdependence of function are obviously recognized. In other words, Hippocrates conceived organization in the body, but his false doctrines of pathology precluded the possibility of a scientific foundation for medicine.

Early Greek medicine was not entirely sacerdotal. Priests, philosophers, and physical trainers practiced medicine as well as physicians proper. But whereas the physicians practiced the healing art, the priest corresponded to the mental or faith healers, philosophers to medical scientists or physiologists, and the physical trainers to bone-setters of later centuries. The physicians and the philosophers, however, were responsible for medical progress.

Hippocrates, the father of medicine, born 460 B.C., flourished in the golden age of Pericles, a contemporary of the most brilliant group of men known to history. He was a practicing physician and a philosopher. By virtue of his dual interest, he clearly separated the two. His greatest contribution to medicine was his rejection of the supernatural. In this he was influenced to some extent by his environment, for at that time the Greeks were in a transition period, falling away generally from their belief in mythology. That his rejection of the supernatural resulted in his other contributions to medicine is within the realm of possibility, for what is more natural than that one, needing support in his anomalous position as champion of natural causes for disease, should undertake to prove the cause, nature, and course of disease?

In his study of disease he emphasized the necessity of accurate observation, describing the facies and the splash bearing his name. He made clear, concise, clinical records, more than forty of which are preserved, and from which it is possible in some instances to make diagnoses. Diseases were considered in their entirety, the course and final outcome being noted. He recorded his deaths, which were relatively numerous. He was the first to properly value prognosis, stating that though cure was the most important consideration, it was well for the physician to be able to predict the outcome of any illness. His methods were those of science, accurate observation, careful records, interest sustained to a conclusion, in an attempt to predict the outcome from the facts available.

Of his treatment little is known except that, recognizing the limitation of diagnosis and of therapy, he insisted on considering the individual rather than the disease and above all things on doing no harm. Treatment to him consisted of assisting nature, for his belief was strong in the "vis medicatrix naturae," environment, diet, bowels, sleep and all the natural functions receiving appropriate attention. Purgatives and bleeding he used most frequently. Treatment was individualistic, the patient's comfort, feelings, and wishes being consulted and considered as far as possible.

His aphorisms alone would have sufficed to bring his name down through the ages, revealing his philosophical outlook on life and his great store of wisdom. Hippocrates not only stands as the father of medicine, but as the greatest medical character of all times. In founding a school of medicine, he took the final step which made his influence permanent. The School of Cos embodied his teachings and ideals. Through it, his medicine and his inspiration were handed on, not only to his pupils, but to succeeding generations. Such was his influence that his teachings held sway almost unchallenged for two thousand years, while some of his principles guide us even today.

Greek Medicine Subsequent to Hippocrates

The School of Cos became the center of Hippocratic medicine as the School of Cnidus under Euryphon insisted more on accuracy of diagnosis and on vigorous treatment; but lacking instruments of precision and correct fundamental conceptions of disease, vigorous treatment was applied frequently to the patient's serious detriment and ofttimes with disastrous results.

The interest taken in medicine just subsequent to Hippocrates was little short of remarkable. The up-to-date monarch of the day delighted in medical discussion and in medical problems. Mithridates at Pontus became the most famous of toxicologists. Attalus of Pergamus planted a famous poison garden, while the Greek kings of Egypt exhibited unusual interest in all things medical. About 300 B.C. Ptolemy the First established a museum in Alexandria, and that city from that time on became the center of medicine and of learning generally, a fact well attested by the fame of its library. Three great schools of medicine arose subsequent to Hippocrates.

(1) *The Dogmatic School.*—It advocated rational medicine, the cause being the important factor to determine and remove. Galen credits Hippocrates with founding this school; others, Thessalus and Draco, supposedly sons of Hippocrates. Praxagorus of Cos, Diocles, the Alexandrine anatomist Herophilus, and Erasistratus were its leading spirits. They recognized the necessity of basing medicine on physiology. Herophilus (student of Praxagorus) and Erasistratus were the actual founders of anatomy, physiology still remaining in the embryonic stage. Authority in physiology rested in (a) "On the Nature of Man," a treatise written supposedly by Polybius, son-in-law of Hippocrates, and

(b) on "Timaeus," from the hand of Plato. Unfortunately Plato was unsound as a physiologist, and medicine built on his physiology lacked firm foundation and in consequence suffered greatly.

For a thousand years the School of Alexandria flourished. In it were made numerous dissections and many important anatomical discoveries. It is credited with many vivisections on criminals and captives. In anatomy, Herophilus and Erasistratus worked side by side, having a community of interests in anatomy but differing widely on the question of treatment. The former followed Hippocrates, the latter, while operating fearlessly, rejected bleeding as too depleting and adopted extremely small dosage in drug therapy. On the question of treatment, they continued irreconcilable, each founding his own school of therapy.

The shortcomings of the dogmatists, while numerous, can be readily overlooked in the light of their high ideals. They contributed largely to the science of medicine, creating anatomy and establishing as a principle medicine based on physiology. Their weakness lay in their excess of theory.

(2) *The Empiric School* arose in Alexandria, splitting off from the dogmatists about 280 B.C. as the result largely of the extravagant theorizing of the latter. The founders were pupils of Herophilus, Philinus and Serapion by name. They despised anatomy, physiology, and pathology, were uninterested in the cause of disease, claiming that "the cure and not the cause" was the vital question. They accordingly adopted symptomatic treatment, and with it, a correspondingly narrow point of view. They sought specifics and increased markedly the number of remedies without improving treatment.

One great man they produced, namely, Heraclides of Tarentum, born B.C. 230, the greatest therapeutist of ancient times. He might qualify to-day as a pharmacologist. Though an empiricist, he did much to combat the evils of that system. He investigated the clinical effect of drugs, utilizing only those he had personally studied, and he did much to place therapy on a scientific basis. His greatest work was entitled, "On the Preparation and Proving of Drugs," in which he points out the virtues of opium, which he finds useful in sleeplessness, spasm and colic, cough, cholera, and serpent's bites, and locally in the form of poultices in painful ophthalmia. He advocated water for fever and treated brain fever on logical grounds. His principles, had they been followed, would have relegated empiricism to the background and resulted in rational treatment based on experimental therapy.

Aristotle, the greatest of Greek philosophers, was a great exponent of empiricism. As the originator of logic, he was naturally forced to forsake the dogmatists with their innumerable, untenable theories. In fact, so far as medicine is concerned, he devoted himself almost entirely to criticisms of the theories of the dogmatists. Constructively he labored with anatomy, in which field he rivaled even the founders of the Alexandrine School.

The famous tripod, the basis of the empirical system of therapeutics, supposedly made possible the discovery or creation of specifics for symptoms or syndromes. It consisted of (1) observation and experiments (autopsies), (2) contemporary and earlier experience (history), and (3) conclusions based on similar conditions (analogy). At a later date was added "epilogism," whereby past events could be inferred from present conditions.

(3) The third school, *Methodic School,* arose under Roman influence and is described under that heading, which follows immediately.

Roman Medicine

The march of time shifts the scene from Greece and Alexandria to Rome, but Roman medicine, as all medicine until the time of Harvey, was Hellenic, in reality, reflected Greek medicine.

Asclepiades was the first great physician of Rome, incidentally the most successful practitioner of ancient times and the prototype of the fashionable physician. He introduced into medicine a theory important because it subsequently became the foundation of methodism, and at a still later date reappeared in the form of Bruónianism. According to him the body consists of various-sized atoms with intervening channels and pores through which the smaller atoms circulate. Disease consists of relative changes in the size of the pores and particularly in the blocking of pores. He also believed that alterations in the solids of the body could cause disease as well as humeral changes, drew a clear distinction between acute and chronic diseases, and was a great advocate of air as a therapeutic agent.

The Methodic School.—This, the last of the great schools of antiquity, found its origin in the principles enunciated by Asclepiades. Themison, despising the dogmatists in their search for specifics for the cure of symptoms, founded a simpler system of medicine based on the fact that diseases have symptoms in common. Symptoms are the result of the relaxation or contraction of pores, for Themison worked on the principle *contraria contrarius;* and drugs were found, laxatives and astringents, to relax the contracted and constrict the relaxed. These doctrines were brought to their greatest stage of perfection by Thessalus, who introduced alterative treatment and laid great stress on the subject of diet.

The medicine of Rome was the medicine of Galen. It is true that

Celsus, the "Cicero Medicorum," wrote "De Re Medicina," which outlined perhaps better than any other publication the medicine of his time. But Celsus was not merely a doctor. He wrote equally well on many subjects. He tells us that in his day medicine was divided into three fields, "dietetics, pharmaceutics, and chirurgics."

Galen, 131-200, was also a founder of a system—one that combined much of the best of dogmatism and empiricism, and also of methodism, although to the latter he was utterly opposed. Physiologist and anatomist, as well as practicing physician, he wrote prolifically on many subjects. Through him comes to posterity much of our knowledge of Greek medicine.

Public opinion in Rome being adverse to anything quite so brutal as the dissection of the human body, as an anatomist he dissected various animals, thereby laying the foundation for comparative anatomy. He recognized the three coats of arteries, and demonstrated that the vessels did not contain only air. His physiology, like that of the dogmatists, was marred by much theory. Long before the discovery of oxygen he pondered over the question of body heat, declaring that, when that part of air which supports combustion was identified, we would have the secret of life and of body temperature. To him belongs the credit of distinguishing motor, sensory, and mixed nerves, for he recognized their true rôle in the organism.

Galen's medicine rested on anatomy and physiology. "Disease," he says, "is an abnormal affection of the body, giving rise to a lesion of function, and may affect an individual organ, a system, or the body as a whole." He recognized three kinds of causes, exciting, predisposing, and proximate. Symptoms are of three varieties: (1) altered function; (2) vitiated qualities; and (3) results of these two, morbid excretion and retention. He differentiated signs and symptoms. Signs to him might be either diagnostic or prognostic in character.

In his therapy he accepted experience with the empiricists, but recognized the cause as the first indication in treatment, thus upholding the dogmatists in rational therapy. But symptoms also served as indications and could be met sometimes by similars and at others by contraries. In addition, other considerations were important in indications, namely, temperament, season, and environment.

In the history of medicine, Galen alone has vied seriously with Hippocrates. To be sure, he had the advantage of 500 years of progress. For a thousand years his principles and practice, though somewhat modified by mysticism and magic, held sway through the middle ages. For leadership he competed with Hippocrates, but untinctured Greek medicine on being ushered into western civilization proved its superiority with the result that Hippocrates was adjudged the true father of medicine, even as he is today.

Influence of Christianity on Medicine

With the advent of Christianity a mixture of religion and medicine was again attempted with the usual result, lack of progress, which lasted in this instance for a thousand years. Christianity influenced medicine in three ways: (1) by restoration of primitive theories of disease; (2) by restriction of free thought; (3) by religious controversies which monopolized the best efforts of thinkers for centuries.

Arabian Medicine

In the year 632, wild barbarian tribes from Arabia descended upon the Roman Empire and within a century stripped her of her most valued eastern provinces. Imagine the surprise of Europe when the victorious barbarians demanded in the terms of peace the right to collect and purchase Greek manuscripts. But the Arabs were not altogether barbarians. Wild and vigorous by nature, they were nevertheless endowed mentally with great love of learning.

The cradle of Arabic medicine was at Gondisapor, where the Nestorian School was located, and where later there arose one of the most famous hospitals and libraries of medieval times. These people were remarkable as translators and compilators, and through their efforts much that was good in ancient medicine was translated, preserved, and handed down to western civilization.

Although Arabian medicine is replete with interesting anecdotes, no great progress was made. The torch of Greek medicine was kept burning in Arabia while elsewhere it was stifled or allowed to go out. Two only of the many interesting figures of Arabian medicine will be mentioned, Rhazes, "the Experimentator," and Avicenna, "the Versatile."

Rhazes gave the first description of measles and of smallpox. He experimented with drugs both on animals and humans, found metallic mercury markedly toxic for monkeys, and introduced the extensive use of mercurial inunctions. His "Continens" in nine volumes was a storehouse of information for succeeding generations.

Avicenna's "Canon," however, surpassed in popularity all other medical writings of Arabian origin. In it he attempted and partially succeeded in reviving the teachings of Galen and Aristotle. The Canon became the textbook of medicine for the following four centuries.

During the five hundred years that Arabia flourished, hospitals, scientific institutions, academies of learning, and great libraries sprang into existence at Bagdad, Cairo, Damascus, Cordova, and Gondisapor. The first book exclusively devoted to surgery appeared, the work of Albucasis. Drug therapy flourished as never before. The first "Pharmacopeia" was issued from the hospital at Gondisapor. Mesué the Younger in 1015 wrote a book on Materia Medica. In these publications drugs introduced or popularized by Arabian physicians are duly discussed, such as camphor, senna, cubebs, rhubarb, cloves, musk, syrups, rose water, and alcohol. These works served as the basis for the western pharmacopeias and were consulted almost to our own times.

During the dark ages, medicine degenerated into medieval scholasticism. The School of Salerno rose and fell (1000-1200). The thirteenth century appears brilliant mainly because of its somber background. Medicine produced but one outstanding figure prior to Basil Valentine and Paracelsus, namely, Arnold di Villanova, 1235-1312, one of the early members of the faculty of the famous School of Montpellier. Like other great men of early times, he also was versatile, in fact, a doctor in four faculties, medicine, law, theology, and philosophy. His chief claim to our attention, however, is by virtue of his interest in alchemy, and his search for the universal remedy, or the "elixir of life." Alcohol, to his mind, constituted the nearest approach. With it he made extracts of various plants, laying in this way the foundation for our present tinctures.

Medicine of the Renaissance

With the revival of learning came the revival of medicine. At this time the mystics or astrologers were in the ascendency, and the administration of medicine was controlled largely by the signs of the Zodiac. Witches were being industriously hunted down. Alchemy was beginning to play a rôle in the life of the people, especially since alchemists were devoting their attention to medicinal remedies instead of transmutation of metals. In this setting appeared Basil Valentine and Paracelsus.

Basil Valentine, the Benedictine monk of Erfurt, is shrouded in mystery. His works were not published until a century after his death, and by some are considered to be from the hand of Paracelsus. On the contrary, others hold that Valentine actually supplied the ideas so loudly acclaimed by and usually accredited to Paracelsus. Valentine's labors in alchemy resulted in the recognition of salts of antimony, nitrates of mercury, zinc, bismuth, hydrochloric acid, sugar of lead, and in methods of producing sulphuric acid and ammonia. To mercury he ascribes great value, but "the noblest of drugs is the quintessence of antimony."

Paracelsus, 1493-1541, justly or unjustly, receives the credit of being the founder of medical chemistry. He has been called the Luther of Medicine. Bombastic, conceited, abusive, and scurrilous in his attacks on his predecessors and contemporaries, he is difficult to appraise. To some he is a second Hippocrates, to others a mere blatant mountebank. But to Paracelsus or Valentine, one or both, medicine is indebted for its start along chemical lines.

The four pillars of medicine, according to Paracelsus, were philosophy, anatomy, alchemy, and virtue. From the noxious and indigestible the stomach separates the nutritious and digestible and utilizes it. The physician must emulate the stomach. Until he can find that which is chemically desirable, his medicine will be a failure. He believed that a specific remedy, "arcanum," existed for every disease. Simplicity in prescribing drugs was the natural result. He abused the profession shamelessly for their absurd mixtures and concoctions, for he also believed in the quintessence of drugs, possibly a foreshadowing of active principles and alkaloids.

To Paracelsus the world was a macrocosm, all parts of which are represented in man, the microcosm, the most important constituents being sulphur, mercury, and salt. Disease was chemical in origin. Thus, if the archeus of the stomach fails to separate the toxic from the nutritive, or the excretory organs retain them, we have the deposit of tartar on teeth, in joints, or as calculi in various other organs. Tartaric diseases of Paracelsus were apparently the forerunners of "lithemic diatheses."

Antimony he introduced into medicine. Tartar emetic was his favorite prescription. So strongly did he champion it, and so bitter was the opposition, that at one time the University of Paris demanded from its candidates for the doctor's degree a pledge never to prescribe it.

It must be admitted that Paracelsus was strong in his belief in the supernatural, in magnetism, in astral influences, and in every other form of humbuggery known to mankind. Similars, sympathetic ointment, and signatures permanently remove him from leaders such as Hippocrates, Galen, and Harvey. Nevertheless he called attention to the importance of chemistry as the foundation for medical chemistry which, however, disproved most of the beliefs which he so loudly proclaimed.

Van Helmont, greatly imbued at first with the teachings of Paracelsus, studied alchemy in relation to medicine, with the result that he discovered CO_2, and proof of the existence of an acid in gastric digestion. Through refutation of many of the fantasies of Paracelsus, he did much to put medical chemistry and therapy on a sounder basis.

The Beginnings of Scientific Medicine

With Harvey commenced experimental medicine. Demonstration and proof were subsequently demanded, words, customs, authority, and theories failing longer to satisfy the profession. The "Anatomical Exercise on the Motion of the Heart and Blood in Animals," 1628, ushers in a new physiology and the science of medicine. Admittedly, the profession was loathe to accept, but Harvey defended his thesis despite the most bitter persecution, and in so doing demonstrated once and for all the advantages of the experimental method. The discoveries by Pecquet of the thoracic duct, by Rudbeck of the lymphatics, the ocular proof of the circulation in the lung of the tortoise by Malpighi, and the introduction of the microscope by Leeuwenhoek still further established the practice of furnishing experimental proof with any new claim.

But probably medicine profited more from without than from within. Not alone were needed experiment and demonstration but training in methods of thought. This was supplied by Bacon and Descartes, the former formulating "The Principles of Inductive Science," and the latter clearly distinguishing the materialistic from the vitalistic. Galileo was creating the sciences of physics and mathematics while Sanatorius through his assistance was applying the thermometer and the scales to physiology. Borelli was utilizing mechanics and physics in investigations of the mechanics of motion. In other words, science and the instruments of science were coming into general use in medicine as elsewhere. Iatro chemistry, iatro mathematics, and iatro physics were laying the foundation of the new medicine, and men were beginning to specialize in various fields of medicine and its underlying sciences.

Space does not admit of detailed consideration of its various branches, but an attempt will be made to indicate the lines along which the most important of these advanced, while more detailed consideration will be accorded the development of pharmacology in another section of this article.

The Development of Clinical Medicine

Through adopting the outstanding features of Hippocrates, the father of medicine, Sydenham, 1624-1689, became the father of modern clinical medicine. Observation and careful clinical records separated him from his fellow practitioners, and resulted in the differentiation by him of diseases, and the discovery of new diseases, scarlet fever and chorea. In therapy he was an empiricist, but used great intelligence. Progress may be made in three ways: (1) careful histories of disease, with according to him attempts at differentiation of essentials from the non-essential features; (2) fixed treatment founded on experience; (3) searching out specifics in treatment.

He gave a practical tendency to clinical medicine which has been retained to our day. His teachings pervaded the whole realm of clinical medicine, and were accepted and followed by Baglivi in Italy and Boerhaave in Leyden. The former, applying Sydenham's methods of observation, differentiated fevers and described enteric fever which was prevalent in Rome, and enlarged on the part played by tissues in disease. He clearly outlined the clinical effects of coffee, tea, and chocolate, and as a result introduced coffee as a cure for headache originating from fatigue. Boerhaave, though contributing nothing new, inculcated these principles in the work of his students, and became the greatest clinical teacher of his day.

In 1761 Leopold Auenbrugger, a young Austrian physician, published a paper, "A New Invention for Discovering Obscure Thoracic Diseases by Percussion of the Chest." Keen of observation, he utilized inspection (noting lack of mobility), palpation and percussion, and made many fundamental contributions to methods of physical diagnosis. His work, however, attracted little attention until unearthed and reintroduced by Corvissart in 1808. Four years later, 1812, Laennec introduced the stethoscope, which tremendously increased the value of auscultation. Thereafter clinical medicine was fully equipped with methods of physical diagnosis.

Bruonianism.—A new system of medicine was introduced in 1780 by Brown, which was subsequently known as Bruonianism. According to him Life is a state produced by excitability which is constantly being used and constantly replaced. As in a furnace, fire is life, coal is excitability, the draft is the stimulus. Diseases result from too much or too little excitability and stimulus, and are sthenic or asthenic accordingly. Treatment consists of restoring the normal state of excitability by regulating the stimulus. Drugs are stimuli and effectively regulate excitability in the following order: opium, camphor, ammonia, musk, alcohol, all of which are used in asthenic states. On the other hand, bleeding, purgation, cold, low diet, and passive exercise are debilitating and should be used in sthenic states. Brown's treatment was extremely radical, resulted in great injury, and would have brought medicine into general disrepute had it been more generally adopted.

Specialism.—At this period physicians began to specialize in internal medicine.* Prominent among them were Thomas Willis, Sir John Pringle, John Howard, Wm. Heberden, John Fothergill, James Parkinson, Richard Bright, and Edward Jenner of vaccination fame. The names of Parkinson and Bright were attached to diseases they described. In this development should be mentioned the great John Hunter, who,

* According to Garrison, specialism existed among the ancient Babylonians, there being a physician for each disease, so that this movement must be looked upon as the revival of specialism.

though a surgeon, did much for diagnosis. His interest in syphilis, however, was unfortunate. His personal auto-inoculation experiment, though based on the sound principle of experimentation, was premature and retarded progress for many decades so far as syphilis was concerned.

Modern cellular vitalism was the gift of Rudolph Virchow. "It breaks up the old indivisible 'vital force' distributed throughout the whole body or located in a few organs into an infinite number of individual associated vital forces working together yet separately and assigns to them the elementary parts (which latter are considered to be cells) in definite microscopic seal." "Social arrangement or organization is beautifully conceived, each part playing its own rôle, influenced by others, but performing its own function which in turn affects those of other parts."

In the final analysis, it is seen that the fundamental reasons for the lack of progress in medical treatment were: (1) the inadequate state of science, which made it impossible to cope with the complex problems of the human organism, of disease, and of the processes of life; and (2) the incorrect methods which were employed for approaching the subject, theories and speculations predominating rather than observation and experimentation. Our forefathers erred in accepting supernatural agencies as the basis of disease, in employing remedies about which they knew but little for diseases about which they knew less, and in not having true conceptions of either physiological or pathological processes. Their fallacies resulted from dealing with ideas instead of facts.

The introduction of the "experimental method" opened up new channels in medicine through which science has flowed in ever increasing volume. The development of these so-called underlying sciences has made possible scientific medicine.

Present-day Forms of Therapy

Rational Therapy

Rational therapy is a consummation devoutly to be wished—true rational therapy—treatment based on science and fact. It includes all the elements necessary to success in the treatment of the individual case and for the progress of medicine at large. It necessitates a correct diagnosis, a grasp of physiologic pathology, legitimate indications for treatment, and the correction of deranged functions along rational lines. The indications for rational treatment are derived from three sources:

(*a*) *Etiology.*—Removal of the cause constitutes radical treatment and effects cures in conditions in which irreparable damage has not already resulted. This is specific therapy, the ultimate towards which all treatment strives. Unfortunately its application is restricted owing to existing limitations in the science of medicine. All too frequently the cause is unknown, the mechanism and development of clinical manifestations obscure, conditions usually precluding specific therapy. Nevertheless in this field, treatment has made great progress during the last decade.

Specific therapy includes representatives of drug, serum, vaccine, and organotherapy, the group of diseases subject to direct control being constantly on the increase. Thus we have quinine in malaria, mercury and arsenic in syphilis, arsenic and antimony in trypanosomiasis, specific sera for many infectious diseases, desiccated thyroid in myxedema, and pituitary extract in diabetes insipidus. The chemical nature of some of the hormones has been determined, a few have been isolated, and in one instance, namely, thyroxin (the active principle of the thyroid), it has been actually synthesized and demonstrated to have all the effects of the desiccated gland. With thyroxin metabolism can be profoundly affected. Thus it is seen that specific therapy leads to fundamentals and will in all probability constitute the basis of the scientific treatment of the future.

(*b*) *Pathology.*—This is used in its broadest sense and includes functional and chemical as well as anatomical changes. Certain pathological conditions are encountered clinically which demand a definite line of treatment irrespective of the underlying causes. To be sure, the cause may need treatment in addition. Thus, outspoken myocardial insufficiency calls for treatment, per se, independently of whether it is due to myocarditis, secondary to syphilis, rheumatism, arteriosclerosis, nephritis, focal infection, exophthalmic goiter, or to some valvular lesion. The underlying cause may also demand its own treatment simultaneously or at some subsequent time. Similarly uremia calls for a certain line of treatment irrespective of whether it is due to nephritis, polycystic kidneys, or obstruction of the lower urinary tract; and marked acidosis demands its own therapy independently of the underlying diabetes or nephritis.

(*c*) *Symptoms.*—Generally speaking, symptomatic treatment should be avoided except as a last resort when other methods fail. Symptoms are the expressions of deranged function and often blessings in disguise. Their nature and cause should be determined. Treatment should first be directed not to them but to their cause and to the correction of the deranged function. This failing, and particularly where the symptoms occasion great distress or endanger vital functions or life itself, general measures for symptomatic relief may be adopted; but the clinical investigation should continue and due caution be exercised that no harm is done.

Symptomatic treatment is often the easiest for the doctor, but injudiciously applied, is responsible for most of the mistakes and many of the tragedies of practice.

Empirical Therapy

This is based on clinical experience, previous results serving as the guide, the cause and mechanism involved and the reason for cure remaining obscure. The term "purely empirical" carries with it a certain element of reproach. The name has become a term of opprobrium. While it is not the intent of the author to champion empiricism, it should be remembered that "experience is a good teacher," and that the empirical treatment of one period has occasionally become the rational or specific therapy of a later date. In a considerable number of instances clinical experience has furnished irrefutable evidence of the efficacy of the therapeutic measure long before the underlying cause and the character of the disease have been determined. For instance, mercury was used in syphilis, and quinine in malaria before the tryponema and the plasmodium were discovered, while digitalis was used in the treatment of dropsy before the express relationship of dropsy to myocardial insufficiency was recognized. In these and many other instances therapy has outdistanced the other branches of medical science, a matter of commendation and not of reproach so far as treatment is concerned.

Empiricism in therapy is permissible at times, but only if the proof of its efficacy is convincing. Inability to explain is admission of ignorance. Empirical treatment may constitute the starting-point of clinical investigation, but invariably demands controls, accurate observation of results effected, critical judgment, and simultaneously intensive search for the causal factors concerned. Such scrutiny ofttimes reveals ineffectiveness, whereupon the treatment must be abandoned.

Supernatural Therapy

This is based on the primitive conception of disease, and is perhaps the oldest of all forms of therapy. It is primitive, fundamental, and fixed. The credulity of the heathen amuses us; in fact, in our wisdom we smile. Wherein does our own childhood teaching differ? It gives us faith and casts a cloak over reason. Just as our Greek forefathers slept before the temples of Esculapius, so we make pilgrimages to Rome or visits to the shrine of St. Anne de Beaupré. Absent treatment today is as effective as was the sympathetic ointment of Paracelsus. Mental treatment, suggestion, and faith healing are unquestionably helpful at times, but their use should be supplemented by all that science and sound experience can furnish.

Baseless Therapy

This is the "therapy of fancy" of Lauder Brunton. Although medical science has caused the "old vessels which once held human beliefs" to be abandoned, therapy based on these beliefs still persists. Often lack of time or ignorance prevents the busy practitioner from applying the four fundamentals of treatment. Only too frequently the outstanding symptom is treated, headache instead of uremia, or loss of weight instead of diabetes.

At times polypharmacy replaces pathology, undiagnosed conditions being met by mixtures of drugs, the action of any one of which is but poorly understood. Fortunately the inclusion in the curriculum of medical schools pharmacology is rapidly doing away with this practice. Perhaps more than any other factor, the large pharmaceutical firms are responsible for the remnants of polypharmacy which still persist.

Incredible as it may seem, the therapy of many well-trained physicians is directed not by their knowledge of the action of drugs, but by the greed-inspired claims of pharmaceutical houses. Pamphlets dealing with theoretical and scientific considerations somewhat beyond the training of the average physician and outlining new discoveries of merit are placed in the hands of the practitioner for his seduction. Because the information is new and smacks of science, and because he fails to recognize fallacies in supposed correlations presented, he is led into grievous error; to wit, the application of baseless therapy in the belief that he is treating his patient along approved modern scientific lines.

Textbooks of therapeutics are the basis of much baseless therapy. Authority, that which dominated medicine from Hippocrates to Hunter, is still effective. The conscience of the physician is clear despite the disastrous outcome provided authority exists; i.e. the finger can be pointed to the printed page. Fortunately the day of prescribing the name of a drug for the name of a disease is passing with the advent of modern works on pharmacology.

Diagnostic Therapy

So certain and so well understood are the actions of certain drugs, that they are used at times to assist in arriving at a diagnosis. Thus it is possible to determine factors important in diagnosis: (1) Whether or not a certain mechanism is hyper- or hypo-active by observing the effect upon it of standard stimuli. "Believing that excessive reaction to pilocarpin on the one hand, or to epiniphrin (adrenalin) on the other, points to a high tonus (or a high excitability) of the autonomic nervous system in one instance, and of the sympathetic nervous system in the second, Eppinger and Hess ([2]) have made use of injections of these two substances for diagnostic purposes. (2) Whether or not a function is disturbed or a lesion exists, by giving drugs which accentuate or minimize the underlying defects thereby accentuating or removing the symptoms and signs. In this connection (a) atropin and digitalis are utilized in relation to questions of conductivity and heart block, atropin removing partial block, and digitalis increasing it. (b) Nitrites are used in questionable cases of mitral stenosis. (3) Whether or not cure or specific reactions result from the use of specific remedies. Thus in districts where malaria is prevalent, fevers quickly subsiding on the administration of quinine are frequently accepted as malarial, or vice versa. Therapeutic tests are resorted to frequently where the existence of syphilis is in question.

By such means diagnoses can be deduced at times. Thus through knowing the seat of action it is possible to determine the functional state of the mechanism involved, to bring out greater defects, or to remove an etiological factor through the use of etiotropic remedies.

Prophylactic Therapy

The miracles wrought by preventive medicine in the prevention of typhoid fever, smallpox, etc., are made possible through immunity reactions, and do not at the present time come in the province of pharmacology.

On the other hand, specific drug therapy has already achieved great results in relation to protozoal diseases and to local bacterial infections, especially the venereal diseases. Thus, quinine is effective against malaria, salvarsan against syphilis, while mercury ointment prevents the development of syphilis and injections of protargol or argyrol, the development of gonorrhea.

Factors Responsible for Progress in Therapy

Having considered the factors which retarded the progress of therapy, let us attempt to identify and analyze the factors responsible for the remarkable progress of recent years. Innumerable influences have borne on the problem, but the more important can be selected and analyzed. Some of them are too broad to be dealt with other than in a general way, while some which apply directly to pharmacology will be considered in more detail. These factors may be enumerated as follows:

(1) The most important factor perhaps is the advancement of science generally. Without science and its methods, medicine would have remained an art.

(2) The development of pharmacology whereby remedies, whose actions are understood, are directed to the correction of derangements in physiological functions.

(3) The chemical basis of pharmacology; the recognition of the relationship of pharmacological action to chemical constitution of drugs and the development of remedies on this basis.

(4) The development of specific chemotherapy and experimental therapeutics whereby remedies are scientifically developed and directed towards the removal of specific causes of disease.

(5) The discovery of microorganisms and their relation to disease. This is directly responsible for the development of bacteriology and immunology and for the development of preventive medicine, the most important advance in medicine of all times. It has also revolutionized surgical practice, bringing all structures within the province of the operator through the application of aseptic and antiseptic principles.

(6) Recognition of the rôle played in the organism by glands of internal secretion, their relationship to metabolism and growth in health and disease, and the development of endocrinology and organotherapy.

(7) The adoption of a functional conception of disease with the consequent direction of treatment toward restoration of function.

(8) Organization of medical effort (schools, hospitals, medical institutions, and societies) and adequate channels of communication.

An attempt will be made to outline the more important advances along these lines, and the effects of each of these factors upon medicinal doctrines and practice. Obviously it is impossible to do more than select outstanding examples in each field. These will be dealt with in some detail, however, in order to reveal the development of principles.

(1) Advancement of Science and Progress of Medicine

Progress has come through the advancement of science. The Greek mind was active, inquisitive, and speculative, the age dark scientifically though brilliant perhaps philosophically. The Greeks had facts, isolated but not correlated. Experimentation was possible, but lacking laws of science they could neither appreciate its value nor did they possess its methods.

Let us visualize the difficulties confronting Hippocrates. Let us suppose him confronted by a case of malaria. The patient complains of chills, fevers, sweats, and aching in his bones and muscles. Malaria has never been described and none of his colleagues has ever encountered a similar case. He studies the patient and confirms the temperature changes with his hands. He offers a purgative or bleeds him and keeps him in bed. The symptoms continue. How can he proceed? Examination of the blood is impossible, for he has no microscope, and nothing is known of the character of the blood, of corpuscles, red or white, or of plasmodia. How is he to know that the mosquito has caused the infection? No one has discovered insects as carriers of disease. How is he to know of cinchona which grows in far-off Peru? Quinine has not yet been isolated. Can he transfer the disease to animals? Syringes have not yet come into existence, experimental production of disease has never been attempted, and the maltreatment of an animal might cost him his life. Pathology is unknown and if in the event of death of his patient he obtains an autopsy, he has no normal control. What, then, must he do to get at the whole truth?

It would be necessary to: (1) invent the microscope; (2) invent methods of studying blood slides, and establish the normal blood picture with which to compare the findings of his patient; (3) discover the plasmodium of malaria; (4) recognize mosquitoes as hosts and determine their rôle as hosts; (5) prove the possibility of transmission from mosquito to man and work out the life cycle of the plasmodium; (6) select cinchona from the thousands upon thousands of plants, and in this particular instance it would have involved the discovery of the new world; (7) isolate quinine, for which procedure must be developed the science of chemistry; (8) create protozoology and experimental pathology. Since it has taken the best efforts of science and medicine twenty-five centuries to accomplish these things, we can scarcely hold Hippocrates responsible for failing to handle the case scientifically.

Medicine is science and can only grow with science generally. Hippocrates was honest. Recognizing existing limitations, he preferred not to go too deeply into the question of diagnosis but to treat the individual if not the disease; to assist the "vis medicatrix naturae." We fail to recognize that the average citizen of today has a larger opportunity of casually acquiring medical science than was possible to Hippocrates through a long life of arduous labor.

Lauder Brunton ([3]), writing in 1880, says, "Unfortunately we do not know medicine as we do chemistry and physics. We have medical sciences, for physiology, pathology, and pharmacology are justly beginning to lay claims to the title; but medicine itself, the recognition and cure of disease, is still an art and not a science," and as proof thereof he instances the same disease, malaria. "We know that if a man pass through certain districts, and more especially if he sleep in them, he is likely to be attacked with a fit of shivering which often lasting some time will be succeeded by a burning fever, and then by profuse sweating, after which he will feel comparatively well until the next day, when another shivering fit will come on at the same hour, and run the same course as the first. We know that, by warning the man against the dangerous locality, or by making him adopt certain precaution, take cinchona alkaloids, if he cannot avoid the place, we may be able to prevent the disease; by administering one large dose of quinine before the paroxysm, we may stop its approach, and by continuing the remedy we may prevent its recurrence altogether. But we are ignorant of the nature of malaria as we trace the course of these paroxysms whatever it may be. We do not know how it acts upon the bodily mechanism so as to cause them. We have no notion of the manner in which quinine counteracts the malarial effects."

And this was scarcely forty years ago. Physiology, pathology, and pharmacology have more claim to the title of science now, than then. Medicine itself, the recognition and cure of disease, is rapidly becoming science. The recognition and treatment of malaria is science—applied physiology, pathology, and pharmacology.

Today we know the cause and the cure of malaria. Brunton,* together with thousands of other physicians, had at hand the instruments necessary for the solution of the problem in 1880; Hippocrates did not in 460 B.C. Both were equally honest in every respect. Each acted in accordance with his light, with the state of science and of cosmic consciousness.

But have we reached the ultimate in our conception of malaria and its cure? What is fever? What is a chill? Why does segmentation of the plasmodia result in fever? What relation have dehydration and sweating to chills and fevers? Is quinine necessary? What radicle of quinine is responsible for the destruction of the plasmodium and will it suffice? Innumerable questions confront us just as they did the Father of Medicine and Lauder Brunton. These, the future and science will solve. All medicine truly rational is science, or fast becoming so.

(2) The Development of Pharmacology

Although drugs come down from antiquity, the science, mechanism, and seat of their action is of quite recent date. Bichat, dissatisfied with the prevailing opinions of pathology and treatment, devoted his short life

*These statements are not intended as derogatory to Sir Lauder Brunton. His name is mentioned in this connection, first, because of his pharmacological writings from which an excerpt is here presented, and secondly, because he represented the highest type of physician of his day and contributed abundantly to the sciences of pharmacology and therapeutics.

to the former. Fired by his spirit, his pupil Magendie took up his work and did for treatment what Bichat had done for pathology, namely, laid the cornerstone of an underlying science. Perhaps more important than the results themselves were the methods of his experimentation. His object was to determine the seat of the action of a drug. Utilizing upas, which contains strychnine, he attempted to prevent it reaching the cord and again applied it directly, finding in the first instance that it did not cause convulsions but that in the latter it readily did. The first pharmacological experiment, therefore, was the demonstration of the action of strychnine on the cord.

This appears a matter of simplicity today, but was a new conception in Magendie's day. He first used upas subcutaneously, getting convulsions in three minutes. The prevailing explanation concerning absorption and action of upas was that it was absorbed from the wounds into the blood, was carried to the heart and thence to all organs including the nervous system, where its special action was exerted. It was in his method of proving this explanation that Magendie founded pharmacology. He did not take it for granted, he demonstrated and proved it. As these constitute the first pharmacological experiments, it seems advisable to present them.

(*a*) *Channels and Rate of Absorption.*—Injections into pleural and peritoneal cavities resulted immediately in the appearance of symptoms, into an isolated loop of intestine, after six minutes, into a full stomach, after one-half hour. Absorption occurred from the large bowel, bladder, and vagina, but was slower as it was also from the stomach isolated by ligatures at the cardia and pylorus.

(*b*) *Proof that Poison Acts Through the Circulation.*—Injection into the jugular vein was much more quickly followed by convulsions than injection into the femoral arteries, for in the latter the peripheral circulation must be made before the blood reached the heart and eventually the cord. To rule out the so-called sympathetic action suggested by his contemporaries, he isolated the limb except for the blood vessels, injected the drug, and obtained the convulsions. This experiment he repeated successfully after severing artery and vein and connecting their divided ends by goose quills. He thereby ruled out lymphatics and nerves.

(*c*) *Proof of Seat of Action in Cord.*—Injections were made into carotid artery, no convulsion resulting until sufficient time had elapsed for the drug to complete the circulation and reach the cord, whereby the brain as the seat of action was ruled out. The destruction of the cord by a probe prevented the appearance of tetanus, dorsal cord destruction preventing tetanus of forelegs, lumbar destruction, tetanus of hind legs.

Following the exposure of the cord by operation, direct application to the cord caused immediate tetanus. Thus for the first time was revealed not only the seat of action, but also the channels of absorption and transportation, and the mechanism of action.

He next attempted to apply his discoveries clinically. Nux vomica, which was on the market, acted much as upas, and this he utilized in a case of paralysis with remarkably good results. He found later, however, that it had already been used by M. Fourquier, but its use was based on Magendie's experiments.

This remarkable investigation was followed by another by Claude Bernard (4), who was a pupil of Magendie. Sir Benjamin Brodie (5) had demonstrated in 1812 that curare, an arrow poison used by the Indians in the valley of the Amazon, paralyzed voluntary muscles, and that even after apparent death the heart continued to beat and the blood to flow as evidenced by the spurting of blood on section of an artery.

Bernard took up the work in 1844. Three possibilities obtain, an effect on the muscle itself, on the peripheral nerve, on the central nervous system. The effect on the muscle itself could be ruled out by eliciting response by a galvanic current subsequent to curarization. The absence of response in applying the current to the nerve located the seat of action in the nerve or muscle. Was it nerve trunk or nerve-ending? Muscles and nerve were soaked in a curare solution and it was found that on immersing the nerve trunk alone, normal reactions followed stimulation, whereas following immersion of the muscle no response could be elicited. The seat of action, therefore, must be found in the nerve-endings in the muscle. Following this, he demonstrated that the drug acted locally, for after isolating the limb of a frog by ligation and injecting curare subcutaneously, the ligated limb responded in normal fashion to stimulation despite the fact that the rest of the body was paralyzed.

Little has been added to our knowledge of the action of curare since these experiments of Bernard. To be sure, Lauder Brunton subsequently showed the effect of curare on the cord itself and its slight effect in inhibiting conduction through sensory nerves. The neural-muscular junction has become somewhat better defined and we know that the nerves and end-organs have no medullary sheath and hence are exposed to drug action. The nerve-end organs are complex structures containing nerve fibrils, which pass into the true end-organs or nerve plates, which in turn send branching filaments into the muscle cells. We know that curare interposes to centrifugal impulses resistance at a point below the nerve fiber and the actual termination in the muscle, but the exact seat is still not known. The union of curare with the nerve is chemical or physico-chemical in character, the drug finally being freed and excreted if death has not supervened. The curare action is due to the quaternary nitrogen group, a property held in common with tetra-methyl and tetra-ethyl amines.

Magendie and Claude Bernard inaugurated a new epoch in therapy. Their investigations revealed the possibility of ascertaining accurate information concerning the seat and mechanism of action of drugs, their methods constituting the foundation on which pharmacology now rests.

Crum, Brown and Fraser ([6]) in 1868 attacked pharmacology from a somewhat different point of view; namely, the relation of pharmacological action to chemical constitution. Their work elucidated the subject of the anchoring of drugs by cells. It was they who first determined the chemical character of curare. They fixed the responsibility of its action on the quaternary nitrogen and proved that this action was held in common with all other quaternary ammonia bases. Their claims were subsequently confirmed by Brunton and Cash. Brunton devoted much time to pharmacology and scientific therapy, investigating the action of an "ordeal poison," casca, on the gastrointestinal tract, heart, and circulation, and the action of digitalis on heart and circulation. He also studied the diuretic action of digitalis. On pharmacological grounds he introduced into medical practice the use of vasodilators.

Schmiedeberg exercised a profound influence on the development of pharmacology, to which he devoted his long life. He introduced a new method of pharmacological study, namely, the action of drugs on the frog's heart, which resulted in a much clearer conception of cardiac action and the influence on it of drugs. In addition, he also emphasized the chemical side of pharmacology and its relation to physiological chemistry, discovering the synthesis of hippuric acid from glycocoll and benzoic acid, and determining the formula of histamine and nucleic acid. Above all else he influenced others, his pupils perhaps more than any other group being responsible for establishing the science of pharmacology, Hans Meyer of Vienna, John J. Abel of Baltimore, and Arthur Cushny, formerly of the University of Michigan, now of London, all leaders in the new science.

In America pharmacology has made great strides. Horatius C. Wood ([7]) of Philadelphia, a pioneer in this field, bore the load single-handed in the earlier days, carrying out pharmacological and therapeutic researches on nitrites and hyoscine, writing prolifically on all matters pertaining to the use of drugs and on many other fields of medicine. With the coming of Abel and of Cushny, chairs of pharmacology were created and its future in this country became assured.

So rapid has been its progress that the action of drugs has been made the basis not only of treatment but also of determining the state of activity of certain systems. One example may be given which reveals in a remarkable way on the one hand the complexity of the mechanisms involved in physiological functions, and on the other the exactness with which the seat of action of drugs can be determined.

Through the researches of Gaskell, Langley ([8]) and others, much light has been shed upon the structure and functions of the sympathetic nervous system. Although it presides over many of the vital functions, the importance of its rôle has but recently been ascertained. In disclosing these revelations, drugs have been of the greatest assistance, and have resulted in the use of the so-called pharmaco-dynamic tests.

In opposition to the animal nervous system, which is under the control of the will, stands the vegetative system ([9]) through the efferent branches of which are supplied organs whose function is not so controlled. The vegetative system consists of two varieties of nerves, the sympathetic and the autonomic or craniosacral (Fig. 1). Almost all the internal organs are supplied by fibers from each class which act antagonistically, thereby resulting in tonicity of a smooth muscle, and normal function of glandular structures.

Excessive activity on the part of either system results in a rather characteristic train of manifestations. Since their actions are antagonistic, stimulation of one system produces effects analogous to inhibition of the other. The vegetative system as a whole is influenced by nicotine, which at first stimulates and later paralyzes all its ganglia and post-ganglionic fibers. On the other hand, certain drugs affect only one system or the other. Thus epinephrin acts only on the sympathetic nerve-endings, exciting them, and hence produces the same effect on the various organs as stimulation of their sympathetic nerve supply. Epinephrin therefore causes vasoconstriction (coronary and pulmonary excepted), strengthening and accelerating the heart, dilating the pupils, and increasing secretion of the salivary glands, while on the functions of the stomach, intestines, and bladder, where the sympathetic normally inhibits, it causes relaxation.

Certain other drugs affect the autonomic exclusively without influencing in any way the sympathetic system. The drugs acting on the autonomic system are atropine which paralyzes it and pilocarpin and muscarin which stimulate it. Thus muscarin and pilocarpin cause miosis, slowing of the heart, contraction of bronchial muscles, violent contraction of the intestine, and secretion of true glands, while atropin in each instance causes the reverse of these effects.

By the therapeutic application of epinephrin, atropin, and pilocarpin, much can be learned concerning the functional state of mechanisms

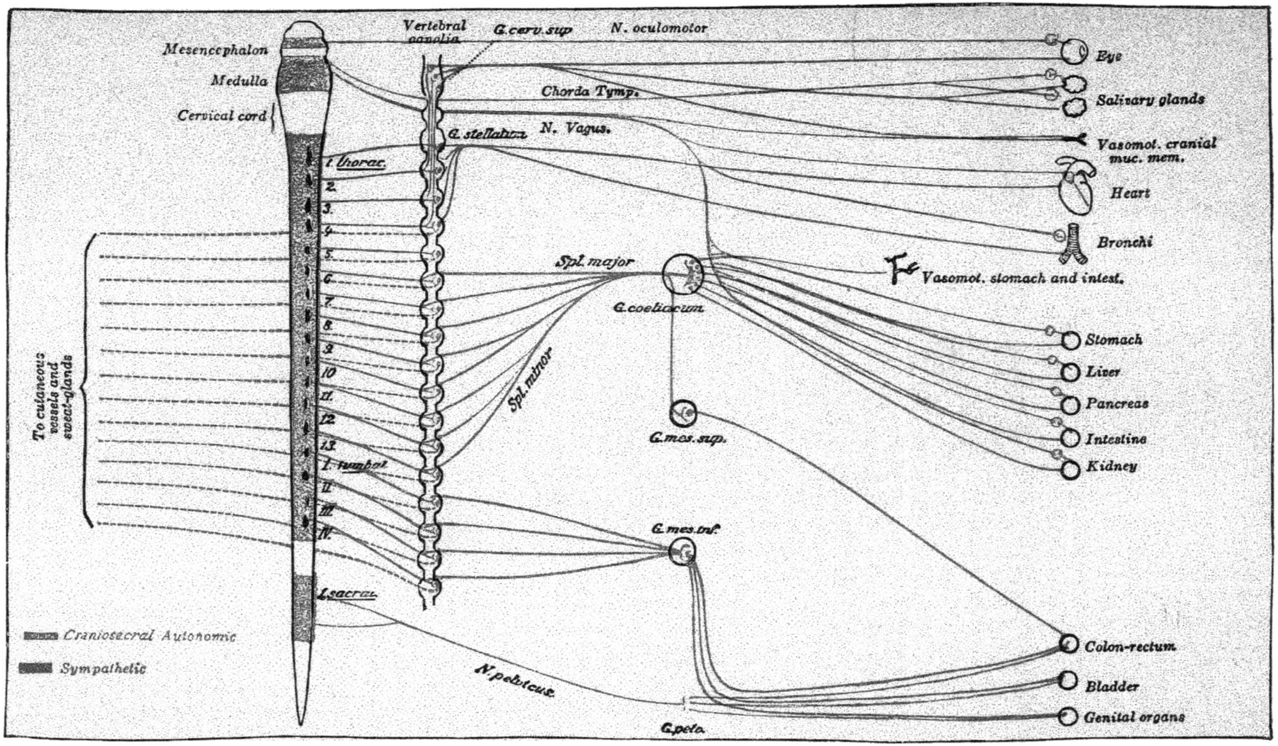

FIG. 1

DIAGRAM OF THE AUTONOMIC OR VEGETATIVE NERVOUS SYSTEM. THE SYMPATHETIC INNERVATION IS IN RED AND THE CRANIOSACRAL AUTONOMIC IN BLUE.

(After H. H. Meyer and R. Gottlieb, "Die Experimentelle Pharmakologie," published by Urban & Schwarzenberg, Berlin.)

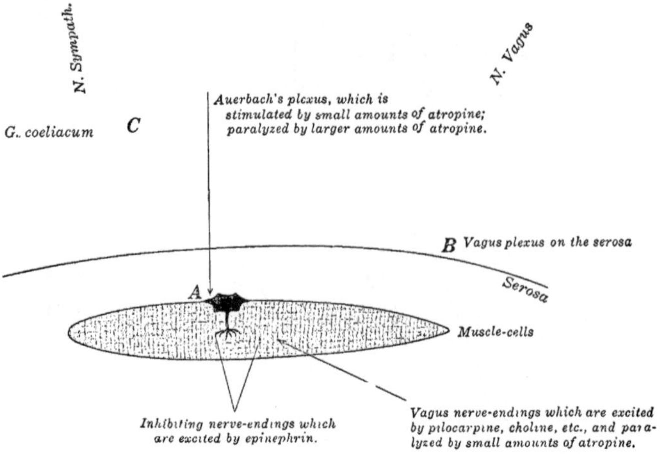

FIG. 2 DIAGRAM OF THE INNERVATION OF THE INTESTINE.

After Meyer and Gottlieb, "Die Experimentelle Pharmacologie,"
Urban and Schwarzenberg, Berlin.

P. 839]

innervated by these systems. Through their use the responsibility of sympathetic or autonomic systems for certain manifestations can be determined. According to the preponderance of the sympathetic or autonomic systems generally, individuals are classified as sympatheticotonic or vagotonic. It is true, however, that these pharmacological facts have led to speculations in clinical medicine which on the whole have caused confusion rather than clarity.

The effects of these drugs can best be exemplified by consideration of their action on the muscles of the intestine. Movements of the intestines are of three kinds; (a) pendulum, which results in division, mixing, and moving about of intestinal contents; (b) true peristalsis, with contraction above and relaxation below, the result of distention or chemical stimulation; resulting in the moving downward of the intestinal contents; and (c) rolling movements, violent contractions of the small intestine involving considerable stretches of it, described by Meltzer and by him ascribed to increased vagus tone with simultaneous inhibition of the splanchnic sympathetic. These movements are under the control of Auerbach's plexus or Langley's "enteric system," stimulation coming through the vagus and hypogastric and inhibition through the splanchnics. (Fig. 2.)

Drugs which act upon the autonomic and sympathetic systems markedly affect intestinal movements, pilocarpin, muscarin and physostigmine stimulating contraction which may be violent and tonic in character, and atropin inhibiting contraction through paralysis of the vagus terminals. These results are effected by direct action on the vagus terminals and not through Auerbach's plexus and the sympathetic terminals. Auerbach's system is composed of branches from the vagus and sympathetic, and acts automatically and independently. On stimulation it accelerates and strengthens normal waves of contraction, but does not result in tonic contractions or cramps. On this plexus, atropin exerts in small doses at first a stimulating and later in larger doses a paralyzing effect, just as do nicotine and strychnine.

The sympathetic system is the inhibitor, acting antagonistically to the plexus and to the vagus nerve. It is subject to stimulation by nicotine and epinephrine, both of which cause relaxation of the intestinal wall. The innervation of the muscles, together with the seat and character of the action of various drugs are graphically depicted in Fig. 2.

The action of atropin is interesting because of the existence of two points of action. Thus, therapeutically, it may cause either relaxation of spasm or increased normal peristalsis, depending on the condition of tonicity obtaining at the time of administration. In lead poisoning and vagotonia, for instance, where tonicity is greatly increased through stimulation of the vagus, atropine causes relaxation through its action on the vagus. Through the relaxation of spasm, normal intestinal movements and activity supervene. In this manner atropin may act as a purgative or a supplement to other purgatives in the conditions of increased intestinal tonicity resulting in constipation. On the other hand, administered when increased tone or spasm is absent, atropin tends to increase peristalsis through its influence on Auerbach's plexus. Thus is explained pharmacologically, a fact long recognized clinically, namely, that belladonna or atropin in small doses are valuable in conjunction with purgatives in some spastic types of constipation. In large doses they paralyze the intestines. The dose, therefore, must be adapted to the existing condition and must remain small if intestinal peristalsis is desired.

(3) The Chemical Basis of Pharmacology *

One approaches this subject with trepidation, yet with hope. Much is known in a fragmentary way; there are isolated instances of the effects of constitution on pharmacological action. Definite laws can be laid down in some instances as to the character of changes in action, resulting from changes in constitution along determined lines. Still in a broad practical sense but little is known about it at the present time. We have but a vision of the " promised land."

As the atom and molecule are fundamental to the understanding of chemistry, so cell and molecule are fundamental to chemotherapy. In the progress of science, naturally form received attention first, later function, and lastly constitution and chemical reactions. The body consists of cells of different sizes, shapes, and groupings, all of which are affected by disease. The cells perform functions of diverse nature in relation to which there exists great interdependence of activity. Their functions are also affected by disease. The cells live. Their life depends upon chemical activities, and the function is associated with or controlled by chemical reactions, and these in turn are affected by disease.

From the standpoint of chemotherapy, the living cell and the chemical molecule are brought into relation. The cell must be looked upon as a participating seat of microchemical reactions. In it are chemicals undergoing reactions resulting in the development of forces; to it are being added constantly new chemicals resulting in modification of reactions and of forces. Products result which are valuable to the cell, and hence are

* Two excellent works exist on this subject, "Die Arzneimittel-Synthese," by Sigmund Frankel, Julius Springer, Berlin, 1906, and "The Chemical Basis of Pharmacology," by Francis and Fortescue-Bricksdale, Edward Arnold, London, 1908.

retained, or to other cells, when they are transported elsewhere, or which are simply by-products or end-products, in which event they are thrown out from the cell for excretion. The living cell is a series of electric cells or a laboratory, in which reactions are going on constantly, and in which forces are being created. The medicament is a new chemical reagent and the effect of these new chemical molecules on the natural process is the factor to be determined.

In order to obtain a comprehensive grasp of these activities of a cell and of the effect of new extraneous chemical molecules upon them, it is necessary to understand both factors; namely, the constitutional reactions and normal activity of the cells on the one hand, and on the other the constitution and relationships of the new chemical molecule added.

The key to pharmacological action of a drug is found in the chemical constitution and activities underlying and associated with cell function. Unfortunately this is where medical science is lacking. Knowledge of the ultimate physics and chemistry of cells is wanting. Consequently, at present, investigation in chemotherapy is limited in character, permitting only modification relative to the extraneous chemical molecules and the study of the effects of these changes in modifying gross physiological functions.

From the foregoing, it is obvious that in order to act upon the cells, contact or incorporation is essential. In this connection Ehrlich ([10]) has emphasized the importance of distribution of chemicals and in the same connection has introduced his conceptions which involve chemoceptors. The distribution varies with different drugs and is more or less accepted by the profession as a matter of course. On the other hand, it constitutes a vital process which is a determining factor in pharmacological action. Localization, seat of action, and channels of excretion are not matters of chance, but are determined by the chemical constitution of the medicament. In order that a drug may act on the cell, it must be anchored by a receptor.

Cells possess receptors of several types, nutritive-ceptors, chemoceptors, and immuno-ceptors. Foods, drugs, and toxins contain haptophore groups which, in the event they fit the receptors, attach the molecule to the cell. But some differences exist in the mechanism involved with these varying substances. The nutritive molecule is assimilated by the cell. The molecule of toxin is capable of setting up processes of immunization which result in excessive production of receptors which are thrown off into the circulation, where they constitute antibodies capable of uniting with and rendering inert the toxic molecule. Chemoceptors unite with haptophores of drugs and thus render them capable of action, but they are not found as a rule in excess, that is, they do not exist as antibodies, free in the circulation. It also appears that the receptors may be only partially occupied by the drugs, in which condition they are still susceptible to union with closely allied drugs; i.e. atoxyl and arsenious acid. Thus a trypanosome may be resistant to atoxyl and its affinity for arsenic blunted, yet if it be subjected to a surcharge of arsenious acid, it is affected. It is possible in other instances that some radicle or side chain constitutes the haptophore group and is responsible for fixation, as for instance the acetyl group (CH_3CO) in arsacetin, which renders the latter effective in atoxyl-fast strains. On the other hand, receptors may be completely fixed by one drug, and also by closely allied drugs, for instance, trypanosomes made fast for both atoxyl and arsenious acid may be fast also for antimony.

The physical and chemical properties of the cell and of the medicament determine the presence or absence of affinities. The nature of these affinities or receptors is important. The variants must be considered; (*a*) the chemical, and (*b*) the protoplasm of the cell, the relation being mutual or reciprocal.

(*a*) *Chemical Factors.*—From the chemical viewpoint, many factors must be considered. Variation in valence markedly affects the chemical properties. The fundamental observation in Ehrlich's work consisted in recognizing that it was trivalent and not pentavalent arsenic which destroyed trypanosomes. The striking difference in the toxicity of Hg_2Cl_2 and $HgCl_2$, and of CO_2 and CO affords ample proof of the importance of valence.

The chemical constitution or formula is another determining factor. Knowledge of the empirical formula is necessary but does not suffice. Complications arise in the possibility of different arrangements of the atoms in the molecule. Thus two substances may have the same empirical formula, the same number of C, H, and O atoms, but yet be different in every respect. Thus $C_2H_4O_2$ represents acetic acid, but it also represents formic ester, two very different substances. Chemistry teaches us that C_3H_8O may represent two substances, $OHCH_2CH_2CH_3$, normal propyl alcohol, or $(CH_3)_2CH{\cdot}OH$ isopropyl alcohol, and that these substances have different chemical and physical properties. Properties depend on chemical grouping within the cell, so that knowledge of structural formulae is also necessary.

Pasteur demonstrated that there were several kinds of tartaric acid, $C_4H_6O_6$, dextro, laevo, meso, and racemic. He demonstrated that atoms may have different space arrangements, and in so doing he founded stereoisomerism. The stereoisomeric arrangement also markedly affects chemical and pharmacological properties. As the molecule of hydrocarbons increases in size and the complexity multiplies, the possibilities for different substances increases tremendously, thus $C_{13}H_{28}$ offers more than 800 possibilities. Consequently the difficulty of assigning constitutional formulae has become increasingly great. But structural formulae are essential as the basis of study of pharmacological action. Radicles play a great rôle as haptophores or as powers affecting chemical reactions. Affinities are "constitutional" properties in the terms of Ostwald.

Solubility is of the utmost importance. Toxicological measures frequently consist of attempts to render solutions of drugs insoluble, and antidotes frequently owe their efficacy to their power of precipitating the poison before its absorption. Unless in solution, incorporation in the cell is most difficult. Incorporation is necessary for action.

The methods of administration of certain drugs are determined by the factor of volatility, thus chloroform and ether owe much to their volatility, which permits a ready means of administration, and also considerable control.

(*b*) *The Protoplasm of the Cell.*—The chemical structure of the molecule of most drugs is simple compared with that of the cell. It is the protoplasm of the cell that offers the chief difficulty in solving the problem of the action of drugs. Proteins are so infinitely complex that attempts to consider them chemically are not profitable at present. The chemistry of the living cell is beyond the science of today. At present, however, our main interest centers on the living cell, and particularly on the properties of cells which make them subject to influence by drugs. What constitutes the chemoceptors? A silk fiber stains with picric acid, a nerve fiber takes up methylene blue intravitam, a certain nerve responds to an alkaloid. Ehrlich discards the possibility of surface attraction and of absorption in staining of fibers and limits consideration to two factors, (a) insoluble salt combinations as advanced by Knecht, and (b) solid solutions of van't Hoff as outlined by Witt. In the first instance lanugic acid from wool fiber and nucleic acid of nuclear substances may precipitate basic dyestuff from solutions. Methylene blue as a vital stain is thus thrown down by the plant as the insoluble tannate. An example of solid solution is seen in silk stained with rhodarium which fluoresces. This must be a solution since rhodarium is not fluorescent except in solution. It is assumed, therefore, that the dye forms a homogeneous mixture with the silk fiber; i.e. it is in the form of a solution. "The same dye often produces different tints in various kinds of fibers. This is analogous to the fact that the same substance often dissolves in different solvents in entirely different tints."

The factors which determine the formation of the dye are properties of both the drugs and the cell. Mutual relationships must exist. It is impossible to separate them absolutely as factors apart, since mutual forces are encountered in the drugs and in the cell.

(*a*) *Colloidal State.*—What relationships exist in the living cell? In gelatin there are "vesicular and sponge-like gels." In the former, the liquid phase exists in the form of separate droplets, each surrounded by a continuous film of solid phase. In the latter, the two phases are reversed, the solid phase is in the form of a network of threads, while the liquid phase is continuous. The former is the ordinary gel from which fluid can be expressed only with the greatest difficulty; the latter, obtained through the action of formaldehyde, is a gel from which water is readily expressed. This problem has been elucidated by the system of solvents so nicely demonstrated in the work of Clowes Bayliss ([11]) who says, "Protoplasm in the living state has the properties of a liquid system, containing, however, particles of solids and amounts of immiscible liquids in a freely moving state." The relationship of dyes and drugs to the various phases must enter into consideration of pharmacological action.

(*b*) *Surface Condensation or Adsorption.*—The structure of protoplasm is such as to present large surfaces which furnish excellent ground for the play of surface forces so important in life processes. Drugs may be held in contact with cells by adsorption.

(*c*) *Changes in Cell Membrane.*—The surface layer of cells frequently present relatively limited permeability, through which the cell is protected from other cells and from surrounding fluids. The character of this membrane and its permeability plays a rôle in the action of chemicals. Solvents of this membrane make ingress possible.

(*d*) *Velocity of Diffusion.*—The passage of substances into a cell must be considered a factor in some instances. Thus Straub showed that muscarin in the heart of aplysia had no effect when the concentration within the cell reached the concentration outside of the cell. Only during the period of concentration in the cell was the drug active. Naturally, in addition, the physical and chemical properties such as solubility, volatility, surface condensation, or adsorption and electrical charges are important.

Velocity of diffusion, solubility, and volatility of drugs, colloidal states, surface condensation, and electric charges of both drugs and cells all play a rôle in determining fixation, rate of absorption, physiological action, and excretion of the drugs by the cell.

The cell protoplasm plays a great rôle in solubility and hence in making substances available. The narcotic value of a drug depends principally on its solubility in lipoid substances. Generally speaking, "the most powerful narcotics are those which are most soluble in oil and least soluble in water." Lipotropic substances are also neurotropic. The Overtun-Meyer theory of narcosis attempts to explain the entrance of drugs to the nerve cells on this basis: "They gain access to the cells of the cerebral nervous system owing to their solubility in cell lipoids in which these cells are particularly rich." Gradations in narcotic power are due to the presence of groups which increase the partitive coefficient; i.e. which render the derivatives more soluble in such fatty substances. Physical, as well as purely chemical factors play a rôle. In the cell proteins, lecithins, salts and water exist in a physicochemical combination, and the drugs affect this physicochemical equilibrium. This conception is constantly attracting more attention. A chemical may be anchored to a cell very quickly, yet it may not manifest its effect immediately, for instance, tetanus toxin is anchored eight minutes subsequent to intravenous injection, at which time antitoxins are usually ineffective and fail to protect, though given simultaneously with the toxin they protect perfectly.

These theories explain the presence of the drug in the cell, but not its mechanism of action. According to Oscar Loew, general poisons react on protoplasm in four ways: oxidation, catalysis, salt formation, and substitution.

The first includes oxidizing agents such as H_2O_2 and ozone, permanganates, etc. The catalytic agents are represented by the aliphatic narcotics. Iodine in relation to metabolism is considered by some to act as a catalizing agent only. Salt formation is dependent upon the amphoteric character of protein, and involves acids bases, alkaline earths, and salts of heavy metals. The fourth group includes a large number of substances capable of reacting with aldehydes and amines, such as hydroxamines, phenyl hydroxamines, hydroxylamines, anilines, free ammonia, phenols, especially the amido phenols, and HCN and H_2S.

Amines particularly are active, primary amines other than of the aliphatic series being more active than secondaries, which in turn are more active than tertiary. Thus NH_2 groups are important radicles in basic dyes, OH in acid dyes, where they are known as auxochromes. These active radicles react with labile groups of living protoplasm and thus affect the living cell. These labile groups disappear with the death of the cell, subsequent to which such reactions cease. Loew believes that "toxicity increases *pari passu* with reactivity."

Ehrlich launches many arguments against synthesis in cells, and states that, in his belief, it rarely occurs in relation to substances foreign to the cell. He admits, however, that it does occur in relation to vinylamine, which produces a peculiar papillary nephritis, an ethyl amide group entering the protoplasmic molecule.

Specific or special poisons act only on certain classes of organisms. In this group he considers toxins and antitoxins, specific poisons, alkaloids, and indirect poisons which interfere with oxidations such as HCN. In the mind of the writer, no reasons exist for placing alkaloid and specific poisons in this special class.

In selective action two factors naturally suggest themselves; namely, (a) reactions which play such an important rôle in relation to staining, and acid and basic dyes, and (b) the degree of oxygen saturation. Unquestionably these are determining, or at least secondary factors in many instances.

In relation to pharmacological action and absorption and excretion it is interesting to revert to an observation made by Ehrlich, and which he refers to repeatedly; i.e. that the sulphonic group introduced into neurotropic substances renders them inert from the point of view of the nervous system. The introduction of a sulphone group, SO_3H ($=SO_2$), renders many substances inert; i.e. it changes the distribution of the drug in the organism.

Sulphonation also plays a rôle in relation to excretion of drugs. Thus phenolphthalein, $C_2H_{14}O_4$

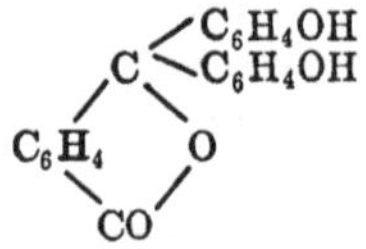

when introduced into the body is excreted by both liver and kidneys. If chlorine is introduced in the phenol rings [12] [13]

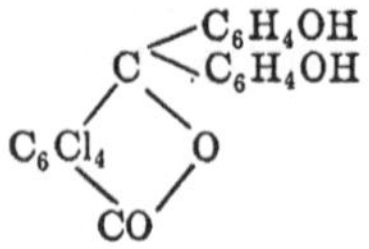

it is excreted entirely by the liver. If, on the other hand, it is sulphonated [14]

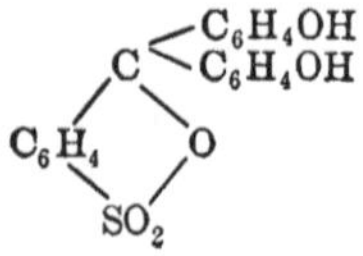

it is excreted entirely by the kidneys. Sulphonation, therefore, has resulted in a different channel of excretion, and in one of the most striking instances of specificity known to medical science. Sixty to eighty per cent. of the drug on intravenous injection is excreted in one hour by the normal kidney. In this connection a striking affinity exists for the dye by the renal cells; so striking that practically all of the dye is taken up by the kidney in the course of an hour. But the dye is not fixed. Here, then, we have an affinity without action on the cell, the drug being picked up and excreted. The explanation is difficult. Unquestionably many other similar instances exist in relation to excretion.

Instances of Chemical Constitution Controlling Pharmacological Action

In 1859 Stahlschmidt ([15]) demonstrated that strychnine loses its tetanizing action when a methyl group is introduced and the new compound assumes a curare-like action. Crum, Brown, and Fraser in 1868, in view of the ammonium base formed in this reaction, investigated other similar bases derived from alkaloids, brucine, morphine, and thebaine, and discovered that all quaternary ammonia bases exert a curariform action, paralyzing motor nerve-endings. This was the beginning of rational synthetic pharmacology and called attention to the relation of pharmacological action to chemical constitution.

Ehrlich ([16]) in 1898 enumerated five important instances selected from the whole field of therapy where a relationship was established between chemical constitution and pharmacological action. (1) The antipyretic action of aniline and amido phenol derivatives is definitely related to the amount of pure amido phenol ($NH_2C_6H_4OH$) split off in the organism. Prevention of the splitting off of this substance by substitution as in amido-acetophenon ($NH_2C_6H_4COCH_3$) renders the substance ineffective as an antipyretic.

(2) Antipyretics become ineffective through the introduction of salt-forming acid radicles such as SO_3H and CO_2H. Thus the antipyretic action of acetanilid, $C_6H_5NHCOCH_3$ is destroyed by the introduction of acetic acid, CH_3COOH, which results in $C_6H_5N(COCH_3)CH_2CO_2H$. Similarly the sulphone derivative, $C_6H_5NHCOCH_2SO_3H$, no longer affects temperature. Phenacetine

$$C_6H_4 \langle {OC_2H_5 \atop NHCOCH_3}$$

likewise is no longer an antipyretic if sulphonated or carbonated. The reason for this is found in the prevention of splitting, resulting in free p-amido phenol,

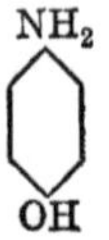

which is essential for antipyretic action.

(3) In the pyridin series, C_5H_5N, the hydrated products act more strongly than the parent substances.

(4) The benzoyl radicle (C_6H_5CO) is the anesthesiophore group of cocaine, and many of its substitution products. Cocaine, $C_{17}H_{21}NO_4$, breaks up on hydrolysis as follows:

$$C_{17}H_{21}NO_4 + 2\ H_2O = C_9H_{15}NO_3 + C_6H_5COOH + CH_3OH.$$

If the ecgonine methyl ester is substituted by other radicles than benzoyl, for instance, succinic acid ($C_4H_6O_4$), the resulting chemical has no anesthetic properties. Substitution, leaving the benzoyl radicle intact, has been the basis of many of the cocaine substitutes.

(5) Recognition of the relation of ethyl groups to hypnotic action of drugs resulted in the preparation of more effective hypnotics. The more ethyl groups in di-sulphonic bodies, the more active becomes this property. In sulphonal there are two, $(CH_3)_2\ C\ (SO_2C_2H_5)_2$, and in trional three, $CH_3(C_2H_5)C(SO_2C_2H_5)_2$. They are also present in amylene hydrate and ethyl urethane. The ethyl group is also active in phenacetine, $C_2H_5OC_6H_4NHCOCH_3$, in holocaine,

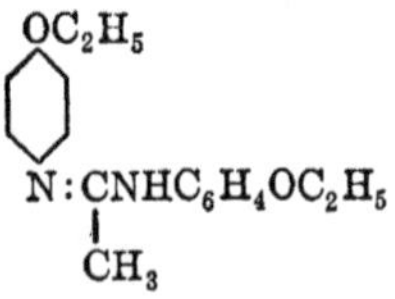

Thus alcohol itself exerts a soporiferous action, as do the alcohol radicles in various hypnotics, sulphonal, trional, amylene hydrate, and in certain anesthetics.

Obviously, it is impossible to more than touch upon certain rules or generalities * relating to the subject. The aliphatics as a group are not as active pharmacologically as the aromatic hydrocarbons, which are also, in addition, more reactive from the chemical point of view.

* For detailed discussion of the chemical basis of pharmacology, the reader is referred to the excellent volume of Francis, and Fortescue Bricksdale, which is the best publication of its kind known to the writer. From it are taken many selected examples of the relation of pharmacological action to chemical structure here presented.

Aliphatic Hydrocarbons

Lauder Brunton called attention to the fact that the action of the aliphatic series is chiefly on nerve centers, first stimulation, then narcosis, and predominantly on sensory nerves. The lower members of the fatty series, especially, are preponderantly stimulating and anesthetic to nerve centers. Schmiedeberg recognized two classes: (a) the alcohol and chloroform group, which includes most of the narcotics of the aliphatic series, gaseous and fluid hydrocarbons, the monatomic alcohols, their ethers, ketones, aldehydes, and their halogen derivatives; (b) the ammonia derivatives, which exercise a convulsant action on the cells of the cord. Conversion from trivalent to pentavalent nitrogen is accompanied, as already stated, by marked changes in physiological effect, a curare-like action replacing the convulsant.

The introduction of alkyl groups into aliphatic compounds generally increases the physiological effect. But, as the molecule increases, the solubility and volatility decreases, and the compound becomes relatively inert. As a rule, substitution of the H of the hydroxyl by an alkyl group results in an ether, an entirely different substance with different properties and increased volatility. Under such conditions ethyl alcohol is converted into ethyl ether, $C_2H_5OC_2H_5$, while glycerine becomes the glycerine ester, which has narcotic properties. On replacing the H atom of ammonia with alkyl groups, amines (primary, secondary, and tertiary) result with decreased toxicity, but as the tertiary amines are converted into ammonium compounds the toxicity is markedly enhanced. An alkyl group entering a carboxyl group, converting the organic acid into an ester, naturally confers new properties; thus, oxalic acid yields the narcotic di-ethyl-oxylate.

The ureids are important in the animal economy and in therapy. Uric acid represents dibasic ureids, the end stage of nuclear metabolism. Xanthine,

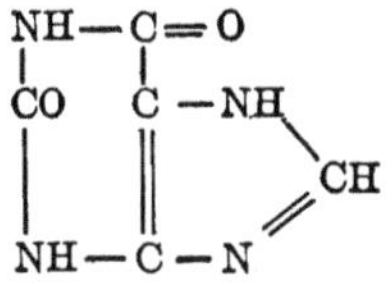

one of the intermediate products, is somewhat inert. By the introduction of methyl groups, one, two, or three, into the amide radicles, new pharmacological properties appear. Thus we obtain theobromine,

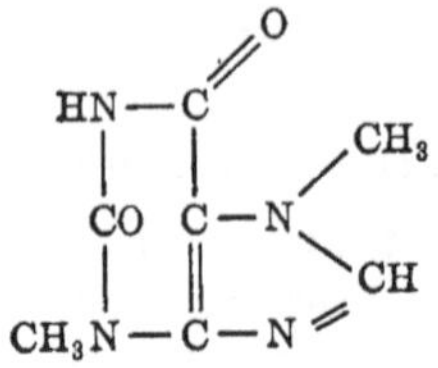

and caffeine,

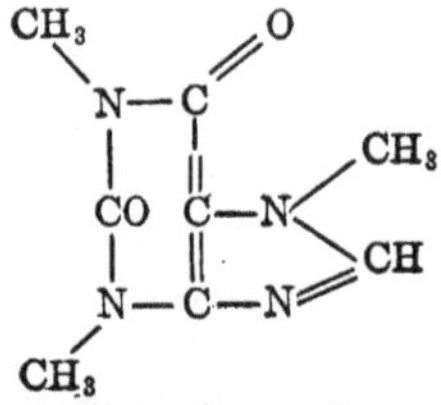

both of which are excellent diuretics and cardiac stimulants.

Unsaturated open chain hydrocarbons are more toxic than the saturated, and are extremely reactive. The double bond offers enlarged opportunities for reaction. Toxicity is multiplied many fold. To this class belongs neurine,

$$(CH_3)_3N(OH)CH:CH_2$$

a dehydration product of cholin, which is itself not markedly toxic.

Aromatic Hydrocarbons

Generally speaking, these are more reactive, have more marked pharmacological action, and tend, as pointed out by Brunton, to affect motor rather than sensory nerves, and to produce convulsions and paralysis. Benzene acts on cerebral centers producing somnolence and also paresis of muscles and tremor. Diphenyl and its compounds tend to be more inert. Napthalene is relatively more toxic and is said to slow respiration and decrease metabolism.

Substitution of H of the ring nucleus of benzene by alkyl groups tends to decrease reactivity and toxicity, and to modify pharmacological properties. In anilines it increases toxicity, while in phenols it increases the antiseptic value and decreases toxicity. Alkyl substitution of the OH of phenol renders the new compound practically inert, while the same procedure in resorcin results in increased toxicity. Alkyl substitution in the NH_2 group of anilines depresses the convulsant action, whereas in benzamides and salicylamides it increases it. Alkyl substitution in the carboxyl chains of aromatic compounds changes the character of the substance, thus salicylic acid becomes the methyl ester, methyl salicylate, or oil of wintergreen. Phenols become inert ethers. Substitution may occur in the H atoms of the ring or in the groups which substitute. H. Kendricks and Dewar laid down a rule that the introduction of H into cyclic bases invariably increases pharmacological action and toxicity. Dujardin, Beaumetz, and Bardel studied the influence of side chains on benzene compounds and concluded that: (a) those with OH are antiseptic; (b) those with amide or acid amide groups are hypnotic; (c) those containing both an amide and alkyl group are analgesic. These rules must not be taken as absolute, but they hold in the majority of cases and constitute an intelligent basis for changes in structure.

The influences of certain changes in relation to benzene seems, perhaps as well as any other example, to demonstrate the effect of structure on function:

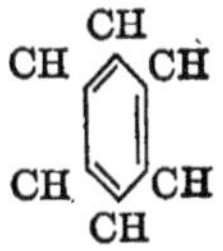

(benzene) produces somnolence and lethargy;

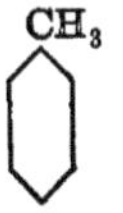

(toluene) is antiseptic;

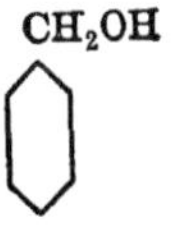

(benzyl alcohol) is a local anesthetic;

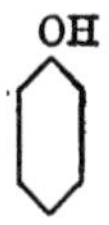

(phenol) has acid properties and is antiseptic and toxic;

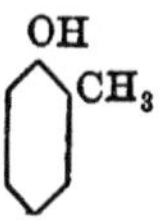

(cresol), the substitution here has increased the germicidal efficiency, while the toxicity is not increased, at least not in the same ratio. Cresoles possess advantages as antiseptics.

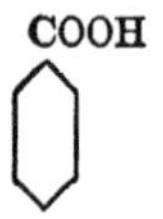

(benzoic acid), is non-toxic and slightly antiseptic;

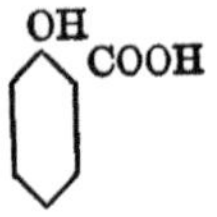

(salicylic acid) is mildly toxic, antiseptic, and has specific properties against streptococcus infection (fever, pain), the corresponding meta and para derivatives having neither of these properties;

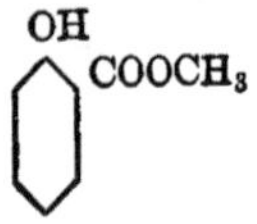

(methyl salicylate) has the same general properties as salicylic acid. Substituted methyl radicles yield other substances with similar properties, methyl oxymethyl (mesotan), mono glycol (spirosal),

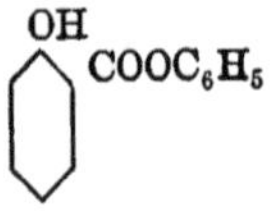

(salol). Such phenyl salicylates on decomposition yield active phenols for local action. Consequently their use has been attempted as intestinal antiseptics. Instead of the phenyl group, naphthyl may be substituted.

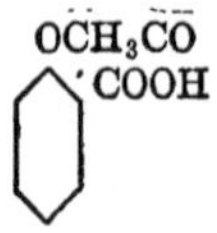

(aspirin) has the same general effect as salicylic acid, but the analgesic and antipyretic effects are greater, and the local irritating effect is less marked. Salicin, $C_{13}H_{18}O_7$, yields on hydrolysis, a glucoside and saligenin,

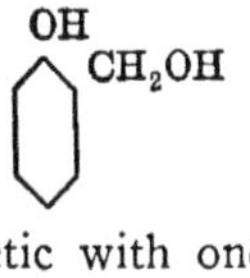

(saligenin) is a local anesthetic with one-half the toxicity and twice the anesthetic effect of benzyl alcohol, according to Hirschfelder.

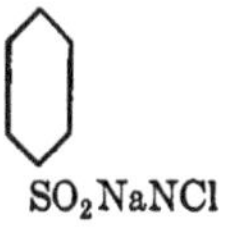

(benzene sodium sulpho chloramine, or chloramine-B) in which the NCl group is held responsible for its marked antiseptic property.

Heterocyclic Hydrocarbons and Alkaloids

The important members of this group are:

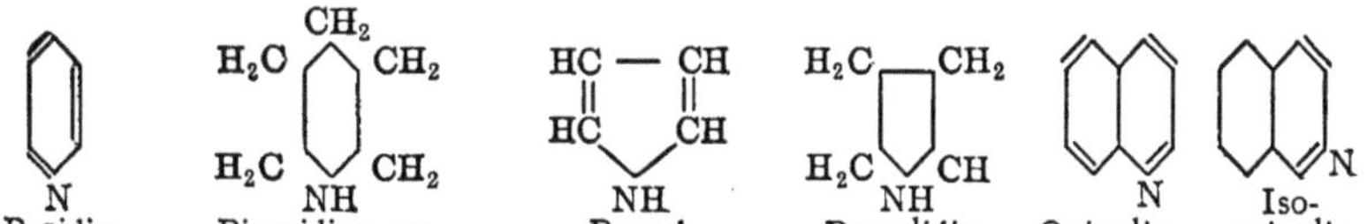

Pyridin | Piperidine or hexa hydro pyridine | Pyrrol | Pyrrolidin | Quinolin | Iso-quinolin

These enter into the consideration of the chemistry of alkaloids, and therefore are of great medical interest.

Pyrrol somewhat resembles benzene in its action. Pyridin is the nucleus, thus

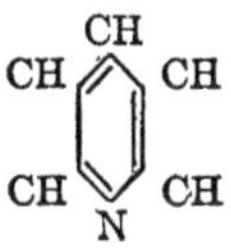

and is least toxic, while piperadine and pyrrol, and pyrrolidin are more active. The larger the chain, the more active the compound, as a rule. The entrance of an alkyl group definitely increases activity, tetra-methyl pyridin being several times as potent as pyridin itself, and exhibiting somewhat different action. Quinolin is closely related to pyridin.

Alkaloids are complex nitrogenous substances with basic properties, possessing a pyridin or a condensed pyridin nucleus.

Atropine, $C_{17}H_{23}NO_3$.

Atropine,

$$H_2C-CH-CH_2$$
$$N-CH_2CHO-CO\cdot CH \begin{matrix} CH_2OH \\ \diagdown \\ C_6H_5 \end{matrix}$$
$$C-C-CH_2$$

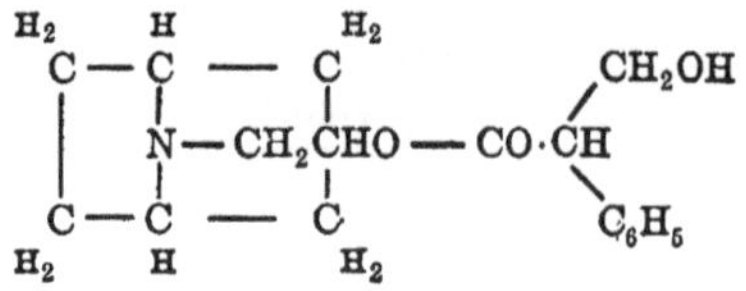

is an ester. When hydrolized it yields tropine, a condensation of piperadine and pyrrolidin rings, and tropic acid:

$$C_{17}H_{23}NO_3 + H_2O = C_8H_{15}NO + C_9H_{10}O_3.$$

Tropine has the formula,

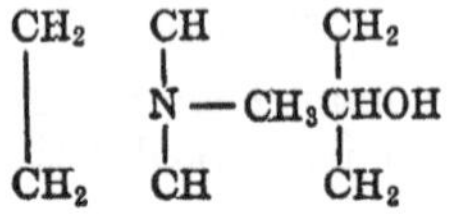

$$CH_2 \quad CH \quad CH_2$$
$$N-CH_3CHOH$$
$$CH_2 \quad CH \quad CH_2$$

tropic acid,

$$C_6H_5CH \begin{matrix} CH_2OH \\ \diagup \\ \diagdown \\ COOH \end{matrix}$$

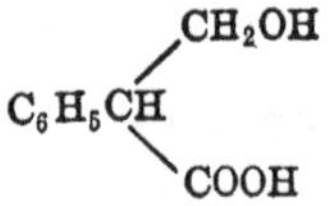

Tropine differs from ecgonin by one carboxyl group (*vide infra*), consequently, atropin and cocaine are very closely related chemically. As a matter of fact, they give almost identical constitutional effects so far as cerebrum, heart (vagus terminals), temperature, blood pressure, and eyes are concerned. Atropin, however, paralyzes the nerves to unstriped muscles and secreting glands, while cocaine has a more marked anesthetic effect and causes in addition peculiar foamy degeneration in the liver cells of mice, first recognized by Ehrlich.

The substitution of other acids for tropic acid may be made, resulting in other tropines. Thus homatropin is a tropine of mandelic acid,

$$C_6H_5CH \begin{matrix} OH \\ \diagup \\ \diagdown \\ COOH \end{matrix}$$

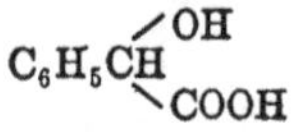

The relation of tropic and mandelic acid is evident. The more rapid onset, and the shorter duration of action of homatropin, is due to more rapid absorption and excretion.

Cocaine, $C_{17}H_{21}NO_4$, is represented by:

$$CH_2-CH-CH\cdot COOCH_3$$
$$N \quad CH_3 \quad CHO\cdot C_6H_5CO$$
$$CH_2-CH-CH_2$$

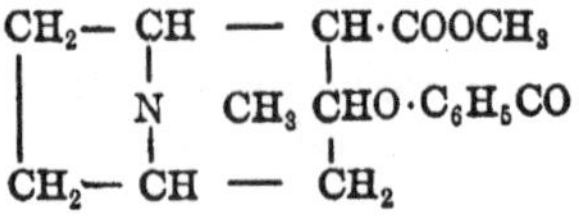

(benzoyl ecgonium methyl ester). On hydrolysis it splits up into a base, ecgonine, methyl alcohol, and benzoic acid:

$$C_{17}H_{21}NO_4 + 2H_2O = C_9H_{15}NO_3 + C_6H_5COOH + CH_3OH.$$

Ecgonine, as already stated, is closely related to tropine, and has the formula:

$$\begin{array}{ccc} CH_2 - CH & \!\!\!\!-\!\!\!\! & CH \cdot COOH \\ | & N \cdot CH_3 & | \\ | & | & CH \cdot OH \\ CH_2 - CH & \!\!\!\!-\!\!\!\! & CH_2 \end{array}$$

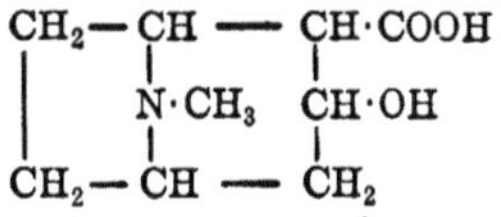

The most important pharmacological attribute of cocaine is its power of producing analgesia and anesthesia. This is not due to the ecgonine group, but usually to the "presence and relative position of the two substituting groups. The (CH_3COO) group is essential to the action of cocaine as activating the carboxyl group. The importance of the benzoyl group is shown by the fact that in its absence no anesthetic effect occurs," and moreover many other substances containing it, exert the same effects. "In ecgonine derivatives it cannot act without simultaneous replacement of the carboxyl group by a COOR group, and the presence of the two groups alone in such a simple substance as benzoic methyl ester, $C_6H_5COOCH_3$, is sufficient to produce local anesthesia."

As already indicated, Ehrlich referred to the C_6H_5CO group as the anesthesiphore radicle. The $N(CH_3)$ group is an "auxotox," and on it, depends the liver degeneration. Thus it is possible to analyze cocaine into its more important radicles and to explain rationally its various properties on the grounds of its chemical constituents.

Opium Alkaloids.—Opium contains several alkaloids, the more important being morphine, papaverin, codeine, narcotine, narcine, and thebain. Their properties have been known for a long period. Recently, through the work of Macht ([17]), our knowledge of their nature, mechanism, and cause of action has been greatly enhanced.

Macht began his studies by investigating the action of the opium alkaloids individually, and in combination with each other on the respiratory tract. He demonstrated (a) that, on the bronchi, narcotine and papaverin are dilators, as are also morphine and codeine, but to a less extent. The other alkaloids have no such effects. Morphine and narcotine act antagonistically; (b) that morphine and codeine are sedative or depressant, while narcotine, papaverin, narcine, and thebain are stimulating to the respiratory centers; and (c) that the combined action of opium alkaloids is a combination of their individual effects.

He later studied quantitatively the analgesic effects of the six principal opium alkaloids and found the effective dose to be: morphine

(10 mg.), papaverin (40), codeine (20), narcotin (30), narcine (10), thebain (10), respectively. On combining morphine and narcotin, meconates (narcophin), the analgesic power is greater than the arithmetical sum of the effects of its constituents. Therefore, true synergism exists in this combination.

Later studies followed dealing with the action through the sacral autonomics of several of these alkaloids and other drugs on the ureter. An effort was then made to determine the relation of the action of these alkaloids to their chemical structure. Morphine belongs to the pyridine phenanthrene group,

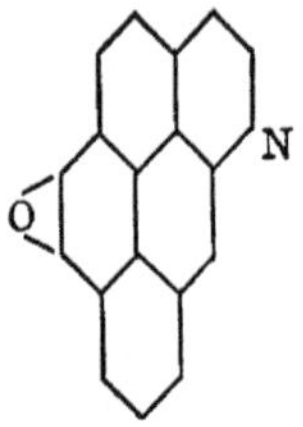

papaverin and narcotin to the benzyl isoquinolin group,

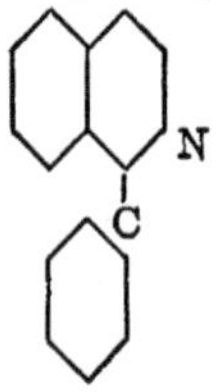

Morphine was found to increase contraction and tonicity, and papaverin to inhibit contraction and to induce relaxation. In combinations such as pantopon, the benzoyl isoquinolin radicle action predominates. This group was therefore investigated, with the result that the relation of the relaxation to the combination of a double nucleus; namely, the combination of an isoquinolin with a benzyl component was discovered. The isoquinolin radicle itself does not produce relaxation. The benzyl group, therefore, was considered responsible for the inhibitory and sedative action of papaverin and narcotin. Confirmation was obtained in the action of peronin, which is a benzyl morphine. Unlike morphine and its other derivatives, it produces inhibition. An hypothesis was advanced that the inhibitory action of papaverin on the ureter is due to the benzyl constituent and that the stimulating action of morphine is due to the piperidin constituent. Extension of the work to the gall bladder yielded confirmatory results, but the contraction of the gall bladder produced by morphine and analogous bodies is slight compared with that of the ureter.

Recognition of the rôle played by the benzyl group in the relaxation of unstriped muscles led him to further investigation of the properties of the benzyl nucleus, and to the discovery of its value as a local anesthetic. Benzyl alcohol or phenmethylol has the formula, C_7H_8O or

$$\text{CH}_2\text{OH}$$

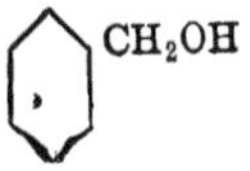

In nature it occurs in jasmine and as an ester in the balsams of Peru and of Tolu. Compared with the well known local anesthetics it possesses powerful local anesthetic properties, and at the same time is relatively non-toxic. Clinically in one to four per cent. solution it is an effective safe local anesthetic.

The esters, benzyl acetate

$$\text{CH}_3\text{CO}_2\text{H}_2\text{C} \overset{\text{CH}\quad\text{CH}}{\underset{\text{CH}\quad\text{CH}}{\big\langle}}\text{CH}$$

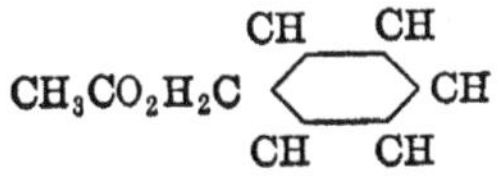

and benzyl benzoate

$$\text{H}_5\text{C}_6\text{CO}_2\text{H}_2\text{C} \overset{\text{CH}\quad\text{CH}}{\underset{\text{CH}\quad\text{CH}}{\big\langle}}\text{CH}$$

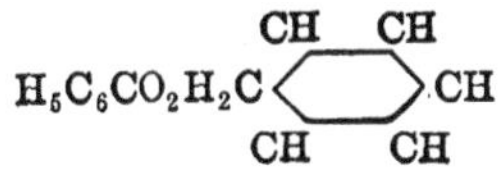

were next studied, and found to act much like papaverin. They are metabolized, are low in toxicity, and have been employed by Macht with excellent results in conditions of excessive peristalsis of smooth muscle.

Macht, through analyzing the structure of various alkaloids, has succeeded in determining the properties of the various groups, and through the recognition of the importance of the benzyl group has placed in the hands of the profession a valuable local anesthetic, and two general sedatives capable of overcoming undue contraction of smooth muscles.

Quinine, $C_{20}H_{24}N_2O_2$. Quinolin

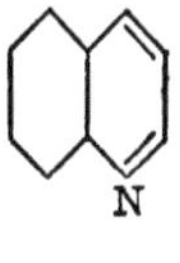

is the structural skeleton of the active principle of quinine and also of nux vomica. It is an antiseptic, and decreases metabolic rate. But it is irritating to the gastric intestinal tract, and cannot be used internally. It, and its isomers, have many properties in common with pyridine. Quinine is oxymethyl cinchonin with the formula as ascribed by Skraup:

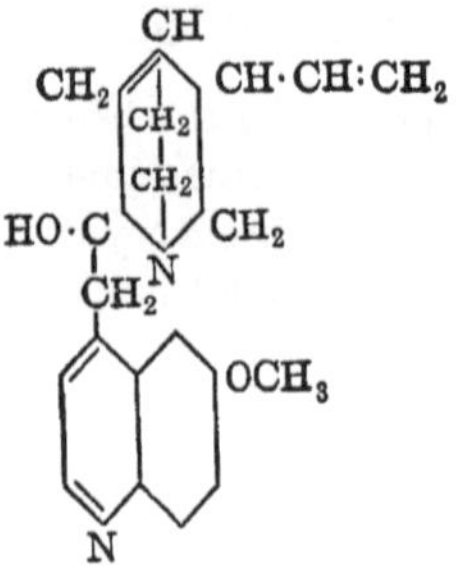

Quinoline itself has but little antipyretic action in malaria, has but little effect on the parasite, and in pneumonia has no effect on the fever.

At the present time it has not been determined in which radicle the potency of quinine resides. It is not thought to be in the quinoline constituent. Discussion has been centered about the vinyl ($CH:CH_2$) group in the side chain. Hunt ([18]) has shown, however, that the alteration of the vinyl group in quinine to CH_2CH_3 or to $CHOH{\cdot}CH_3$, and $CHCl{\cdot}CH_3$ does not appreciably influence its effect against infusoria.

Cupreine has come into some prominence in medicine because of its effect in pneumonia. Quinine is methyl cupreine. Morgenroth demonstrated that in pneumonia of mice ethyl hydroxy cupreine exercises an effect little short of specific.

Influence of Metabolism

Drugs after administration may undergo great alterations. Given by mouth, changes occur frequently before the tissues are reached. In the mouth there is no change, as a rule. In the stomach the free HCl tends to increase the solubility of basic substances, and to break down anilides. In the intestine the bile and pancreatic juice cause saponification of fats, and esterification also increases the solubility of some organic acids. Generally speaking, the drugs are changed in such a way that they become less toxic.

The chief changes, however, occur in the blood and tissues. Synthesis, oxidation, and reduction are the three processes best understood. In synthesis, combinations occur with sulphonic, glycuronic, and glycocollic acids, the end-results being most frequently urea and its derivatives, glycuronates, sulphocyanides, and sulphocarbolates. These processes are of great importance in the process of detoxification. Oxidation affects many drugs in the same manner as it does foodstuffs, the end products being CO_2 and H_2O. Partial oxidation facilitates further oxidation. The primary alcohols oxidize to aldehydes and acids, the secondary to ketones, while tertiary alcohols tend to break down into simpler compounds. The nature of the process is but incompletely understood. In the aromatic hydrocarbons the ring is usually left intact, oxidation affecting the groups substituting the H atoms of the ring. Benzoic acid frequently results, combines with glycocoll, and is excreted as hippuric acid. Oxidation of hydrogen in the beta position sometimes yields beta oxybutyric acid, diacetic acid, and acetone.

Reduction is effected in the body with more difficulty and instances are relatively rare, but chloral is reduced to the corresponding alcohol and excreted as a glycuronate, and some nitro-bodies are reduced to corresponding amines.

Vital Force has been a subject of controversy for long periods. With a clearer understanding of various forces, the types of forces are disappearing. Radiant energy is now classed as a branch of chemical science, and chemical and electrical energy are probably one and the same form of energy. In considering, as one must, the mutual relationship of the drug and cell, involved in pharmacological action, it appears that we have many theories involving facts of very diverse nature. In all probability a combination of forces plays a rôle. Barger and Dale ([19]) say, "The least unsatisfactory view seems to us to be that which regards the existence of stimulant activity as dependent on the processes of some chemical property, the distribution, and, in the main, the intensity of activity as due to a physical property."

(4) Specific Chemotherapy and Experimental Therapy

The surest and usually the shortest approach to the specific treatment of any condition is through the experimental reproduction of the disease in animals and through the subsequent application of experimental therapy. Science is built on experimentation. Nature's secrets are well shielded. Facts must be pried from her through experimentation, scientific methods constituting a fulcrum. But in the human, only the most limited experimentation is possible. Human life is too valuable, only in desperate conditions are desperate remedies justified. But desperate conditions do not permit of recovery as a rule even though the treatment be correct in principle.

The value of human life has retarded progress in therapy by blocking the channels through which science ordinarily flows. In consequence the physician is limited in his practice to well established, usually time-honored, partially effective, non-harmful measures. His responsibility is heavy, and he adheres to the ancient principle, "primum non nocere." Science is not built on isolated observations, but on laws established through the study of behavior in repeated experiments under conditions accurately controlled.

Although desperate remedies are rarely justified, they are frequently needed. Once laws governing their action have been established, the element of danger can be quantitatively determined, and in some instances practically eliminated. These laws can only be established through ascertaining the proximity of death, which means that death itself must result in certain instances. This obviously eliminates human experimentation from consideration, and hence, we resort to lower animals. With the experimental disease, all the tools of science are made available, the only limitations existing being those of the investigator.

Aside from pharmacology, experimental therapy centers about three major fields, specific chemotherapy, immunotherapy, and organotherapy. Each of these constitutes an independent branch of science.

Specific Chemotherapy of Trypanosomiasis

This field of science was created almost entirely through the labors of Paul Ehrlich ([20]), which culminated in the introduction of salvarsan (" 606 "), and of neosalvarsan. The character of the work involved, the underlying principles covered, and the factors leading to practical results can be best presented by quotations from his preface in his masterpiece, " Spirilloses and Their Treatment." " A medicinal substance can only act upon the bodily system into which it has been incorporated. The object of the researches was to find a distinct curative type and to improve it more and more by means of transformation and substitution. Whereas, formerly the substances were offered to the medical man by the chemist for testing purposes, the conditions could now be reversed, and the chemotherapeutist could give the chemist points which lead to the desired recovery of genuine curative substances." In this way he substituted science for chance. " It was far more a question of putting the principles of action of medicine on a therapeutic basis, the study of what I should like to describe as the therapeutic biology of parasites. The success of my work depends upon the conception of chemoceptors obtained in these researches." In relation to syphilis, he further says, " It was only by knowledge of the parasite which causes the disease, and through the possibility of transferring it to animals, that experimental chemotherapeutic work is rendered possible, while the specific blood reaction is indispensable in determining the genuine curative action."

The discovery of trypanosomes ([21]) as the cause of disease in animals, surra of camels by Evans (1880), nagana by Bruce, dourine by Rouget (1894), and their occurrence in humans, by Dutton (1901), and their etiological relationship to sleeping sickness by Castellani (1903), led to the experimental production of these diseases in animals and to attempts at their cure.

Laveran in 1903 demonstrated that arsenious acid exerted a marked toxicity on trypanosomes, but was incapable of effecting á cure in infected animals. Thomas ([22]) of the Liverpool School of Tropical Medicine used atoxyl in experimental trypanosomiasis with good results, and sought other forms of arsenic, less toxic for the host. He considered atoxyl to be the sodium salt of the anilid of meta-arsenic acid, with the formula

$$
\bigcirc \!\!\! \rangle NH - \underset{\underset{ONa}{|}}{\overset{\overset{ONa}{|}}{As}} = O
$$

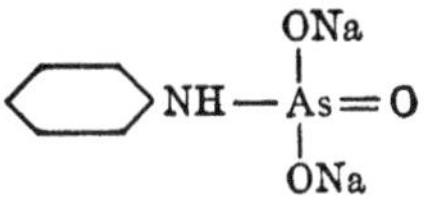

Ehrlich, who had previously tried and discarded atoxyl in his studies on trypanosomiasis, interested himself in it again subsequent to the report of Thomas and Brienl ([20]). With the assistance of Bertheim ([20]), he investigated atoxyl chemically, being puzzled by certain of its reactions. He finally concluded that it was not an anilide of meta-arsenic acid, but the sodium salt of para-amino-phenyl-arsénic acid,

$$
NH_2 \langle\!\!\!\bigcirc\!\!\!\rangle \underset{\underset{ONa}{|}}{\overset{\overset{O\ddot{N}a}{|}}{As}} = O
$$

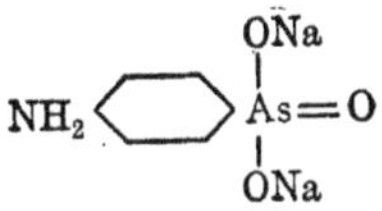

This discovery was of the greatest significance to medical science, and constituted the basis of the work which resulted in the development of chemotherapy. Thomas made definite progress by establishing the value of atoxyl, and in calling attention to the desirability of searching for arsenicals with greater toxicity for parasites and with decreased toxicity for the host. Ehrlich, on the other hand, found the key to greater progress in recognizing the true nature of atoxyl. The first conception of it, as a fixed analid, admits of no great changes in the molecule, whereas its true formula reveals the possibility of the preparation of a whole series of compounds. The NH_2 group can be acetylated, benzoated, can be substituted by halogen or by hydroxyl radicles. In this way arsacetin resulted with the formula,

$$
COCH_3NH \langle\!\!\!\bigcirc\!\!\!\rangle \underset{\underset{OH}{|}}{\overset{\overset{OH}{|}}{As}} = O,
$$

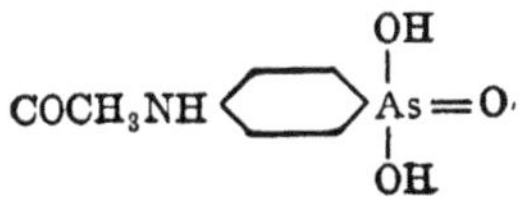

This was found to possess decided advantages over atoxyl, being more stable and somewhat less toxic, while equally parasititropic. It was used clinically in sleeping sickness with fair results.

Ehrlich's efforts were next directed to determining the method in which atoxyl acts. In vitro it was not strikingly toxic to trypanosomes, but after administration serum containing it, it was extremely toxic acting in dilution of 1/120,000 according to Koch. Ehrlich conceived the idea that the increase in toxicity after administration was due to reduction of the arsenic; i.e. that the arsenic became trivalent instead of pentavalent. In this connection, the following facts were established:

$$NH_2 \langle \rangle \overset{O}{\underset{OH}{As-OH}}$$

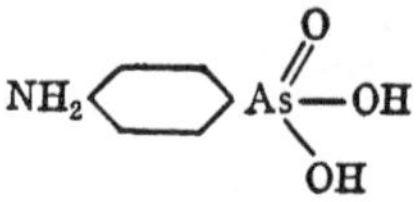

(atoxyl) does not kill in five per cent. solution in one hour;

$$OH \langle \rangle \overset{O}{\underset{OH}{As-OH}}$$

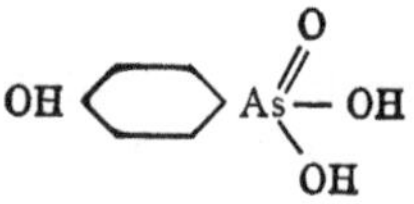

(p. oxyphenyl arsenic acid) kills in one to two per cent. solution;

$$\langle \rangle As=O$$

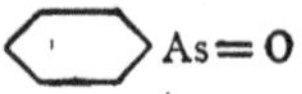

(arsenoxide) kills in 1/100,000 in one hour;

$$OH \langle \rangle As=O$$

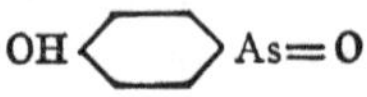

(paroxyphenyl arsenoxide) kills in 1/1,000,000 in one-half hour. Reduction has resulted in increased toxicity, as it has done in many other instances, CO being more toxic than CO_2 and HCN than HCNO. Ehrlich decided that the toxic body concerned in the death of the parasite was not atoxyl but the reduced form of

$$OH \langle \rangle As=O$$

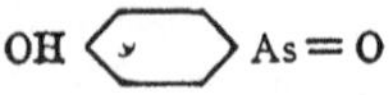

Salvarsan can be made directly from atoxyl. It is easier, however, to start with paroxy-phenyl-arsenic acid

$$OH \langle \rangle \overset{O}{\underset{OH}{As=OH}}$$

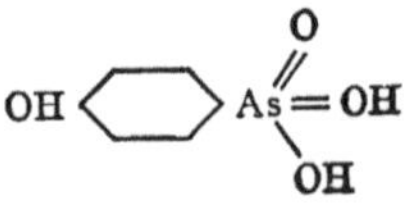

When properly treated with nitrous acid, this yields a compound, meta-nitro-paroxy-phenyl-arsenic acid,

$$NO_2 \quad\quad O$$
$$HO\langle\ \rangle As\!\!=\!\!OH$$
$$\backslash OH$$

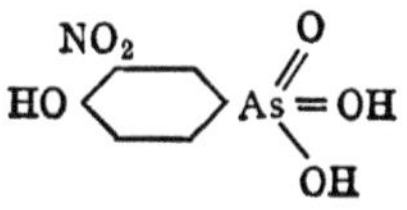

On further reduction, this yields meta-amido-paroxy-phenyl-arsenic acid,

$$NH_2 \quad\quad O$$
$$HO\langle\ \rangle As\!-\!OH$$
$$OH$$

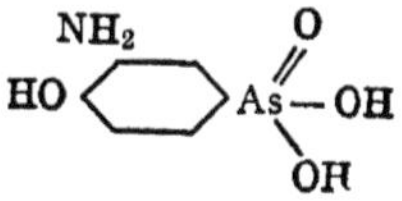

and later meta amido-para-oxyphenyl arsinic oxide.

$$NH_2$$
$$OH\langle\ \rangle As\!=\!O$$

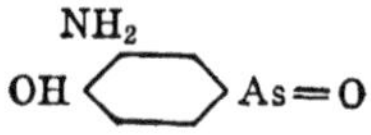

which in turn can be further reduced to dioxy-diamido-arseno benzol,

$$NH_2 \quad\quad\quad\quad NH_2$$
$$OH\langle\ \rangle As\!=\!As\langle\ \rangle\!-\!OH$$

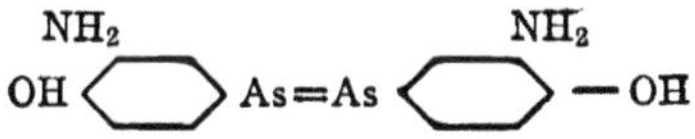

The reduced form $(R - As = As - R)$ is much less toxic for the host than $R - As = O$.

Salvarsan is marketed in vacuum tubes in order to prevent oxidation, which readily occurs on exposure, and results in great increase in toxicity. By the addition of hydrochloric acid, it is readily converted into the acid salt, NH_2HCl. By the addition of NaOH, it is neutralized, and forms the alkaline base

$$NH_2 \quad\quad\quad\quad NH_2$$
$$NaO\langle\ \rangle As\!=\!As\langle\ \rangle ONa$$

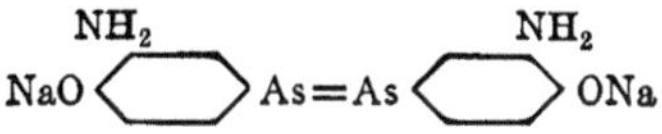

which is the form in which it is administered. It is locally irritating, and therefore given now exclusively by the intravenous route.

Neosalvarsan, or " 914," was later introduced by Ehrlich, being somewhat less toxic, and decidedly less irritating locally. It is obtained from salvarsan by the addition of formaldosulphoxylate. A sulphoxyl group has the formula SO OH, is derived from the sulphoxyl acid (H·SOOH), and corresponds to the carboxyl group COOH. Salvarsan combines with sodium formaldosulphoxylate (HCOHOSNa), which is a condensation product of H_2SO_2 (sulphoxylic or hyposulphurous acid) and formaldehyde (HCOH).. Neosalvarsan has the formula,

$$\underset{\text{OH}}{\overset{\text{NH}_2}{\bigcirc}} \text{As} = \text{As} \underset{\text{OH}}{\overset{\text{NHCH}_2\text{O--OSNa}}{\bigcirc}}$$

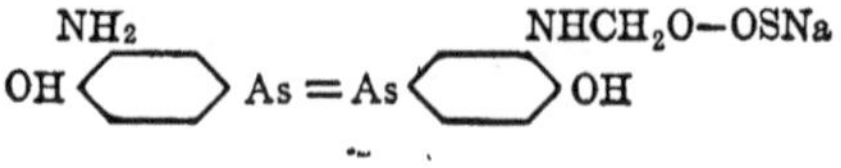

and being readily soluble in water and locally non-irritant, may be injected subcutaneously or intramuscularly.

The work of Ehrlich constitutes one of the most remarkable achievements of modern medicine. It furnished mankind with a useful remedy, demonstrated in a most practical way that pharmacological action is dependent upon chemical structure, founded chemotherapy, and revealed the methods whereby the creation of specific treatment is made possible. He aimed at a cure in one dose for syphilis, a " Therapia sterilisans magna." In this he did not altogether succeed, but he produced the most effective remedy yet found for syphilis and blazed the way for future progress.

Ehrlich's Experiments with Trypanosomes.—Ehrlich's own animal experiments were conducted on trypanosomes, and it was from these studies that he acquired the principles which resulted later in such great discoveries.

Mice and rats are readily infected with many species of trypanosomes, notably T. brucei, T. evansi, T. gambiense, and T. equiperdum. Only one who has worked with trypanosomiasis in mice can appreciate the opportunities it offers. No more ideal conditions for experimental therapy can be desired. A given strain will result in death of the animals with clock-like regularity as to time. The severity of the infection can be readily ascertained by the number of organisms in the blood, as can also the rate of disappearance of the organisms as the result of therapy. In addition, large numbers of animals can be handled at one time, the only facilities needed being jars or cages, syringes, glass slides, and a microscope. The technique is simplicity itself.

Successful treatment furnishes one of the most spectacular phenomena ever witnessed in the field of therapy. A seriously infected animal lying on its side, too weak to move, and with as many as two or three million wriggling trypanosomes swarming in each cubic millimeter of blood, may, as the result of a single treatment, return within one or two hours to absolute normality so far as can be determined. With the disappearance of clinical evidence of disease, the organisms disappear entirely from the blood. This transformation within an hour from death's door to normality must be seen to be appreciated.

The principles established, and the laws discovered by Ehrlich, are as follows:

(1) No organism is affected by a drug unless it is incorporated in the organism, or in Ehrlich's own words, "Corpora non agunt nisi fixata," which, as applied to chemotherapy, must be interpreted, "parasites can only be destroyed by those materials for which they have a certain affinity, thanks to which they are anchored by the bacteria." In this connection, he assumed the presence of chemoceptors.

(2) Remedies affect both the host and the parasite, "only those substances can be employed as medicaments in which organotrophy and parasitotrophy stand in proper relation."

(3) By accepting the best remedy available, it is possible through modification of its constitution to change its properties, and further through experimentation and control it is possible to increase parasitotrophic and decrease organotrophic properties. Thus in using atoxyl as the basis, the potent part of the molecule was sought. Trivalent arsenic was recognized as the essential factor. Experimentation proved the possibility of increasing the toxicity of the arsenic of the molecule for the parasite, and by working on the benzyl end of the molecule its toxicity for the host was decreased. Three objects were attained, (a) diminished toxicity, (b) increased action on the parasite, (3) increased stability of the combination.

(4) In chemotherapy experience teaches what types of changes in the molecule are desirable, in other words, the constitution of a chemical determines its action, and the laws governing organotrophic and parasitotrophic properties can be recognized and utilized. The investigator, therefore, must direct the work of the chemist, suggesting changes in molecules as they are deemed desirable, and not testing drugs made at random by the chemist.

(5) Closely allied organisms differ in pathogenicity, in the acuteness of the resulting disease and in their resistance to a given therapy, while different strains apparently causing the same disease also may differ from each other in the same respects. For example, T. lewisi and T. nagana are both trypanosome infections. In rats, nagana kills quickly and produces a fatal disease, which, however, responds readily to treatment with arsenic; whereas T. lewisi, which occurs naturally in rats, does not as a rule prove fatal, and is totally resistant to arsenicals. In sleeping sickness in Togoland, many cures were reported with arseno phenyl glycin, whereas the disease as encountered in the Congo was much more resistant.

(6) Cures are the more readily obtained the earlier the treatment is instituted.

(7) Relapses, generally speaking, are more difficult to cure than original infections.

(8) Treatment unsuccessful in the first instance is usually unsuccessful in repetition.

(9) Repeated non-curing treatments frequently result in progressively decreased effects on the parasite. This condition Ehrlich calls "Festigkeit," which indicates that the strain has become fast, tolerant, or resistant to the drug.

(10) Repeated non-curing treatments with some preparations result in the development of hypersensitiveness on the part of the host to the medicament. This was demonstrated by Kline, Eckard, Ullrich, and by Scherschmidt.

(11) As the ultimate cure by one dose is desirable and best, a "therapia sterilisans magna" should be sought.

Ehrlich's work was some years in progress. Collaborators working clinically, especially in Africa, assisted in recognizing and establishing some of these laws so that clinical as well as laboratory experience contributed to the solution of the problems. Some of the principles enumerated were recognized independently by other investigators.

It is interesting to note that among thousands of preparations investigated by Ehrlich and others, only four groups of drugs have been found which are strikingly effective in trypanosomiasis. These are as follows:

(1) Certain arsenicals, arsenious acid, atoxyl, arsacetin, arsenophenylglycin, salvarsan, and neosalvarsan.

(2) Certain azo dyes; (a) trypan blue,

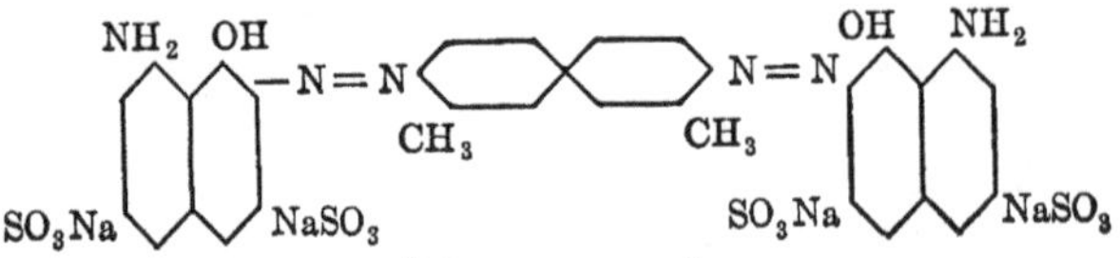

(b) trypan red,

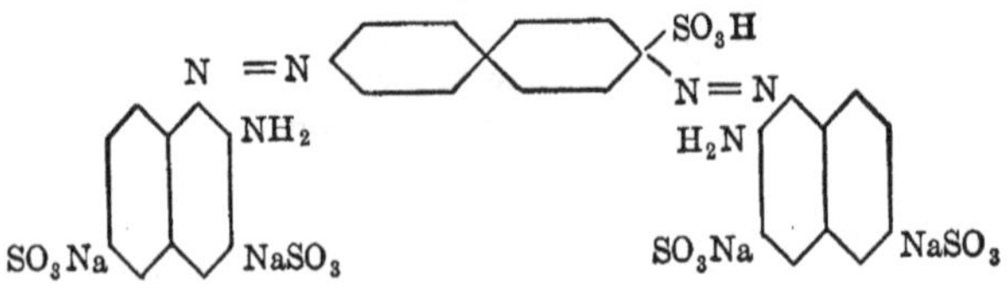

(3) Certain triphenyl methane basic dyes, parafuchsin, pyronin, and methyl violet,

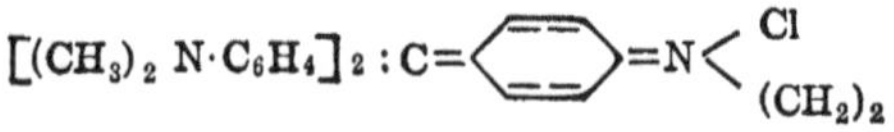

(4) Certain antimony preparations—antimony tartrates of potassium and sodium, tartar emetic, $K(SbO)$ $C_4H_4O_6 + \frac{1}{2}H_2O$, p. amino phenyl stibinic acid (corresponding to atoxyl),

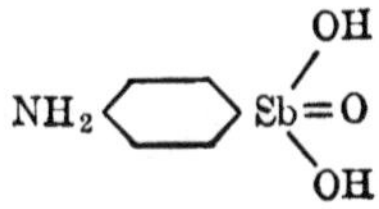

Aniline antimonyl tartrate,

$$Sb \overset{C_4H_4O_6}{\underset{OHC_6H_7N}{<}}$$

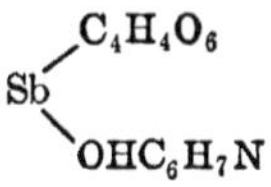

Triamids of antimony, thio glycollate,

$$Sb - \overset{SCH_2CONH_2}{\underset{SCH_2CONH_2}{\overset{SCH_2CONH_2}{<}}}$$

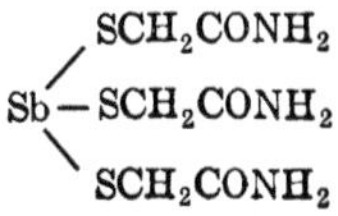

Sodium antimony thioglycollate,

$$Sb \overset{SCH_2COONa}{\underset{SCH_2COO}{<}}$$

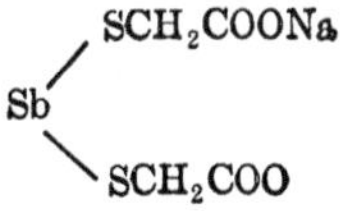

In 1909, before salvarsan was introduced, Dr. Abel and the writer became interested in chemotherapy and carried out experiments throughout 1910 and 1911. Our interest centered chiefly on the effects of antimonials and arsenicals in trypanosomiasis, though, as will be seen, later we also worked with spirilla and spirochetae. The trypanosomes used were: (1) T. brucei, which is responsible for the tsetse fly disease which affects horses, mules, donkeys, and cattle in Africa; (2) T. evansi (strains from India and Mauritius), which produces diseases of camels and cattle; (3) T. equiperdum, which affects horses, producing dourine, instances of which are not infrequent in this country. The experimental animals employed were rats, rabbits, and dogs, some of which were under observation for a year to eighteen months.

Prior to these studies, antimony had been tried by others, Cushny first suggesting its use. Sodium and potassium salts of antimony, tartrates (Thomson and Plimmer), p. amido phenyl stibinic acid (Breinl and Nierenstein), sodium antimony malate, ethyl antimonyl tartrate (Collie, Thomson, and Cushny), and aniline antimony tartrate (Laveran); of these, tartar emetic proved effective, but very irritating locally.

The substitution of an alkyl radicle as in ethyl antimonyl tartrate resulted in definite improvement in this respect, no local reactions whatever following its use, and cure being effected in seven of the thirteen rats treated.

In our work two new compounds of antimony were prepared, the triamide of antimony thioglycollate, and sodium antimony thioglycollate. These chemicals were tested in regard to their efficacy as trypanocidal agents in several series of inoculated rats, rabbits, and dogs.

The difference in the virulence in the diseases produced by these strains of trypanosomes is striking; T. brucei and T. evansi killed rats regularly in 72 to 84 hours, while that of Mauritius and of Dourine were much less virulent, a week or even a month elapsing before death in some instances. The greatest success was obtained with the triamide of antimony thioglycollate and with sodium antimony thioglycollate.

The time elapsing between the date of inoculation and the beginning of treatment is the most important factor in determining the results obtained. The longer the period before the institution of treatment, the less the degree of success from the point of view of ultimate cure; the shorter the period, the greater the success. These drugs administered 24 hours before inoculation failed to protect, but given at the time of the inoculation prevented the development of the disease in every instance. With the more virulent trypanosomes, after the lapse of 24 hours, at which time organisms were beginning to appear in the blood, absolute cure was effected, but after 48 hours or more, permanent cure was infrequent. It is possible to drive the organism from the blood, so that subinoculations fail. By intermittent graded doses it is possible to banish the organism for prolonged periods, weeks and months, but on the withdrawal of treatment, they reappear, and the disease rapidly runs its course unabated. This can be accomplished with animals which would otherwise die in the course of an hour or two. During the time that the blood is free, the animal appears perfectly normal in every respect, but when treatment is continued the animal after some months finally succumbs to the effect of the antimony.

Two problems present; namely, what becomes of trypanosomes, and how do relapses develop?

Examination of the blood subsequent to treatment reveals morphologic changes in the trypanosomes. They become slower and tardy in their movements. Their bodies become constricted, and they take on a more granular appearance such as is commonly seen in them after death, and subsequent to the death of the host. They undergo involution. They finally become immotile; the flagella often become detached or adherent to the centrosome. The process is associated with a leucocytosis as a rule, and frequently débris from the organisms can be demonstrated in the leucocytes. Fever is present in some of the larger animals during the period of blood infection, and this may disappear promptly upon their disappearance from the blood.

Many investigators have studied the tissues of various organs in the attempt to find a lodging-place for the trypanosomes during the period in which the blood is free. Emulsions of various organs have been inoculated into animals and controlled by utilizing in others injections of blood from the heart. The claim has been made that the liver and bone marrow harbor the organism during this period, and that inoculations from these tissues are frequently successful at the time that the inoculations from the heart blood fail. Others question this, and feel that the further removed from relapse, the more frequent the emulsions from organs fail, and that only immediately subsequent to treatment, and just before relapse, is it possible to get positive results from organs, at which time the blood is also positive if a sufficient amount is investigated.

Ehrlich believes that there exists during this period a true immunity. This immunity is specific for the single strain concerned, and the immunity reaction may be utilized for the differentiation of strains. Subsequently, when this immunity wears off, generally speaking, reinoculation results in infections analogous in every respect to the original infection. In this connection, Terry has utilized the method to prove that surra of India and surra of Mauritius are not identical. He cures surra of India in a mouse, and then injects a mixture of surra of Mauritius and surra of India, and proves to his satisfaction that the animal develops only surra of Mauritius. Provided this is true, it is perhaps the most striking instance of drug specificity known to medical science.

Relapses are difficult to explain, but the following hypotheses have been suggested:

(*a*) That on treatment, some of the organisms are driven into hiding in some of the internal organs, where they are not subjected to the action of the drug. Subsequently they reappear in the circulation and cause reinfection.

(*b*) That not all trypanosomes are equally susceptible to the influence of drugs, and that the more resistant organisms persist. This is strongly suggested by studies of the action of drugs on trypanosomes in hanging drop preparations. After the vast majority of organisms are killed, it is not at all unusual to find isolated trypanosomes still very active.

(*c*) That trypanosomes undergo cycles in development, and that they are more resistant in some parts of the cycle than in others.

Drug Resistance

Tolerance.—During the course of the work with trypan red and arsenicals Ehrlich and his collaborators found that non-curative doses, which at first sufficed to cause disappearance of the organisms from the blood, lost this power subsequently in the same animal. Larger doses at first gave some effect, but eventually even maximal doses failed to have demonstrable effect on trypanosomes. This strain on passage through another animal of the same species remained resistant for many generations. This phenomenon Ehrlich called "Festigkeit." It was this resistance which particularly interested him, and caused him to continue his work with trypanosomes, and it was the study of drug resistance which led to the fundamental conception of chemotherapy responsible ultimately for the introduction of "606." This tolerance on the part of trypanosomes holds only for the particular type of remedy used, arsenic, antimony, or dye substance, but once firmly established, it holds for other members of the same group. Thus, a strain which is resistant to fuchsin is also immune to the related basic dyes, but not against azo dyes, arsenicals, or antimonials. Similarly, a strain resistant to arsacetin is also resistant to atoxyl. The resistance to atoxyl is easiest obtained, next, to arsenophenylglycin, and finally to tartar emetic.

In relation to arsenic resistance, a peculiar phenomenon is observed. A strain may be made resistant to atoxyl, without being resistant to arsenious acid, arsenophenylglycin or antimony. In the attempt to make this strain resistant to arsenious acid, resistance to antimony, or better to tartar emetic, develops. Another striking peculiarity is the development of a temporary resistance to tartar emetic in producing an arsacetin fast strain without developing resistance to arsenious acid. Apparently resistance to arsenious acid is accomplished by resistance to most arsenical derivatives. According to Ehrlich's conception, the trypanosome has many chemoceptors. In relation to arsenic and its acetyl derivatives, there exists at least two. The formation of one (the arsenoceptor) by atoxyl does not interfere with the acetylceptor which can be brought into play in relation to arsacetin.

It is difficult to see why it is easier to obtain resistance to tartar emetic by first establishing tolerance for atoxyl. In relation to resistance, it is interesting to note that with the antimonials employed by Abel and the writer, no resistance developed, except perhaps in relation to the donkey. In rats, many treatments with many passages did not result in the slightest diminution of the effect of the antimonials employed.

The Rôle of the Host.—A drug resistant race produces a disease similar in every respect to that of the non-resistant race. The resistance itself remains the same through many generations (thousands) in as many as 100 passages through the same species. Passage through another animal usually does not affect the resistance; thus a strain, atoxyl resistant in the mouse, remained unchanged in 46 subsequent passages through rats, no treatment with atoxyl having been given in the meantime. In transfer to another animal, the disease runs its natural course in that animal and the strain regains, as a rule, its original sensitiveness to the drug in question.

In working with the donkey, Brienl and Nierenstein encountered resistance to atoxyl which persisted in transferring the strain to the rat. In our work, we found in two rats, which were infected from blood of the donkey under treatment with antimony, a temporary resistance to antimony. Unquestionably the resistance to the drug is most marked in the animal in which the resistance is established, but a lesser degree of resistance is sometimes encountered in passage to a new species. Resistance is a property of the strain but is most marked in the species in which it was created.

Naturally, in relation to arsenic tolerance, the arsenic eaters, the mountaineers of Styria, come to mind. Whether or not heredity plays a rôle in this has never been determined. By some the increased tolerance is ascribed to lessened absorption, by others to increased excretion. That it exerts a decreased effect on the gastrointestinal mucosa has, however, been definitely determined.

Specific Chemotherapy of Spirilla

Hata ([24]), working in Ehrlich's laboratories, carried on work on spirilla, utilizing the same drugs that Ehrlich used in his work on trypanosomes. His investigations dealt with the spirilla of relapsing fever, of chicken spirillosis, and of syphilis.

Spirilla of Relapsing Fever.—The effect of each chemical was first studied in the test tube, the drug dissolved in water or alcohol being added to a blood-containing spirilla mixture diluted with physiological salt solution or isotonic sugar solution to a constant quantity. Usually a dilution of the blood of thirty- to forty-fold was attained. The motility of the spirillae was investigated at the end of one hour, immotility being interpreted as death.

The animal experiments were carried out with mice and rats with an attenuated virus, but with equal infections so far as possible in all cases; i.e. one in which the organism could be found in the blood of the animal on the following day and in about equal numbers, this necessitating constantly greater dilution for the same quantity injected, since virulence increases with constant passage. The amount of blood necessary for this varied with different strains, and with different conditions. Nevertheless it was possible to obtain a fairly constant infection. The disease, as its name indicates, presents frequent relapses, provided the animal does not die in the first attack. Animals were grouped in series according to the mortality of the untreated condition, inasmuch as continuous passage through one specifies invariably results in increased virulence. Chemicals were administered on the day after inoculations, and the blood studied microscopically thereafter for a period of 60 days, since relapses occur as late as 50 days.

In some instances test tube and animal experiments give similar results but not invariably. Obviously the animal experiments yield the truer criterion for practical results. The most striking results were obtained with arsenicals. The three arsenicals, atoxyl, arsacetin, and arsenophenylglycin, were practically inert against the spirilla. Arsenophenol was itself more effective, while its derivative, dioxy diamido-arseno-benzol, both as acid and alkaline salt was wonderfully effective. The effect in the test tube is but slight, solutions of 1/10,000 being necessary to kill the spirilla. Organisms subjected to 1/10,000 solution of the drug, if still motile, cause the disease but with a modified course. With dilution of 1/100,000 the disease develops immediately. Permanent cure, however, could be effected on the first day following inoculation by doses well below the danger line.

Hata determined the toxicity of dioxy diamido arsenobenzol for various animals with the following result:

Animal	*Application*	*Dose tolerated*
Mouse	subcutaneously	1 : 300 per 20 gms.*
	intravenously	1 : 300 " 20 "
Rat	subcutaneously	0.2 gram per kg.
Hen	intramuscularly	0.25 " " "
	intravenously	0.08 " " "
Rabbit	subcutaneously	0.1 " " "
	intravenously	0.15 " " "

* 1 c.c. of 1/300 soln.

Animals vary somewhat in susceptibility to both the disease and the drug. But by taking a series of animals it is possible to arrive at a fair average in relation to both. The important desideratum to determine is the relation of the curative dose to the dose tolerated. Thus for mice Hata found the following in relation to permanent cure:

Dose	*One Treatment*	*Two Treatments*	*Three Treatments*
1 : 600	100 per cent.		
1 : 700	100 " "		
1 : 800	100 " "		
1 : 1000	75 " "	100 per cent.	
1 : 1500	18 " "	75 " "	100 per cent.
1 : 2000	16 " "	66 " "	100 " "
1 : 3000	0 " "	0 " "	33 " "

This result is important as indicating the increase in effectiveness in repetition of the treatment. Better results were not obtained with more than three treatments.

The dose curative as related to the dose tolerated was represented by $\left(\frac{C}{T}\right)$. The following results were obtained with single and repeated injections:

With single injections, 300/800 or 1/2.7
With two injections, 300/1000 or 1/3.3
With three injections, 300/1500-2000 or 1/5 to 1/7.

He also found that double the curative dose did not entirely protect animals which were inoculated 24 hours subsequently, although the course of the disease was modified. Rats, he found, tolerated relatively large doses, and the $\frac{C}{T}$ was more constant (0.06 to 0.08 gms. per kg.), completely sterilized and was well tolerated in all instances.

As the result of his work it was evident that relapsing fever in mice and rats could be readily cured by single doses of these arsenicals, without untoward effects of any kind.

Experiments with Spirillosis of Fowls.—Spirillosis of chickens is easily cured by arsenicals. Uhlenhuth and Gross demonstrated the effectiveness of atoxyl, and Uhlenhuth and Manteufel that of atoxyl acid mercury. The blood of canaries on the third day was diluted 15 to 20 times with salt solution so that it showed about 20 spirilla to the field, and of this mixture 0.5 c.c. was injected intramuscularly. In Hata's work, treatment started on the second day, at which time the blood was but lightly infected. Untreated animals showed a mortality of thirty-three per cent. The drugs tested were injected into the pectoral muscles, and the blood of the animal was examined subsequently at frequent intervals. Many arsenicals gave good results, the best, however, being obtained with diamino-dioxy-arsenobenzol. A curative dose afforded considerable immunity. The relative value of various arsenicals is indicated in the following table compiled by Hata:

Atoxyl	0.03/0.06	C/T = ½
Arsacetin	0.03/0.1	1/3.3
Arsenophenylglycin	0.12/0.4	1/3.3
Arsenylic acid Hg.	0.04/0.1	1/2.5
Dioxydiamido arsenobenzol	0.0035/0.2	1/58
Amido phenol arsenoxyd	0.0015/0.03	1/20

Specific Chemotherapy of Spirochetes (Syphilis)

The brilliant success attending the use of arsenicals in experimental trypanosomiasis and spirillosis attracted to them widespread attention which resulted in their being tried in syphilis. Atoxyl was studied in relation to syphilis in apes by Metchnikoff ([25]), Salmon, and Uhlenhuth and his collaborators, and in syphilitic keratitis of rabbits by Uhlenhuth ([26]) and Levaditi ([27]). The results were most encouraging. In the meantime clinical studies with atoxyl were started at the suggestion of Salmon, by Lesser ([28]), Lasser, Qwanga, and von Zeissl, all reports indicating that its effect was considerable. Other arsenicals were tried, arsacetin by Neisser ([29]), arsenophenylglycin by Alt, and cacodylates by Murphy in this country.

Ehrlich and Hata applied themselves to the investigation of syphilis, using the same methods which had proved so successful in their other chemotherapeutic studies. The work was carried out on rabbits in which two forms of syphilitic diseases can be produced, namely, keratitis and syphilis of the scrotum. The efficacy of the treatment was determined by noting the effects on the lesions, and was further controlled through Wassermann studies.

Syphilis of the scrotum was first produced in rabbits by Osiola and later by Truffi ([30]). A fragment of cornea from experimental luetic keratitis is transplanted under the skin of the scrotum. In approximately two weeks a small patch of infiltration appears which increases in size to that of a bean, then breaks down, becomes encrusted, ulcerates, and presents an infiltrated raised margin. In the untreated animal, the chancre persists for as long as four or five months at times, but it is difficult to obtain a uniform disease such as one obtains in trypanosomiasis. The Wassermann becomes positive and remains so. The condition is one admirably adapted to chemotherapeutic studies, the Wassermann reaction, provided care is exercised in the selection of the inoculated animals, furnishing an excellent and reliable means of control for the general condition, while the local lesion, the chancre, lends itself to ordinary clinical investigations and to the determination of the presence or absence of treponema.

Selected infected animals were subjected to intravenous treatment in varying dosage with the different arsenicals. With diamido dioxy-arsenobenzol, Hata found that "*the spirilla can be destroyed absolutely and immediately by a single injection,*" and that "*no relapses occur,*" and that the local lesion subsequently dries up rapidly and disappears. This solved from an experimental viewpoint, at least, the treatment of syphilis. From an experimental basis the "therapia sterilisans magna" was attained.

The Introduction of Salvarsan into Practice.—The next investigation concerned the clinical value of salvarsan, as the preparation was now called. Ehrlich determined to subject it to critical tests to prove or disprove its value before introducing it into general use. He says, "many thousands of patients must be treated before the preparation should be available for general introduction. For even if a preparation has been tested in the most careful way by means of experiments on animals and has been recognized as good, this naturally does not prove that it is also applicable for human beings." Idiosyncrasy to drugs plays considerable rôle in relation to human therapy, but is apparently a negligible factor in animals. Salvarsan was therefore subjected to crucial tests in some of the leading clinics, its value established and its dangers ascertained prior to its being offered to the profession.

Special commendation must be accorded Ehrlich, not only for his brilliant work in chemotherapy, but also for the sound clinical judgment exhibited in the method adopted in introducing salvarsan into practice. It was first used in selected cases in the best clinics, under the closest supervision, its effects being carefully followed. Later it was used in types showing complications, and its contraindications and untoward manifestations determined. Eventually satisfactory methods of administration and dosage were determined so that, on coming into general use, excellent results were obtained from the first, and accidents were extremely infrequent.

These studies have the greatest significance in medicine. They have not only yielded efficacious specific treatment for syphilis, relapsing fever, and sleeping sickness, but have revealed the possibilities of actually creating specifics for disease, and have demonstrated beyond question the advisability of determining further the relation of pharmacological action to chemical constitution.

Specific Chemotherapy in Protozoal and Bacterial Diseases Contrasted

It is in the field of protozoan infection that chemotherapy has wrought such brilliant results. The plasmodium of malaria, the trypanosome of sleeping sickness, the treponema of syphilis, the spirilla of relapsing fever and of chicken spirillosis, all yield to specifics. But in infectious diseases only a beginning has been made, there being but one or two drugs in the entire pharmacopeia which may be said to exercise a specific effect on infectious diseases. (Vide infra.)

The explanation for the relative failure of drugs in infectious diseases is not apparent. Syphilis offers the best opportunity of revealing the secret as it is so closely allied to infectious diseases. For many years syphilis was considered an infectious disease due to Lustgarten's bacillus. The lesion produced is an infectious granuloma similar to that seen in tuberculosis and leprosy. Not until 1905 was the spirocheta pallidum discovered as its cause, by Schaudinn and Hoffmann.

Later this organism was reclassified and named treponema pallidum. The treponema are very closely related to spirilla which in turn are closely related to bacteria.

It is difficult to determine where protozoa end and where bacteria begin. The animal and vegetable kingdom merge in such a way that doubt often arises as to which is concerned. Reliable criteria are wanting. A comparative study of the borderline infections is of the greatest importance.

Immunity reactions interest the bacteriologist and serologist. The work on trypanosomes furnished the laws of chemotherapy which eventually lead to a cure for syphilis. The treponema, which is surpassed in versatility only by the B. typhosis, has already been brought under control. The writer is sanguine enough to expect similar results in infectious diseases when the combination of genius, perseverance, chemistry, biology, and organizing capacity of an Ehrlich is brought to bear on the problem.

(5) Infection and Antiseptics

The discovery by Pasteur of microorganisms as the cause of disease has revolutionized many of the principles and much of the practice of therapy. Immunotherapy, however, is sharply defined from pharmacology. It deals, at present, largely with infection and with specific immunity reactions. These, undoubtedly, are physiochemical in origin, but from this point of view are, as yet, but little understood. Because of the definite line of cleavage, immunity treatment will not be discussed here.

Pharmacology deals with bacteria borne diseases at but a few points, the more important being: (1) in the treatment of pneumonia; (2) in the treatment of rheumatism; (3) in the treatment of diseases of the genito-urinary tract; and (4) in antiseptic surgery, particularly in the use of the Carrel-Dakin treatment.

(*1*) *Pneumonia.*—Morgenroth and Halberstaedter demonstrated the efficacy of ethyhydroxy cuprein against the pneumococcus. In experimental pneumonia its effect is little short of specific and much greater than that of quinine. All strains of pneumococci are inhibited by it in vitro in dilution of 1/100,000. Some promising results have been secured in practice, but its application is limited owing to a tendency to produce blindness and on the whole its use so far has not been satisfactory.

(*2*) *Rheumatism.*—Much discussion has centered about the question of "specificity of action" of salicylates in rheumatism. Salicylates unquestionably lower the fever and remove the pain in the majority of cases of acute rheumatic fever. On the other hand, the incidence of endocarditis is not diminished. On the latter account, it has been argued that salicylates have no specific action, but so far as their effect on fever and pain is concerned they have a definite action and in many instances they shorten the course of the attack

(*3*) *Diseases of the Genito-urinary Tract.*—Certain chemicals manifest antiseptic action against local infection in the body. Thus hexamethylamine in acid urine unquestionably affects the colon bacillus and exerts a curative action in pyelitis and cystitis. Other chemicals, notably argyrol, protargol, and certain dyes influence the course of gonorrhea. These, however, do not belong in the same category with salvarsan and syphilis.

(*4*) *Antiseptic Surgery.*—Following the work of Pasteur and the adoption of the germ theory, Lister applied antiseptic principles to surgery. Aseptic surgery, in reality a form of preventive medicine, proved so effective that upon it was laid the greater stress, antisepsis in consequence not receiving the attention it actually merited.

But with the advent of war, came the need for antiseptic surgery. For reasons quite obvious, asepsis was inapplicable. Lister's doctrine and methods were tried, but with disappointing results, which at first were ascribed to technical inadequacies, but later to incorrect principles. In fact, eminent authorities insisted that sterilization of war wounds was impossible, and that "the treatment of suppurating wounds by means of antiseptics is illusory, and that belief in its efficacy is founded upon false reasoning." Lister's clinical observations and experiences were forgotten, replaced by theories and experiments in vitro, which failed to approach the actual conditions confronted.

The problem was attacked by Carrel ([31]) and Dakin ([32]) on simple and logical grounds, to wit, the utilization of a substance, non-irritating to the tissues and of sufficient bactericidal power to kill all microbes of all varieties present in the wound, for in the beginning at least, surgical infection is local in character. Dakin set about finding such a substance, and Carrel devoted himself to finding the most effective manner of applying it.

The problem was chemotherapeutic in nature. Methods such as were employed by Ehrlich were adopted. Various antiseptics were tried until the most desirable were determined, and these were then modified to best meet the conditions.

The Chemotherapy of the Newer Antiseptics

The germicidal action of free chlorine and the hypochlorites is well known. In medicine this action has been obtained through the use of chlorine water, chlorinated lime, Labarraque's solution (solution of chlorinated soda) and Javelle water (solution of chlorinated potash).

Hypochlorite solutions are relatively permanent, provided they are alkaline, but the degree of alkalinity encountered in Labarraque's solution, for instance, is destructive to the tissues and skin as well as to bacteria. The problem chemically consisted of retaining the bactericidal, while deleting or minimizing the tissue-destroying properties of the preparation.

Tissue destruction was found to be dependent to a large extent on the alkalinity. Therefore, the usual solution of chlorinated soda, made from chlorinated lime and monohydrated sodium carbonate, was neutralized with boric acid to the degree of alkalinity determined by experiment to be least irritating to the tissues. This was found to be at a point where, on adding powdered phenolphthalein, no color reaction occurred, while the addition of one per cent. alcoholic phenolphthalein solution still resulted in a red flash, the color quickly fading. Such a solution can be used without marked irritation to well vascularized tissues. The skin, however, proves an exception which necessitates the use of petrolatum as a protective agent.

Raschig had already shown that the addition of ammonia to hypochlorite solution resulted in the formation of chloramines. Dakin ascribed the antiseptic power of resulting compounds to the NCl grouping, since, "The parent substances from which these chloramines are prepared, whether substituted or containing chlorine attached to carbon, show no such action." A series of substances containing the NCl grouping with sulphur, benzine, naphthalene, and other radicles were investigated with the following important conclusions:

"(1) Almost all the substances examined containing the NCl group possess very strong germicidal action.

"(2) The presence in the molecule of more than one NCl group does not confer any marked increase in germicidal power.

"(3) The germicidal action of many chloramine compounds is, molecule for molecule, greater than that of sodium hypochlorite.

"(4) The chloramine derivatives of naphthaline and other di-cyclic compounds of the sulphochloramide type closely resemble the sulphur aromatic chloramines in germicidal action.

"(5) Bromamines are less effective as germicides.

"(6) Derivatives of proteins prepared by the action of sodium hypochlorite and containing NCl groups are strongly germicidal. Blood serum inhibits their germicidal action to much the same extent as it does with sodium hypochlorites and the aromatic chloramines."

Mode of Action of Hypochlorites.—Dakin has duly considered the mode of action of hypochlorites, and offers the following explanation. When the hypochlorite solution comes into contact with protein, a reaction occurs analogous to the interaction between ammonia and hypochlorites, resulting in the formation of chloramines:

$$H_2NH + NaClO = H_2N{\cdot}Cl + NaOH$$

The bactericidal effect is chemical in nature, due to such a reaction occurring in the protein of the organism itself, or in the medium in which the organism is suspended, in either instance the resulting chloramine being responsible for the death of the microbe. In this reaction, Cl is substituted for the H of the amino group (NH_2), the Cl uniting directly to the N, with the formation of chloramine. In other words, the capacity of hypochlorites to attack proteins and to form compounds with them in which the halogen is directly attached to the nitrogen is responsible for their bactericidal effect.

The destructive action of hypochlorites on skin and tissue is associated with their soda content. Their action on living tissues, according to Guillaumir and Vienne, is modified by the concentration present of other salts, a process known to the tanners as "pickling." Dakin corrected the excess alkalinity, but whatever the explanation, the fact remains that living tissues evidence marked resistance to the destructive action of Dakin's solution.

Mode of Action of Chloramines.—Chloramines kill organisms more readily or at a lower molecular concentration than corresponding hypochlorites, from which it may be argued that the compound as a whole exercises some toxicity. They react with amino-acids, peptones, and proteins in the same way as hypochlorites, thus chloramine T. (p. toluene sodium sulphochloramid) reacts with glycin in the following manner:

$$CH_3C_6H_4SO_2Na : NCl + CH_2(NH_2)COOH = CH_2(NHCl){\cdot}COONa + CH_3C_6H_4SO_2NH_2$$
$$CH_2(NHCl)COONa + H_2O = H_2CO + CO_2 + NaCl + NH_3$$

Peptones and proteins probably react in a manner similar to amino-acids, but more slowly. It appears that chloramines can act as chlorinating agents upon important constituents of living cells, and this may play an important rôle in their antiseptic properties.

As a result of these facts, Dakin drew the following tentative conclusions:

(1) The fact that proteins contain N in a form capable of attracting Cl from chloramines, is probably a factor in the germicidal action of chloramines.

(2) The superior germicidal action of chloramines over hypochlorites is due to special toxic action of the chloramine molecules, or "possibly, to selective chlorination of particular cell constituents."

Carrel's problem cannot be better summed up than has been done by himself. Speaking of his method, he says, "The method, therefore, is based upon the employment, rigorously controlled by the microscope, of an approved agent, under conditions of contact, of concentration, and of duration, established by direct experiment upon infected wounds."

In order to determine its effectiveness, an antiseptic must be considered from the following points of view: "its capacity of irritating tissues, its toxicity, its solubility, its power of penetrating the tissues, and of being absorbed by them, and the manner in which it reacts with product and other constituents of the tissues."

Each of these factors received special consideration and was made the subject of experimentation. Because of their important rôle in the action of antiseptics, proteins were considered in all their work, microörganisms being suspended in blood serum instead of water while determining the antiseptic properties of drugs. The importance of this is indicated in the following table compiled by Carrel and Dehelly from experiments of Dufresnes on the action of antiseptics on bacteria.

Antiseptics	*Without blood-serum*	*With blood-serum*
Acid carbolic	1 : 250 —	1 : 50 —
" "	1 : 500 +	1 : 100 +
Acid salicylic	1 : 2500 —	1 : 100 —
" "	1 : 5,000 +	1 : 250 +
Hydrogen peroxide	1 : 3,500 —	1 : 1,700 —
" "	1 : 8,000 +	1 : 2,000 +
Iodine "	1 : 100,000 —	1 : 1,000 —
" "	1 : 10,000,000 +	1 : 2,500 +
Bichloride of mercury	1 : 5,000,000 —	1 : 25,000 —
" " "	1 : 10,000,000 +	1 : 50,000 +
Nitrate of silver	1 : 1,000,000 —	1 : 10,000 —
" " "	1 : 10,000,000 +	1 : 25,000 +
Hypochlorite of soda	1 : 500,000 —	1 : 1,500 —
" " "	1 : 1,000,000 +	1 : 2,000 +

The sign (+) indicates that the culture is positive, and the sign (—) that it remained sterile.

The power of penetration was determined by immersion in antiseptic solution of small blocks of infected tissues, followed by incubation and subsequent cultures. In this manner it was found that hydrogen peroxide, for instance, failed to sterilize blocks of infected liver when cubes larger than one millimeter were employed, B. welchii being the infecting organism.

The effect on tissues was ascertained in the following manner: Dakin's solution, Eau de Javel, and Labarraque's solution, all of equal strengths (0.5%), were placed in containers. To each was added a fragment of skin from a stillborn babe. At the end of two hours, the fragments in Javel's and Labarraque's solutions were greatly swollen, and the epidermis readily detachable; subsequently they became transparent, and in ten to twelve hours were completely dissociated. The tissue in the Dakin's solution after twenty-four hours was in a condition similar to that existing in the other solutions after two hours.

The antiseptic solutions were next studied in infected wounds themselves. "When hypochlorite of soda is applied to a wound in such a manner that its degree of concentration remains constant, and the duration of the application is prolonged, the microbes disappear." It was determined that this result was not due to spontaneous sterilization, to mechanical washing away by the instilled liquid, or to alkalinity of the solutions. Toxicity was determined by subcutaneous and intravenous injections into animals.

The action of the antiseptics on living wounded and healthy tissue was next investigated. "Dakin's solution possesses a concentration which allows one to make use of the differences of resistance presented on the one hand by microbes, free anatomical elements and necrosed tissue, and on the other hand, normal tissue equipped with a circulation. It destroys the first and does not damage the second." The factors considered in their work in this connection were the condition of the wound, the measurement of wounds, the cicatrization of infected wounds, and the cicatrization of aseptic wounds, the influence of the drug being determined in each instance.

The following preparations, after intensive study in war surgery, have proved of value as local antiseptics: surgical solution of chlorinated soda (Carrel-Dakin), chloramine T., and dichloramine T.

The Carrel-Dakin solution in concentrations up to 0.4 or 0.5 per cent. is applied by practically continuous irrigation according to methods developed by Carrel which, however, are too technical to be discussed in this connection. Chloramine T. sodium paratoluenesulphochloramide, in one-half per cent. aqueous solution, is used in the same way. It has the advantage of greater solubility, convenience of preparation, and less local irritation, but lacks the solvent action of the hypochlorites. It can be prepared up to eight per cent. by solution in chlorcosone or chlorinated paraffin oil. Dichloramine T., or paratoluenesulphondichloramide, is but slightly soluble in water and hence is used exclusively in oil (chlorinated eucalyptus oil or chlorcosone). It is more irritant and also more solvent than chloramine T.

Surgical Experience with These Antiseptics

Abundant proof has accrued as to the value of these newer antiseptics. Opposed by some, enthusiastically received by others, they have been "weighed in the balance" in war surgery, and have not been "found wanting." Like all other remedies, they have their indications and contraindications.

In all cases, general surgical principles should first be applied. In fact, some surgeons still believe that the débrisement operation, mechanical cleansing, and physiological rest, are all that are necessary. But of those who have tried débrisement alone, and Carrel-Dakin's treatment alone, and the combination of the two, the majority recognize great virtues in these antiseptics.*

The chief value of these antiseptics is found in the treatment of infected wounds where the infection is near the wound surface or superficial in character. The exudate present appears to enhance somewhat the antiseptic action, and to prove a source of protection against tissue destruction on the part of the solution. Thus superficial abcesses, infected burns, infected abdominal wall wounds, and amputation stumps where suppuration already exists, respond particularly well. Sterilization of the ulcer with Dakin's solution immediately increases the chances for "takes" in skin grafts.

On the other hand, clinical experience has proved that in fresh uninfected wounds and in the presence of great cicatrization Dakin's solution is of but little value and harmful at times. In the former, Dakin's solution results in the destruction of tissues, especially to those poorly vascularized, such as cartilage and tendons. Nerves, on the other hand, are but little affected. In deeply infected, markedly cicatrized or stratified wounds, the treatment usually fails utterly.

In applying the treatment, certain cardinal considerations must be borne in mind; namely, contact of the solution with every part of the wound, mechanical cleansing of the wound with the removal of all foreign bodies, the use only of solutions properly prepared and of proper strength, and finally, absolute adherence to the technique described until

* These statements emanate from the large experience of my surgical colleague, Dr. J. F. Corbett, who has utilized these antiseptics extensively in war surgery and in the wards of the university hospital.

such time as experimental and clinical proof is furnished of the superiority of modifications. Only by strict observance of these directions can the best results be obtained.

(6) The Rôle Played by Glands of Internal Secretion

Metabolism.—Eternal as the everlasting hills, metabolism goes on, the basis of life and all its phenomena. While "men may come and men may go," like Tennyson's brook, it goes on forever. Species are cast in various molds, generations appear and disappear, youth is followed by age, yet through it all running along on predetermined lines goes metabolism. Where there is life there is chemical reaction, and regulating this are the endocrine glands, the glands of internal secretion.

Protoplasm from the physician's point of view is not matter. The cell is the seat of vitality, of chemical exchange, of growth, of function, and of life. The assimilation of nutriment, growth, reproduction of kind, inflammation, degeneration, regeneration, exercise of function, motion and emotion are all matters of chemistry. Species, genus, and time of life are accidents determined by heredity, while size, weight, and sometimes appearance, are matters of metabolism, which in the individual is controlled by the internal secretions and also by the nervous system.

Physiological alchemy held sway for centuries and introduced many fundamental ideas. Exact sciences, physiology and physical chemistry, are rapidly replacing it, bringing light into darkness.

The basis on which the science of nutrition rests was laid in 1780 by Lavoisier. Lusk ([33]) says of him, "He was the first to apply the balance and thermometer to the investigation of the phenomena of life," and he declared, "La vie est une fonction chimique." He established the true character of the "dephlogisticated air" of Priestley, and through researches on animal heat and on respiration established the relationship of oxygen to bodily functions. He quantitatively determined in man the oxygen used per hour, the influence of temperature on the quantity used, the relation of oxygen to digestion and to exercise, thus establishing the relation of oxygen absorbed and CO_2 excreted to food, work, and temperature.

Liebig ([34]) became interested in nutrition, and studied biology along chemical lines. Voit, inspired by his work, devoted himself to problems of nutrition, but particularly to the rôle played by nitrogen in protein metabolism. He calculated the nitrogen content of food, determined its excretion in the urine, and showed the relationship of urea output to nitrogen intake. He suggested to Pettenkoffer ([35]) the need of an apparatus by which the total carbon excretion might be measured, a problem which they undertook jointly. The respiration apparatus was completed in 1862. Voit next "computed from the substances oxidized in the body the quantity of heat which should have arisen from the destruction of these substances." Thus was established indirect calorimetry.

Rubner in 1894, working in Voit's laboratory, made accurate determination through calorimetric methods of the heat value of urea and of dry urinary solids, through which were established biological standards for the caloric values of proteins, carbohydrates, and fats. In 1894 he built the first successful respiration calorimeter which actually measured heat production in the dog, and in so doing established direct calorimetry.

Atwater, while in Germany, was associated with Voit and Rubner. In 1877 he investigated the dietary requirement. In 1894, through the assistance of the American government, he and Rosa started the construction of a respiration calorimeter for man, which was completed in 1897.

Through the labors of Lusk, Benedict, and Dubois ([36]), calorimetry has been made applicable to clinical medicine and practical therapy. Indirect calorimetry is coming into general use in the larger clinics. For comparative purposes a normal control is always essential. This for clinical studies is found in the rate of basal metabolism, which is expressed in calories per hour per square meter of body surface. The variation from the normal average is expressed in terms of percentage above and below normal.

In this manner developed the science of nutrition, whereby is revealed the function, value, and fate of food. Through gas analysis, determinations of heat production and analysis of excreta, the possibility was revealed of determining quantitatively the rôle played by various foods, such as proteins, carbohydrates, and fats in metabolism and their relationship to heat and energy production, to growth, and to the processes of building up and repairing of tissues. With increase in the knowledge of metabolism, of physiological chemistry, and of medicine in general, the relation of disturbances of metabolism to disease became manifest. Detailed studies of these disturbances is shedding much light on both the processes of normal metabolism and that of disease.

In metabolic studies attention centered in the mechanisms involved in digestion, storage, and assimilation of foods, in their fate and function under varying conditions, and in the factors affecting metabolic processes generally, such as oxidation, cleavage, deamidization, reduction, and synthesis.

Nutrition and Food Values

In the space allotted, it is impossible to attempt more than an outline in a general way of the more important phases of nutrition, the rôle played by the glands of internal secretion, and the use of glands or their products in organotherapy.

Foods are utilized by the body as, (a) material for construction of body substance, (b) to make good the losses incurred in the wear and tear of life, i.e. maintenance, (c) to supply energy for life's activities, and (d) to supply heat. The foods required are carbon, hydrogen, nitrogen, oxygen, sulphur, phosphorus, chlorine, iron, salts, and water. Some of them must be prepared, since higher organisms have not the same capacity as the lower of building up their own food from simple chemical compounds. The carbon and hydrogen produce energy through oxidation; nitrogen is utilized for repair of structures containing nitrogen, and secondarily for energy; oxygen is needed for oxidation of carbon and hydrogen and is the chief source of energy; sulphur is necessary for growth, and repair of structure containing sulphur; phosphorus, for growth and repair of structures containing phosphorus; iron for hemoglobin; salts for osmotic pressure; and water for facilitating solution, and for carrying off waste products in excretion. The nitrogen and carbon must be in forms as complex as amino-acids and the sugars respectively. The classes of foodstuffs are ordinarily carbohydrates, proteins, and fats, the caloric values of which have been accurately determined. But calories do not always suffice; these may be supplied in abundant quantities without maintenance or growth.

It is just at this point that recent advances have been made. In addition to caloric values, there are other factors known as accessory factors. These are of two kinds: (a) originating from without, bausteine and vitamines, (b) arising from within, hormones or internal secretions.

Bausteine, or Building Stones.—Proteins from different sources differ chemically and biologically. Newer knowledge of the structure of these highly complex nitrogenous compounds makes possible a new conception of protein metabolism. The nitrogen must be in the form of a molecule at least as complex as an amino-acid before it can be utilized in the body. Such units constitute building stones, or "bausteine." The work of Osborne, and Mendel ([37]), and of McCollum ([38]) in this country and of Abderhalden ([39]) in Germany introduces a new conception of nutrition and also a broader conception of the function of the cell in its capacity to synthesize.

Proteins are broken down in digestion into amino-acids. These are absorbed, circulate as building stones, and are utilized by the cell in the building up of new protein. For maintenance certain amino-acids are necessary; for growth, still others are needed. In so far as a protein possesses in its molecule the building stone needed, just so far can it be utilized for maintenance or growth. For example, if only proteins deficient in cystin (a sulphur-containing amino-acid) are furnished the body, the production of new cystin-containing bodies will be difficult and limited by the supply in the food ingested. Through feeding artificial food mixtures to mice the importance of certain bausteine have been demonstrated, tryptophane for maintenance and glycin and lysin for growth. For maintenance the addition of tryptophane is necessary to zein, carbohydrate, and fat diet and also to completely hydrolyzed (enzymatic) proteins. For growth of mice, milk must be added to mixtures of pure caseinogen, fats, carbohydrates, and salts, and lysin to certain other food mixtures. The body can, however, synthesize glycocoll.

Similar requisites probably exist in the field of lipoids. Thus cod liver oil, so long utilized in nutritional diseases of childhood, is shown to facilitate growth in mice in artificial food mixtures when lard fails. This is another instance of sound empiricism which is now being rationalized.

Vitamines.—For normal metabolism vitamines are necessary. Little is known of their character or of their mechanism of action. In their absence diseases appear. Reintroduced to the diet after prolonged absence, they sometimes result in cure. Lack of fresh vegetables and fruit juices may result in scurvy, lack of rice polishings in beriberi, while absence of eggs, meat, and milk in the diet is responsible for pellagra. These are known as deficiency diseases, and their treatment consists of the addition of appropriate foods to the dietary.

Funk ([40]), who first recognized the existence and importance of vitamines, has attempted their isolation. To the vitamine of rice polishings, he has ascribed the formula $C_{26} H_{20} O_9 N_4$ and believes it to be a tetrabasic acid. But inasmuch as its formula closely resembles that of nicotinic acid ([41]) (an inert substance from this point of view) further work is necessary. Hopkins ([42]) feels that the true vitamine is still unknown. It belongs to the " water soluble A " class of McCollum.

Hormones, Internal Secretion.—The work of Starling and Bayliss ([43]) resulting in the recognition of hormones or internal secretions opened up a new chapter of physiology and revealed the existence of another factor in metabolism which is of the greatest importance to medicine. The endocrine glands manufacture substances which act as catalysts and markedly affect metabolism. Under- or over-production of them results in the development of diseases of metabolism; thus, the absence of thyroxin leads to myxedema; of the secretion of pancreas (islets of Langerhans) to diabetes; of tethelin to infantilism; of the extract of the posterior lobe and pars intermedia of the pituitary to diabetes insipidus;

of the parathyroids to tetany; and of some secretion of the adrenals to Addison's disease. On the other hand, excess of thyroxin leads to exophthalmic goitre and of tethelin to gigantism or acromegaly.

These secretions are chemical entities, one of them, thyroxin, having already been synthesized and used therapeutically. Future therapy will probably use synthetic drugs to replace these internal secretions in the diseases of metabolism in which they are deficient.

In relation to metabolism, attention should be called to the "specific dynamic action of protein." In studies of basal metabolism, it has been found that proteins stimulate the rate of metabolism more than carbohydrates. Some of the amino-acids, for instance glycin and alanin, exhibit this property. It is supposed to be due to the direct stimulating action of some of the intermediary acids such as lactic and peruvic.

Little is known concerning the effect of drugs on metabolism, but since the synthesis of thyroxin has already been accomplished, it would appear that the day of drug control of metabolism is at hand. The influence of caffeine and strychnine has been determined by Edsall and Means ([44]) and Higgins and Means ([45]) and of adrenalin by Sandiford. Opium is said to slow the rate of metabolism. The effects of these drugs on metabolism are in all probability due to their effects on the neuromuscular system, whereby acceleration on the one hand and inhibition on the other occur. Cacodylate of sodium has been utilized clinically to control the increased rate of metabolism in exophthalmic goitre; arsenic and phosphorus in therapeutic doses are both said to check oxidation and to favor nutrition in growth.

Growth

A new science of growth is in the making. Life is a sequence; embryonic life, birth, infancy, childhood, adolescence, maturity, and senility follow each other unless death intervenes. Growth characterizes the young. According to Lee, it consists of only three processes: multiplication of cells, enlargement of cells, and deposition of intercellular substance. Great variations from the mean are uncommon, and until recent years have not been subject to explanation. But investigation in the field of growth, nutrition, and hormone actions, is doing much to elucidate this subject.

Growth is a function of the cell. Two or perhaps three fundamental factors are concerned; namely, growth impulse, nutrition, and accessory factors such as hormones and vitamines. The first we do not understand, it is life itself. Nutrition is controlled by laws of physiology, of chemistry, and physics. The importance of the accessory factors are just beginning to be recognized. Growth is regulated for each species, the same food in the same amounts fed to different species resulting in different rates of growth.

Metabolism or nutrition in the young organism differs in some respects from that of adult life. Additional processes are at work involved in changes in character of tissue, such as ossification of bone and union of epiphyses. But the chief difference lies in growth or the creation of new tissues, which involves the building up of new proteins. The ordinary foodstuffs play the same rôle as in adults. Maintenance can be procured in mice on the same artificial food mixtures utilized in the nutrition experiments for growth, but the bausteine, tryptophane, glycin, and lysin are absolute requisites for growth. The addition of small quantities of lactalbumen and of edestin to zein, fed to mice, increases growth out of all proportion to the amount added.

The glands of internal secretion play a great rôle in growth as well as in nutrition. The addition of thyroid extract to the food of the cretin revolutionizes not only his metabolism but his growth, and with it his appearance, his physical and mental development. According to Brailsford Robertson ([46]), tethelin, a substance obtained from the anterior lobe of the pituitary, plays the leading part in the control of growth. The pituitary came under suspicion naturally in this connection owing to the intimate association of gigantism, infantilism, acromegaly, and obesity to tumors of the hypophysis. Other glands such as the thymus and the gonads unquestionably are concerned also to some extent.

Energetics

Energy is the capacity for doing work. Energy characterizes life. The ultimate source of energy is the sun; the immediate source for the living body is its nutriment. Various classes of food have different food values, but equal heat values do not of necessity have equal free energy values, for energy is of two kinds, bound and free, only the latter being available for actual work. The total energy is constant, the bound tends to a maximum, therefore the free tends to diminish. Some foods are more easily metabolized than others, and their energy is quickly available. Free energy, the ability to do, is the object of life.

In life, physical forces are controlled largely by chemical transformations. Energy results from chemical exchange and is comprised of two factors, " intensity " and " capacity " factors. Chemical energy can be converted into other forms without passing through heat, just as it does in a battery. Faraday demonstrated that the quantity of electricity obtained from a Voltaic cell is proportional to the amount of chemical change. Bayliss ([47]) believes that chemical energy is the quantity of a substance "capacity factor" multiplied by its chemical potential, or "affinity," and that the capacity factor of chemical and electrical energy is proportional, and further, that the intensity factors are also proportional. In other words, he agrees with Faraday in regarding electrical force and chemical affinity as one and the same thing.

The transformation from chemical to dynamic energy appears to the writer a fruitful field for investigation. The chemistry of nutrition is relatively well understood, but the conversion of chemical forces into energy and activities so vital to life are poorly understood. Heats of combustion do not entirely suffice. They do not render accurate information as to the energy available in the organism. Bayliss says, for example, that it is necessary to know if, calorie for calorie, carbohydrates have a greater energetic value than fats. Such information would render dietetics of infinitely greater value.

The problem is difficult, but fundamental. One great difficulty is the number of factors to be considered and the consequent complexity.

The amount of metabolism controls the amount of oxygen needed. The amount of oxygen needed controls the work of the lungs and heart, respiration and circulation. Thus the fast heart of exophthalmic goitre and of fever is due to increased rate of metabolism, and the slow pulse encountered during starvation in the diabetic is probably due to a decreased rate of metabolism.

Influence of the Nervous System

In early embryonic life, nutrition is carried on without the existence of a demonstrable nervous system, but at an early stage of development the nervous system begins to exert an important influence on the processes of growth and development. This is most strikingly evidenced, perhaps, in the function of growth in anterior poliomyelitis. The mind naturally turns to the question of trophic nerves. Unquestionably, interference with the nerve supply to a muscle may be followed by atrophy, but the atrophy is not of necessity due to the nutritional disturbance occasioned directly by lack of proper nerve supply. Herpes zoster is difficult to explain otherwise than on the basis of direct influence of the nervous system involving metabolism of the part supplied. The possibility of direct nervous control of metabolism cannot be denied, but on the other hand, proof of the same is still lacking. The growth of tissue in Locke's solution outside of the body proves the possibility of nutrition and growth aside from nervous influences.

The blood supply to a part unquestionably plays a determining rôle in its metabolism, and thus indirectly at least the nervous system is important. It is possible that vasomotor control is a principal factor through regulation of blood supply.

The question of the rôle of the nervous system is deserving of the greatest consideration. The intimacy between the sympathetic systems and the ductless glands suggests related functional activity. Before the days of " hormone activity " attempts were made to correlate the activities of the various endocrine glands through nervous channels. Difficulties encountered in establishing such relationships made it necessary to look elsewhere, with the result, the discovery of hormones.

Emotions

Similarly emotions, fright, anger, and pain, which heretofore have been looked upon as nervous or mental attributes, have assumed within later years a much broader aspect. One hormone at least is of great importance in this connection. Additional information concerning the function of the sympathetic system and endocrine glands must precede a solution of many questions of nutrition and metabolism.

Since the nervous system is one of the controlling factors in the function of the endocrine organs, it must of necessity play a leading rôle, at least indirectly. In the absence of the nervous system, normal function is impossible.

The endocrine glands play a leading rôle in the control of metabolism, nutrition and growth, and bodily dynamics. The most important are the thyroid, suprarenal, and pituitary glands. The influence of drugs in this connection, though marked, has never been satisfactorily explained from a fundamental point of view. The influence of adrenalin and to a lesser extent of strychnine and caffeine in removing the feeling of physical exhaustion as the result of prolonged work is intimately associated with the question of dynamics and energetics. The work of Cannon ([48]) and Crile ([49]) on internal secretions and emotions brings the problem into the limelight and indicates its importance. In these fields, fundamental processes are being revealed and the foundation of science being laid on which will be built the medical treatment of the future.

The Relation of Thyroid Function to Metabolism and Disease

So long as the thyroid is normal in size and function, it is of no particular interest to the practicing physician. Meckel in 1806 noted that it enlarged during menstruation and pregnancy, which suggested a close relationship between it and the female gonads. The first important contributions to our knowledge of the thyroid were made by practicing physicians. In the posthumous writings of Parry ([50]), 1825, a fashionable physician of Bath, is a description of eight cases of " Enlargement of the Thyroid Gland, in connection with Enlargement or Palpitation of the Heart." In describing the first cases, 1786, he writes, "The eyes were protruded from the sockets, and the countenance exhibited an appearance of agitation and distress, especially on any muscular movement." The pulse rate was 150. In speaking of the heart, he says, "It was so vehement that each systole of the heart shook the whole thorax." The salient features, the rapid, overacting heart, the exophthalmos, the struma, and the anxiety are all clearly depicted. It is extremely interesting to note that the dynamic and stress features are portrayed in the original description. Graves ([51]), a great clinical teacher, and Basedow ([52]), a general practitioner, also described the same disease in 1835 and 1840, respectively; Graves' original description being, "A lady, aged 21, became affected with some symptoms which were supposed to be hysterical. . . . After she had been in this nervous state about three months, it was observed that her pulse had become singularly rapid." Basedow was the first to attempt a physiological explanation of the manifestations of exophthalmic goitre.

Many years later, in 1873, Gull ([53]), another noted English physician, described the condition known as myxedema, and in 1877, Ord ([54]) established its relationship to thyroid activity. Some six years later, Kocher ([55]) described a cachexia strumapriva occurring in thirty per cent. of cases after the removal of thyroid in goitre, but this was a year after the Reverdins had described the same condition under the name, "myxedema post opératoire." Still later, von Brunn established the relationship of cretinism to decreased thyroid activity. The early experimental work blocked, rather than aided, progress until the functions of the parathyroid were established and this factor covered in experimental surgical procedures.* Schiff ([56]) and Horsley ([57]) both demonstrated that transplantation of the thyroid prevented the effects of removal. Finally came the discovery of Murray ([58]) and of Howitz that feeding of the gland results in the cure of myxedema.

The thyroid is an extremely vascular ductless gland, a single organ composed of two lateral, frequently unsymmetrical masses or lobes connected by a transverse median band or isthmus. Its nerves are probably all derived from the sympathetic and accompany the arteries to the gland. The true thyroid develops as an unpaired hollow outgrowth from the foregut, ventrally to the branchial arches and in the middle line. It has its origin therefore from the epithelium of the buccal cavity.

Function of the Thyroid.—It exercises an important control over the processes of nutrition of the body, and especially over the nervous system.

* Schiff described the results of complete thyroidectomy in animals in 1859.

How is the control exerted? Several opinions have been held: (1) The thyroid elaborates an internal secretion characterized by a large iodine content which is given off to the blood and lymph, is transported to the tissues, and there exercises a regulating function. This is borne out by excision of the organ, and by pathological processes leading to its destruction as evidenced by the development of cretinism, myxedema, and thyreopriva, and by the close parallelism existing between hyperplasia of the thyroid and clinical manifestations of toxicity. (2) The thyroid secretion neutralizes or destroys toxic substances arising in metabolism in the same manner that the liver overcomes the toxic properties of ammonia through converting it into urea. Following removal of the thyroid, toxic substances accumulate, cause toxic manifestations and result in death. For support of this hypothesis, proof is entirely lacking. (3) Still another view was put forward by Cyon, and is deserving of some consideration. On account of its extreme vascularity, he believes that it acts as "a vascular shunt, or flood gate to protect mechanically the circulation in the brain." This is reflexly effected through the hypophysis cerebri, and the vagi. This theory, though unacceptable in its entirety, recognizes the relation of the thyroid and its internal secretion to distribution and the total blood supply. In the present state of knowledge, it is probable that the thyroid does control blood supply, not directly, but secondarily through control of the rate of metabolism. It is metabolism which controls the work of the heart. The vascular phenomena of exophthalmic goitre may be looked upon as resulting from correlated influences on the vasomotor mechanism. The heart works at its maximum, and the peripheral circulation is thrown wide open to provide a maximum blood supply.

The point of contact or seat of action of the internal secretion has not yet been determined. Whether thyroxin acts directly on the cells of the body, or through their nerve supply still remains to be settled.

The body is like the social organism at large; "no man liveth unto himself alone." The function of the thyroid is internally related to the function of the body as a whole. Disturbance of its function disarranges function as a whole. Medicine has adopted an anatomical viewpoint in relation to disease. But for a true grasp of disease and its manifestations, this functional conception is a requisite.

In treatment of diseases of the thyroid, the fundamental question is not so much whether it is an adenoma, colloid goitre, or exophthalmic goitre, but whether or not the active principle of the thyroid is overstimulating or failing to stimulate metabolism; in other words, whether we are dealing with hypo- or hyper-activity or perversion of function.

Obviously it is desirable to know the nature of the active principle of the thyroid and the mechanism of its action. Recent work has shed much light on the former subject.

Chemistry of the Thyroid.—Kocher, with his vast clinical experience in goitre, surmised that the thyroid contained an iodine combination because of the clinical effects of iodine preparations on goitres. In 1896, Baumann ([59]) isolated a colloid substance which he called iodothyreoglobulin, demonstrated its organic character, that the gland contained several milligrams of iodine, and further that the thyroid was several times richer in iodine than any other tissue of the body. Subsequently, through the work of Ostwald, the protein nature of the compound was revealed. The desiccated gland was found to be largely composed of this material, and its activity was in proportion to its iodine content.

The brilliant work of Kendall ([60]) has resulted in the isolation of the active principle of the thyroid in crystalline form, and in the recognition of its chemical nature. In describing the compound, Kendall says, "Analysis has shown that it contains an indol group with the iodine undoubtedly attached to the benzene ring," and "that on the carbon atom adjacent to the amino group of the indol ring there is an oxygen atom." He ascribes to it the formula,

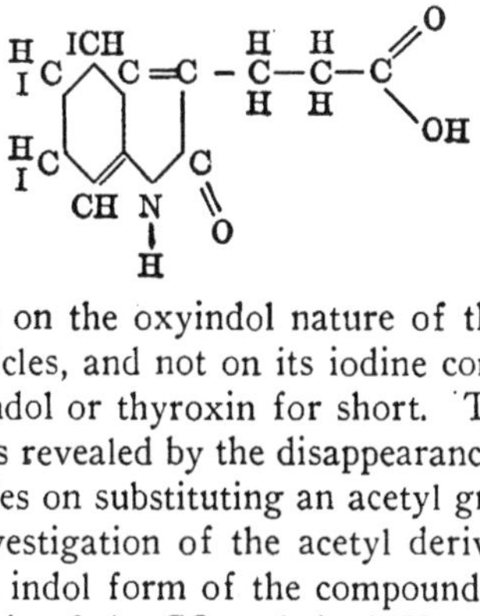

He lays emphasis on the oxyindol nature of the compound, and on the CO and NH radicles, and not on its iodine content. The substance was named thyroxyindol or thyroxin for short. The importance of the CO and NH groups is revealed by the disappearance of the characteristic physiological properties on substituting an acetyl group for the H of the amino radicle. "Investigation of the acetyl derivative showed that in alkaline solutions the indol form of the compound no longer exists, but that there is hydrolysis of the CO and the NH groups, resulting in the opening of the ring and the formation of COOH and NH_2,

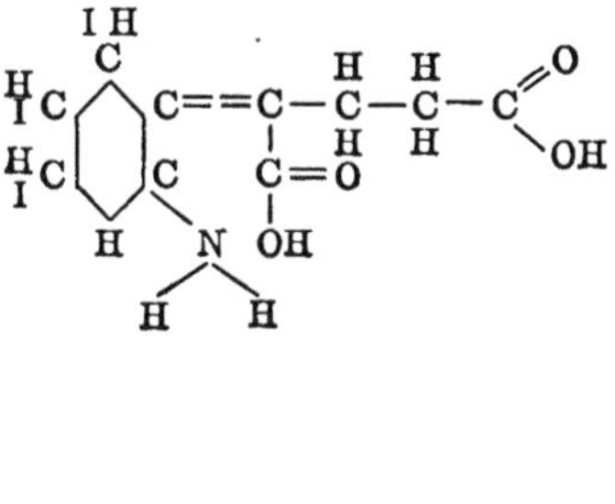

Further investigation showed that the thyroxin behaved in the same way, and that it exists within the body not in the closed ring form such as is present in indol, but in the form of COOH and NH_2."

This obviously accounts for the failure of physiological activity on substituting an acetyl group for the H of the amino radicle. Kendall further calls attention to the analogy between the open and closed forms of thyroxin, and the open and closed forms of creatin and creatinin, and states that the same relation exists between amino-acids, per se, and the form in which amino-acids exist, united in protein. He considers the CONH and the $COONH_2$ nuclei important desiderata in the production of energy in protein metabolism. Synthesis of the product has been accomplished, the resulting compound exhibiting all the chemical and physiological properties of the substance isolated from the gland.

The question naturally arises, does the thyroid synthesize thyroxin, or does it serve merely as a storage and distributing center as the liver does, for instance, in relation to glycogen and dextrose?. The available facts are: (1) the iodine is found in the gland in large quantities; (2) that the quantity is variable, even in health; (3) that it exists in colloidal state as a protein combination, iodothyreoglobulin; (4) that this latter is not a chemical entity; (5) that the desiccated gland varies in its iodine content and its activity is dependent quantitatively upon its iodine content; (6) that the iodine content of the thyroid varies in disease; (7) that a definite chemical entity, thyroxin, has been isolated from the gland in crystalline state; (8) that thyroxin counteracts the effects of thyroidectomy in animals, and in extremely small quantities causes striking improvement in human cases of myxedema and of sporadic cretinism; (9) that its effect in raising metabolism is quantitative in character, reaching its maximum after an appropriate dose, only after some days, and persisting for some weeks after a single injection; (10) that its activity is not dependent entirely on its iodine content. Whether the hormone of the thyroid is synthesized or merely stored in the gland has not yet been determined, and must be left to the future to decide.

Little is known as to the mechanism of action of the thyroid. The smallness of the dose of thyroxin and its marvelous effect in accelerating metabolism naturally suggests catalysis. Catalytic differs from enzymatic activity in that the latter is destroyed at relatively low temperature, and is as a rule markedly specific in character.

The characteristic actions of a catalyst are: (1) that it accelerates chemical action; (2) that relatively small quantities suffice, and beyond certain limits further increase in the catalyst does not further accelerate the action; (3) that it acts only by its presence, and it does not itself participate in the reaction (with certain exceptions), or at least it does not form part of the resulting system in the final equilibrium; (4) that it acts over and over again, and that as a rule it is destroyed or "removed from the sphere of action in the form of constituents of some of the subsidiary reactions"; (5) and that when the system is one that reaches a definite equilibrium under the conditions of the experiment, the position of this equilibrium is unaffected by the presence or the amount of the catalyst, which merely hastens the time taken by the process and this in proportion to its concentration up to a certain point.

Two important things are shown by these facts; namely, that the catalyst does not supply or remove energy from the system, and that it accelerates both the hydrolytic and synthetic components of a reversible reaction. Thyroxin fulfills most of these requirements, in that it increases the rate of metabolism, acts in small quantities, increasingly more with somewhat larger quantities, acts over a period of some weeks from a single dose so that in all probability it acts repeatedly, and finally, in that it does not modify the type but only the rate of metabolism so far as can be ascertained. Against its catalytic activity can be argued the slowness with which its effect is exerted, the maximum not being reached for several days, and the evident dynamic effect in increasing the energy of the individual. The latter, however, is secondary; not the result of the increase of the chemical reaction, per se, but of the restoration of normal function as the result of normal metabolism.

The seat of action of the active principle of the thyroid is still a matter of discussion. Is its function carried on in the gland through the nervous system, or in the cells of the body generally? It seems probable that the gland acts as a storehouse, and gives off the active principle which acts, as Plummer believes, on the cells of the body generally, both directly and indirectly.

The gland itself is subject to control. It is influenced by other glands of internal secretion, and also by the sympathetic nervous system. The work of Cannon, in which overactivity of the thyroid was obtained through continuous stimulation of the sympathetic, through transplantation of the phrenic into the cervical sympathetic, established the importance of the sympathetic system in relation to the function of the thyroid.

Clinically, the anamnesis of exophthalmic goitre is usually a history of prolonged nervousness. Its clinical manifestations include many and marked evidences of the involvement of the sympathetic. Barker says, "Among the symptoms largely referable to the autonomic nervous system are included: (a) the eye signs; (b) the cardiovascular phenomena; (c) the cutaneous phenomena; (d) the digestive disturbances; (e) the respiratory disturbances; and (f) the urogenital symptoms."

Similarly, infection, local or general, exercises a marked influence on the thyroid, and upon metabolism. This knowledge is born of clinical experience which reveals the closest connection between acute or chronic infections and manifestations of Graves' disease.

Before discussing the diseases of the thyroid, a survey of the clinical manifestations following the removal of the thyroid and those of Graves' disease cannot fail to impress one with the significance of the rôle of the thyroid. In fact, the contrast was in large part responsible for the present-day view, that the thyroid itself, through overactivity, is a primary factor in Graves' disease. Kocher has tabulated the following facts:

Cachexia Thyreopriva	*Graves' Disease*
Absence of atrophy of the thyroid gland.	Swelling of the thyroid gland, usually of a diffuse nature. Hypervascularization.
Slow, small, regular pulse.	Rapid, full, and at times irregular pulse.
Cold skin without flushings.	Irritable vasomotor system.
An uninterested, quiet stare without expression of life.	Anxious appearance, angry expression.
Narrow palpebral aperture.	Wide palpebral aperture, exophthalmos.
Slow digestion and excretion, poor appetite, requiring little food.	Abundant excretions, an excessive appetite, with increased needs of food.
Retarded metabolism.	Increased metabolism.
Skin is thick, opaque, folded, dry, and scaling.	Skin is thin, transparent, finely injected, and moist.
Short, thick fingers with broad ends.	Long slender fingers with pointed ends.
Sleepy.	Wakeful and disturbed sleep.
Dulled sensation, apperception, and action.	Increased sensation, apperception, and action.
Lack of thoughts, interest, and emotion.	Flight of ideas, psychic excitation even to hallucination, mania, and melancholia.
Slow, awkward muscular movements.	Constant activity and haste.
Stiffness of the extremities.	Tremor, and increased mobility of joints.
Delay in growth of bones, often with deformities. Bones thick and soft.	Slender skeleton with here and there soft bones.
Constant chilliness.	Unbearable feeling of heat.
Slow, deep breathing.	Superficial breathing with imperfect inspiratory expansion.
Increase in weight.	Loss of weight.
Aged appearance, even of young people.	Youthful appearance, especially at the onset.

Hypothyroidism.—There are three types of hypothyroidism. The first described was spontaneous myxedema. As already indicated, surgical removal of the thyroid in goitre led to the recognition of myxedema "post opératoire" while later, cretinism was recognized and also its relationship to the thyroid. According to Osler, credit is due to Felix Simon for recognizing that these were all one and the same disease, and all due to loss of function of the thyroid gland. They have in common nutritional disturbance, mental retardation, changes in tegumental structures, and edematous or mucous deposits.

Myxedema may occur spontaneously or subsequent to operative removal of the thyroid. The name myxedema was employed because of the peculiar edematous-like swellings observed in the cutaneous and subcutaneous and other tissues. These swellings differ from ordinary edema in that they are firmer, and do not pit on pressure, and in that histologically they show a mucin-like material.

The disease is characterized, according to Ord, who established its etiology, by marked increase in the general bulk of the body, a peculiar firm swelling or edema of the skin, which does not pit on pressure, dryness and roughness of the skin (which, together with the swelling, tends to obliterate the normal lines of the face, thus resulting in a peculiar physiognomy which is often pathognomonic), and finally, imperfect nutrition of hair and nails. The features become coarse and expressionless, and the skin takes on a pallid, waxy appearance. In addition to physical changes, there is generally marked mental retardation, suggesting stupidity, at times lethargy and somnolence. Slowness in movement is also striking. Patients complain bitterly of being cold. This is worse in cold and less troublesome in warm weather.

The onset is insidious, slowly progressive, resulting eventually in most instances in the bodily changes already described and in asthenia, loss of capacity for work, and a susceptibility to marked mental changes, involving suspicions, delusions, hallucinations, and occasionally dementia. Instances of both hyper- and hypo-activity of the thyroid have been noted from time to time. Myxedema has also been encountered subsequent to exophthalmic goitre, and in the later stages of adenoma of the thyroid.

The postoperative condition is infrequent in this country. After complete thyroidectomy it occurs in seventy-five per cent. of cases according to Kocher, who advises that at least one-quarter of the gland be left if possible. Its features are identical with those of myxedema proper. It follows operations in which a large proportion of the gland is removed, and occasionally in less marked resections in patients who have exhibited dysthyroidism.

Skeletal changes such as are seen in cretinism are rare except in cases developing in youth subsequent to one of the febrile diseases. Through studies of the rate of basal metabolism, decreases of from ten to thirty per cent. are revealed. Formerly such studies were possible only in special institutions, but now that indirect calorimetry has been made simple and reliable, studies of metabolic rate are being made in many clinics throughout the country.

Cretinism.—Of this there are two forms, the sporadic and the endemic, only the former occurring in America. The condition may be congenital, due to absence of the gland, or acquired, due to atrophy, resulting from one of the febrile affections. It is encountered not infrequently. It is characterized by bodily and mental retardation and by certain skeletal deviations which are more or less characteristic, and which indicate that the thyroid secretion plays a rôle in relation to growth and mental development.

Recognition of the condition is usually not made before six months of age, while the disease is well marked at the end of the first or in the second years. The head is deformed in sporadic cases, long in the antero-posterior diameter (dolichocephalic). The body is undersized, dwarfed, pudgy, and the abdomen protuberant. The face is that of an imbecile, the mouth open, the tongue large and protruding, and the bridge of the nose sunken. The fontanelles close late, and the epiphyses unite with the long bones late or not at all. The hands and feet are thick and stubby. Dentition is delayed. Marked weakness exists, so that the child cannot support itself. The skin is thick, pallid, and waxy, the hair thin, and subcutaneous pads such as are seen in myxedema occur at times, especially about the cheeks. Mentality is markedly retarded, and in some instances imbecility develops.

Once the condition has been seen it is readily diagnosed as a rule. The facial expression, the skin changes, the protruding abdomen, and the physical and mental retardation at once suggest cretinism. Metabolic studies reveal a lowered metabolic rate, decrease of ten to forty per cent. below normal.

Treatment of Myxedema and Cretinism.—The progress in the treatment of myxedema exemplifies the rapidity of the development of the science of therapeutics. Results regarded as impossible a century ago, as marvelous two decades ago, are accepted as a matter of course today. Just as salvarsan overshadows the mercury treatment of syphilis, so thyroxin supplants older methods, owing to its efficacy, its rapidity, and the manner in which it lends itself to quantitative study and control. To revert to the terminology of proprietary medicine, "the results are startling." In some instances individuals are made over overnight. No more brilliant therapy exists in the healing art today than in deficiency of the thyroid gland.

The fresh gland, desiccated powder, aqueous and glycerine extracts are all efficacious in the majority of cases of myxedema. Numerous preparations of gland are marketed, but the most convenient are the desiccated gland and the glycerine extract. The powdered gland is given in 0.065 gm., or one grain, doses three times a day in the beginning and increased to 0.651- gm., or 10 to 15 grains per day. Unpleasant symptoms, irritation of the skin, restlessness, tachycardia and delirium, and in some instances tonic spasms sometimes accompany its use. In the majority of instances no untoward effects are encountered. Within a few weeks the marvelous changes referred to above appear. The skin becomes soft, warm, and natural, the edema disappears, and the face is that of another individual. No less striking is the change in character and deportment; from the slow, cumbersome, sluggish victim of myxedema, there emerges a normal, wide-awake individual.

Following the initial intensive treatment, subsequent intermittent treatment with small doses is necessary in most cases of myxedema, and in all cases of cretinism. Relapse usually follows prolonged absence of the drug.

Treatment with thyroxin is a matter of science. It deals with accurate measurement of the drug, of the rate of metabolism, of the time element, and with the control of effects. After determining the metabolic rate, the dose is calculated according to the percentage decrease of metabolic rate. The number of milligrams of thyroxin required is treated with 10 per cent. NaOH, diluted with distilled water and administered intravenously. With marked lowering of metabolism (25-30%), 10 to 15 milligrams are used, while with a slight decrease (10-20%) 5 or sometimes 10 milligrams are used. Each milligram, according to Plummer, raises metabolic rate two per cent. Metabolism usually reaches its maximum on the 8th or 12th day, maintains a plateau, and then gradually decreases. However, the writer has observed a rise from below twenty-seven per cent. to normal metabolism in five days on administering five milligrams in a single dose intravenously.

Although the maximum effect on metabolism is not immediate, that on the patient may be. Cases, typical in every respect, may be absolutely revolutionized within twenty-four hours. Plummer, who was the first to use thyroxin, relates his great surprise on his first visit, subsequent to treatment. He doubted his own eyes. On the other hand, metabolic rate may be brought to normal without striking concomitant clinical results, as in one of our own cases.

Large quantities of urine, sometimes amounting to several liters, are not infrequently passed during the first twenty-four hours, and with the polyuria, the edema or myxedema of the skin and subcutaneous tissues disappears. Palpitation is apt to be a striking phenomenon. Headache is frequently a marked symptom, and occasionally vomiting. In the majority of cases the patient appears to be, feels, acts, and is a different individual. The skin resumes its softness, perspiration is reëstablished, and the patient feels warm again, sometimes after being cold for years.

The time relationship between this recovery of the patient and the return of metabolism to normal is a matter of great interest, but no explanation is yet apparent. Subjective and objective improvement may precede the maximum metabolic rate by at least a week.

The treatment in cretinism is identical in every respect, except that smaller doses are employed. A cretin treated with thyroxin by us was converted within a short period from a slow stupid imbecile to the liveliest and most interesting youngster in the ward, the result of two injections of 2 mgms. each.

Hyperthyroidism.—Before considering hyperthyroidism clinically, it is well to obtain a view of its experimental aspects. Two general methods have been employed in its production:

(1) The administration of thyroid. In sufficient doses, toxicity appears in all animals, but is most readily produced as a rule in the human. Carnivorous animals are least affected. In man, loss of weight is one of the most constant manifestations, the result apparently of increase in metabolism. Skin changes are common, especially sweating, which is accompanied by a general feeling of warmth. Tachycardia is of common occurrence as are also restlessness, irritability, excitability, and insomnia. Trembling is frequent, and gastrointestinal disturbances common. These symptoms are observed not infrequently in the clinical use of the desiccated gland, and lead to its discontinuation. Motthafft's patient, mentioned by Hewlett, a fat man of 43 years who took about 1,000 tablets in the course of five weeks, developed rapid respiration, slight fever, glycosuria, and bilateral exophthalmus, in addition to the usual manifestations listed above. This is perhaps the nearest approach on record to the experimental production of exophthalmic goitre. Exophthalmus is also reported by Beclère.

In animals, emaciation, increased appetite, thirst, digestive disturbances, and exophthalmus have been produced. Glycosuria has resulted in some instances. Increased metabolism is a constant feature. Similar effects have followed the administration of iodine to patients suffering from disease of the thyroid; loss of weight, nervousness, tachycardia, and tremor being the most common manifestations. These are not ordinary evidences of iodism such as are seen in normal individuals, and they probably result from the effect of iodine on the diseased thyroid.

(2) Thyroid stimulation through the sympathetic nervous system. Cannon and his associates have produced hyperthyroidism in a manner which sheds considerable light on the mechanism involved. The phrenic was cut in the neck in cats and its peripheral end was anastomosed into the central end of the cut cervical sympathetic. Subsequent to union, stimuli from the constantly active diaphragm supplied the sympathetic with constant stimulation. Increased excitability, tachycardia, diarrhea,

exophthalmus, and high rate of metabolism were induced. The symptoms bore a striking relationship to those of hyperthyroidism.

Before leaving the subject of the effects of the thyroid on metabolism and growth, the brilliant studies of Gudernatsch should be mentioned. This investigator fed thyroid to tadpoles, and showed that this resulted in stunting of the growth of the animal, but in early metamorphosis. The limbs appeared early, and the tail disappeared earlier than normal, long before the tadpole had attained the size at which this usually occurs. These results are in keeping with our general ideas concerning the direct relation of the thyroid to growth of the soma and gonads.

Exophthalmic Goitre.—Hyperthyroidism is most frequently associated with exophthalmic goitre or toxic adenomata. The former is a disease characterized by goitre, exophthalmus, tachycardia, tremor, nervousness, and increased metabolic rate, associated with a perverted or hyperactive state of the thyroid gland.

The condition has been looked upon by many as a pure neurosis, because of the prominence of nervous manifestations in the anamnesis, and in the disease itself, and because of its development in many instances after nervous and emotional strains. At present it is usually accepted as a disease of the thyroid, the result of hyperactivity. The gland in exophthalmic goitre suggests great activity, extreme vascularity, with increased proliferation and with the production of newly formed spaces and absorption of the colloid material, which is replaced by a more mucinous fluid. The importance of the thyroid itself is borne out by partial thyroidectomy, which yields much better results than any other treatment as yet suggested. With the removal of thyroid substance the metabolism returns rapidly to normal, and the symptoms disappear. If too much thyroid tissue is removed evidences of myxedema develop, which in turn can be removed by administration of the desiccated gland or thyroxin. On the other hand, the disease can be produced experimentally through nervous influences as demonstrated by the work of Cannon. It must be admitted that at the present time the seat of the primary change has not been determined.

The disease is one of adult life, rarely appears before puberty, and affects females more than males. Its course may be acute, but is usually chronic. The main clinical manfestations will be considered in some detail, especially their pathogenesis, in order to learn something of the mechanism involved in the disease.

Barker classifies the symptoms of Graves' disease as follows: (1) the goitre or struma; (2) symptoms referable to the autonomic nervous system, including (a) eye signs, (b) the cardiovascular phenomena, (c) the cutaneous phenomena, (d) the digestive disturbances, (e) the respiration disturbances, (f) and the uro-genital symptoms; (3) metabolic disturbances; (4) symptoms referable to other endocrine glands; (5) cerebral symptoms; and (6) blood changes.

The gland is usually enlarged symmetrically, but not necessarily so. It is extremely vascular, as evidenced by thrills and bruits. Its low iodine content is difficult to explain except on the basis that the gland ordinarily stores iodine, which function is lost in hyper-activity.

In typical cases metabolism is greatly increased, in some cases fifty to eighty per cent. above normal. This increase is exaggerated by extreme nervousness, by bodily and mental overactivity. These are probably but factors in a vicious circle. The skin is usually warm and moist, and fever is not at all uncommon. In addition to total metabolism, change occurs in relation to carbohydrates and proteins.

Tissue catabolism is marked, resulting in increased nitrogen excretion and in loss of weight. Nitrogen equilibrium is difficult to maintain. Alimentary glycosuria is common. The explanation for this is not clear, but the work of Cramer and Kraus suggests the possibility of it being a deficiency in the glycogenic function of the liver.

The possibility of the tachycardia being due to stimulation of the accelerator nerves of the heart is not at present entertained. In all probability it is but a part of the cycle involved in increase in metabolism. The heart is overactive in order to supply sufficient blood to the over-metabolizing tissues generally. The rapid circulation, the overacting heart, the high systolic and low diastolic pressure, the high pulse pressure, capillary pulsation, and vascular erythema are all incidental features involved in the effort to supply sufficient blood. The development later of myocardial insufficiency, of dilation and arrythmias are but natural sequences of overuse. If the cardiac control is of nervous origin this is probably secondary to metabolic states.

The exophthalmus is probably due to relaxation of the extra ocular muscles or to spasm of the smooth muscle fibers described by Müller. Their function in contraction is to protrude the eyeball and pull back the lids, and it is carried out through fibers from the cervical sympathetic. The possibility of localized edema of the orbit seems unlikely to the writer, though the presence of fat as the explanation of the failure of disappearance of exophthalmus after cure in long-standing cases appears quite reasonable.

The tremors are unexplained, unless they are accepted as evidence of the tense overwrought nervous system or secondary to concomitant involvement of the parathyroids. The nervous manifestations indicate that the nervous system is involved in the process primarily or secondarily. They appear early, as a rule, and occasion great discomfort to the patient. As already indicated, they frequently result from the administration of thyroid. Increased metabolic rates, such as are encountered in febrile conditions, are not infrequently also accompanied by similar nervous symptoms (Barker).

The disease is one of several years' duration. After persisting several months, symptoms may disappear to reappear again at a later date. Clinically, the effect of infections is most striking. Thus a mild attack of tonsillitis may occasion an acute marked exacerbation of the Graves' disease which in some instances disappears as the local condition clears up, or more frequently subsides slowly in the course of a few weeks or months. Similarly, emotions and nervous strains are prolific sources of acute exacerbation.

Plausible explanations can be found for the clinical manifestation in typical cases. But atypical cases abound. In the early stages of the disease, the diagnosis is most difficult at times. In the same individual, striking evidences for over- and under-function of the thyroid are not at all infrequent. One or another feature may be strikingly exaggerated or entirely wanting. It is the inability to explain the bizarre combinations of clinical findings in the individual case that makes the clinician skeptical of theories and chary of accepting one chemical entity as the active principle of the thyroid. Correlations of laboratory investigations with clinical studies serve to increase this skepticism at times. Normal, or even decreased metabolic rates are encountered at times with clinical pictures very suggestive of Graves' disease or of thyrotoxicosis.

There is a feature of Graves' disease that baffles expression. It is revealed in the facial expression, in the incessant restlessness, the overwhelming nervous strain, and in the pent-up feeling. It is kinetic, dynamic, a hidden fire. I am always reminded by a case of this kind of a motor car, gear in neutral, brakes set, but with the engine still running. Even at rest, the throb of life is evident, combustion is going on, energy is being dissipated or is felt, but it is not being utilized; and back of it all one recognizes that fuel is being consumed, that energy is wasted, and that the engine is being subjected to useless wear and tear. Such factors must be approached through studies in energetics, dynamics, and kinetics, living forces as yet but little understood.

Treatment of Hyperthyroidism

(*a*) If we accept the theory of overactivity of the thyroid as the cause of exophthalmic goitre logically, in the absence of effective methods of control of its action, we are forced to turn to partial removal of the gland. Practically this procedure yields the best results. But since operations cannot be lightly undertaken, every effort must be made to obtain results in other ways until such time at least as the operation appears imperative.

The important features are absolute rest in bed, and freedom from visitors. An ice bag is placed locally over the thyroid, and another over the heart if it is tumultuous. Digitalis, or strophanthus are indicated for myocardial insufficiency. Many drugs have been advocated, but few give outspoken results. Cacodylàte of sodium is used hypodermically for the lowering of metabolism, although proof of such an effect is lacking. We have observed marked decrease in metabolic rate coincident with its employment but whether it is the general treatment (rest, diet, etc.) that played the greater rôle has not yet been determined.

(*b*) Milk of dethyroidized goats has been tried as has also serum of animals into which human thyroid extract has been injected. Some good results have been reported from both these methods, but they have not sufficient effect to bring them into general use.

(*c*) Dietary measures; a low caloric diet with a more than proportionate decrease in proteins, is desirable for a short period at least.

(*d*) Local injections of urea solution into the thyroid gland is followed by improvement in some cases.

(*e*) Removal of foci of infection exercises a beneficial effect at times.

Ligation of vessels suffices in many cases, but in the majority of instances the results are purely temporary. Partial excision, as practiced by many surgeons, gives much the best results. Recovery is rapid, and complete in many cases. Excision of the superior cervical sympathetic ganglia has also been practiced; the slight ptosis resulting, serving to alleviate the staring expression associated with the exophthalmus.

Two procedures practiced by surgeons in relation to thyroid operations are worthy of mention: (1) the practice in certain clinics of observing the effect of the visit to the operating room, and the postponement of the operation in the event of undue excitement, with marked exacerbation of symptoms; and (2) anoci association, which was introduced by Crile in an effort to protect the nervous system generally from the shock of the operation. These indicate the importance which the nervous system plays in the experience of the surgeon.

The thymus, which is enlarged in a considerable percentage of thyroid cases, has been subjected to systematic X-ray treatment. The results as a whole have been disappointing. Systematic and prolonged treatment of both thymus and thyroid has yielded some brilliant results.

Here again in the treatment of thyroid disease the basis for future drug therapy is being laid. With increasing knowledge of metabolism chemical control of these processes will be sought. Means of chemically increasing the rate of metabolism have already been attained. The problem of finding chemicals capable of slowing the rate of metabolism now confronts us.

(7) Treatment Based on a Functional Conception of Disease

A functional conception of disease as a basis of treatment is rapidly attaining a foothold in medicine. From the vast field presented, only one example will be considered. This, however, will be discussed in considerable detail, since through such a procedure the various principles underlying this form of treatment can be presented.

Myocardial Insufficiency

The function of the heart is to keep the blood circulating, sending it: (1) to the lungs where it rids itself of its CO_2, and takes up oxygen; (2) to the tissues where it supplies oxygen and nutriment, and takes up waste material; (3) to the gastrointestinal tract where it receives nutriment; and (4) to the organs of excretion which remove waste products. The heart must efficiently maintain circulation, which involves a sufficient minute volume output and an adequate blood pressure. The " factor of safety " or reserve force of the heart is great. The guiding principle of treatment is restoration of reserve force. The muscle power of the heart is the chief concern of the therapeutist.

Harrington Sainsbury ([61]) emphasizes this in a most charming and forceful way in the prologue to his little volume " Principia Therapeutica," in a dialogue between the pathologist and internist, parts of which the author was wont to use in beginning his course of lectures in therapeutics.

Path.: " The apothecary tells me there is a long bill on account,—digitalis, strophanthus, sparteine, and Heaven knows what more, for I could not outstay the tale of the remedies employed. Friend, what had you in mind, and what was the real task before you, could you but have seen? See here, this aortic valve, which you rightly diagnosed to be narrowed, it scarcely admits a thin pencil—and the valves, if you can call them such, fused and thickened as they are, and hard as a piece of Roman mortar; they do not look exactly amenable to treatment; did you think to soften them? And this heart muscle, its fibers stretched and degenerate, what hope was there? Doubtlesss you proposed to make new fibers to overcome the destruction? What a commentary upon the drug list is here! "

Phys.: " Not mine the fault, for, as you say, I did not spare the drugs, but proceed—this case of stenosed aorta which you have so accurately described, was taken from the body of a woman. Can you favor me with her age?"

Path.: "Seventy-six."

Phys.: "Precisely, and her history tells, I think, that though always ailing, her symptoms did not point definitely to failing heart until after her sixty-seventh year. The rigid valves are so thickened that the orifice is reduced to a mere chink. Could you perhaps give a date to this calcification?"

Path.: "That would be difficult; it is certainly not of yesterday."

Phys.: "The change has clearly been of slow development, and I think you will admit that its first beginnings may date back many years, perhaps to infancy, and that in this extreme form, it must have existed for many months."

Path.: "Agreed."

Phys.: "And yet symptoms have been so surprisingly absent. But you are well aware, this is no isolated occurrence, and cases as extreme as this have been entirely latent through a long life, and have proved compatible even with seeming good health. This was so in a case which I have in mind, in which the patient, also a woman, again reached the age of seventy-six."

Path.: "Need we elaborate this portion of the argument?"

Phys.: "Willingly I pass on, but first let me very briefly insist upon the inference; viz., that this specimen declares vitality, not mortality. Here, for instance, is a vital organ irreparably damaged at the fountain-head, so to speak, and yet the patient outlives her three-score years and ten.

"By what means? You have called attention to the dilated chambers of the heart and to the stretched and degenerate fibers of the muscular walls; you have confirmed these degenerations by the microscope, and you have admitted, I think, that these same changes give clear evidence of long standing, and that some of them, e.g. the dilations, must reach back in their beginnings to the first changes in the damaged valve; thus you have borne witness to an inadequacy, declared, and long prepared. Not by virtue of these, but in their despite, has life been prolonged, and yet the patient attains to the age of seventy-six. By what means?

"Surveying the whole case, and placing upon the one side the work to be done, the mass of blood to be moved, the obstruction to be overcome, and upon the other, available forces of the heart muscle, we must confess, I grant it, that the latter *appear* wholly unequal to the task. Yet the sum of it all is a long life. Will you think me unreasonable if I claim this heart is an instance of triumph, not of failure?"

Myocardial insufficiency arises from many causes. In its chronic form it is caused by: myocardial changes or lesions; lesions of the valves; lesions affecting the vascular fields of the efferent arteries; overexertion; poisons, especially alcohol (beer); adherent pericardium; goitre, and Graves' disease. Numerous anatomical bases such as coronary sclerosis, interstitial myocarditis, fragmentation and segmentation, parenchymatous degeneration, fatty or amyloid degeneration, and lesions affecting the bundle of His can be ascribed as the underlying cause. Hypertrophy or dilation, or both, may exist. Hypertension, alone or in combination with nephritis, is frequently associated with the myocardial insufficiency. But irrespective of the nature of the cause, or of the lesion, or of associated complications, *the important desideratum is restoration of myocardial function.*

But what are the functions of the heart muscle? They depend on its cardinal properties, which are five in number, contractility (inotropism), conductivity (dromotropism), irritability (bathmotropism), rhythmicity (chronotropism), and tonicity. Cardiac function may be disturbed in relation to all or one or a combination of these properties recognition of which markedly affects the efficiency of treatment, since treatment can be directed especially, in some instances, towards one or more of these derangements. Digitalis in therapeutic doses affects tonicity, conductivity, and contractility. In toxic doses irritability is greatly increased and rhythmicity markedly disturbed.

A word might be said concerning renal function in myocardial insufficiency, since it must be considered in the treatment of this condition.

Myocardial Insufficiency and Renal Function ([62]).—Myocardial insufficiency may occur independently, but in a large proportion of cases it develops in association with nephritis. It is often impossible, on purely clinical lines in an individual case, to decide whether the kidney or heart is primarily responsible for the clinical picture encountered. In this connection renal functional studies are of the greatest assistance.

Marked renal insufficiency may result from pure chronic passive congestion. Very exceptionally, clinically and experimentally, the functional studies reveal a decrease in function equaling that seen in the most severe grades of nephritis. Since the congestion to effect this must be of a most extreme grade death is imminent on account of the heart. As a rule, in myocardial insufficiency, with a symptomatic and urinary picture identical with that seen in a moderately advanced nephritis alone, or in nephritis associated with a cardiac break, renal function as indicated by both excretory and retention tests is surprisingly good. When low renal function is followed by an increased phthalein output, the amount of increase gives a fair approximation of the extent of cardiac improvement.

In this connection also urea and total non-protein nitrogen studies are of great value. In pure passive congestion, an increase in total non-protein nitrogen above 50 mg. to 100 c.c. of blood is extremely rare. In only three instances among several hundred cases studied has the author encountered it. Foster has lately reported three more instances. Blood creatinine is rarely significantly increased in pure passive congestion of the kidney. The finding of normal nitrogen figures, therefore, is of considerable diagnostic significance. A phthalein rapidly returning to normal associated with a low level of blood total non-protein nitrogen and urea speaks strongly for passive congestion as the underlying process.

Treatment of Myocardial Insufficiency.—Myocardial insufficiency constitutes a pathological indication for treatment, and calls for treatment notwithstanding other conditions present. The principles underlying this treatment are rest, limited diet, limited salt and fluid intake, depletion through bleeding, purgatives, diuresis or paracentesis, and support of the heart. In addition, certain symptoms may call for special attention.

In many instances the general treatment is more important than drug therapy. On the other hand, drugs are of unquestionable value, frequently playing an important rôle. In this article, detailed consideration can be allowed only drug therapy.

Rest.—This is essential and must be complete at first, absolute rest of short duration. In long continued chronic myocardial insufficiency, absolute rest is of course impossible. A back rest often affords great comfort. An additional reason for absolute rest is found in the serious consequences which may attend exercise in a patient under the influence of digitalis.

Diet.—This must be restricted in three ways as to (1) the quantity taken at one feeding, (2) the salt content, and (3) water intake. Rest for the stomach as well as for the heart must be insisted on. Do not overfeed. This is a good rule, often broken.

Fluids.—The intake of water and fluids should be restricted, the more the edema, the greater the restriction. A special fluid chart, indicating the fluid intake and the urinary output should be kept in all cases with marked edema. The total fluid intake should be limited to 1 to 1.5 liters a day at first; more fluid being allowed as diuresis is established and edema disappears. Enormous quantities of water may be lost in the course of a few days, a decrease of 20 to 30 pounds in the course of 5 to 6 days not being infrequent. In one of the author's cases, 70 pounds were lost in one week, anasarca disappeared, and the phthalein output increased from sixteen per cent. to normal.

Sodium Chloride.—Widal has shown how important is the restriction of sodium chloride. In the diet the salt content must be small. An absolutely salt-free diet is practically impossible, and is not necessary. It is next to impossible to obtain a salt content less than 1 gm. a day. Milk contains 0.16 per cent. sodium chloride, so that any diet containing milk of necessity contains some salt.

So great restriction of salt is often not advisable over prolonged periods. The guide to the amount allowed is found in the ability of the kidney to excrete it. Where fair amounts are excreted, and particularly where its concentration in the urine is good, more can be allowed. Many patients are kept on a salt-free diet long after the necessity of it has passed. Great quantities of salt are excreted as a rule with the clearing up of edema and anasarca. Prolonged use of salt-free diet may lead to deprivation of the tissues of sodium chloride.

Methods of Depletion.—Bleeding, tapping of the pleural, pericardial, or abdominal cavities, diuresis and purgation, may all be indicated at times. Sweating is contraindicated owing to the strain involved upon the heart.

Bleeding.—Venesection is indicated in acute dilation of the heart, particularly of the right heart.

Purgation.—This is employed in practically all cases of outspoken myocardial insufficiency. It is useful for the removal of water, for the removal of putrefactive material from the intestine, and also for the relief of intestinal distention. It may be employed without fear even where asthenia is marked and the pulse feeble. Hydragogues should be used. Magnesium sulphate 16 to 48 grams (½ to 1½ ounces) given in concentrated form each morning on an empty stomach is the most satisfactory method of inducing purgation in the majority of cases. This usually results in two or three large fluid stools each day. When this is not well borne by the stomach, i.e. when it occasions nausea and vomiting, 1 or 2 compound cathartic pills each night or compound jalap powder 1 to 3 gms. (15 to 40 grains) or compound elaterin powder 3 to 6 gms. (1/20 to 1/10 grain) in alcohol is sometimes efficacious when other methods have failed. Enemata may occasionally be necessary.

After the anasarca disappears, milder purgatives or laxatives such as cascara and liquorice powder may be required for regulating the intestines.

Diuresis.—This is usually obtained through the use of digitalis. Where this is not effectual, recourse is had to one of the caffeine diuretics. Theocine is most satisfactory, 0.2 gm. (3 grains) t.i.d. for one day. The effect is noted and the drug repeated on alternate days if necessary.

Support of Heart.—Digitalis is the drug par excellence in this connection. Introduced by Withering in 1785 for the relief of dropsy, it has become our mainstay in the treatment of myocardial insufficiency. Its relation to circulatory disturbances was emphasized by John Ferrier, 1799. Although a great amount of work has been done on this subject, little is yet known in a practical way concerning the chemistry of the active principles of digitalis. Undoubtedly, the future will furnish synthetic chemicals which ultimately will replace digitalis. But in the meantime, striking results can be obtained through its intelligent use.

Myocardial insufficiency constitutes the indication for its use regardless of the nature of the underlying lesions. Auricular fibrillation demands an intensive digitalis therapy, and indeed it is in cases of auricular fibrillation that we see its most striking effects. Its best diuretic effect is seen in dropsy dependent upon circulatory changes in the kidneys. In the acute myocardial involvement of acute febrile diseases, the usefulness of digitalis is rather limited. Once circulatory collapse supervenes, results are meager. Earlier in the disease, before blood pressure is markedly depressed, good results can be obtained especially in cases developing fibrillation. Toxic manifestation should be carefully watched for in such conditions.

Digitalis is manifold in its action. It acts on the heart muscle * itself, increasing its irritability, tonicity, and strength of contraction; on the bundle of His, decreasing conductivity; on the vagus, slowing the rate; on the vascular system through the vasomotor center; and directly on the vessel walls inducing vasoconstriction and increase in blood pressure. It slows the heart, increasing its force and the output per beat, and per minute, and tends, in passive congestion resulting from myocardial insufficiency, to shift the blood from the venous side, where it has collected, to the arterial side of the vascular system. In therapeutic doses it results in improved circulation through the kidney (a relative vasodilating effect upon the renal vessels being claimed), diuresis resulting. It finds its greatest value in cases of mitral disease with marked edema and small, rapid, and irregular pulse, although it is of value in all cases of myocardial insufficiency despite the nature of valvular lesion.

Digitalis should be administered in courses and its use should be intensive from the beginning, irrespective of the preparation used. A single course may suffice, but repeated courses are usually indicated. In auricular fibrillation intensive treatment is indicated at first and subsequently, after compensation is reëstablished, more or less continuous or

* In this connection the work of Schliomensun is extremely illuminating. (*Arch. f. Path. u. Pharm.*, LXIII.) An alcoholic phosphatid was extracted from the hearts of animals receiving digitalis therapy, which when injected into a second animal produced all of the biological reactions of digitalis. This, he claims, indicates a direct combination of digitalis with the heart muscle. Similar extracts from other tissues of these animals failed to yield such a product, indicating that the substance was specific to heart muscle.

tonic treatment. In this condition small doses can be taken almost continually, or at frequent intervals for months or years. Patients may feel well on this regimen, who otherwise do badly.

The preparations of digitalis are numerous, but four stand out preeminently. These are the powdered leaf, the tincture, the infusion, and digipuratum. Each preparation has its advocates. Results can be obtained with any of them provided the preparation is an active one and that it is properly administered to suitable cases.

The preparations most commonly used in the wards of our hospital are the infusion and the tincture. The infusion is given every 3 or 4 hours for 48 hours. The infusion is an aqueous extract and contains relatively more digitonin than the tincture. As a diuretic it is particularly valuable. It should be prepared fresh, a new supply being obtained once a week. The tincture is also excellent. It is an alcoholic preparation, containing relatively more digitoxin, digitalin, and digitophyllin than the infusion. It is administered in 1 c.c. doses every 3 or 4 hours for 48 hours. It is usually combined with tincture amygdali amari or some other bitter and administered well diluted.

The powdered leaf is given in 0.065 to 0.1 gm. (1 to 1½ gr.) doses every 3 or 4 hours for 48 hours. Digipuratum is a standardized preparation of digitalis in tablet form each corresponding to 0.065 to 0.1 gm. (1 to 1½ gr.) of the digitalis leaf. Four tablets are given during the first 24 hours, three the second, two the third, and one the fourth. It is an active preparation and well standardized, but much more expensive than any of the foregoing preparations which are equally efficacious, provided they are properly standardized. Digipuratum is also marketed in ampules in liquid form. This preparation can be given intravenously or intramuscularly without marked irritation. The ampule contains 1 c.c. which corresponds to 0.1 gm. of the leaf.

The doses given above represent the routine of the hospital. It cannot be too strongly emphasized, however, that digitalis should not be measured in grams, grains, or hours, but by results. The chief requisites are an active standardized preparation and proper indications. The former is readily obtained and is unquestionably of the greatest importance.

Standardization of Digitalis.—Two methods are in common use, the frog and the cat method. The frog method consists of injecting the digitalis preparation into the anterior lymph sac of a frog (Rana pipiens) and determining the amount necessary to bring about systolic standstill in one hour. The results are expressed in heart tonic units. This conveys no impression as to the activity of the preparation unless one knows what constitutes a heart tonic unit. According to Houghton, a heart tonic unit is ten times the normal fatal dose per gram of frog; to Edmonds it is the amount per 20 gm. weight of frog necessary to bring about systolic standstill in one hour, while according to Hale, it is the amount necessary per gm. of body weight. A heart tonic unit may therefore vary 400 per cent. according to what constitutes the standard. Nevertheless, the standardization is of value if one accepts any standardized preparation and learns how to use it intelligently. The frog method is not satisfactory for the standardization of a dilute preparation, such as the official infusion, since such large quantities must be introduced into the lymph sac that absorption is often not complete at the end of an hour.

The cat method of Hatcher ([63]) is simple and satisfactory. The preparation to be tested is slowly run into the femoral vein of a cat until death results. The number of c.c. per kg. of cat constitutes a cat unit. The technic as employed by the author in standardizing the infusion is as follows:—the cat is given just sufficient ether to permit a cannula being placed in the femoral vein. By means of a burette or a syringe 10 c.c. of the filtered infusion is injected in the course of five minutes, and 1 c.c. every two minutes thereafter until death. The total amount is noted, and the amount per kg. of the cat unit is calculated.

The following emphasizes the importance of standardization. Leaves from various sources (German, English, and American) obtained for the hospital pharmacy infusions were prepared according to the United States Pharmacopoeia. Macht ([64]) and the writer found that some of these infusions required only 6 to 7 c.c. per kg., whereas others required 10 and 12, and one (the German leaf) required 23 c.c. per kg. to kill the cat. A variation of 400 per cent. was therefore found in leaves in the hospital pharmacy. Before leaving Baltimore, the writer introduced American grown digitalis (Wisconsin leaf) into general use in the wards. Standardized American grown digitalis (Minnesota, Washington, and Oregon) was used extensively by the Medical Corps of the Army.

Eggleston ([65]) has recently claimed that 0.143 cat units per pound of body weight constitutes the amount necessary for maximal therapeutic effects. The additional claim is also made that this full amount can be given in 24 rather than in 48 hours, one-half being given in the first dose, one-third 4 to 6 hours later, and small doses at 4-hour intervals until the calculated amount is reached. Doses up to 50 c.c. of the infusion now in use in our wards have been given as the initial dose without untoward effect. This method has been thoroughly tested in my wards during the last three years by Drs. White and Morris ([66]) utilizing standardized American grown digitalis.

"Our impression is that the Eggleston method is a valuable addition in digitalis therapy, that it gives confidence in the use of the drug, and that the shorter time necessary for securing digitalis effects should give the method wide use. Results are frequently obtained within twenty-four hours.

The method must be used with care to select cases in which these effects are desired. Cases of acute or chronic infections, with the probability of the presence of endocardial infections, should be given the method, if at all, only after careful study, because of the possibility of embolism and, quite as important, in our opinion, the possibility of associated myocardial changes predisposing to block."

The method requires careful study of the patient before, during, and after its administration, and since it produces powerful and clear-cut effects, should be used with extreme care and judgment. The digitalis effect is often secured within 24 hours.

Since there are so great variations in the potency of digitalis, it becomes imperative for its intelligent use that the physician be familiar with the potency of the preparation which he is administering. The only other alternative is to push the drug until the therapeutic effect is obtained, provided it is a case suitable to digitalis therapy.

In order to do this, one must have well in mind what constitutes the therapeutic stage of digitalis treatment, and what criteria are to be accepted as indicating the desired digitalis effect. Slowing of the pulse is sometimes erroneously accepted as the criterion. It should not be, since slowing of the pulse does not always occur in the therapeutic stage, and since slowing of the pulse is not attained by digitalis in certain types of myocardial insufficiency. Thus Edens ([67]) states that slowing does not occur when hyperthyroidism is present, in acute myocarditis, in idiopathic hypertrophy, or in the small heart of tuberculous diathesis. In such conditions the toxic manifestations appear before slowing occurs.

When the patient is closely followed, the therapeutic stage is often accompanied by the first toxic manifestations, which are usually readily recognized. The following should be closely observed: (1) the urinary output in relation to the intake, since diuresis usually characterizes the therapeutic stage and oliguria the toxic stage of digitalis; (2) the outline of the heart; (3) the character of the heart beat and heart sounds; (4) the symptomatic condition of the patient with respect to dyspnea, cyanosis, and edema; (5) the effect on blood pressure and on the character of the pulse; and (6) the effect on cardiac function as revealed in electrocardiograms the inversion of the T wave occurs in the therapeutic stage, but block and other arrythmias indicate toxicity.

The time element in digitalis therapy is important. It is unusual to get digitalis effects from any preparation given by mouth in the ordinary dosage in less than 36 to 48 hours, more frequently 48 to 72 hours. Digitalis given today does not manifest its action until the day after tomorrow. Where immediate effect is necessary recourse may be had to strophanthin, and where the need is less urgent, Eggleston's dosage may be employed, provided the case is otherwise suitable.

Digitalis is cumulative in its effects and consequently should be given in courses. When the desired amount is prescribed, the digitalis should be stopped and the effect noted. The toxic effects are nausea and vomiting, vertigo, syncope, and diminished urinary secretion. The pulse may become either slow (vagus effect) or fast (increased muscle irritability). Irregularities may develop; a bigeminal or trigeminal pulse is rather pathognomonic of the toxic state. Auricular fibrillation may develop. Sudden cumulative effects are said to occur, but the more closely a patient is watched, the less sudden as a rule are the toxic effects of digitalis. Nausea and vomiting, which herald toxic action, often go unheeded.

The effect on blood pressure is deserving of comment, since digitalis in animal experiments leads to increase in blood pressure. Little or no influence on blood pressure is seen clinically. In some cases a rise is encountered, but more frequently a gradual fall in pressure is seen, which is often synchronous with unquestionable clinical improvement. Naturally rest, diet, purgation, and depletion also play a rôle in determining the effect on blood pressure.

Substitutes for Digitalis.—For routine use no drug can replace digitalis. Strophanthin, however, is unquestionably the best substitute, and in certain conditions it is preferable. Strophanthin is the most valuable preparation, the tincture of strophanthus comparing in no way with the tincture of digitalis.

Strophanthin is given in 0.25 to 0.5 mgm. doses intravenously and in 0.25 to 1 mgm. doses intramuscularly. Local massage for 15 minutes at the point of injection obviates the local irritant effect otherwise encountered. When used in 1 mgm. doses, it cannot be repeated within 24 hours; a dose of 0.5 mgm. may be repeated in 12 hours, although in the majority of cases it is unnecessary. Doses of 0.25 mgm. should be repeated in 8 to 12 hours. Strophanthin is given as is digitalis in courses of 2 to 3 days' duration.

Warning is necessary concerning its use where digitalis has been already administered. As already stated, digitalis requires 24 to 36 hours to demonstrate its effect. The addition of 0.5 mgm. strophanthin at the end of a course of digitalis may precipitate alarming toxic manifestations. On the other hand, strophanthin is admirable when used in the beginning of a course of digitalis as follows; a patient suffering from acute dilatation of the right heart may be bled, 0.5 mgm. strophanthin given intramuscularly, and then a course of digitalis started in the ordinary way. From this procedure an almost immediate digitalis effect is secured and maintained.

Strophanthin acts pharmacologically and therapeutically much as digitalis, but has somewhat less effect in vasoconstriction. It constricts the splanchnic terminals, as does digitalis, but not the vessels of the extremities and cerebrum, which may even undergo slight dilatation at times. Considerable controversy has been waged over its effect upon the coronaries. Digitalis constricts the coronaries and, therefore, decreases the blood supply to the heart muscle. Loeb claims that strophanthin here exerts a dilating influence. Voegtlin and Macht using arterial rings find a constricting influence for digitalis and a dilating effect for strophanthin. The chief effect of both drugs is identical, however; in shifting the blood from the venous to the arterial side of the vascular system.

The time necessary for the manifestation of their physiological effect is the chief point of difference. The strophanthin effect is almost immediate, whereas digitalis requires 24 to 36 hours. Strophanthin is, therefore, used in preference to digitalis where the need is urgent.

Caffeine or some member of the caffeine group is sometimes substituted for digitalis where the latter fails. When slowing results from its use, the pharmacological effect resembles that of digitalis. However, the pulse rate is more frequently accelerated than retarded. Unfortunately, its use is commonly attended with the development of palpitation, insomnia, and sometimes nausea, vomiting, and delirium. These untoward effects often appear as early as the effect on the heart, consequently caffeine is seldom employed in this connection.

But these purin derivatives are excellent diuretics. According to Schroeder, they exert a specific effect on the cells of the renal tubules and consequently they are often employed in myocardial insufficiency not as a substitute for digitalis, but as a synergist from the point of view of renal secretion. Theobromine has a more constant renal effect than caffeine, and is frequently used in 0.7 to 0.5 gm. t.i.d., or in the form of sodio-salicylate of theobromine 1 gm. t.i.d. The most valuable preparation of the caffeine group, however, is theocin, which is administered in 0.2 gm. (3 grain) doses three times a day for one day. It exerts less cerebral effect and consequently does not result so frequently in insomnia. It can be repeated on alternate days if its effect disappears rapidly. Where the diuretic effect of digitalis is lacking, our own practice is to turn to theocin, which is given in addition to digitalis and in the manner just indicated.

Certain other remedies sometimes substituted are perhaps worthy of mention. Squill is of value at times. It has a very mild digitalis effect, and is an excellent diuretic. It is given as the tincture (0.3 to 1 c.c.) or as the syrup (2 to 4 c.c.). Neimeyer's or Addison's pills which contain one grain each of calomel, digitalis, and squill is a valuable preparation. Apocynum as the fluid extract (1 c.c.), convallaria as the tincture (0.3 to 1 c.c.), and adonidin 10 to 20 mgm. are occasionally used, but are of very doubtful therapeutic value. Spartein sulphate 0.065 to 0.13 gm. is rarely employed. Cactus grandiflorus is absolutely inert and should be deleted from the pharmacopeia.

Adjuncts to Digitalis Therapy.—Anemia is not at all infrequent in myocardial insufficiency. Iron and arsenic are here of the greatest value. Strychnia is occasionally of value. Alcohol in small doses for its psychical effect is employed at times, in those accustomed to its use, when craving is great.

The value of charts, quickly conveying the effect or need of treatment from the standpoint of the kidney is worthy of emphasis. At a glance, one accustomed to their use grasps the condition of renal activity.

The Symptomatic Treatment of Myocardial Insufficiency

At times certain symptoms become so pronounced as to call for special treatment in addition to the general treatment described above.

(1) *Edema* is usually controlled by rest, diet, restriction of fluids and salts and by digitalis alone, or together with one of the caffeine bodies. Where these fail, or where the anasarca is extreme so that pressure interferes with the action of the heart or lungs, tapping of the cavities concerned is necessary. Where edema of the extremities is so severe as to threaten gangrene, drainage may be employed with success.

(2) *Dyspnea.*—The cause of the dyspnea should be determined. If mechanical, paracentesis may be indicated or special attention to diet if there is pressure from intestines filled with gas. The back rest may bring great relief. For orthopnea, morphine 10 mgm. and atropine 0.5 mgm. often brings relief. When these fail, and when marked dilatation of the right heart is found, venesection and strophanthin answer best.

Formerly nitrites were much used in dyspnea associated with hypertension. The dyspnea is now considered as evidence of beginning myocardial weakness and calls for digitalis and not for vasodilators.

(3) *Arrhythmias.*—Digitalis has a marked effect on rhythm. This

must be constantly in mind since many arrhythmias encountered clinically are of digitalis origin, and the treatment consists in the removal, not in the administration of the drug.

Auricular fibrillation is the condition in which digitalis produces its most brilliant effects. "The overstretched auricular muscles are unable to make concerted contractions and instead enter into a state of tremulation or fibrillation." These irregular impulses are transmitted to the ventricle, producing a confusion of rhythm, or absolute irregularity. The output of the heart is markedly decreased, and its efforts ineffective. The main effect of digitalis is lessened conductivity, but an influence is also exerted on the irritability of the muscle. Improvement in rhythm is often accompanied by prompt and decided increase in blood flow.

Digitalis is indicated in auricular flutter. Fibrillation is frequently induced which disappears on the removal of digitalis, leaving a normal rhythm in its stead. Partial heart block is exaggerated by digitalis which intensifies the degree of the block and tends to result in a complete block. Unless digitalis is needed for other reasons, it should be withheld. Atropine, on the other hand, may be effective in the removal of this form of block. Since in complete heart block interference with conductivity is sufficiently complete to effect total dissociation in auricular and ventricular rhythm, digitalis can do no harm. It renders ventricular contraction more effective and tends somewhat to decrease its rate and consequently is of value. Extra-systoles are the result of increased myocardial irritability and hence tend to be increased rather than decreased by the drug. Digitalis, if indicated, can be used effectively despite their existence. Extra-systoles should be treated by general hygienic measures. Sinus arrhythmia likewise is exaggerated by digitalis because of the stimulation of the vagus.

(4) *Hypertension.*—This is best met through general measures such as rest, sleep, diet, and depletion. The medicinal lowering of blood pressure is best effected through the use of digitalis. Other vasodilators and blood pressure lowering drugs are rarely indicated. The use of nitrites should be restricted to conditions in which there is localized arteriosclerosis or arterial spasm in a vital part as in angina pectoris, and to cases in which, as a result of high blood pressure, a vascular accident such as apoplexy is feared. It must be admitted, however, that nitrites occasionally result in benefit when used in conjunction with digitalis, and when digitalis along with general measures have failed. If used at all, the onset and duration of their action should be borne in mind. The results of Wallace and Ringer ([68]) in relation to these desiderata are shown in the following tables:

Drug	*Dose*	*Time of beginning action*	*Time of max. effect*	*Duration of action (min.)*	*Max. extent of action*	*Maximum extent of action (mm. Hg.)*
I						
Amyl nitrite	3 min.	1	3	7	15	
Nitroglycerin, 1 per cent. sol.	1 1/2 min.	2	8	30	15	In normal subjects
Sodium nitrite	1 gr.	10	25	60	14	
Erythrol tetranitrate	1/2 gr.	15	32	120-240	16	
II						
Nitroglycerin	1/30 gr.	2	8	35	32	In arterio-sclerosis
Sodium nitrite	2 gr.	15	45	120	53	
Erythrol tetranitrate	2 gr.	30	60	180	60	

(5) *Palpitation and Cardiac Distress.*—Occasionally the gastrointestinal tract is at fault, and its responsibility should be investigated. Local treatment may suffice. The ice bag is frequently the most potent source of comfort. Small blisters and belladonna plasters are of value at times. Internally, potassium iodide is frequently employed with success. Tincture aconite may also help at times.

(6) *Gastric Symptoms.*—Nausea and vomiting are commonly encountered. They frequently yield rapidly to the general treatment already described. Their origin must always be determined since their appearance after instituting digitalis therapy should suggest the possibility of responsibility of digitalis. The treatment may be withdrawal of digitalis. Similarly Epsom salts may be responsible.

All food should be stopped for 12 hours if nausea and vomiting become extreme, and nothing should be allowed by mouth except crushed ice. Later, milk and lime water are allowed in small amounts. Gastric sedatives such as sips of cold effervescing drinks, champagne, apollinaris water or an ordinary syphon are often of value. Bismuth 1 to 2 grams, creosote 0.1 c.c., dilute hydrocyanic acid 0.065 c.c., cocain hydrochloride 5 to 10 mgm. or a mixture of tr. nux vomica 0.3 c.c. and soda bicarbonate 0.1 gram may be tried. Counter-irritation in the form of a mustard plaster to the abdominal wall is occasionally helpful.

Naturally in myocardial insufficiency associated with chronic nephritis, nausea and vomiting may be evidences of uremia. All of the above methods may be tried without success while some general sedative acting centrally, such as chloral 0.3 gram every 4 hours or morphine 10 mgm., may bring relief. Persistent nausea and vomiting, particularly if associated with a markedly enlarged and pulsating liver, is an extremely serious complication, often ending fatally.

(7) *Cough.*—The cough is usually due to circulatory changes in the lungs and responds to the cardiac treatment. Expectorants are as a rule contraindicated.

(8) *Hemoptysis.*—Though most alarming to the patient, hemoptysis in myocardial insufficiency is seldom serious. The patient should be assured that the hemorrhage is salutary and does away with the necessity of doing a venesection. Assurance, absolute quiet, and an ice bag over the chest usually suffice. When the patient is markedly upset, a small dose of morphia is often desirable.

(9) *Edema of the Lungs.*—This is an extremely serious complication and calls for quick action. The patient should be bled 400 to 600 c.c. Morphia 15 mgm. should be given hypodermically. Atropin 0.5 mgm. is used at times, but morphine is of greater value.

(10) *Insomnia.*—This is frequently a very troublesome symptom. A good back rest with side supports often allows a comfortable sleep in a sitting posture. Any of the following hypnotics or sedatives can be tried—paraldehyde 2 to 8 c.c. in capsules, sulphonal 0.6 to 2 gms., Hoffman's anodyne 2 to 4 c.c., spts. of chloroform 0.3 to 0.6 c.c., spts. of camphor 1 to 3 c.c. alone or 2 c.c. in combination with ether 2 c.c., veronal 0.3 gm., barbital or barbital sodium 0.6 to 1 gm. or urethane 1 to 2 gm. Where these do not give relief it is better not to waste valuable time. Morphia 10 to 15 mgm. alone or in combination with atropine 0.5 mgm. should be given hypodermically.

In these various ways conditions arising from myocardial insufficiency are met. The means used are successful in so far as they influence function. They can have little if any effect on structure. They do in many cases so modify function that discomfort is converted into comfort, dangerous crises averted, and life prolonged with a reasonable degree of daily activity.

(8) Medical Organization

Specialization more than any other single factor serves to advance a science. A coterie of workers devoting "whole time" to the advancement of a subject brings to it that concerted continuous thought and effort so necessary for success. The field of pharmacology is being tilled and cultivated by an ever-increasing group. Chairs of pharmacology assure the development of this subject. Similiarly, institutions such as the Speyer House and the Rockefeller Institute and Hospital have contributed greatly to progress. The methods adopted by Ehrlich, Flexner, and Cole in relation to trypanosomiasis, syphilis, relapsing fever, meningitis, poliomyelitis, and pneumonia are those most needed in medicine. Cole and his co-workers have exercised the type of critical judgment and employed the numerous controls so necessary for sound progress yet so uniformly lacking in most therapeutic investigation.

Pharmacological societies and publications, the natural outcome of the development of the science, in turn, have played a great rôle in its further development.

What is Needed for the Advance of Therapy

Since doctrines control therapy, treatment will improve as medicine advances. This involves the adaptation to medicine of all that is applicable in science. All progress in the fundamental branches eventually advances practice. The healing art must give place to the healing science.

Sound training in the fundamental sciences, in medicine and in pharmacology, constitutes the therapeutist's greatest asset. The doctor must feel the responsibility of treatment as well as of diagnosis. The same thought and individual effort accorded diagnosis must also be accorded treatment. Individualistic diagnosis must not be followed by book treatment. Common sense individualized, and not book authority, is needed in treatment.

Pharmacology is young. Science, like history, is built by individuals. Individual effort in research is the basis of progress in pharmacology. Dosage must be reduced to a matter of certainty. In the absence of chemical entities, standardization of drugs and units are greatly needed, otherwise accuracy of dosage is impossible. Treatment should always be conducted after the manner of a scientific investigation. The remedy and dosage once decided, throughout treatment, careful observations must be made with adequate record of results. Daily notations, keeping in mind the disease and the treatment, markedly increase the physician's capacity as a therapeutist. Graphic methods of record such as electrocardiograms and fluid balance charts are most desirable.

Leadership on the part of leaders of medicine is needed. Therapeutic nihilism or failure to utilize useful remedial measures on the part of teachers of medicine engenders neglect of therapy in the mind of the student. Organized effort is necessary to combat the growing evils of advertising on the part of proprietary pharmaceutical interests. The physician must see to it that treatment rests on the basis of science, and not on the claims of drug houses.

It is interesting to note that progress in therapy has been associated with a marked decrease in the number of drugs used. The application of science has revealed true values as a result of which the majority of drugs have fallen into disuse. There is, however, great room for further progress along such lines. New drugs are needed, but for each one adopted many should be discarded.

The complexity of the human organism, of life processes and to a less extent of drugs demands breadth and depth in investigation, the details of which are usually beyond one individual. Group investigation is as greatly needed as group practice. In chemotherapy, chemistry and experimental medicine are represented, but chemical detail is usually best handled by chemists and therapeutic detail by physicians. Each deserves the best individual effort of a specialist. The master mind must deal with the fundamental conception and with close scrutiny of all details rather than with their actual execution. This involves organization and great expenditure of time. In America one of the greatest needs of modern medicine is a national institute for pharmacological research.

BIBLIOGRAPHY

(The articles listed include the more general and collective summaries and relatively few of the more specific articles quoted in the text.)

1. WITHINGTON, E. T.: Medical History from the Earliest Times. London, 1894.
   GARRISON, F. H.: An Introduction to the History of Medicine. Philadelphia, 1917.
   BAASS: Author of the History of Medicine. New York, 1910.
2. BARKER, L. F., and SLADEN, F. J.: Tr. Ass. Am. Phys., 1912, XXVII, 484.
3. BRUNTON, L.: Goulstonian Lectures: Pharmacology and Therapeutics. London, 1880, 10.
4. BERNARD, C.: Compt. rend. Soc. de biol., Paris, 1850, XXX, 1533; 1856, XLIII, 825.
5. BRODIE, B.: Phila. Trans., 1812, 205.
6. CRUM, BROWN, and FRASER: Trans. Roy. Soc. Edinb., 1869, XXV, 151.
7. WOOD, H. C.: A Treatise on Therapeutics, 1876.
8. LANGLEY, J. N.: Jour. Physiol., 1898, XXIII, 240.
9. MEYER, H. H., and GOTTLIEB, R.: Pharmacology, Experimental and Clinical. Philadelphia, 1914, 139.
10. EHRLICH, P.: Studies in Immunity. Bolduan, New York, 1910, 404.
11. BAYLISS, W. M.: General Principles of Physiology. New York, 1915.
12. ABEL, J. J., and ROWNTREE, L. G.: Jour. Pharm. and Exper. Therap., 1909, I, 231.
13. ROWNTREE, L. G., HURWITZ, S. H., and BLOOMFIELD, A. L.: Johns Hopkins Hosp. Bull., 1913, XXIV, 327.
14. ROWNTREE, L. G., and GERAGHTY, J. T.: Arch. Int. Med., 1912, IX, 284.
15. STAHLSCHMIDT: Poggendorff's Annalen, 1859, CVIII, 523; quoted from Crum, Brown and Fraser.
16. EHRLICH, P.: *Loc. cit.*

17. MACHT, D.: Jour. Pharm. and Exper. Therap., 1915, VII, 339; 1916, VIII, 1 and 451; 1917, IX, 121, 473, and 351; 1917-18, X, 95; 1918, XI, 389 and 419; 1919, XII, 255.
18. HUNT, R.: Arch. Internat. de Pharmacodyn., 1904, XII, 448.
19. BARGER, G., and DALE, H. H.: Jour. Physiol., 1910-11, XLI, 19 and 51.
20. EHRLICH, P.: The Experimental Chemotherapy of Spirilloses, Ehrlich, and Hata, translated by Newbold. New York, 1911.
21. LEVERAN, C. L. A., and MESNIL, F.: Trypanosomes and Trypanosomiasis. Paris, 1912.
22. THOMAS, H. W.: Brit. Med. Jour., 1905, I, 1140.
23. ROWNTREE, L. G., and ABEL, J. J.: Jour. Pharm. and Exper. Therap., 1910-11, II, 101 and 501.
24. HATA, S.: The Experimental Chemotherapy of Spirilloses, Ehrlich, and Hata, translated by Newbold. New York, 1911.
25. METCHNIKOFF: Ann. de l'Inst. Pasteur, 1907, XXI, 753.
26. UHLENHUTH, P., HOFFMAN, E., and WEIDANZ, O.: Deutsch. Med. Woch., 1907, XXXIII, 1590.
27. LEVADITI, C., and YAMANOUCHI, T.: Compt. rend. Soc. de biol., Paris. 1908, LXIV, 911.
28. LESSER, E.: Deutsch. Med. Woch., 1907, XXIII, 1076, 1313, 1559.
29. NEISSER, E.: Deutsch. Med. Woch., 1908, XXXIV, 1500.
30. TRUFFI, M.: Centralb. f. Bakt., 1908-09, XLVIII, Abt. I, 597, and LII, Abt. I, 555.
31. CARREL, A., and DEHELLY, G.: Infected Wounds, translated by Childs. New York, 1917.
32. DAKIN, H. D., COHEN, J. B., DAUFRESNE, M., and KENYON, J.: Proc. Roy. Soc. London, 1915-17, LXXXIX, 232.
33. LUSK, G.: Science of Nutrition. Philadelphia, 3d ed., 1917.
34. LIEBIG, J.: Die organische Chemie in ihrer Anwendung auf Physiologie u. Pathologie, 1842.
35. PETTENKOFFER: Annal. de Chem. Pharmakol., Supplement 2, 1862.
36. DUBOIS, E.: Arch. Int. Med., 1915, XV, 793-939; 1916, XVII, 855-1010; 1917, XIX, 823-931.
37. OSBORNE, T. B., and MENDEL, L. B.: Trans. Fifth Internat. Congress of Hygiene and Dermograph; Jour. Biol. Chem., 1912, XII, 81.
38. McCOLLUM: Jour. Biol. Chem., 1912-13, XIII, 209.
39. ABDERHALDEN, E.: Synthese der Zellbausteine in Pflanze und Tier. Berlin, 1912.
40. FUNK, C.: Jour. Physiol., 1911-12, XLIII, 395.
41. BARGER, G.: The Simpler Natural Bases, 1914, 112.
42. HOPKINS, F. G.: Jour. Physiol., 1912, XLIV, 425.
43. STARLING, E. H., and BAYLISS, W. M.: Lancet, 1905, II, 339, 423, 501, and 579; Proc. Roy. Soc. London, 1904, LXXIII, 310.
44. EDSALL, D. L., and MEANS, J. H.: Arch. Int. Med., 1914, XIV, 897; Trans. Am. Phys., 1914, XXIX, 69.
45. HIGGINS, H. L., and MEANS, J. H.: Jour. Pharm. and Exper. Therap., 1915, VII, 1.
46. ROBERTSON, T. B.: Jour. Biol. Chem., 1916, XXIV, 416.
47. BAYLISS, W. M.: Principles of General Physiology, 1918, 29.
48. CANNON, W. B.: Am. Jour. Physiol., 1914, XXIII, 356.

49. CRILE, C. W.: The Origin and Nature of the Emotions. Philadelphia, 1915.
50. PARRY, C. H.: Collections from the unpublished medical writings of the late Caleb Hillier Parry. London, 1825.
51. GRAVES: London Med. and Surg. Jour., 1835, VII, 516.
52. BASEDOW: Wochnschr. f. de ges Heilk., 1840, VI, XIII, and XIV.
53. GULL: Trans. Clin. Soc. London, 1873-74, IV, 180.
54. ORD: Medico-Chirurgical Trans., London, 1878, LXI, 57.
55. KOCHER, T.: Arch. f. klin. Chir., 1883, XXIX, 254.
56. SCHIFF, M.: Arch. f. exper. Path. u. Pharm., 1884, XVIII, 25.
57. HORSLEY, V.: Brit. Med. Jour., 1890, I, 287.
58. MURRAY, G. R.: Brit. Med. Jour., 1892, I, 449.
59. BAUMANN, E.: Muench. med. Woch., 1896, XLVI, 309.
60. KENDALL, E. C.: Trans. Assoc. Am. Phys., 1918, XXIII, 324.
61. SAINSBURY, H.: Principia Therapeutica. New York, 1907.
62. ROWNTREE, L. G.: Trans. Cong. Am. Phys. and Surg., 1913, IX, 23.
63. HATCHER, R. A., and BRODY, J. G.: Am. Jour. of Pharm., 1910, LXXXII, 360.
64. ROWNTREE, L. G., and MACHT, D. I.: Jour. Am. Med. Assoc., 1916, LXVI, 870.
65. EGGLESTON, C.: Arch. Int. Med., 1915, XVI, 1.
66. WHITE, S. M., and MORRIS, R. E.: Arch. Int. Med., 1918, XXI, 740.
67. EDENS, E.: Deutsch. Arch. f. klin. Med., 1911, CIV, 512.
68. WALLACE, G. B., and RINGER, A. I.: Jour. Am. Med. Assoc., 1909, LIII, 1629.

A Desk Index of Oxford Medicine will be issued following publication of the last volume.

In the meantime, use the Table of Contents at the beginning of each chapter.

CHAPTER XXIII

EDEMA

By GEORGE D. BARNETT

Table of Contents

Historical

Dropsy has been an outstanding problem since the beginnings of medicine. It is mentioned in the Ebers papyrus and on the clay tablets of medical prescriptions of ancient Assyria. Modern nutritionists have noted with satisfaction the report that 2,300 years ago Heraclitus, disgusted with mankind, retired to the mountains, lived on vegetables and herbs alone, acquired dropsy and died. The Hippocratic writers have a good deal to say about it, classifying it, regarding it as a liquefaction of the tissues brought about by some malady of the spleen and treating it by laxatives and by abdominal puncture, when there was much ascites. Others among the ancients thought dropsy due to a disorder of the liver, as often it doubtless was. Saliceto in 1275 mentioned an association with scanty urine and hardened kidneys, but otherwise the medieval writings are not enlightening. Even Sydenham, who gives so vivid a description of cardiac edema, does not mention a suspicion that the heart might be at fault. In the XVIII Century Morgagni found valvular defects in many cases of dropsy but did not carry the matter farther. Withering knew no distinction between cardiac and renal dropsy and was disappointed that cerebral and ovarian dropsies did not yield to the foxglove. Not until two hundred years after Harvey was edema recognized as a symptom common to many disease pictures, and this we owe to Corvisart, to Laennec and especially, to Bright.

A rational consideration of the mechanism of dropsy also began early in the last century, when the rise of clinical physiology brought numerous suggestions, such as the lymphatic obstruction hypothesis of Broussais, the increased capillary filtration of the Ludwig school and Heidenhain's idea of augmented lymph secretion. Present concepts date from 1896 when Starling[31] first pointed out clearly that a balance between hydrostatic and osmotic forces determines fluid movement through the capillary walls and is, consequently, concerned primarily in edema formation. For fifty years the hypothesis has served those who have wished to understand edemas. There have been some clinical discrepancies, and the recent studies of electrolyte and water balance[10, 27] have made it plain at least that we have not arrived yet at a complete knowledge of the physiology of edema. A brief consideration of some of the factors that influence fluid distribution in the body will permit an understanding of some of the mechanisms concerned.

The Physiology of Fluid Distribution

Edema is a local or general increase in the interstitial fluid of the body. Normally the interstitial compartment is separated from the blood plasma by the capillary endothelium, a membrane through which water and crystalloid substances pass with ease, but which is largely impermeable to colloids, chiefly the proteins of the plasma. It is separated from the intracellular fluid by the cell walls, which are permeable to water but not freely so to electrolytes, to proteins or to most other solutes. Membrane permeabilities within the body probably are never absolute; normal interstitial fluid probably contains a small amount of protein[33], and the conditions under which variations in permeability may occur frequently are not understood. The interstitial fluid constitutes the immediate internal environment of the body cells, and its volume and the total osmolar content of its dissolved substances are maintained at quite constant levels by gain or loss of fluid from or to the vascular or cellular compartments and indirectly, by excretion or retention of water or solutes by the kidneys[10, 17].

Fluid transfer through the capillary walls is of especial importance in the edema problem. Normally the effective hydrostatic pressure, which maintains a constant flow from capillaries to tissue spaces, is the capillary pressure minus the tissue pressure, and the effective osmotic pressure, which moves fluid in the opposite direction, is the osmotic pressure of the plasma colloids, chiefly proteins, minus the osmotic pressure of the proteins in the tissue fluids.* For further discussion and diagrams see Vol. III, Chapter X of Oxford Medicine.

The Starling Equilibrium

It was this balance of hydrostatic against osmotic forces that Starling postulated in 1896, and its validity as the immediate mechanism by which fluids are moved through membranes in the body is beyond question. Landis[21] has shown that the actual measured pressures conform to the hypothesis; Schade[29] has demonstrated the mechanism in a laboratory model, and Peters[27] reminds us that the fact, that extracellular fluid has been shown to have the composition of an ultrafiltrate of plasma, is even more substantial proof of its validity. Apparent discrepancies are recorded occasionally in the literature, but no data are given which include measurements of the effective hydrostatic and osmotic pressures.

Possible Changes That Favor Edema Production

There are many possible changes in the Starling equilibrium in the direction of edema production. If the flow of lymph from a region be obstructed, the increasing tissue pressure will decrease the outward flow from the capillaries until it equals the return flow inward, and during this period edema fluid will accumulate. Decrease in the effective colloid osmotic pressure may result from diminished plasma protein concentration or from increased protein in the tissue fluids, due almost always to increased permeability of the capillary endothelium. Hypoproteinemia has many possible causes, which Rytand[28] has outlined (Table I).

TABLE I

PHYSIOLOGICAL CAUSES OF HYPOPROTEINEMIA

A. Loss and destruction of body protein
   - I. Urine (Bright's disease)
   - II. Ascitic fluid (cirrhosis with paracenteses)
   - III. Tissue (cachexia)
   - IV. Fetus (pregnancy)

* The effects of hydrostatic pressure are obvious. The nature of the osmotic action is perhaps clarified by noting that the protein molecules within the capillary, by their mere presence and because they cannot escape, obstruct the outward diffusion of water and dissolved crystalloids, but in the fluid of the tissue spaces there is nothing to obstruct their diffusion inward. The net flow due to the plasma proteins is, therefore, inward. By this concept the osmotic force, which moves fluid, is derived from the universal kinetic energy of molecular movement and need not be regarded as a mysterious "attractive" or "drawing" force exerted upon water molecules by dissolved substances. By another similar concept the net diffusion of water and crystalloid molecules is inward, because they are in higher concentration outside than inside the capillary.

B. Retarded formation of serum protein
  I. Lack of dietary protein
    (a) Absolute total dietary insufficiency
      (1) Starvation
      (2) Pyloric obstruction
      (3) Diarrhea
    (b) Relative total dietary insufficiency
      (1) Pregnancy
      (2) Hyperthyroidism
      (3) Diabetes mellitus
    (c) Dietary protein deficiency
      (1) Low protein diet
      (2) Pancreatic disease

  II. Altered states of the body
    (a) Normal
      (1) The newborn
    (b) Abnormal
      (1) Hepatic disease
      (2) Bright's disease
      (3) Beriberi

  III. Unexplained

Increased capillary permeability may result from the damaging effect of a local or general toxic agent, and capillary dilatation from any cause probably produces some degree of protein leak. So a rise in tissue temperature from the application of heat, from fever or even from hot weather may increase tissue fluids. Nervous impulses, normal or abnormal, also may increase capillary permeability both by simple vasodilatation and probably also by a neurochemical mechanism.

Increase in the effective capillary hydrostatic pressure may occur if there is obstruction ahead in the veins, or because of increased capillary volume if there is arteriolar dilatation or increased total plasma volume. Less obvious are the effects of electrolytes, especially sodium salts, which may have a profound effect on water distribution in the body[10].

Salt Effects

Physiological variations in the volumes of the three fluid compartments (vascular, interstitial, intracellular) are not normally very great. Fluid usually enters the blood stream from the gastrointestinal tract. Selective absorption of water and salts in the intestinal villi and prompt renal excretion of excesses of one or the other combine to make the electrolyte concentration changes in the plasma minimal. Whatever added volume of fluid remains in the plasma increases the hydrostatic pressure and decreases the colloid osmotic pressure in some degree, and both of these changes lead to increased outflow from capillaries to interstitial fluid. Thus salt solution retained for even a short time is distributed rapidly throughout the extracellular compartment. Large amounts will increase any edema already present, or the process may combine with pathological factors to produce an initial clinical edema. Sufficiently vigorous and prolonged administration of salt and water may even cause slight edema in normal subjects. If experimentally or as a result of pathological conditions the interstitial fluid becomes hypertonic, there will be an osmotic flow of water into it from the intracellular fluid, and conversely, if interstitial fluid becomes hypotonic, its volume will shrink by osmotic transfer of water into the cells. The occurrence of such a loss of edema without change in weight of the patient has been described.

It should be noted here especially that the transfer of salt solution from plasma to tissue spaces is to be regarded as a simple consequence of the shift in the Starling equilibrium acting throughout the vast capillary membrane, and that it implies no peculiar ability of the tissues to attract or to retain salt. Flow of fluid in the opposite direction also occurs with equal ease whenever the balance shifts to require it. This usually involves renal excretion of salt and water with reduction in plasma volume and capillary hydrostatic pressure and increase in plasma colloid osmotic pressure. The kidney can excrete excess salt or excess water as the occasion demands, and slight hypotonicity or hypertonicity probably can be an adequate stimulus, but beyond this the conditions under which body fluid volumes are regulated and how they are regulated by the kidneys is not understood completely. Some of the factors involved are the volume of blood flow to the kidneys, the number of active glomeruli and the acceptance or rejection of water or electrolytes by the tubule cells[29(a)]. It is here that certain of the hormones are active.

Hormone Effects

An antidiuretic substance is elaborated by the pituicytes of the neurohypophysis and may be identical with the pressor hormone pitressin. It controls effectively the polyuria of diabetes insipidus and participates in the normal fluid balance. The steroid hormones of the adrenals and gonads are concerned also with electrolyte and water balance[35] and thus indirectly with the edema problem. In Addison's disease deficiency of the adrenal cortical hormone leads to a low level of the sodium salts in the plasma, to dehydration, to low plasma volume and to shock. Replacement therapy with cortical extract or desoxycorticosterone may then so increase the salt and water content of the extracellular fluid that general edema results. The action of the adrenal cortical hormone is upon the renal tubules, promoting reabsorption of sodium salts. Most of the hormones of the ovary and testis are said to promote retention of water and sodium salts[36], but their mode of action has not been established. Lack of thyroid hormone brings about in some manner an increase in soluble colloid material, probably mucoprotein, in the interstitial fluid. The effective colloid osmotic pressure of the plasma is reduced and edema results. Fluid retention is seen also at times during insulin therapy, rarely with slight but definite edema, especially in patients recovering from coma. Excessive infusions of salt solution as well as some lowering of the plasma proteins from a dietary cause not related to insulin are responsible frequently. A true hormonal action here is doubtful.

Compensation for Varying Capillary Pressure

Hydrostatic pressure in the capillaries varies widely in different parts of the body. In the standing position gravity increases the pressure greatly in the legs, and pressures are believed to be low in the capillaries of the lungs and of the liver. Since the colloid osmotic pressure of the plasma is presumably about the same throughout the circulation, the question must arise as to how a balance can be obtained. Partial answers are available. In the liver a high protein content of the tissue fluid lowers the effective colloid osmotic pressure and is evidenced by high protein figures in liver lymph[32]. It has been suggested that this is protein newly formed in the liver. In the lower extremities lymph flow is greater, indicating that outflow from the capillaries is maintained there at a higher level. Local increase in capillary permeability is another possible adjustment to offset low capillary hydrostatic pressure, but good evidence of such a compensation is lacking. It is of some teleological interest to note that in the lungs the low capillary pressure is strikingly adapted to the maintenance of dryness in the alveoli.

Imbibition of water by the colloids of the tissue cells under the influence of environmental changes has been considered important in edema formation, but edema fluid is essentially interstitial, and the chief known changes that take place in intracellular fluid volume are osmotic, the result of differences in concentrations of electrolytes inside and outside the cells. The contribution of colloid imbibition to edema is small, and the occasions of its participation are not known.

Clinical Edemas

Edema is nearly always a pathological finding, although occasionally small local accumulations of excess tissue fluid may be recognizable in normal individuals. A transient, slight swelling of the eyelids and periorbital tissues may be present in some persons on arising in the morning, and others may show a slight edema of the ankles on prolonged quiet standing.

The interstitial space is very distensible, and weight curves in certain patients show that it can accept as much as eight or ten liters before edema appears. Bedside recognition of minimal edema is occasionally uncertain, and opinions may differ in a given case. The phenomenon of pitting, by which we commonly demonstrate subcutaneous edema, is merely the displacement of freely movable fluid in the intercommunicating tissue spaces, but sufficient pressure maintained sufficiently long will produce pitting in the normal subject, and the borderline between normal and pathological pitting thus is not sharp. Edema that has been present a long time is apt to become hard and to pit with difficulty. This is said to be due to connective tissue proliferation. In myxedema there is said to be a nonpitting edema, but if the fluid resides in the intercellular spaces and not in the tissue cells, the term is without meaning. True non-pitting edema, other than the weight increase usually called pre-edema, probably is non-existent.

The Edema of Circulatory Failure

Cardiac edema usually is a late manifestation of heart failure. Frequently it is noticed first as a slight swelling above the shoetops, present in the evening and gone the next morning, and examination at this time will show distention of the neck veins, which also disappears promptly with rest. Often preceding this edema there has been a long period of increased load upon the left ventricle, such as hypertension, aortic valve disease, with gradual asymptomatic hypertrophy and dilatation, later dyspnea, and with physical findings due to pulmonary congestion or frank pulmonary edema. This common clinical sequence from the left ventricle through the lungs to the systemic veins strongly supports the backward-failure hypothesis of cardiac insufficiency with its corollary that the edema of heart failure is due immediately to the increased intracapillary pressure which must follow venous congestion. Starling proposed this mechanism[32], and many investivations have served to confirm it. Landis and others [21] have shown that even a small rise in venous pressure is sufficient to cause measurable amounts of fluid to accumulate in the tissues and recently Landis and associates[22] have reported that, after experimental cardiac damage of several kinds in dogs, exercise produces elevation of venous pressure, whereas in normal dogs it is reduced by similar exercise. It seems proven, therefore, that a chief immediate cause of the edema of congestive heart failure is increased hydrostatic pressure in the capillaries, and that the effective increase is at first that which occurs during exercise.

Some decrease in plasma proteins is not an uncommon finding in heart failure and is the sum of several items[15]. The diet is often low in protein, and with severe congestion loss in the urine may be considerable. Late in heart failure there is usually a significant increase in blood volume[22] in which both hydremia and increased permeability due to anoxia may contribute to the lowered plasma protein percentage, and finally the congested liver may be unable to produce new protein at an adequate rate. Although the plasma protein levels are never very low, any decrease will contribute to the accumulation of edema fluid.

Increased permeability of the capillary walls as a result of anoxia is mentioned often as a factor in cardiac edema. Landis has demonstrated that lack of oxygen will make the endothelium more permeable, but the degree of anoxia in his experiments is greater than that usually found in any but terminal stages of heart failure. A necessary result of increased permeability would be a high concentration of protein in the edema fluid. Reported values vary considerably but do not indicate any significant leakage of protein. The protein concentrations found in cardiac edema fluids also do not show any correlation with the duration of the edema. So it must be concluded that the integrity of the capillary wall is rarely much impaired.

Increase in the sodium salt content of the body will bring about an increase in extracellular fluid volume in cardiac patients as well as in normals and thus will promote edema formation. With failure of the circulation there may be a marked reduction in blood flow to the kidneys[38] with impaired excretion of sodium salts and water. This would increase an edema already present, but that such a mechanism is ever active early in the course of heart failure is unlikely.

Hydrothorax of some degree is almost a constant part of the edema of late heart failure. Its appearance earlier and more extensively on the right side is an old clinical observation which has had several explanations such as the pressure of the enlarging heart on the right pulmonary vein or stasis in the azygos vein. Dock believes that like other cardiac edema it is localized by gravity, as there is a longer return course of blood from the right lung than from the left. Right lateral decubitus thus will favor its accumulation.

Pulmonary Edema

Intracapillary pressure is considerably lower in the lung than in the systemic circulation, and the Starling balance thus should be displaced in favor of dryness in the alveoli. The ability of the pulmonary capillaries to absorb fluid from the air cells is in fact extraordinary. Drinker[12] cites the experiment of Colin, who in 1873 poured 21 liters of water into the trachea of a horse in a period of 3½ hours without ill effect.

Acute pulmonary edema[12, 24] occurs commonly in patients with heart failure. Its association with long-standing overwork of the left ventricle is so striking that the conclusion seems justified that left ventricular failure with increased pressure throughout the pulmonary circulation is an important mechanism in its production. Welch[41] suggested such an explanation in 1878 and supported it with animal experimentation, but Wiggers[43] was unable to produce pulmonary edema in dogs, in which very high capillary pressures were maintained for thirty minutes, and believes that back-pressure alone rarely can account for acute pulmonary edema in man. The frequent occurrence of attacks of acute pulmonary edema during the night, when left ventricular recuperation should be greatest, has been an enigma. Acute myocardial strain from disturbing dreams has been suggested, but a more likely cause is a nocturnal increase in blood volume in the lung as a result of rest[22]. Systemic venous congestion is relieved and reabsorption of tissue fluid may occur. The bout of dyspnea, which often begins the attack, also may favor transudation by lowering intrathoracic pressure.

Other factors may be active also in the production of acute pulmonary edema. Drinker believes that increase in capillary permeability may have even greater influence than pressure changes. The lung capillaries are particularly sensitive to oxygen lack, and since their endothelial cells receive their oxygen from the air, any interference with the air supply may initiate local or general pulmonary edema. Alveolar transudation then further decreases the oxygen supply, and a vicious cycle becomes active, endothelial anoxia — transudation — increased anoxia.

Nervous influences are active also. The nervous mechanism may be excited directly as in the pulmonary edema which occasionally accompanies skull fracture or encephalitis, or reflexly as in the "albuminous expectoration" of paracentesis. The frequent brilliant therapeutic effect of morphine in acute pulmonary edema is to be ascribed to the sedation of nervous impulses. The mode of action of neurogenic influences is unknown, but a local pulmonary neurochemical mechanism has been suggested.

The edema produced by inflammation or by irritant gases presumably is identical with the edema of inflammation elsewhere.

It is evident that a variety of elements may contribute to produce alveolar transudation in the lungs and that clinically the situation may be complex and not subject to exact analysis.

The Edemas of Nephritis

The edema of acute nephritis usually is slight and may escape notice altogether. A little puffiness about the eyes and of the face is common, and there may be a small amount of subcutaneous edema elsewhere. Widespread edema has been reported rarely, but many such cases may include edema from an early nephrotic stage or from the heart failure which is seen occasionally in acute nephritis. Exact determination of the cause of the edema is sometimes difficult.

The nature of the edema of acute nephritis is in some doubt. That there is widespread vascular damage is plain from the occurrence of hematuria and of retinal hemorrhages, and it is evident that the capillary wall must have lost in some degree its efficiency as a membrane semipermeable to the plasma colloids. Edema fluid resulting from such a breakdown would have of necessity a high protein content, and here the reported figures are not in agreement. However it will be noted that the figures of Warren and Stead[37] for acute nephritis are higher than they found in the edema fluid of heart failure and considerably higher than those reported for the edema of nephrosis. Capillary damage is, therefore, probably a principal part of the mechanism.

The most striking edema of renal disease is the widespread and persistent edema characteristic of the active (subacute) or nephrotic stage of glomerulonephritis and in the other nephroses with high albuminuria. It is of interest that Bostock[4], a chemist who worked on Bright's edematous patients, reported: "I think I may venture to say that the serum generally in these cases contained less albumin than in health, although I am not able to state precisely the amount of the difference". Clinicians long believed that loss of protein in the urine led to a watery condition of the blood which favored transudation, and not until Epstein's valuable contribution in 1917 were the Starling concepts used to explain this edema. Epstein[16] pointed out that the plasma proteins, depleted by excessive loss of protein through the kidneys, were no longer able to bring about the normal return of fluid from the tissue spaces to the blood. Clinical observations have confirmed abundantly the correctness of this interpretation, and the plasmapheresis experiments of Leiter and of Barker and Kirk have been further elucidating. They show that by lowering the plasma protein in dogs a level is reached at which edema occurs with great regularity, and the animal recovers completely, when the plasma protein level is restored to the normal range. The edema of nephrosis differs somewhat from this experimental edema, because the protein lost in the urine is principally albumin instead of the mixed albumin and globulin of plasma. The globulin fraction of the remaining plasma proteins is, therefore, greater than normal. Globulin molecules are large and exert less osmotic pressure, gram for gram, than do molecules of albumin; so the level of total plasma protein, at which edema may occur, is a variable one and will depend on the albumin-globulin ratio. There is also at times a lack of correlation between the amount of protein losses and the plasma protein level. In some patients the plasma protein concentration may be low after relatively small losses in the urine, while in others large losses may cause only slight lowering of plasma levels. Variations in the ability to replenish plasma proteins seems probable.

Spontaneous disappearance of the edema may take place, while the plasma proteins are still low, and such findings are cited to discredit the Starling hypothesis. These discordant data, however, never include measurements of effective osmotic or hydrostatic pressures. Furthermore it should be remembered that in the nephrotic edemas the Starling equilibrium may be operative at a low level.

Low colloid osmotic pressure because of low plasma protein is balanced by low hydrostatic pressure because of increased tissue pressure. Loss of edema may well begin in response to slight lowering of the hydrostatic pressure at very low levels of plasma protein. Even slight diuresis, the mechanisms for which are not clearly understood, might be an initiating factor. Warren, Merrill and Stead[39] point out that the increased tissue pressure due to edema is an important factor in determining the size of the plasma volume in patients with low plasma protein levels. The decrease in colloid osmotic pressure of the plasma is compensated for by the increase in tissue pressure, usually permitting the patient to maintain an adequate blood volume.

Finally in nephritis we may have the edema of heart failure, including acute pulmonary edema, as a part of the clinical picture. This is seen most often late in the disease, when heart failure results from the long-standing hypertension. When heart failure supervenes during or closely following the active stage of a glomerulonephritis, clinical distinction between renal and cardiac responsibility for the edema may be impossible.

In the treatment of nephrotic edema restriction of salt may be of value, but the results are often unsatisfactory and erratic[6]. Attempts to raise the plasma protein level by a high protein diet are also disappointing, and by increasing the work of the kidney may be harmful. On the other hand diets too low in protein may add more edema to the picture. The use of human plasma albumin[34] intravenously may be effective when available, but large amounts are necessary, retention of about 75 grams of albumin being required to bring about an increase of one per cent. in the plasma protein level, and with continuing albuminuria a lasting effect cannot be expected. The substitution of other colloids has been practiced extensively, such as acacia or pectin. While they are effective in reducing the edema, they are known to diminish protein formation in the experimental animal, and their ultimate fate in the body may entail other disadvantages[2]. Their hazards appear to outweigh their usefulness. With a low salt diet water need not be restricted and may have some diuretic action. Other diuretics such as the purines and the organic mercurials are used often, but opinion is divided as to their harmfulness in the presence of kidney disease. For the relief of stubborn extreme edema Southey tubes may be used, and serous transudates, when large, likewise are best removed by paracentesis.

Nutritional Edema

In many states of malnutrition considerable edema may be seen. Lack of vitamins in the diet, a low protein ration, failure to absorb or to utilize vitamins and proteins because of bowel disease are common etiological pictures. Liver function often is below normal with impaired protein formation and low plasma protein levels. In the United States during the depression years many cases of beriberi with edema were seen, identifiable chiefly by the history of inadequate diets, the presence of peripheral neuritis and of greatly dilated hearts which returned to normal size promptly under vitamin B_1 therapy. The edema in these patients is largely that of heart failure, but some reduction of plasma albumin is common, and in some instances vasomotor paresis may augment intracapillary pressure. The starvation edemas seen so abundantly in prison and concentration camps form a striking and appalling group. Lack of adequate protein intake and eventually the utilization of amino acids for body fuel instead of protein synthesis combine to produce low plasma levels of protein. An accompanying anemia may contribute to the edema by increasing capillary permeability.

Whether the edema and ascites of Laennec's cirrhosis belong in the nutritional group is not fully settled. The toxic agent responsible for the hepatitis is unknown, but a dietary factor is suspected. Portal obstruction alone does not produce ascites in experimental animals and probably not in man. A low plasma protein level is a constant finding in the stage of ascites and is the result of impaired protein formation in the damaged liver and later the result of the loss of protein into the ascitic fluid. Usually the albumin-globulin ratio is diminished or reversed, and while edema levels are not reached, the loss of plasma colloid osmotic pressure plus the increased capillary pressure from portal obstruction will account adequately for the ascites as well as the leg edema. Partial obstruction of the vena cava by the ascites is often mentioned as a factor, but evidence of obstruction of the venous return from the legs usually is lacking. Treatment of the edema and ascites of portal cirrhosis with diuretics is unsatisfactory, and treatment directed toward the relief of the underlying liver disease also is discouraging in cases which have progressed to this stage.

Obstructive Edema

Edema resulting from obstruction to veins or lymphatics is common. Unilateral or unequal edemas of the legs are most frequently the result of venous obstruction from thrombosis or varicosities. Edema from the pressure of an enlarging uterus or a malignant tumor also is not infrequent. Whether or not occlusion of a vein will cause edema depends upon the amount of collateral circulation available and upon the presence or absence of other factors which might contribute to edema formation. In experimental animals edema seldom occurs after ligation of even large veins such as the femoral or the inferior vena cava, and in man such edema may be transient, disappearing with the development of collateral channels. In cachectic individuals even moderate degrees of venous obstruction, such as may result from an unusual position in bed, may result in edema. Here low plasma proteins are a frequent contributing factor. In patients with congestive heart failure venous thrombosis may occur as a result of stasis, and local edema due to minor thromboses is seen not infrequently.

The edema of lymphatic obstruction has a characteristic appearance. There is no redness or cyanosis of the skin, and having attained a certain moderate degree, it may remain at that level for long periods. This corresponds to the mode of its production. Tissue drainage via the lymphatics being stopped, the outflow from the capillaries will equal the return flow into them, and there will be no occasion for further increase of tissue fluid. In very long-standing lymphedema the skin and subcutaneous tissues are apt to show some hypertrophy and induration.

There are many conditions in which lymphatic obstruction occurs. Lymphangitis may cause temporary or at times permanent obliteration of lymph channels, or they may become occluded by invading cancer cells. Surgical removal of groups of lymph nodes is followed often by regional edema. In tropical elephantiasis the lymphatics are blocked by filaria. In addition a good many cryptogenic cases of lymphedema are seen[3], including the rare familial edema of Milroy and a group of somewhat similar sporadic lymphedemas, occurring especially in women. Some of these are believed to have resulted from old pelvic inflammatory disease[13]. The pathogenesis is not known. (See also Oxford Medicine, Vol. II, Chapter XIV–C, Swellings of the Limbs due to Local Causes.)

Inflammatory, Toxic and Allergic Edemas

The presence in the tissues of substances toxic to the vascular and tissue cells produces edema regularly as a part of the reaction. Burns, bites, chemical irritants of various sorts are the common exciting agents, and a humoral toxic agent probably is active also in tissues that are especially sensitive to allergic antigens and to certain physical agents such as heat, cold and mechanical stimulation. Common to all of these reactions is an early hyperemia, presumably with increased intracapillary pressure and an increased permeability of the capillary wall as evidenced by the high protein content of the edema fluid. The cloudy swelling of inflammatory tissue cells is evidence that some increase in the volume of the cells must occur also. The edema that may persist after active inflammation has subsided is due to the lowering of tissue pressure which follows stretching of the tissues.

Of particular interest is the group of skin reactions with wheal formation that are produced by heat, chemical irritants, mechanical stroking and probably at times by neurogenic impulses. Lewis[23] has presented evidence that a substance resembling histamine is liberated in the skin in response to each of these agents, and that the same mechanism is common to the action of all of them. In the case of remote response to nerve impulses such as that in herpes zoster and some urticarial lesions Dale[9] has suggested that liberation of acetylcholine at the arteriolar nerve endings may play a rôle, producing both vasodilatation and increased capillary permeability. There is a large group of cases of asthma, urticaria and angioneurotic edema, in which specific allergy may not be demonstrable, and in which psychic and nervous influences frequently precipitate the attack. In these a neurochemical mechanism seems not unlikely. The rare local edemas occurring in diseases of the central nervous system probably would belong in the same group.

The Clinical Investigation of Edema

The cause of most edemas can be determined by means of a good history and physical examination and a routine urine analysis. In the study of cases of obscure edema the following measurements may be of value; (1) total plasma protein concentration, (2) fractionation of plasma albumin and globulin, (3) colloidal osmotic pressure of plasma, (4) blood volume, (5) blood and urine chlorides, (6) hematocrit determination, (7) quantitative protein in the urine, (8) weight curve of patient, (9) venous pressures.

Fairly satisfactory clinical methods are available for total plasma protein determinations based on the parallelism between protein content and specific gravity[19]. Present clinical methods for albumin-globulin fractionation are unsatisfactory but may be of some value, particularly in determining changes from time to time. Colloid osmotic pressure measurements are rarely available clinically, and are worth little unless done by special workers Blood volumes usually are determined clinically by convenient dye methods, whose inaccuracies are many and well known.[27]

BIBLIOGRAPHY

1. ADDIS, T.: Proteinuria, Transact. Assoc. Am. Phys., 1942, LVII, 106.
2. ADDIS, T.: Unpublished observations.
3. ALLEN, E. V.: Lymphedema of the extremities, Arch. Int. Med. 1934, LIV, 60
4. BRIGHT, R.: Reports of Medical Cases, I, 83, Longman, Rees, Orne, Brown and Green, London, 1827.
5. BYROM, F. B.: The nature of myxedema, Clin. Science, 1934, l, 273.
6. CHRISTIAN, H. A.: Types of edema and their treatment, New England Med. Jour., 1935, CCXIV, 418.
7. CHRISTIAN, H. A.: Some changing views about edema and diuresis, Canad. Med. Assoc. Jour., 1937, XXXVII, 29.
8. COLLER, F. A., DICK, V. S. and MADDOCK, W. B.: Maintenance of normal water exchange, Jour. Am. Med. Assoc., 1936, CVII, 1522.
9. DALE, H.: Chemical factors in control of circulation, Lancet, 1929, I, 1179.

10. DARROW, D. C.: Tissue water and electrolyte, Ann. Rev. Physiol., 1944, VI, 95.
11. DRINKER, C. K. and FIELD, M. E.: Lymphatics, Lymph and Tissue Fluid, Williams and Wilkins, Baltimore, 1933.
12. DRINKER, C. K.: Pulmonary Edema and Inflammation, Harvard University Press, Cambridge, Mass., 1945.
13. ELLIS, L. B.: The causes and treatment of edema, New England Jour. Med., 1941, CCXXIV, 1060.
14. ELLIS, L. B. and WEISS, S.: Edema associated with cerebral hemiplegia, Arch. Neurol. and Psych., 1936, XXXVI, 362.
15. ELLIS, L. B.: Hypoproteinemia in patients with cardiac edema, Med. Clin. North America, 1933, XVI, 943.
16. EPSTEIN, A. A.: Causation of edema in chronic parenchymatous nephritis, Am. Jour. Med. Sci., 1917, CLIV, 638.
17. GAMBLE, J. L.: Extracellular Fluid, Harvard Medical School, 1941.
18. HARRISON, T. R.: Failure of the Circulation, 2nd. edition, Williams and Wilkins, Baltimore, 1939.
19. KAGAN, B. M.: Estimation of the total protein content of plasma, Jour. Clin. Invest., 1938, XVII, 373.
20. LANDIS, E. M., ANGEVINE, M. and ERB, W.: Passage of fluid and protein through capillary wall, Jour. Clin. Invest., 1932, XI, 717.
21. LANDIS, E. M.: Capillary pressure and capillary permeability. Physiol. Reviews, 1934, XIV, 404.
22. LANDIS, E. M., BROWN, E., FAUTEUX, M. and WISE, C.: Central venous pressure in relation to cardiac "competence", blood volume and exercise, Jour. Clin. Invest., 1946, XXV, 237.
23. LEWIS, T.: Clinical Science, Illustrated by Personal Experiences, Shaw and Sons, London, 1934.
24. LUISADA, A.: Pathogenesis of paroxysmal pulmonary edema, Medicine, 1940, XIX, 475.
25. McMASTER, P. D.: The lymphatics and lymph flow in the edematous skin, Jour. Exp. Med., 1937, LXV, 373.
26. PETERS, J. P.: Body Water, Charles C. Thomas Springfield, Illinois, 1935.
27. PETERS, J. P.: Water exchange, Physiol. Rev., 1944, XXIV, 490.
28. RYTAND, D. A.: Edema with hypoproteinemia, Arch. Int. Med., 1942, LXIX, 251.
29. SCHADE, H.: Grundzüge der Oedempathogenese, Ergeb. der inn. Med. u. Kinderheilk., 1926, XXXIV, 1.
29(a). SMITH, H. W.: The excretion of water, Bull. N. Y. Acad. Med., 1947, XXIII, 177.
30. SODEMAN, W. A. and BURCH, G. E.: The tissue pressure in subcutaneous edema, Am. Jour. Med. Sci., 1937, CXCIV, 846.
31. STARLING, E. H: On the absorption of fluid from the connective tissue spaces, Jour. Physiol., 1896, XIX, 312.
32. STARLING, E. H.: Fluids of the Body, Arnold Constable, London, 1909.
33. STEAD, E. A., Jr. and WARREN, J. V.: The protein content of extracellular fluid, Jour. Clin. Invest., 1944, XXIII, 283.

34. THORN, G. W., Physiologic considerations in the treatment of nephritis, New England Med. Jour., 1943, CCXXIX, 33.
35. THORN, G. W. and EMERSON, K., Jr.: Rôle of gonadal and adrenal cortical hormones in the production of edema, Ann. Int. Med., 1940, XIV, 757.
36. THORN, G. W., NELSON, K. R. and THORN, D. W.: A study of the mechanism of edema associated with menstruation, Endocrinology, 1938, XXII, 155.
37. WARREN, J. V. and STEAD, E. A., Jr.: Edema fluid in acute nephritis, Am. Jour. Med. Sci., 1944, CCVIII, 618.
38. WARREN, J. V. and STEAD, E. A., Jr.: Fluid dynamics in chronic heart failure, Arch. Int. Med., 1944, LXXIII, 138.
39. WARREN, J. V., MERRILL, A., Jr. and STEAD, E. A., Jr.: The role of extracellular fluid in the maintenance of plasma volume, Jour. Clin. Invest., 1943, XXIII, 635.
40. WEISS, S. and WILKINS, R. W.: Cardiovascular disturbances in nutritional deficiencies, Ann. Int. Med., 1937, XI, 104.
41. WELCH, W. H.: Zur Pathologie des Lungenödems, Virch. Arch., 1878, LXXII, 375.
42. WIDAL, F. and JAVAL, A.: Les variations de la permeabilité du rein par la chlorure de sodium et de l'urée dans le mal de Bright, Compt. rend. Soc. de Biol. de Paris, 1903, LV, 1532.
43. WIGGERS, C. J.: Physiology in Health and Disease, 4th ed., Lea and Febiger, Philadelphia, 1944.

September 1, 1947.

The following pages will be used at a later date.

CHAPTER XXIV

THE REGULATION OF BODY WATER AND ELECTROLYTE IN HEALTH AND DISEASE

By DANIEL C. DARROW and EDWARD L. PRATT

TABLE OF CONTENTS

Without a considerable knowledge of the physiology of body water and electrolyte, physicians cannot properly treat dehydration, edema, acidosis, alkalosis and shock, or plan a rational therapy when all or part of the fluid requirement must be given parenterally, or electrolyte has been lost in large amounts in sweat, urine and gastrointestinal secretions.

Previous concepts of the physiology of body fluids were dominated by two postulates which are now known to be erroneous. First, cellular membranes were regarded as practically impervious to sodium and potassium, and second, only alterations in extracellular electrolyte were thought to be accessible to fluid therapy. During the past fifteen years analyses of the tissues of experimental animals and determinations of the balances of water and electrolytes in patients have demonstrated that intracellular fluids undergo fairly rapid changes in composition which alter profoundly the acid-base equilibrium of extracellular fluids. Furthermore, the changes in composition of intracellular fluids, particularly the loss of potassium and the alterations in the concentration of electrolytes in body fluid, affect the function of cells.

The Relation of Extracellular to Intracellular Electrolyte

In order to enable the physician to visualize the quantitative relationships between extracellular and intracellular electrolyte, a schematic representation of the composition will be presented[1]. The extracellular fluids will be considered to have the composition of an ultrafiltrate of plasma. The intracellular concentrations will be represented as those of rat and cat muscle. Both concentrations will be expressed per kilogram of water. Data are available which indicate that the intracellular compositions of the muscle of young and mature cats are essentially the same and that human muscle has about the same composition as that of other mammals. The intracellular composition of the various tissues is similar to that of skeletal muscle. Some of the changes in intracellular composition, which will be described, are known not to develop to the same extent in other tissues, but similar changes probably take place. Since the intracellular fluid of muscle comprises about 70 per cent. of the total intracellular fluids, the errors are not significant in depicting the relationship between extracellular and intracellular fluids for the body as a whole.

Charts I and II illustrate the relationships of extracellular and intracellular fluids of one kilogram of tissue in babies and adults. The extracellular concentration of sodium is represented on the ordinate for extracellular fluids, while the intracellular concentration of potassium is represented on the ordinate for intracellular fluids. The abscissae indicate the volumes of water in each kind of fluid. The amount of extracellular sodium and intracellular potassium is indicated by the respective areas. The amounts of the various electrolytes contained in each compartment are indicated by the concentrations multiplied by the volumes.

It will be seen that total water per kilogram of tissue is slightly greater in infants than in adults. For the first months of life extracellular water in infants is about 30 per cent. of the body weight. Although the intracellular water of adults may be slightly less than 45 per cent. of the body weight, this figure is suitable for all ages. Actually, the total body water varies appreciably in normal individuals. The chief differences are accounted for by variations in the proportions of fat. Since fat is deposited with relatively little water, fat individuals contain relatively less water per unit of weight. However, the quantitative relationships between the two types of fluid are essentially the same in normal individuals except for the variations with age.

Since the changes in body water and acid-base equilibrium are explained chiefly by variations in water, sodium, potassium and chloride, the discussion will emphasize the rôle of these constituents. First, the total intracellular sodium is about 7 mM per kilogram and approximately equivalent to total extracellular bicarbonate or one fourth of the total extracellular sodium excluding the sodium of bone salts[2, 3]. The sodium in bone salts need not be considered again, since this sodium does not alter the sodium available to the rest of the body except when bone salts are being deposited or removed. This factor is small in any short period since there is 1 mM of sodium for each 30 mM of calcium in calcified material.

Normally, intracellular sodium is variable, since sodium can be transferred from intracellular to extracellular fluids and vice versa. The charts show the usual high normal value for intracellular sodium. In normal individuals the variations are chiefly in the direction of lower values. Since the transfer between the two phases of body fluid apparently is accomplished without change in extracellular chloride, the effect on extracellular fluids is to alter the amount of sodium available to form bicarbonate. If total body electrolyte does not change, transfer of extracellular sodium to intracellular fluids decreases the concentration of bicarbonate in extracellular fluids, and transfer of intracellular sodium to extracellular fluids increases the concentrations of bicarbonate in extracellular fluids. Hence the shift of sodium between the two compartments is an important mechanism for diminishing the variations in extracellular bicarbonate. In abnormal conditions changes in the distribution of sodium explain the development of disturbances in acid-base equilibrium. In many clinical situations this mechanism functions in addition to the usually described buffers of the blood and must be considered in the explanation of the effects of balances of

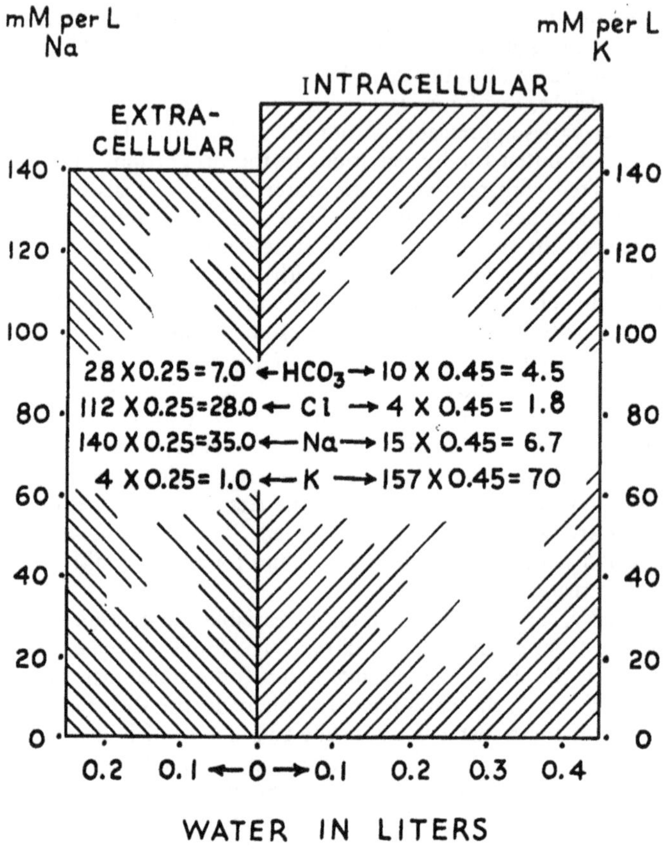

CHART I. Diagram of body fluid of 1 kilogram of tissue in infants. The concentration of sodium and potassium is represented on the ordinates for the extracellular and intracellular fluids respectively. The volumes are represented on the abscissae. The total contents are given by the concentration multiplied by the volumes.

electrolyte on the acid-base equilibrium and the distribution of body water.

Second, intracellular potassium in normal animals may be about 10 per cent. lower than the values shown on the charts. This variation may occur without appreciable alteration in body water or acid-base equilibrium. The charts show the high normal figure since this is the

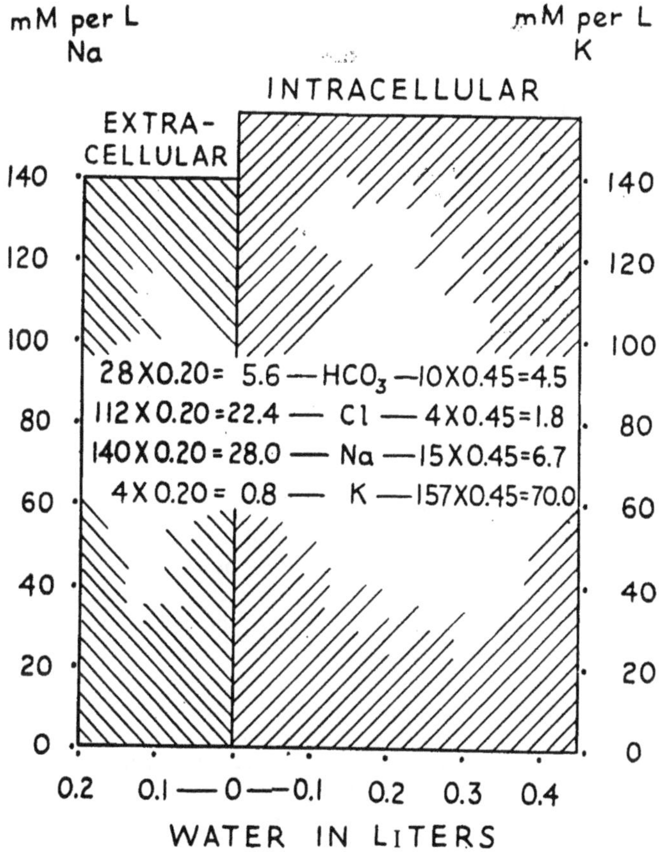

CHART II. Diagram of body fluid of 1 kilogram of tissues in adults and children. For description, see Chart I.

one usually found in rats and cats. Changes in intracellular potassium may occur without detectable changes in intracellular sodium, though there usually is a reciprocal relation between intracellular sodium and potassium.

Third, under abnormal conditions as much as one half of the intracellular potassium of muscle may be replaced by about two thirds of the equivalent amount of sodium. This change in intracellular electrolyte was first discovered in rats subjected to diets low in potassium[4, 5] or receiving repeated injections of desoxycorticosterone acetate[6, 7]. As will be pointed out later, this type of deficit of potassium develops as a result of decreased intake of potassium and increased output in urine, stools, gastrointestinal secretions and sweat. Deficit of potassium may result also from processes leading to release of this ion from the cells.

Fourth, there is a predictable relationship between the acid-base equilibrium and the composition of muscle under certain circumstances[2]. Chart III shows the relationship between the concentration of bicarbonate in serum and the intracellular sodium and potassium of 157 grams of fat-free muscle solids. Since this amount of fat-free solids is associated with 450 grams of intracellular water, the chart shows the intracellular composition for the same amount of intracellular fluids as charts I and II show for 1 kilogram of tissue. The relationship was demonstrated for rats subjected to any one of the following conditions: (1) loss of chloride or primary metabolic alkalosis, (2) loss of sodium or primary metabolic acidosis and (3) primary deficit of potassium. Since water and other ions were abundantly available, the chart is based on conditions in which the kidneys would adjust body water and electrolyte to a deficit of only one of the ions, sodium, potassium or chloride. The relationship may be regarded as a biological adjustment or steady state for these conditions. The adjustment must be considered a biological one since a chemical equilibrium or steady state would be achieved in several hours and not require several days. The chart is useful in illustrating the sort of changes which the body will tend to develop with a deficit of one of these ions when the kidneys are able to maintain a relatively constant composition of the body fluids.

The chart is based on data from rats where the relationship is readily demonstrated. Clinical studies show that the relationship is manifested in humans. In dogs[8] it is difficult to induce alkalosis in response to potassium deficiency, though the same changes in cellular composition result from deficit of potassium.

It will be seen that deficit of chloride and deficit of potassium produce the same changes in both extracellular and intracellular fluids. At biological adjustment a deficit of one of these ions leads to deficit of the other. Intracellular sodium may reach several times the normal value and several times the equivalence of the bicarbonate of extracellular fluids. This relationship is important first, because alkalosis will

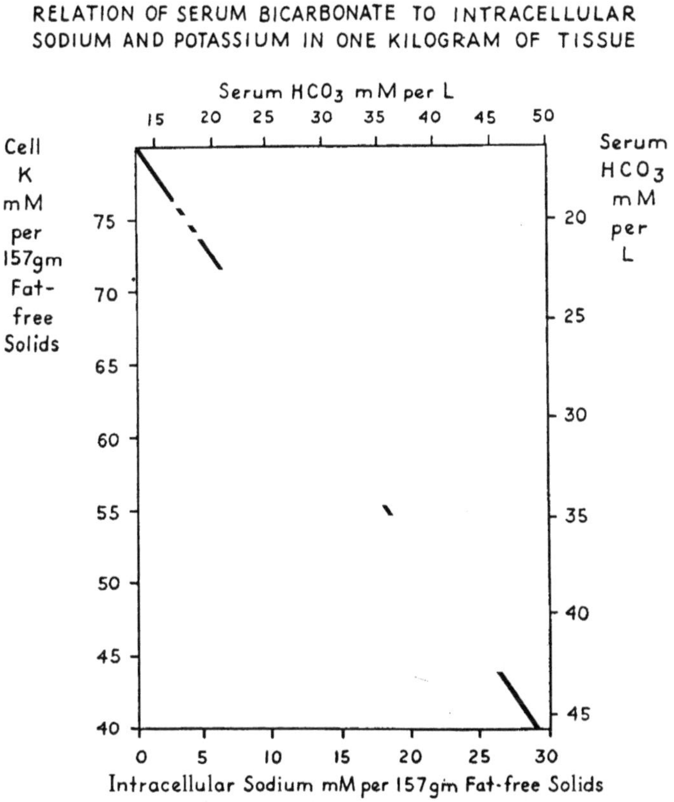

CHART III. Relation of the concentration of serum bicarbonate to intracellular sodium and potassium of muscle. The line shows the relation of intracellular sodium to potassium; the bicarbonate concentrations on the ordinate are the best fit for intracellular potassium, while those on the abscissae are the best fit for the intracellular sodium. The values for intracellular sodium and potassium are for the same amount of intracellular fluid used for 1 kilogram of tissue in Charts I, II and IV.

tend to persist if potassium cannot be replaced, and second, because deficit of potassium will result in alkalosis even in the presence of abundant sodium chloride. Examples of both of these events will be cited later. On the other hand acidosis produced by loss of sodium alone leads to deficits of this ion not only in the extracellular fluids but also in the cells. It is this combined deficit that measures the amount of sodium bicarbonate that must be retained in order to restore the concentration of bicarbonate in serum. Thus acidosis resulting from loss of sodium without loss of potassium will have an extracellular deficit equal to the decrease in bicarbonate concentration multiplied by the volume of extracellular water, i.e. $(25 - 5)\ 0.25 = 5$ mM of sodium per kilogram of body weight, if the serum bicarbonate is 5 mM per liter. In addition, there would be a deficit of about 7 mM of sodium in the cells making a total deficit of about 12 mM per kilogram of body weight.

Clinically, chloride is relatively deficient, if the concentration in serum is low, but the loss may occur alone or in conjunction with deficit of potassium or as a result of deficit of potassium. Low concentration of bicarbonate indicates a loss of sodium from extracellular fluids unless there is an accumulation of other ions displacing bicarbonate. However, the decrease in bicarbonate does not reveal the state of intracellular sodium, since if there is deficit of potassium, there may be high intracellular sodium in the presence of acidosis. Deficit of potassium can be proved only by demonstrating a greater relative loss of potassium than nitrogen during the development of the condition or a greater relative retention of potassium than nitrogen during recovery. If body water and circulation are relatively normal, deficiency of potassium is likely to be accompanied by low concentration of potassium in serum.

The physiochemical factors controlling the acid-base equilibrium of the blood have been discussed adequately in a recent paper by Singer and Hastings[9] and in textbooks[10]. The present discussion will, therefore, emphasize the relationship of the changes in acid-base equilibrium of the blood to alterations in the composition of extracellular fluids and the accompanying changes in the cells.

Changes in the acid-base equilibrium may be defined as deviations from normal in the reaction or pH of the blood. The pH is determined by the ratio of the carbon dioxide to the bicarbonate of plasma. The concentration of carbon dioxide depends on the partial carbon dioxide pressure of arterial blood which is normally equilibrated with the carbon dioxide of residual alveolar air. Hence, the carbon dioxide tension is subject to the regulation of pulmonary ventilation by the respiratory center. The concentration of bicarbonate in plasma is dependent on the amount of cations available to form bicarbonate at the particular carbon dioxide tension with the particular amounts of blood electrolytes and organic buffers. The cations available to form bicarbonate are regulated by the kidneys. Inasmuch as we are chiefly concerned with the content of water and electrolyte in body fluids, we shall neglect the relatively small changes in the buffering effects of the plasma proteins, red cells and phosphate and emphasize the contents of the tissues in sodium, potassium and chloride. These ions are the chief factor determining the major clinical disturbances in the amount of cations available to form bicarbonate. The cations available to form bicarbonate are the algebraic sum of the total cations minus the plasma anions excluding bicarbonate, i.e. $(Na + K + Ca + Mg) - (Cl + HPO_4 + \text{proteins} + \text{sulphate} + \text{lactate} + \text{keto acids}———)$. For many purposes the changes in cations available to form bicarbonate in the body as a whole are adequately defined by the balances of sodium plus potassium minus chloride.

Metabolic Acidosis

Metabolic acidosis is primary decrease in the cations available to form bicarbonate. It may be produced by relative increase in the concentration of anions or relative decrease in the concentration of cations. An increase in anions may arise as a result of ingestion of acidifying salts or through the endogenous production of organic acids owing to exercise, anoxia, hemorrhage, keto acids in starvation ketosis and diabetic acidosis or the retention of phosphates and sulphate in renal insufficiency. A relative deficit of cations may result from losses of intestinal secretions, biliary secretions or through abnormal renal excretion.

The changes in intracellular electrolytes in metabolic acidosis are only beginning to be studied. Deficit of sodium alone, such as is illustrated in chart III, apparently is relatively rare. It has been shown that feeding protein milk to premature infants leads to retention of chloride and little change in body sodium[11, 12, 13]. The change in the acid-base equilibrium and the balances demonstrates that practically all the intracellular sodium is transferred to the extracellular fluids under these circumstances. The resulting change in intracellular composition must be about the same as is illustrated for deficit of sodium in chart III. Acidifying salts such as ammonium chloride and calcium chloride probably produce similar changes. In one baby subjected to protein milk feeding for six days, the balances showed losses of intracellular potassium during the last three days. It is likely that acidosis resulting from loss of sodium first leads to deficits of sodium in the extracellular and intracellular fluids and later, losses of potassium may develop. Under these circumstances sodium may be transferred back into the cells and aggravate the acidosis. Thus acidosis beginning as primary sodium deficit tends ultimately to produce depletion of potassium and water.

Metabolic acidosis usually is accompanied by deficits of water, sodium, potassium and chloride. When there is acidosis and deficit of potassium, intracellular sodium apparently remains normal or may even be somewhat high but not as high as when there is a similar deficit of potassium and no acidosis. The difference between the deficits of sodium and potassium and the deficit of chloride is a measure of the relative deficiency of cations available to form bicarbonate. Since the deficit of potassium may be greater than total normal extracellular bicarbonate plus normal intracellular sodium, most cases of acidosis cannot be treated rationally with sodium chloride and sodium bicarbonate alone. If intracellular potassium remains low, the amount of sodium in excess of chloride required to restore extracellular bicarbonate would be more than the normal excess of sodium over chloride including intracellular sodium. The changes in tissue composition in metabolic acidosis indicate clearly that replacement of potassium as well as sodium and chloride is necessary in most cases.

Metabolic Alkalosis

Metabolic alkalosis is produced by primary increase in sodium available to form bicarbonate in plasma. Although metabolic alkalosis may be produced by relative excess of sodium, it usually results from relative deficit of chloride. The commonest cause is loss of gastric juice by vomiting or suction drainage after operations. If sufficient water is available to permit renal adjustment, potassium will tend to be lost from the cells, and sodium will partially replace the intracellular deficit of potassium. If the plan of therapy offers no opportunity for the body to replace the deficiency of potassium, alkalosis may continue despite the administration of sodium chloride, because the biological adjustment to deficit of potassium leads to maintenance of alkalosis by the kidneys. A similar reaction by the kidneys explains the development of alkalosis as a result of primary deficiency of potassium. In either case recovery from alkalosis requires the replacement of potassium as well as chloride.

Respiratory Acidosis

Respiratory acidosis results from primary increase in serum carbon dioxide tension. Probably the most frequent cause is depression of pulmonary ventilation owing to narcosis, injury to the respiratory center or paralysis of the muscles of respiration. However, both acute and chronic respiratory acidosis may be produced by diseases of the lungs leading to thickening of the alveolar walls, exudates, bronchiectasis and emphysema. Since oxygen diffuses less rapidly than carbon dioxide, the arterial blood becomes less saturated with oxygen than normal when carbon dioxide accumulates. Presumably, there is no change in body electrolyte in uncompensated respiratory acidosis.

Respiratory Alkalosis

Respiratory alkalosis results from primary decrease in carbon dioxide tension. It is produced by excessive pulmonary ventilation such as occurs during exercise, fever and disturbances in the respiratory center as a result of infections of the central nervous system, tumors and drugs (salicylates). Overventilation may occur in hysterical patients or as a result of anoxia in cardiac failure and at high altitudes. Uncompensated respiratory alkalosis presumably results in no change in body electrolytes.

The *disturbances in acid-base equilibrium* have been discussed above as if only the carbon dioxide tension or the cations available to form bicarbonate were altered. Actually the alteration of one of these variables leads to compensatory variations in the others. In metabolic acidosis the respiratory center responds to the low pH by increased pulmonary ventilation which reduces the carbon dioxide tension. The reduction is not sufficient to produce a normal pH in the blood. In metabolic alkalosis the respiratory center may reduce pulmonary ventilation, but the reaction is limited because anoxia tends to be produced and again stimulates increased respirations.

On the other hand, the kidneys may alter the cations available to form bicarbonate in both respiratory acidosis and alkalosis. In respiratory alkalosis the serum bicarbonate may be reduced fairly rapidly, but as long as the disturbance in pulmonary ventilation persists, the blood pH remains normal or slightly alkaline. However, after the kidneys have reduced the available cations, the respiratory center may recover and respond normally. The patient then will suffer from true metabolic acidosis. Since recovery from the effects of drugs such as salicylates may be rather rapid, respiratory alkalosis is likely to go through a phase of metabolic acidosis during recovery.

In respiratory acidosis the kidneys may increase the cations available to form bicarbonate to quite high figures (45 mM per liter). The blood pH remains more acid than normal, and arterial blood shows diminished oxygen saturation. In respiratory acidosis due to lung disease recovery of lung function is unlikely to be sufficiently rapid to produce true metabolic alkalosis.

It is not known whether compensated respiratory alkalosis and acidosis lead to changes in cell sodium and potassium. It is likely that such is the case and that compensated respiratory acidosis produces increase in cell sodium and decrease in cell potassium. Compensated respiratory alkalosis is likely to lead to loss of intracellular as well as extracellular sodium.

Disturbances in body water and electrolyte involve changes in the volume and electrolyte concentration which are just as important as the changes in acid-base equilibrium. Dehydration usually involves decrease in body electrolyte, and loss of electrolyte tends to cause losses of water. If the losses of electrolyte are proportionately greater than the losses of water, there is a decrease in the concentration of electrolyte in serum. This type of disturbance may be called hypotonic dehydration.

Hypotonic Dehydration

Methods are available for study hypotonic dehydration due to loss of electrolyte with little change in body water[14]. Loss of extracellular electrolyte without significant change in body water produces decrease in the concentration of sodium and chloride in serum, while the concentration of proteins in serum and red cells in blood are increased. The plasma volume is markedly reduced. The animals look sick, refuse to eat and are weak. The volume of urine decreases, the rate of glomerular filtration is reduced to quite low figures, the non-protein nitrogen rises. Water and sodium are excreted more slowly than normal[15]. The cardiac output is strikingly reduced[16]. It can be shown that the volume of extracellular water decreases while the volume of intracellular water increases. The changes in distribution of water are dependent on the adjustment of the osmotic pressure in the intracellular fluids by shifts of water rather than by losses of electrolyte from the cells. The animals are in a shock-like state and do not withstand bleeding as well as normal animals[17]. The clinical picture is essentially the same as that of the usual dehydration seen in patients. The experiments are important because they emphasize that the central feature of hypotonic dehydration is loss of extracellular electrolyte.

For practical purposes hypotonic dehydration may be considered to result from the loss of proportionately more electrolyte than water, although rare cases may involve little or no deficit of water. With low concentrations of electrolyte in serum the cells of the body contain more water than is normal. Statistically the increase in intracellular water in experiments involving losses of extracellular electrolytes is only about two thirds as much as would reduce the electrolyte concentration of the intracellular fluids of muscle as much as the reduction of extracellular concentration[18]. In chronic states in patients the relationship has not been studied but may be somewhat different. In any case the disturbances in circulation, renal function and muscular strength are dependent not only on the reduction in extracellular water and plasma volume but also on the decrease in electrolyte concentration[16]. Hypotonic dehydration produces the picture of medical shock and responds to replacement of electrolyte, but the response is somewhat better when blood or plasma as well as electrolyte is given[19].

Hypertonic Dehydration

Hypertonic dehydration results, when the loss of water is proportionately greater than the loss of electrolyte. This leads to increase in the concentration of electrolyte in serum[20]. It can be shown that relatively pure increase in extracellular electrolyte produces increase in extracellular water and dehydration of the cells[14]. Patients with hypertonic dehydration may show symptoms of shock, but circulatory failure is much less prominent than in hypotonic dehydration. The patients are likely to show hyperpnea, mental symptoms and fever[20]. Patients and experimental animals with hypertonic fluids show evidence of cerebral damage; death is likely to be preceded by high fever and arrest of respiration.

As will be pointed out later, symptoms develop when serum potassium rises to about twice the normal concentration. When the level of serum potassium increases, the concentration of potassium in cells rises[5]. However, if animals are given diets high in potassium, the compositions of the cells remain essentially normal. If rats are given water containing potassium chloride at greater concentrations than can be excreted by the kidneys, they refuse to drink. If potassium chloride is injected into the peritoneal cavity, the concentration in the serum rises in proportion to the amount injected. Accompanying this rise there is an increase in the intracellular potassium. If the potassium does not produce fatal intoxication in 60 to 90 minutes, the rats survive. If they live for about 18 hours, compensatory excretion leads to low normal potassium in the muscle. From these facts it can be seen that high intracellular potassium probably does not occur except when extracellular potassium is also high.

Edema

The term edema should be limited to expansion of extracellular water and electrolytes. As will be pointed out later, edema may develop from disturbances in the exchange between the capillaries and interstitial fluids. However, the large expansions of extracellular fluids are accompanied by evidences of failure of the kidneys to excrete sodium. The expansion of water in extracellular fluids may be so great that half of the body weight is extracellular. The edema may be accompanied by acidosis, alkalosis or low electrolyte concentrations. Although increase in electrolyte concentration usually leads to further expansion of body fluids so as to reduce the electrolyte concentrations, hypertonic concentration may be found in edematous patients. While the actual composition of the intracellular fluids in the presence of edema has not been studied, it is usually assumed that the intracellular structures are well preserved. However, there is no reason to doubt that the cells undergo the same sort of changes in composition, when the concentrations and acid-base equilibrium of the plasma are altered, as has been shown to be the case, when there is no increase in extracellular volume. Thus, hypotonic edema should produce increased hydration of the cells, while hypertonic edema should lead to dehydration of the cells. There is also evidence that low electrolyte concentration in patients with edema leads to circulatory failure similar to that seen in hypotonic dehydration. Renal function and circulation may be improved by raising the electrolyte concentration by giving sodium chloride and sodium bicarbonate. It is likely that some of the cases of edema show the changes in intracellular composition illustrated in chart III, when there is a disturbance in bicarbonate concentrations produced by a primary relative deficiency of one ion.

Changes in Tissue Composition

With the above background, based largely on studies of experimental animals, the changes in tissue composition in certain conditions in patients will be discussed briefly. It must be realized that actual values for patients are difficult to obtain, and that the methods are subject to errors not involved in tissue analyses. The composition of tissue of patients can be inferred by measuring the losses during development of the disturbance or by measuring the retentions during recovery. Since it has seldom been possible to determine the skin losses, the balances usually are incomplete. However, this lack of complete balance does not preclude approximate estimations of the changes in body composition.

The experiments on animals indicate that the magnitude of the losses of extracellular electrolyte in patients probably never is greater than one third of the normal content, i.e. about 9 mEq of Cl and 12 mEq of Na per kilogram of body weight in babies or 6 and 10 in adults. This conclusion is based on the fact that losses that are this great in cats and dogs lead to symptoms that simulate those seen in the sickest patients. Loss of half of the extracellular electrolyte apparently was more than the animals could withstand[14]. The experiments on potassium deficiency in animals indicate that only as much as half of the potassium of muscle may be replaced by sodium. Neglecting deficits in other tissue, this would indicate that the maximum deficit of potassium could be about 24 mM per kilogram of body weight. It is unlikely that values greater than 17 will be found in patients.

Infantile diarrhea produces deficits of water, sodium, potassium and chloride which show considerable variations in the absolute and relative

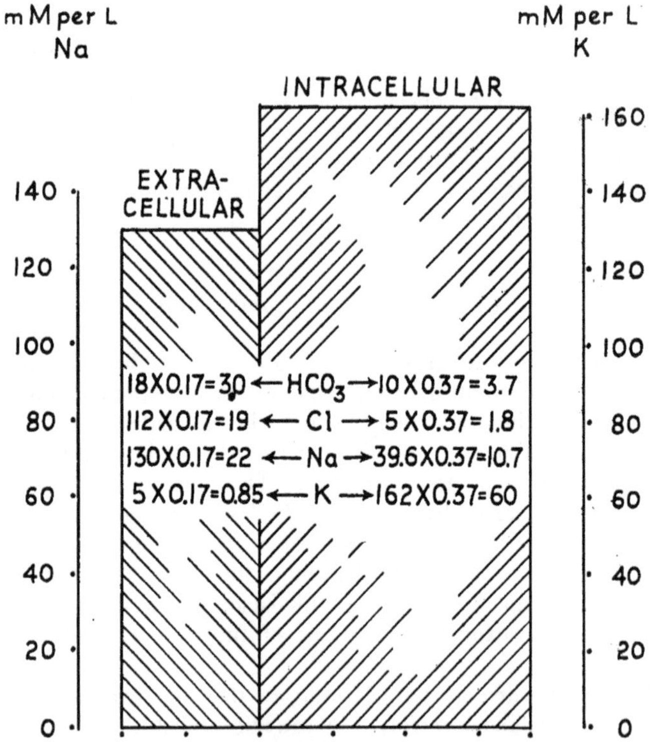

CHART IV. Diagram of 1 kilogram of tissue in infantile diarrhea. The deficits are 125 gm. of water, 9 mM of chloride, 9 mM of sodium and 10 mM of potassium.

losses of these constituents. The plasma may be hypotonic or hypertonic. Metabolic acidosis usually is present in the severe cases. The balances during recovery in 8 severe cases showed average retentions per kilogram of body weight of 125 grams of water, 9.2 mM of chloride,

9.5 mM of sodium and 10 mM of potassium. The effect of such deficits on the body composition of a normal infant is shown in chart IV. Since the deficiency of sodium for the body as a whole is equivalent to the deficiency of chloride, the acidosis is explained by transfer of extracellular sodium to the cells. This conclusion is evident from the fact that the low concentration of bicarbonate indicates relative deficiency of sodium in extracellular fluids.

The deficiency of potassium is equivalent to about one seventh of the total estimated intracellular potassium content of normal babies or to about the equivalent of one fourth of the normal extracellular sodium. Although intracellular sodium is abnormally high, the intracellular sodium is not as great as the deficit of potassium would predict in chart III. The deficiency of potassium is sufficient to explain the acidosis developing with no relative deficit of sodium in relation to chloride. The acidosis in infantile diarrhea is, therefore, dependent on deficit of potassium occurring in patients with deficiency of water, sodium and chloride.

The studies do not show the actual changes in tissue composition in infantile diarrhea, since the state of nutrition of the patients usually is greatly disturbed. The older literature showed that babies dying of diarrhea have a great loss of intracellular structures which apparently leave extracellular fluids relatively large in relation to body weight[21]. However, the authors have analyses of muscles that confirm the changes in intracellular composition indicated by the balance studies. Since the diagram is based on the estimated losses subtracted from a hypothetical normal composition, it does not indicate the changes in tissue composition that are produced by undernutrition. The diagram should, therefore, be considered to represent the composition only in a well-nourished baby with acute diarrhea. The deficit of extracellular water and electrolyte is about one fourth of the normal content. Intracellular sodium is about double the normal value. The deficit of water in the cells is a little greater than that of extracellular fluids.

Inspection of the diagram enables one to visualize the results of various types of treatment. If the infants are treated with sodium chloride and water alone, the deficit of potassium will persist and sodium will enter the cells owing to persistence of the deficiency of potassium[2]. If sufficient water is available to permit renal adjustment, high intracellular sodium and low intracellular potassium leads to alkalosis. High concentration of bicarbonate in serum also aggravates the tendency to development of low serum calcium[22]. All these disturbances will disappear when food with its high content of potassium can be absorbed. Indeed the success of treatment with solutions containing sodium chloride and sodium bicarbonate depends on sufficiently rapid recovery to permit feeding.

If sodium chloride is given with insufficient water to permit renal adjustment, acidosis may persist or be aggravated. Case 3 of a previous study illustrates this course of events[23]. The patient was admitted for severe diarrhea which had been treated at home by the addition of small amounts of sodium chloride to a milk mixture that gave too little water for a baby with diarrhea. On admission the concentrations of bicarbonate and chloride in serum were respectively 7 and 123 mM per liter. During recovery no sodium and chloride were retained while 13 mM of potassium and 100 gm. of water per kilogram of body weight were added to the body. Since the diarrhea would have led to losses of sodium and chloride at home, if sodium chloride had not been added to the food, this treatment had prevented deficits of these ions. The acidosis probably had been aggravated by transfer of sodium to the cells since sufficient water was not available to permit renal adjustment. The persistent deficit of potassium explains the transfer of sodium to the cells. On entry into the hospital the patient suffered chiefly from deficit of water and potassium leading to acidosis and hypertonic dehydration. The picture was the result of treating diarrhea with sodium chloride and insufficient water. A similar picture is seen frequently when acidosis is treated with saline and insufficient water free of electrolytes.

Adults with diarrhea have not been studied by methods which demonstrate the actual deficits of water and electrolye. Nevertheless, it has long been known that adults lose large amounts of water, sodium, potassium and chloride in dysentery and cholera[24]. The importance of losses of potassium is indicated by the observation of paralysis following the treatment of cholera[25]. This paralysis was relieved by the intravenous injection of potassium chloride. Similar observations have been made in sprue[26]. There can be little doubt that diarrhea in adults leads to striking deficits of potassium as well as of sodium and chloride and water and that the changes in tissue composition are similar to those of infants.

About twenty years ago Atchley and others[27] showed that *diabetic acidosis* is associated with losses of potassium as well as sodium and chloride. Holler and others[28, 29, 30] observed paralysis during recovery which was accompanied by low concentrations of potassium in serum and was relieved by potassium salts. The authors found that the retentions during recovery in a severe case of diabetic acidosis in an 8-year-old girl were 100 grams of water, 8 mM of chloride, 12 mM of sodium and 6 mM of potassium per kilogram of body weight. The serum concentrations of phosphorus decrease somewhat more strikingly during recovery from diabetic acidosis than those of infants with diarrhea. The changes in tissue composition in diabetic acidosis apparently resemble those of infantile diarrhea except for the hyperglycemia and ketosis. Recent observations[31] indicate that the elevation of blood sugar expands extracellular fluids and dehydrates the cells owing to its osmotic effect. Since the glucose is only found in the extracellular fluids, it can exert its osmotic effect only in these fluids. A blood sugar of 550 mgm. per 100 ml. has about one tenth as great osmotic pressure as that of normal plasma. These facts must be taken into account in judging the decrease in serum electrolyte concentrations in diabetic acidosis.

The acidosis of *renal failure* has not been studied adequately from the point of view of changes in both extracellular and intracellular composition. Nephritic patients frequently show low serum concentrations of bicarbonate, chloride and sodium, but the intracellular changes accompanying these changes are not known. The usual explanation of the serum electrolyte changes is failure of the kidneys to conserve sodium chloride and preserve the acid-base balance in advanced hyposthenuric nephritis. Certain patients with chronic nephritis have shown weakness which is relieved by potassium salts. These patients have low concentrations of potassium in serum[32], and analyses of other nephritic patients with acidosis have shown low potassium in muscles[33]. The logical explanation is that the kidneys are unable to conserve potassium. These findings suggest that deficit of potassium may aggravate acidosis through transfer of extracellular sodium to the cells in patients who already have low concentrations of sodium and chloride in serum. Thus the acidosis of nephritis may depend on deficits of both sodium and potassium without deficiency in water. However, when there is oliguria, the concentration of potassium in serum may rise to levels associated with disturbances in the heart[34, 35, 36]. Indeed, potassium intoxication is one of the events leading to death in experimental anuria[37] and in some cases of nephritis[38]. The intracellular fluids of such patients probably are high in potassium.

All the disturbances produced by loss of extracellular water and electrolyte may result from the immobilization of water and electrolytes at the site of an *exudate* or *tissue injury*. Burns and crushing injuries to muscles are examples of disturbances of this type which involve no loss of water from the body[39]. It has been shown that the fluids that accumulate at the site of injury contain all the essential elements of extracellular fluids and plasma. Although the fluids are not lost from the body as a whole, the water and electrolytes are not available to the rest of the tissues. Thus, it is not surprising that traumatic shock with immobilization of extracellular water and electrolytes shows the same clinical phenomena of peripheral circulatory collapse, oliguria and anoxia of the tissues as are encountered in medical shock produced by losses of extracellular electrolytes and water.

When the circulation is interrupted or impaired by *shock* or *exposure to cold*[40, 41], the intracellular fluids of the muscles lose potassium and gain sodium. As was pointed out earlier, transfer of extracellular sodium to the cells produces metabolic acidosis when there is failure of renal adjustment of body electrolyte. The cellular loss of potassium raises the concentration of potassium in serum. If renal function is adequate, the potassium will be excreted in the urine.

A similar exchange of potassium for sodium in the cells takes place in *anoxia* and explains the rise in the concentration of potassium in serum in peripheral vascular collapse. High concentrations of potassium in serum are found frequently in diarrheal dehydration and diabetic acidosis before treatment is initiated despite the fact that the intracellular fluids are deficient in this ion. This sort of reaction, leading to urinary excretion of potassium, explains in part the loss of this ion in these and other similar conditions. However, the chief interest lies in the fact that internal shifts of sodium as well as loss of sodium from the body act together to produce acidosis.

Alkalosis usually is produced by primary deficit of chloride resulting from *vomiting*. The authors have determined the retentions during recovery in 4 cases of congenital hypertrophic stenosis. In all there was evidence of abnormally high intracellular sodium before treatment. Three patients retained moderate amounts of potassium during recovery, while one did not. Danowski and others[42] have shown by balances that more potassium is retained during recovery than can be accounted for by the retention of nitrogen. Apparently some cases of alkalosis due to deficit of chloride get enough potassium from food to prevent deficits of this ion, but others develop large deficits of potassium as well as large losses of chloride in relation to sodium[43]. It should be remembered that the presence of high intracellular sodium in alkalosis indicates that the relative excess of sodium over chloride in the body as a whole is much greater than that which is revealed by analysis of the serum for chloride and sodium. The large amount of intracellular sodium explains the slow response of some cases to administration of sodium chloride. The fact that potassium deficit persists means that, in accordance with the relationships depicted in chart III, the kidneys will not excrete sodium so as to increase the bicarbonate in the serum until cellular potassium is replaced.

Prolonged *gastric suction* after operations provides the conditions for the development of alkalosis with potassium deficiency. The removal of gastric fluid depletes the body of more chloride than sodium and produces alkalosis. The administration of sodium chloride facilitates the excretion of potassium by the kidneys. While sodium chloride usually is administered in sufficient amounts to replace extracellular electrolyte, the development of potassium deficiency alters the renal function so that metabolic alkalosis persists. Patients subjected to gastric suction are likely to develop low concentrations of potassium in serum. Clinical improvement follows replacement of potassium as well as sodium chloride[44, 45, 46, 47].

McQuarrie and others[48] first called attention to certain cases of *Cushing's syndrome* which have alkalosis refractory to administration of sodium chloride and ammonium chloride but responding to potassium salts. The serums show not only high concentrations of bicarbonate but low chloride and potassium. Kepler and others[49, 50] studied one patient who recovered from alkalosis after removal of an adrenocortical tumor but again developed alkalosis when metastases became manifest. Analyses of the muscle of these cases probably would show low potassium and high intracellular sodium. The patients suffer from primary deficit of potassium produced by certain adrenocortical steroids which increase the excretion of potassium by the kidneys. The same picture can be produced by repeated injections of desoxycorticosterone acetate[2] and less readily by diets low in potassium. The experimental animals receiving desoxycorticosterone show high intracellular sodium and low muscle potassium together with marked alkalosis of the serum[2]. The administration of cortisone and adrenocorticotropic hormone involves loss of potassium and alkalosis. Part of the effect of operations in producing losses of potassium may be increased stimulation of the adrenal cortex[47].

Edema represents chiefly expansion of the extracellular water and electrolyte. The mechanism promoting the formation of edema, which acts locally in the exchange of the fluid between the capillaries and the interstitial fluids are as follows: increased hydrostatic pressure in the capillaries in heart failure and venous obstruction, decrease in serum protein concentration in nutritional edema, nephrosis, nephritis and liver diseases, the presence of abnormal amounts of proteins in interstitial fluids in allergic reactions, myxedema and acute nephritis and decreased absorption of fluids by the lymphatics in some diseases. Ultimately the volume and concentration of body fluids are controlled by the kidneys. Disturbances in the excretions of sodium play an important rôle in the genesis of edema which is discussed in a subsequent part of this chapter.

The Expenditure of Water and Electrolyte

The intake of water and electrolyte must equal the losses. For this reason knowledge of the physiological factors controlling expenditure enables the physician to plan rationally an intake that meets these demands. The important pathways of expenditure of water and electrolyte are (1) the lungs and skin, (2) the gastrointestinal tract and (3) the urine.

Losses from Lungs and Skin

The losses from the lungs and skin may be divided into the insensible losses occurring when there is no sweat and those involving activity of the sweat glands. The insensible water loss excluding sweat is roughly correlated with heat production so that 42 grams are lost for each 100 calories produced[51]. When there is no sweat, a small amount of electrolyte is also lost from the skin, but this is negligible for most purposes.

Stool Water

Stool water is dependent chiefly on the residue of the diet which, in general, is proportional to the caloric intake. During fasting stool water is negligible unless there is diarrhea. Normal fecal water is about 4 grams per 100 calories of the diet and is such a small part of the total water expenditure as to be negligible for most purposes.

Kidney Excretion

The volume of urine must be sufficient to remove the excretory load presented to the kidneys. The substances presented for excretion are chiefly the end products of protein metabolism together with other osmotically active substances of which electrolytes are the most important. Renal load is proportional to the metabolic mixture being burned or the intake. Although different diets contain variable amounts of protein and electrolytes, the ordinary diets of patients are sufficiently alike to permit an approximate estimation of the renal load from caloric intake. During fasting the renal load consists largely of the end products of protein metabolism together with electrolyte freed by the breakdown of tissues. The metabolic mixture during fasting probably varies somewhat with age, the nutritional state and the length of fast. When all other food is omitted, administration of glucose reduces the renal load not only to the extent that protein is spared but also by abolishing ketosis which requires excretion of these acids together with electrolyte[52, 53]. Minimal protein metabolism is attained by giving 4 to 5 grams of carbohydrate per 100 calories metabolized. In other words the renal load during fasting is proportional to the caloric expenditure except that the load is diminished to a minimum by the administration of glucose. The concentration of the urine determines the volume of water required to contain a given load. The volume of urine is, therefore, dependent on the ability of the kidneys to form urine of varying specific gravity, on the renal load and the intake of water. Knowledge of these relationships enables the physician to estimate the volume of urine which will contain the substances presented to the kidneys for excretion and to plan an intake that will meet the expenditure.

Chart V shows the urinary volume per 100 calories on the ordinate and the urinary concentration on the abscissa. The area labeled diet gives the urinary volumes for the usual adult diet. The area marked glucose gives the urinary volumes during omission of all food except enough glucose to produce maximal reduction of renal load. Complete fasting requires intermediate volumes. Artificially fed infants fall into the lower part of the area marked diet. Owing to the low content of protein and electrolyte in human milk, the renal load of breast fed infants is almost as low as that indicated by the glucose area.

Chart V may be used to calculate the water requirement as follows: (1) the area appropriate for the diet, fasting or glucose administration is chosen; (2) from the chart, the urinary volume per 100 calories is obtained for an appropriate concentration, usually at a specific gravity of 1.012; (3) the caloric production is estimated from the age, weight, activity and food intake; (4) the volume of urine per 100 calories multiplied by one hundredth of the estimated caloric production gives the total urinary volume; (5) for each 100 calories metabolized 42

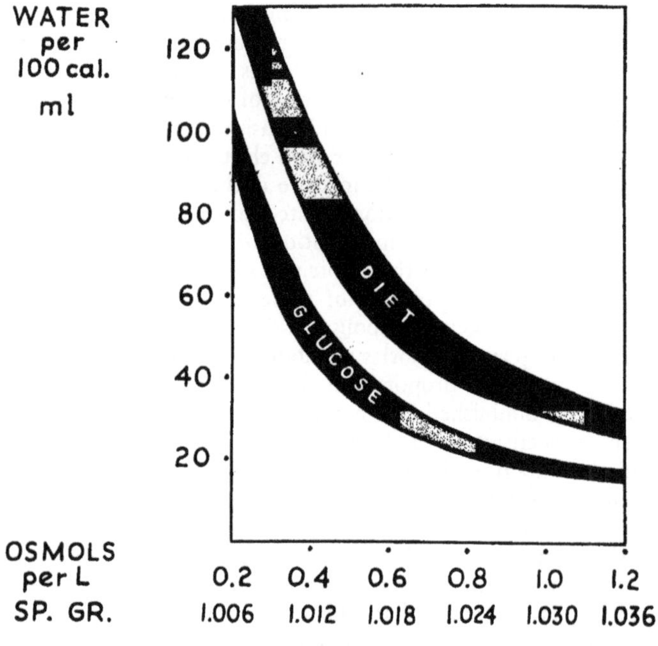

CHART V. Urinary water per 100 calories of food or 100 calories of heat production as related to urinary concentration. The area marked diet gives the renal load per 100 calories of the usual adult diet, while the area marked glucose gives the renal load per 100 calories of heat production, when maximal protein sparing is produced by glucose administration during omission of all other food.

grams of water is required to cover the insensible water losses. The sum of the total urinary volume and the insensible water losses gives the water expenditure excluding sweat, stool water and abnormal losses. Since complete absence of perspiration is unlikely, 15 to 20 ml per 100 calories metabolized should be added to cover total water expenditure in the absence of abnormal losses or large volumes of sweat.

For the normal individual without sweat on a normal diet and having a urinary specific gravity of 1.012, the above calculations indicate that water expenditure is 126 grams per 100 calories or 140 grams assigning a small allowance for sweat and stool water. Since babies metabolize about 100 calories per kilogram of body weight, this figure gives the water requirement of infants per kilogram of body weight. An adult, metabolizing 3,000 calories, would require 3,800 to 4,200 grams or about 54 to 60 grams per kilogram of body weight, if the caloric expenditure is 43 calories per kilogram. If the values are calculated for a urinary specific gravity of 1.024, a baby would require 88 grams per kilogram of body weight, if there is no sweating. An adult would require 2,650 grams or 38 grams per kilogram of body weight. These figures are about minimal except as modified by reduced caloric production or diets giving low renal loads. It should be noticed that calculation of the water expenditure at a specific gravity of 1.012 provides sufficient water for considerable sweat, if the kidneys are able to form a concentrated urine. In the calculation of the water intake it should be kept in mind that the water available for expenditure is equal to the preformed water intake plus the water of oxidation. The latter is about 12 grams per 100 calories metabolized of the usual metabolic mixture. During fasting a small amount of water is made available for expenditure by decrease in tissue water.

The usually prescribed intake of infants is 150 grams per kilogram, which would lead to a urinary specific gravity of 1.008, if there is no sweat or abnormal losses. A similar intake per 100 calories metabolized in an adult would be 4,500 grams. At this level of intake the kidneys could, if so required, provide 62 grams of water per 100 calories metabolized for sweat or abnormal losses or a total of 1,860 for the average adult. This level of intake apparently is appropriate for most infants, since they cannot readily make known their need for water. It may be advisable to prescribe as high an intake as this for children and adults if sweating or abnormal losses are likely to occur. Adults will voluntarily regulate their intake so as to lead to moderately concentrated urine.

Unless there is considerable sweating or abnormal losses, the intake of electrolyte with the diet or freed from breakdown of tissues during fasting is sufficient to replace the losses through the skin, stools and urine. The urine can be rendered practically free of sodium and chloride. Data on the ability of the kidneys to conserve potassium are meager, but it appears that the normal kidney can form a urine which contains potassium at no greater concentration than that of serum. With maximal conservation of electrolyte by the kidneys the urinary losses are about 0.2 mM of chloride and sodium and 0.4 mM of potassium per 100 calories metabolized. The minimal daily losses in a year-old infant are about 2 mM of sodium chloride and 4 mM of potassium. Corresponding losses for an adult would be four- to sixfold.

When food is taken, the stool losses are about 0.1 mM of sodium chloride and 0.4 mM of potassium per 100 calories metabolized. Stool electrolyte is negligible during fasting unless there is diarrhea.

Metabolic studies indicate that the insensible water losses are slightly greater than can be accounted for by the calorie production under ordinary circumstances in infants[54], children[55] and adults[51]. This finding indicates that a moderate amount of sweat usually is being formed. An average estimate is 10 grams of water 0.5 mM of sodium and chloride and 0.2 mM of potassium per 100 calories metabolized. The average sweat losses in adults would be 300 grams of water, 15 mM of sodium chloride and 6 mM of potassium per day.

Allowance of water and electrolyte for growth is of little practical significance inasmuch as the usual diet provides abundant water and electrolyte. The daily retentions during the first year of life are 10 grams of water, 0.6 mM of sodium, 0.4 mM of chloride and 1.6 mM of potassium. During periods of rapid growth the retentions may be twice these values and from the third to tenth year about half as great.

Summary

In summary, the water requirements can be predicted fairly confidently for normal conditions by the calculations described in the discussion of chart V. The minimal losses of electrolyte are about 1.3 mM of sodium, potassium and chloride per 100 calories metabolized. This indicates that the minimal requirements in the first year are about 0.5 grams of sodium chloride and 0.31 grams of potassium (0.6 grams of potassium chloride). An average adult would require 1.5 grams sodium chloride and 2.9 grams potassium chloride. Usually somewhat larger amounts should be given, since minimal expenditure cannot be anticipated. When all fluids are given parenterally, there is evidence that losses of potassium exceed the minimal losses by a considerable amount. This has been found to be the case when patients are given all fluids parenterally after operations. The amount required seems to be 2 to

2.5 mM per 100 calories metabolized, i.e. about 50 mM K (3.7 grams potassium chloride) per day in the average adult.

Abnormal Losses of Water and Electrolyte

Under normal conditions without sweating about two thirds of the insensible water loss occurs by diffusion through the skin. The rate of water loss from the respiratory tract depends on the volume of respiratory exchange and the contents of water in the inhaled and exhaled air. These are in turn dependent on the temperature and humidity of the environmental air since the exhaled air is about 88 per cent. saturated at body temperature. When there is hyperpnea, the magnitude of the water losses through the lungs is difficult to measure but probably reaches values five times as great as the normal rate[56]. In estimating the importance of the losses of water from the lungs, it should be remembered that an increase in the loss by the lungs may be partially compensated by decrease in the activity of the sweat glands. Water loss from the lungs is not accompanied by loss of electrolyte.

The insensible loss of water through the skin is dependent chiefly on the gradient for diffusion through the skin. This is dependent on the skin temperature if the skin is dry. A small amount of electrolyte is lost from the skin, when there is no sweat, presumably through desquamation, though there may always be a minimal activity of the sweat glands.

Sweat

The factors leading to the production of sweat are discussed in the excellent book by Adolph and associates[57]. In the thermal balance of the body the skin acts like a black body with a temperature of 33.3 degrees centigrade (92° F.). The body gains heat from the environment and objects above this temperature and loses heat to objects and environment below this temperature. Under conditions leading to minimal water losses from the skin about one fourth of the heat loss from the body is accounted for by the insensible losses of water. At an environmental temperature of about 26.7 degrees centigrade (80° F.) body temperature is maintained without sweating and without greater production of heat than that characteristic of rest. At a given temperature the radiant energy of direct sunshine may add as much as 50 per cent. to the heat balance when only the indirect energy from the sky is acting on the body. Sweat is produced normally in amounts sufficient to maintain body temperature when the metabolic production of heat and the positive heat balance from the environment are greater than the losses produced by evaporation of the insensible water and the heat losses through radiation, conduction and convection. At low temperatures the insensible losses cannot be decreased so the heat balance is maintained by increased heat production or prevention of loss by clothing. The efficiency of the evaporation of sweat is not seriously impaired until humidity is greater than 80 per cent. Air currents accelerate the rate of evaporation and the exchange of heat with the environment.

The volume of sweat may reach 2.4 liters an hour in man at hard work at a high environmental temperature. A few measurements on normal infants kept practically nude showed that raising the environmental temperature from 26.7 to 33.3 centigrade (80° to 90° F.) increased the loss of water from the lungs and skin from 48 to 108 grams per kilogram of body weight per day[54]. Presumably at least as much as 60 grams of sweat per kilogram per day was produced at the higher temperature. Adults sitting in the shade at similar temperatures showed comparable sweating per unit of heat production[57]. The calculated losses of sweat in infants with diarrhea studied at comparable temperatures in August in Galveston and Dallas averaged 70 grams per kilogram of body weight per day[23].

When the environmental temperature is higher than 33.3 degrees centigrade (92° F.), all the loss of heat is accounted for by the evaporation of water. Light clothing diminishes the amount of sweat at high temperatures by prevention of loss of drops of sweat from the body surface and decrease of the addition of heat from the environment. At lower temperatures clothing sometimes increases the volume of sweat by decreasing the heat loss by radiation and convection. Mere observation of the skin is inadequate to detect the onset or to estimate the amount of sweat. For a lightly clothed individual at a room temperature of 28.8 to 32.2 (85° to 90° F.) an allowance for the loss of 50 grams of sweat for each 100 calories metabolized apparently is indicated. Since operating rooms are likely to be quite warm and the patient is kept under covers and lights giving off a good deal of radiant energy, water loss in sweat may be considerable during operations. Air conditioning of operating rooms is not a matter of comfort for the surgeons but may be a requisite for low operative mortality. Air conditioning and avoidance of overheating are important therapeutic measures for patients suffering from disturbances in the metabolism of water and electrolyte.

The quantity of electrolyte in sweat has been found to be so variable that any prediction of the composition is difficult and unreliable. For clinical purposes the concentration of sodium and chloride may be assumed to be 25 to 50 mM per liter and that of potassium 15 mM. These values may be somewhat high for normal acclimated individuals. Actually, analyses of sweat indicate that the concentration of sodium and chloride tend to be at about equivalent concentrations and to vary from 5 to 100 mM per liter. There is evidence that acclimatization to hot weather is accompanied by a tendency to excrete a less concentrated sweat[58]. On the other hand, a high rate of sweating usually is accompanied by increase in the concentration of electrolyte. Recent work indicates that the concentration of sodium, potassium and chloride is influenced by adrenocortical hormones. Conn has shown that patients with adrenal insufficiency have high concentrations of sodium and chloride and low concentrations of potassium in the sweat produced in response to heat. In contrast, patients with adrenocortical tumors or ones receiving pituitary adrenocorticotropic hormone or desoxycorticosterone acetate have concentrations of sodium and chloride that are lower than normal, while those of potassium are higher than normal[59].

Gastrointestinal Losses

Abnormal losses of water and electrolyte from the gastrointestinal tract occur as a result of vomiting, diarrhea, escape of fluids through intestinal or biliary fistulae or by aspiration through catheters introduced into the stomach or upper intestinal tract. The approximate losses can be estimated from the volumes and the composition of the fluids lost. Chart VI shows the average concentration of certain gastrointestinal fluids. The volumes may be measured but usually can only be estimated approximately. The effect of the losses of gastrointestinal fluids is discussed ably by Gamble, particularly as they affect the composition of extracellular fluids[60].

As the chart shows, the gastric fluid contains more chloride than sodium and appreciable amounts of potassium. As excreted by the chief cells, the chloride concentration is somewhat higher than that of sodium in serum[61]. The gastric contents are the result of mixing the acid excretion of the chief cells with the neutral or slightly alkaline secretions of other cells. The amount of each kind of secretion is so variable that gastric contents may contain considerably more chloride than sodium or more sodium than chloride. The loss of acid gastric juice leaves the body with relative excess of sodium available to form bicarbonate in extracellular fluids. This type of alkalosis is characteristic of pyloric obstruction[62].

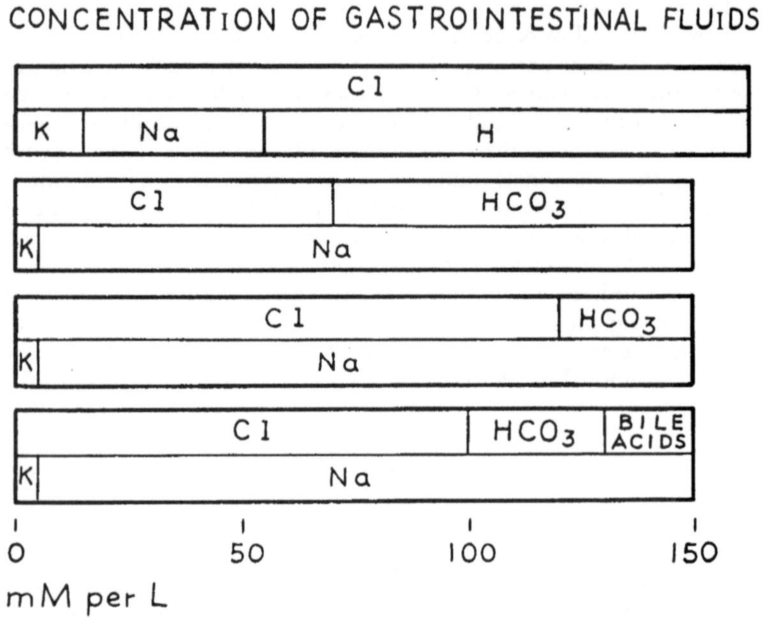

CHART VI. Concentrations of gastrointestinal fluids. From above downwards the following fluids are represented; gastric, external pancreatic, small intestinal and hepatic bile.

In the vomiting of renal failure and as a result of certain infections, the fluid is not acid and may produce no change in acid-base equilibrium or even acidosis. In certain cases of vomiting, typified by periodic vomiting in children, acidosis results not only because the fluid lost is not highly acid but also because starvation leads to non-diabetic ketosis[63]. High intestinal obstruction and loss of fluids by catheters introduced into the upper gastrointestinal tract after operations produce alkalosis because the losses of gastric fluid are greater than the losses of intestinal juices. As originally shown by Gamble, there are appreciable losses of sodium in extracellular fluids even when there is alkalosis. Recent work has demonstrated that considerable deficits of potassium develop. As discussed in the first section of this chapter this loss of potassium results largely from changes in renal excretion. The deficits of potassium following post-operative suction may be so large as to produce serious symptoms[43, 44, 45, 46, 47]. Although gastric juice contains moderate amounts of potassium, it is not great enough to account for the potassium deficits.

Losses of hepatic bile and the external secretion of the pancreas produce acidosis[64]. Drainage from fistulae in the lower part of the small intestines may produce acidosis although intestinal juice is not highly alkaline.

Diarrheal stools vary widely in composition. In some patients the electrolyte concentrations are so small that little decrease in body electrolyte develops despite the loss of large volumes of water in the stools. In other patients the stools contain so much water and electrolyte that the tissues are rapidly depleted of both water and electrolyte. The concentrations per kilogram of stool vary from 12 to 90 mM for sodium, from 10 to 110 mM for chloride and from 10 to 80 mM for potassium[23]. The daily stool losses in severe infantile diarrhea are about 250 grams of water, 16 mM of sodium, 11 mM of chloride and 8 mM of potassium. In adults cholera, severe diarrhea and dysentery probably lead to comparable losses. Sprue and celiac disease do not produce as severe losses of electrolyte except during periods of exacerbation. Practically all types of diarrhea tend to produce greater relative losses of sodium and potassium than chloride. As described in the first section, the resulting metabolic acidosis depends on shift of sodium into the cells owing to deficit of potassium, since sodium and chloride losses tend to be in equivalent amounts.

Gamble and associates[65] and Darrow[66] described a rare type of congenital anomaly of intestinal absorption leading to obligatory watery stools containing more chloride than sodium. The patients suffered from continual alkalosis and deficits of both chloride and potassium. Recent experimental observations indicate that rats subjected to potassium deficiency develop diarrhea in which the stools contain more chloride than sodium[67]. Albright saw a similar development of alkalosis in a patient with diarrhea stools containing more chloride than sodium[68]. It is likely that potassium deficit under certain circumstances alters intestinal absorption.

Renal Losses

A discussion of the rôle of renal losses in disease is difficult, because the kidneys play the chief rôle in the control of the volume and concentrations of body fluids. However, the renal regulation is merely the crucial activity in a complex process integrated by the regulation of the cardiovascular system. The process involves the activity of the vegetative nervous system, the neurohypophysis, the humoral and neural control of the blood pressure and the capillary bed and both parts of the adrenal glands and other endocrine glands[69]. All these influences alter renal function either directly or indirectly or both.

Vascular Movements of Fluids

The movement of substances within the body and the exchange of water, gases and solids with the outside environment is accomplished by the rapidly moving fluids of the vascular compartments. The red cells and the blood plasma are about one fourth of the total extracellular constituents. Although the red cells must be considered intracellular from the point of view of their composition, their function is intimately associated with that of blood plasma. Maintenance of adequate volumes of plasma and red cells is essential to normal function of the vascular system and the kidneys. On the other hand, disturbances in body water and electrolytes are reflected by changes in distribution of the circulation and the concentrations and volumes of plasma. As noted in the first section, loss of extracellular electrolyte leads to decrease in plasma volume, decrease in cardiac output, decrease in blood pressure and diminished renal function. Increase in electrolyte concentration leads to disturbances in cellular activity particularly in the central nervous system. It also increases the rate of glomerular filtration and the flow of blood to the kidneys.

If the rôle of the kidney in controlling the volume of water and electrolyte in the body is neglected, the movement of fluids between the vascular and interstitial fluids is governed by a balanced exchange[70, 71]. The movement of water and diffusable ions and molecules out of the capillaries is favored by the hydrostatic pressure within the capillaries and the colloid osmotic pressure of the perivascular fluids; the movement of these substances into the capillaries is favored by the colloid osmotic pressure of the plasma and the hydrostatic pressure of the perivascular fluids which is maintained by the tissue tension. An example of this balanced mechanism is seen in the portal circulation where low capillary pressure is balanced by high colloid pressure in the perivascular fluids brought about by increased permeability of the liver capillaries to protein. Local alterations in the exchange of fluid may be brought about by changes in the capillary bed. The lymph channels provide an alternate route for the return of vascular fluid getting into the interstitial spaces. The lymph seems to be concerned particularly with the return of proteins from interstitial fluids. The non-renal factors controlling the distribution of body fluids explain most local accumulations of fluid. While theoretically the same factors can explain generalized edema, recent studies show that renal as well as non-renal factors are involved in the genesis of generalized edema.

Kidneys in Relation to Body Fluids

Normally the volume of fluid in the vascular compartment is adjusted to the function of maintaining the exchange of metabolites in vital organs first by redistribution of the circulation according to the need but ultimately by altering the volume of plasma and extracellular fluid[71]. Present knowledge of renal physiology is inadequate to explain how the kidneys maintain the volume and concentrations of body fluid. However, it should be useful to point out certain mechanisms that probably are involved.

According to one theory[72] the distal tubules reabsorb sodium in quantities which are relatively constant under some circumstances. If this be true, the excretion of sodium could be regulated in part by changes in the rate of glomerular filtration and changes in the rate of reabsorption of water and sodium in the distal tubules. Since the reabsorption of water and salt in the proximal tubules is proportional to the rate of filtration, the sodium and water delivered to the distal tubules varies directly with the rate of glomerular filtration. If the amount of water and salt, which reaches the distal tubules, is greater than the rate of distal absorption, sodium is excreted, while if the amount is less than the rate of distal absorption, practically all the sodium will be returned to the body. Since higher concentrations of sodium in serum lead to increased glomerular filtration, a mechanism thereby is provided for regulating the volume as well as the concentrations of extracellular fluids. The weakness of the theory lies in the fact that variations in sodium excretion have been found to occur without change in glomerular filtration, perhaps in part because the methods of measurement introduce alterations in this rate. It is likely, however, that some such mechanism is involved and explains the regulation of the volume and concentrations of extracellular fluids as well as the disturbances in this regulation.

The *neurohypophysis* is integrated into this system since the production of antidiuretic hormone increases when serum electrolyte concentration rises and decreases when serum electrolyte concentration diminishes. The following factors have been noted to be accompanied by changes in the rate of sodium excretion: fluctuations in the rate of glomerular filtration, changes in the venous pressure, changes in the renal blood flow, alterations in the activity of the adrenal glands and the hypophysis and hypoproteinemic states. The exact mechanism by which the body achieves regulation of the volume as well as the concentrations of body fluids apparently involves some combination of these factors controlling the circulation, the neurohypophysis and the kidneys.

Renal excretion may be divided into three phases, the first of which is the formation of a filtrate. With normal glomeruli the amount of filtrate is influenced chiefly by the pressure in the glomerular capillaries which in turn is controlled by the local and general factors regulating the circulation. Glomerular filtration may be diminished by constriction of the renal arterioles which decreases the circulation to the kidneys. This type of reaction occurs in dehydration and shock. At a given extracellular volume, the glomerular filtration is increased by elevation of the concentration of sodium in serum. Glomerular filtration may be diminished by decrease in the number of glomeruli or by diseases of the glomeruli.

Second, about 85 per cent. of the water and electrolyte which is filtered through the glomeruli is reabsorbed by the proximal tubules[72]. The proportion of this reabsorption may vary between 60 to 90 per cent. of the filtered water and electrolyte. Since this operation is proportional to the rate of filtration, most of the reabsorption of water, sodium, chloride and bicarbonate is accomplished by a process which returns a large part of the filtered water and electrolyte to the blood. The evidence indicates that relatively more bicarbonate than chloride is reabsorbed at this stage of urine formation. Normally practically all the glucose is reabsorbed, and most of the urea remains in the urine of the proximal tubules. The osmotic pressure remains the same as that of the plasma since the proximal tubules are freely permeable to water. The loop of Henle seems especially adapted to equalizing the osmotic pressure. The reabsorption of water is dependent on the active transport of sodium and bicarbonate by the proximal tubules. If glucose is not completely reabsorbed, or if large amounts of other osmotically active substances remain, less water and electrolyte are reabsorbed and more are delivered to the distal tubules.

Third, urine is formed from the isosmotic fluid of the proximal tubules by the distal tubular cells which reabsorb water and sodium and reabsorb or excrete other electrolytes and other substances. The various operations are rather specific, and at least the absorption of water and sodium can be carried out more or less independently of each other. Thus, the volume of water reabsorbed is influenced by the antidiuretic hormone of the hypophysis. In the absence of the antidiuretic hormone large volumes of urine of low specific gravity are excreted, while under the influence of this hormone the urine can be maximally concentrated by the normal kidney. By an essentially separate process sodium may be reabsorbed almost completely, or a large part of the sodium reaching the distal tubules may be excreted. The rate of sodium reabsorption is normally regulated so as to maintain the volume and concentration of body fluids. In this process the antidiuretic hormone plays an important rôle[73]. While the necessary modifications of the rate of reabsorption of sodium may be mediated ultimately by adrenocortical hormones, sodium reabsorption is increased by low concentration of sodium in plasma, low filtration rates and high venous pressures. It is also modified by processes regulating urinary acidity. The adrenocortical hormones and to a less extent other related steroids diminish the excretion of sodium[74, 75]. If the venous pressure is raised in one kidney, the tubular reabsorption of sodium is increased in this kidney but not in the other one with unaltered circulation. Since the rate of glomerular filtration remains the same in both kidneys, tubular reabsorption may be altered by the high venous pressure without hormonal influences or changes in the rate of glomerular filtration[76].

The regulation of the acidity of the urine provides the mechanism for excreting unusual loads of acids or alkalis[77, 78]. In this operation, hydrogen ions are exchanged for other cations by a process that is intimately connected with the rate of reabsorption of bicarbonate and carbonate[79, 80]. When the serum bicarbonate is below the normal level, an acid urine is excreted which contains practically no bicarbonate. When the plasma bicarbonate is above 28 mEq per liter, about 28 mEq of bicarbonate are reabsorbed for each liter of glomerular filtrate. While a large part of the bicarbonate reabsorption is accomplished by the proximal tubules, the final regulation is carried out by the distal tubules. Thus sodium and potassium are saved in acidosis, and chloride is saved in alkalosis. The reabsorption of chloride is reciprocally related to bicarbonate reabsorption, and the sum of the two returned to the body is approximately constant for a given amount of glomerular filtrate. Since the reabsorption of cations, chiefly sodium, is related to the sum of chloride and bicarbonate taken back into the body, the electrolyte pattern of the plasma is determined by these processes. Ammonia is excreted promptly in the urine in response to an acid load, but only after one to several days are large amounts of acids excreted by this mechanism. During recovery from acidosis there is a delay in the decrease in ammonia formation so that there is a tendency for body sodium to become higher than normal during recovery from acidosis. With the introduction of large loads of acid to be excreted, sodium is at first lost from the body. Later, excretion of potassium diminishes the losses of sodium but may produce deficits of potassium. Finally, ammonia excretion may achieve a satisfactory conservation of fixed cations[81].

The formation of an alkaline urine enables the kidneys to excrete large amounts of bicarbonate and the equivalent amounts of cations. At high levels of bicarbonate, the urinary pressure of carbon dioxide rises. It is noteworthy that depletion of sodium and potassium as well as chloride leading to alkalosis is accompanied by excretion of an acid urine. Thus, the formation of an alkaline urine is not a simple response to an alkaline plasma but is modified by deficits of water and electrolyte.

The regulation of body potassium by renal excretion only recently has received the attention that it deserves. Potassium can be excreted by the renal tubules since the urine may contain more potassium than can be accounted for by the glomerular filtrate[82]. The tubules are capable also of reabsorbing potassium against a concentration gradient since the urinary concentration may be less than that of the plasma. It is probable that potassium is almost entirely reabsorbed in the proximal tubules or at least reabsorbed to the same extent as the sodium. In this case the usual process is excretion by the distal tubules.

Urinary potassium rises rapidly in response to increase in plasma potassium concentration. Adults can excrete as much as five times the usual daily load of 4 grams. When potassium intake is low, urinary excretion is diminished, but some potassium is found always in the urine.

The kidneys seem to have little difficulty in rendering the urinary concentration at least as low as that of the plasma. Normally the rate of potassium excretion maintains the plasma concentration within narrow limits.

Cellular potassium is maintained by equilibrium with the plasma potassium. Under certain circumstances potassium is released from the cells to extracellular fluids and excreted. Often it is difficult to decide whether the loss is dependent primarily on the release from the cells or increased excretion by the kidneys leading secondarily to cellular loss. A disturbance within the cells, which releases potassium, probably is in part the explanation of potassium losses in alkalosis and in response to desoxycorticosterone acetate and adrenocortical hormones. Disturbances in carbohydrate metabolism in diabetic acidosis and other changes in cellular metabolism in anoxia, shock, dehydration and acidosis produce a similar release of potassium from the cells. Urinary potassium rises so quickly in response to increase in plasma bicarbonate that the initial effect probably is chiefly renal. However, urinary potassium may become quite low in chronic alkalosis after considerable depletion of intracellular potassium. As was indicated previously, excretion of large loads of acid lead to urinary losses of potassium. In part this seems to depend on factors involved in the excretion of large loads of acids. However, acidosis probably also releases potassium from the cells. Indeed, Elkinton and Winkler[83] produced evidence that potassium is released from the cells with loss of body water.

The mechanism involved in the formation of an acid or alkaline urine is chiefly responsible for the preservation of the acid-base balance of the blood and the body content of electrolyte. In alkalosis urine chloride usually decreases owing to increase in urinary bicarbonate. However, it is noteworthy that acid urine is excreted in alkalosis that is accompanied by marked deficit of body electrolyte[84]. The rôle of the relative deficits of sodium and potassium to this phenomenon has not been investigated. Potassium deficit leads to increased reabsorption of bicarbonate and increased excretion of chloride since potassium deficit tends to produce chloride deficit. Similarly, alkalosis due to chloride deficit leads to increased potassium excretion since alkalosis tends to produce deficiency of potassium. Thus not only does the kidney control body composition, but renal function is determined by body composition.

The abnormalities in urine formation involve so many factors that the alterations in renal function of each case may have to be analysed individually. However, it is possible to classify the various defects of urinary excretion into the following types: (1) obligatory water excretion with little loss of electrolyte, (2) obligatory sodium excretion, accompanied by proportionally smaller losses of water and (3) excessive renal reabsorption of sodium and water. In each type disturbances in the regulation of the acid-base equilibrium may develop, and this factor must be evaluated separately.

It is obvious that, if the kidneys excrete water at a greater rate than it is taken into the body, the serum electrolyte concentrations will rise unless electrolyte is excreted also. The body will contain low amounts of water, and the serum will show an increase in concentration of electrolyte. The state of body water and electrolyte is hypertonic dehydration. Obligatory polyuria leading to losses of water and but little change in body sodium and chloride has been described in infants as a result of an anomaly of renal function[85, 86, 87]. The patients are all males, they fail to grow, have fever unexplained by infections and are mentally deficient. The diuresis fails to respond to the antidiuretic hormone. Often the loss of water becomes so rapid that the patients spend practically all their time drinking. The serums show very high concentrations of sodium and chloride without striking acidosis. The continued reabsorption of sodium and chloride in the face of rising serum concentration is the essential feature of the disease. The changes in cellular composition are not known. These patients require low intakes of sodium chloride as well as high intakes of water.

Diabetes insipidus results from deficient production of antidiuretic hormone owing to injury of the neurohyphophysis[88]. The patients usually do not suffer from dehydration, since they develop thirst, which is gratified by drinking large amounts of water. Since the distal tubules seem to function normally with respect to reabsorption of sodium and other electrolytes, there are usually no disturbances in acid-base equilibrium or plasma electrolyte concentration. If the intake of sodium chloride is high, salt is excreted in large volumes of dilute urine. If the intake of sodium chloride is low, the kidneys save sodium chloride and excrete somewhat smaller amounts of dilute urine. The patients seem to suffer chiefly from difficulty in drinking enough water to avoid thirst produced by the obligatory urinary water losses. The symptoms of thirst and the polyuria can be overcome temporarily by injections of antidiuretic hormone or by spraying the hormone on the nasal mucous membranes[89].

Adrenal insufficiency is perhaps the purest type of obligatory excretion of sodium[90]. Although the urinary excretion of sodium and chloride is accompanied by decrease in body water, the concentrations of sodium and chloride in serum are low, and moderate acidosis develops. This indicates that the losses of sodium and chloride are relatively greater than those of water. The patients suffer from hypotonic dehydration. The volume of extracellular fluids is decreased while the cells have high water contents. Although the primary defect in renal function is failure to conserve sodium, the final picture is the result of circulatory and renal failure produced by deficit of extracellular electrolytes. Sodium deficiency is the chief explanation of the diminished circulation, the low blood pressure, the low blood volume, the decrease in the rate of glomerular filtration, the rise in non-protein nitrogen and the failure to regulate the urinary acidity. These disturbances are corrected for the most part as long as body electrolytes are kept normal by the administration of suitable amounts of sodium chloride or a mixture of sodium chloride and sodium bicarbonate[74, 90]. Administration of desoxycorticosterone acetate or cortical extract corrects the absorption of sodium by the renal tubules, and with the restoration of body electrolyte renal function becomes essentially normal.

There is evidence that potassium tends to be retained in adrenal insufficiency, especially when the loss of extracellular electrolytes leads to circulatory changes and diminished glomerular filtration[90, 91, 92]. The muscles under these circumstances may contain excessive amounts of potassium. Some evidence has been assembled that cortical hormones increase cellular water[93]. If this is true, the increase in intracellular water accompanying loss of extracellular electrolytes may not be as great as would be produced by a similar loss in animals with intact adrenals.

Adrenal hormones are necessary for the diuresis of water since intact adrenals or cortical hormones are necessary for the development of the picture of diabetes insipidus[93]. This observation is the basis of the test for adrenal insufficiency showing failure of diuresis in response to a water load[94].

A large part of the picture of Addisonian crisis is explained by deficits of extracellular electrolytes. Adequate supplies of sodium chloride enable the patients to survive and perform the usual metabolic functions, though the response to stress is slow and inadequate. However, it is clear that adrenal insufficiency involves more than disturbances due to loss of body water and electrolytes[74]. Glyconeogenesis from protein and other responses to cortical hormones are not clearly associated with the electrolyte disturbances. Nevertheless, Addisonian patients have striking adverse reactions to relatively small amounts of potassium in food, especially when there are deficits of sodium and chloride. This response has never been satisfactorily explained. Kendall has postulated that the adrenal cortex enables the body to be freed from the vicissitudes of electrolyte metabolism[74].

Although desoxycorticosterone acetate restores renal function with respect to reabsorption of water and sodium, the compound may lead to excessive excretion of potassium. Cardiac injury may result particularly if the intake of sodium chloride is high and that of potassium low[95]. Diets should not be low in potassium or high in sodium chloride when desoxycorticosterone is administered. However, Addisonian patients do better with diets low in potassium and high in sodium chloride when no hormonal therapy is given[96].

The excessive excretion of sodium in hyposthenuric renal insufficiency usually is accompanied by other defects in renal function. While the generalized effects of deficit of extracellular water and electrolytes may develop and aggravate the disturbances in the kidneys, this does not usually take place. The kidneys may continue to excrete sodium and chloride while the serum concentrations of these ions remain low and body water is relatively normal. The body seems to become adjusted to low concentrations of electrolytes. The urine cannot be rendered highly acid, ammonia is not adequately formed in response to acidosis, phosphate and sulphate are poorly excreted, and the urinary concentrations remain constant and low. Since the usual diet requires the excretion of an acid urine in order to preserve body electrolytes, acidosis results. Some cases of chronic renal insufficiency have shown flaccid paralysis accompanied by low serum concentrations of potassium and responding to administration of potassium[32]. The kidneys of these patients apparently are unable to conserve potassium. It is likely that diets high in sodium chloride aggravate this tendency. Some patients with chronic nephritis develop acidosis associated with deficits of both sodium and potassium. The decrease in extracellular sodium is explained, in part, by the transfer of sodium to the cells owing to deficit of potassium, since analyses of the muscles have shown low potassium and high intracellular sodium[33].

In the terminal stages of nephritis, particularly when oliguria has developed, the excretion of potassium is diminished, serum potassium concentration rises, and death may result from potassium intoxication[34, 35]. Along with the elevation of serum potassium, a few patients have shown a flaccid paralysis and weakness with electrocardiographic changes characteristic of high serum potassium and relief of the symptoms when the administration of saline solutions has reduced the serum potassium concentration[35].

If the patients have circulatory disturbances as the results of decrease in the volume or concentrations of extracellular fluids, improvement follows administration of water and sodium chloride. Renal function also may be improved in some cases with low serum electrolyte, if sufficient sodium chloride and sodium bicarbonate are administered to replace the urinary losses despite little effect on the circulation. This effect seems to depend on increase in the urine volume. It is difficult to achieve stable normal concentrations of electrolyte in the serum of many cases of nephritis. If excessive amounts of salt are given, serum electrolyte concentrations may become abnormally high, or edema may be produced or aggravated. Relief from acidosis follows the administration of sodium bicarbonate, but the effect seldom is prolonged. If large amounts of sodium bicarbonate are given to patients with chronic nephritis, a highly alkaline urine is not formed, and alkalosis is produced.

There is evidence that administration of large amounts of sodium bicarbonate in the therapy of peptic ulcer produces renal insufficiency as well as profound alkalosis[97, 98]. The patients lose their appetites and develop lassitude, weakness, headache, nausea and vomiting. Mild stupor, coma or psychic disturbances occur. The non-protein nitrogen rises and returns to normal slowly only after the serum electrolyte concentrations are restored. In some cases the alkalosis seems to have produced permanent renal damage. It is not certain, however, that alkalosis permanently injures the normal kidney, but there is little doubt that it aggravates the pathological process in the kidney already abnormal[99].

Disturbances leading to excessive reabsorption of water and electrolytes tend to produce edema. As was previously indicated, the function of the distal tubules, which provide the mechanism for the reabsorption of water and electrolyte, is the one that is ultimately responsible for regulating the volume and concentrations of body fluids. Particularly in this operation the kidneys are under the influence of the factors controlling the circulation, the neurohypophysis and the endocrines. It is not surprising, therefore, that disturbances in the reabsorption of water and electrolyte by the kidney may arise primarily from generalized circulatory diseases and, even when the kidneys are primarily involved, disturbances involving control of the circulation develop. The circulatory disturbances aggravate the difficulty of renal origin, and changes in the kidneys develop in primary circulatory disorders.

The edema of cardiac failure arises chiefly from circulatory factors leading to increased reabsorption of sodium and water in the distal tubules[100]. Nevertheless, venous stasis augments the capillary pressure and explains some of the accumulation of fluid; low concentrations of albumin in serum may develop and have a similar effect. It is not known whether the tubular absorption is increased owing to high venous pressure in the kidneys, to decrease in the rate of glomerular filtration, to hormonal influences or to a combination of these factors. In any case there is no permanent renal damage, since the kidneys respond normally when the circulation is improved. Other types of circulatory failure probably lead to disturbances in renal circulation which invoke retention of water and electrolyte. Decrease in the effective plasma volume is an important factor leading to increased reabsorption of sodium and water by the kidneys, since the following conditions are associated with this phenomenon: hypoproteinemic states with or without renal disease, hemorrhage, shock, dehydration, exercise, assumption of the posture and certain liver diseases.

The effect of mercurial and certain other diuretics has been thought to depend on decrease in the reabsorption of sodium in the distal tubules. William Wallace and associates have unpublished data which throw light on certain features of the diuresis. In many patients chloride is lost in excess of sodium so that alkalosis develops. When this occurs, mercurial diuretics are likely not to produce further loss of body fluids. Other patients lose sodium and chloride in the proportions found in extracellular fluids and are likely to show continuous diuretic response. Restoration of chloride concentration by ammonium chloride usually restores the diuretic response in the patients developing alkalosis. Although some of the patients developing alkalosis lose body potassium, the losses are not great, and they do not develop in all cases. Apparently the mercurial diuretics produce a disturbance in renal function leading to relative chloride deficits with a minimal tendency to potassium loss. In this type of alkalosis potassium chloride is hardly indicated, since the diet contains abundant potassium, and deficit of chloride is the chief cause of the alkalosis.

Edema is a prominent feature of a number of different types of renal diseases such as acute hemorrhagic nephritis, nephrosis and some types of chronic nephritis. In acute hemorrhagic nephritis increase in the permeability of the capillaries to proteins plays a rôle in the development of edema. In other types of renal diseases cardiac failure occurs. In most types of marked edema regarded as primarily nephrogenic, low concentration of serum albumin develops. It is a frequent observation that diuresis occurs without restoration of the concentration of serum albumin. Nevertheless, diuresis may be quite regularly induced by the repeated injection of purified plasma albumin. While this procedure usually raises the serum albumin concentration, it has not been proved that the diuretic effect is merely a result of mobilizing water and electrolytes from the interstitial fluids. The diuresis may be a response of the tubular cells to the increase in plasma volume and other factors involving the general circulation.

Coller and associates[101, 102] point out that for one to three days after major operations the kidneys fail to excrete sodium chloride in normal amounts, if salt is given, and fail to have a water diuresis in response to a load of intravenous glucose solution. After operations the urine volume is low. Administration of salt solution alone may produce high serum electrolyte concentrations or edema. Injections of large amounts of glucose solution may reduce serum electrolyte concentrations. Unless there is shock, which leads to obligatory expansion of interstitial fluids, or there are deficits of extracellular water and electrolytes, postoperative patients need but small amounts of water and electrolyte. Every effort should be made to prevent shock during operations by transfusion which replaces the blood losses, but if shock develops, additional transfusions should be given[103]. Since deficit of extracellular electrolytes increases the susceptibility to shock, water and electrolyte deficits must be replaced before operations as well as after operations, if electrolyte losses are occurring.

Van Slyke[104] has discussed the disturbances in renal function resulting from shock. The immediate effect is oliguria or anuria. With decrease in the effective circulating volume, peripheral vascular constriction may restore urine flow, if the blood volume is not too low. If the shock is severe, the kidney may be included in the peripheral vascular constriction, and oliguria may result despite the maintenance of a blood pressure as high as 100 mm of mercury. If renal blood flow does not remain low too long, restoration of blood volume will be followed by rapid recovery. However, prolonged anoxia may produce renal damage which is particularly prominent in the loop of Henle and the distal renal tubules. These tubules seem to become indifferent to water and electrolytes, and anuria results from the reabsorption of practically all the glomerular filtrate. Anuria and marked oliguria following shock may lead to death in 2 to 20 days. Although the lesions may produce anuria or marked oliguria for several days, regeneration and recovery often occur. In many cases the recovery will leave permanent renal damage which still is compatible with life[105].

The treatment of renal disturbances accompanying shock should shorten the period of renal anoxia by prompt transfusions of blood and replacement of deficits of water and electrolyte if they are present. When the oliguria is prolonged, recovery is most likely, if body water and the concentrations of electrolyte in body fluids are kept as nearly normal as possible[106]. This end can be attained by initial administration of appropriate amounts of water, sodium chloride and sodium bicarbonate to restore body fluids. Blood volume may have to be sustained by transfusions. During prolonged oliguria sufficient water must be supplied from day to day to replace the obligatory expenditure which will be low owing to failure of urine formation. One must avoid giving enough water to decrease the concentration of plasma electrolyte or enough sodium chloride to expand greatly extracellular fluids. The therapeutic program should be controlled so that body weight remains relatively constant, while enough water and electrolyte are given to keep electrolyte concentrations normal as determined by frequent analyses of the serum. High water intakes will not increase urinary volumes in this type of intrinsic renal damage. Furthermore, low serum electrolyte concentrations may produce general circulatory disturbances which interfere with renal recovery. The opinion that water is effective in oliguria arises from the fact that one kind of oliguria is produced by deficits of water and electrolytes and is treated effectively by replacing the deficits. The fluids may be given by mouth, if there is no nausea or vomiting, but intravenous therapy usually is necessary in severe cases. Diets may be given if they do not induce vomiting or nausea. They should contain practically no protein or potassium. Sufficient glucose or carbohydrate should be given each day to provide maximal protein sparing. This will decrease the rate of release of potassium from the katabolism of tissues. Since proteins and amino acids accelerate the final toxic reaction, they are contraindicated.

During convalescence from oliguria the urine is likely to be low in concentration. In some cases sodium will be poorly reabsorbed, but after some disturbances recovery of sodium reabsorption may occur. while failure of reabsorption of water persists[106, 107]. Since some of these patients have had cerebral symptoms, it is possible that there is injury to the neurohypophysis which leads to deficient production of the antidiuretic hormone. At least in some of these patients increased serum electrolyte concentration has occurred on normal salt intakes. Some patients with calcification of the renal tubules show hyposthenuria with high concentrations of sodium and chloride in the serum[108, 109]. Treatment must consider these possibilities.

Therapy of renal disturbances is based on the calculation of the rate of water and electrolyte expenditure and the changes in body composition that the losses of water and electrolytes have produced. Determinations of the serum electrolyte concentrations usually are necessary, but these do not accurately reveal the intracellular changes. When the urinary specific gravity is fixed at 1.012, about 85 ml of water is required to excrete the load created by metabolizing 100 calories. This indicates that the water intake may have to be as high as 150 ml per 100 calories metabolized. The load may be reduced by diets low in protein, but protein should not be lower than that which will support good nutrition. As was indicated, salt may have to be added, if it is wasted, but in consideration of the effect of high intakes of sodium on the blood pressure and the formation of edema, salt is given with caution.

Finally in considering the factors controlling the expenditure of water and electrolyte, it is necessary to point out that the shifts of water and electrolyte within the body change the amount that is available for expenditure. If there is increase in extracellular fluids owing to the formation of edema or exudates, sufficient water and electrolyte must be retained to maintain the concentrations of extracellular fluids. When such fluids are excreted, a corresponding amount of water and electrolyte is released. These facts must be borne in mind in estimating the requirement of water and electrolyte.

There is such a small amount of water and electrolyte in the body that can be safely used for the obligatory expenditure that small losses produce symptoms of dehydration. The dangers of dehydration have been sufficiently emphasized so that physicians do not knowingly call on body water to cover obligatory expenditure. It is not so generally realized that expansion of body fluids may leave the rest of the body with insufficient water and electrolyte for the renal and circulatory systems to function properly. Burns, exposure to cold, extensive trauma, inflammatory reactions and injury due to ischaemia produce large expansions of fluids at the site of the injury. The fluid accumulated resembles extracellular fluids, and the localization of the water and electrolyte has the same effect as loss of extracellular water and electrolyte[39].

Accompanying the circulatory changes of tissue injury, potassium may be released from the cells and replaced by sodium[40]. The decrease in extracellular sodium produces acidosis which is further aggravated by changes in renal function dependent on the lack of water and electrolyte for the renal and circulatory systems. Part of the benefit of salt therapy in shock is dependent on these changes in the cells and the obligatory expansion of extracellular fluids.

Specific ion effects from the changes in concentration of sodium and chloride are not recognized except that alkalosis may produce or aggravate tetany. However, certain disturbances develop which are attributed to low or high concentrations of potassium in plasma.

Hypokaliemia

The following signs and symptoms have been observed when the serum potassium concentrations are low: (1) weakness and hypotonia of the skeletal muscles progressing to frank paralysis, (2) dyspnea with a gasping type of respirations in which the accessory muscles of respiration are invoked, (3) cyanosis which usually is respiratory but may be cardiac, (4) abdominal distention which probably is dependent on atonia of the smooth muscle; in experimental animals and probably in patients extreme deficiency of potassium may produce paralytic ileus, (5) nausea and vomiting, (6) cardiac enlargement with the appearance of systolic murmurs, (7) increased pulse pressure with Corrigan pulse, (8) elevated venous pressure and signs of cardiac failure. The paralysis of the diaphragm and the abdominal muscles and the functional disturbances in the myocardium account for the major clinical signs and symptoms. The electrocardiographic changes are described later.

Physiologically significant decrease in the concentration of porassium in serum may occur without characteristic signs and symptoms. Nevertheless, most of the symptoms just mentioned occur chiefly when the serum concentration is low. However, while the serum concentration is likely to be low when there is deficiency of potassium in the cells, if there is abundant water available and the circulation is adequate, large deficiencies in the cells occur when the circulation is poor and the serum concentrations of potassium are normal or high. For this reason the specific signs and low serum potassium concentrations will enable the physician to recognize only a minority of the cases of potassium deficiency.

Hyperkaliemia

The following signs and symptoms have been recognized in hyperkaliemia: (1) listlessness and mental confusion, (2) numbness and tingling of the hands and feet with a sense of weakness and heaviness of the legs, (3) cold gray pallor, (4) bradycardia and occasionally, totally irregular rhythm, (5) peripheral vascular collapse with diminished heart sounds and low blood pressure, (6) in a few uremic patients a rapidly ascending, flaccid paralysis with less involvement of the trunk, head and bladder than the arms and legs and (7) cardiac arrest.

Electrocardiograms in Hypo- and Hyper-kaliemia

There are progressive changes in the electrogram which correlate roughly with the concentration of potassium in the serum. These are illustrated diagrammatically in chart VII. When the concentration of potassium is low (below 3 mM per liter), the following alterations have been noticed: (1) slightly prolonged QT interval, (2) decrease in the height and inversion of the T waves, (3) rounded and prolonged T waves which may run into the P waves, (4) depression of the ST segment and (5) possibly, inversion of the P waves, extrasystoles and AV block. The precordial lead CR3 has been the most useful in measuring the QT interval. The height of the T waves has been found to be influenced by the pH, partial carbon dioxide pressure and the concentration of potassium. The changes in the electrocardiogram are reversed by restoration of the concentration of potassium in serum when low concentration of this ion is the cause of the change[110, 111, 112].

The changes in the electrocardiogram accompanying elevation of the concentration of potassium in serum are fairly characteristic. The T waves may become elevated and peaked at concentration of potassium in serum as low as 6.5 to 7.8 mM per liter. These changes are present invariably at concentrations greater than 8 mM per liter. Increase in the duration of the QRS complex develops after the change in the T waves. Increased duration of the PR interval, leading to auricular standstill, then develops. Totally irregular rhythm and heart block develop at concentrations of 10 mM per liter or slightly more[34, 35]

Summary

The purpose of this chapter is to present the physiological basis for fluid therapy. The chief factors to be considered are: (1) the changes

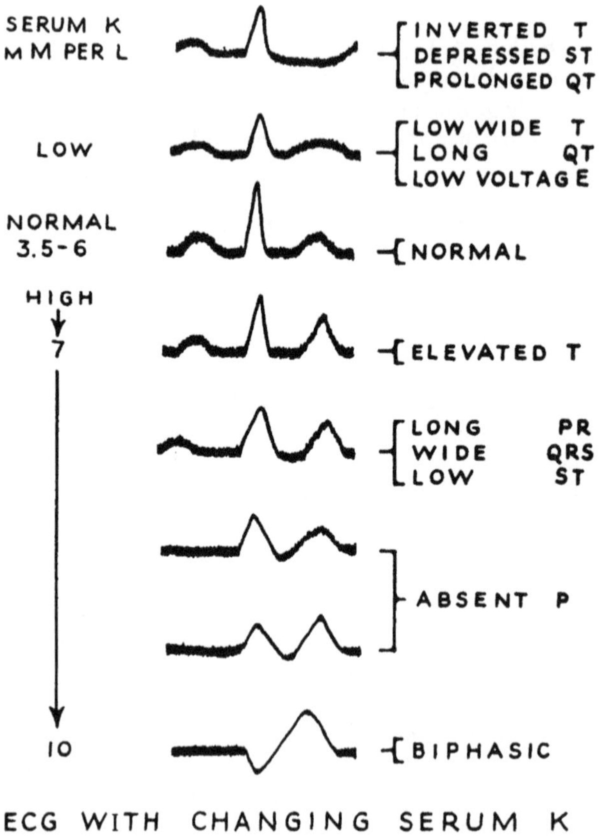

Chart VII. Diagrams of electrocardiogram with changing concentration of serum potassium.

in tissue composition and (2) the rate of expenditure of water and electrolytes. The knowledge of these factors must be applied with due respect to the limitations imposed by the metabolic disturbances of the particular disease. Only the general principles will be outlined in the following paragraphs. The aim of fluid therapy is the restoration and maintenance of normal composition of the body, particularly with respect to water and electrolytes.

When there is no nausea and vomiting, and when oral fluids do not seriously aggravate the losses of fluid from the gastrointestinal tract, the oral administration of fluid or food is the method of choice. If one is attempting to restore electrolyte by mouth, the concentrations of the fluids given seldom should be greater than one third physiological strength. Concentrated salt solutions are likely to produce nausea, vomiting or diarrhea and do not supply enough water without electrolyte to cover the obligatory expenditure as insensible water and as water required for urine formation. The various required ions may be added to beverages or food. The usual intake of potassium for an adult on a full diet is 4 grams of potassium or the equivalent of about 8 grams of KCl. This amount may be safely given orally and usually suffices to replace deficits of this ion. However, more may be given, since it is difficult to induce potassium intoxication by potassium taken orally, except when renal excretion is limited owing to adrenal insufficiency, renal disease or circulatory failure. Children and babies may be given corresponding amounts but dosage should be based on the relative caloric production rather than the relative weight. The usual diets provide enough electrolyte unless there are large deficits or unusual losses.

Parenteral therapy is required when large deficits must be replaced or fluid cannot be taken orally. Electrolyte solutions containing chiefly sodium at physiological concentrations are well tolerated subcutaneously. For slow intravenous injection the fluids may be about three time physiological strength. However, solutions more concentrated than physiological saline should not be used except when it is desirable to raise the serum concentrations. As the sole source of water, physiological saline and other similar solutions do not provide enough water free of electrolyte. When all fluids are given parenterally, the electrolyte concentration in the mixture given over 24 hours should seldom be greater than one third physiological saline. Usually the total requirement of water and electrolytes for twenty-four hours is estimated and added to 5 or 10 per cent. solution of glucose. Such a mixture may be injected slowly into a vein. If the solution is injected slowly, and the amount of glucose does not provide more calories than are being burned, there is little glycosuria.

Certain useful solutions for parenteral therapy are listed in Table I. They are classified according to the chief metabolic need which they meet. The preferred method of administration is indicated by + while

TABLE I

SELECTED LIST OF FLUIDS USED IN PARENTERAL FLUID THERAPY

	Contents per Liter							*Daily Dose*		
	Cl mM	*Na mM*	*K mM*	*P mM*	*Glu-cose gm.*	*Intra-venous*	*Sub-cutaneous*	*per kgm cc.*	*per 100 cal. met. cc.*	*Chief Use**
Appropriate for Water Expenditure										
Glucose	0	0	0	0	50	+	(+)		80-120	Nutrition
Glucose	0	0	0	0	100	+			80-120	Nutrition
Appropriate for Na and Cl replacement										
Saline	154	154	0	0	0	+	+	20-80		Alkalosis
1/7 M.Na Lactate	0	143	0	0	0	+	+	20-60		Acidosis
Na Lactate Na Cl	101	148	0	0	0	+	+	20-80		Acidosis
M. Na Lactate ..	0	1000	0	0	0	(+)		4-8		Acidosis
3.75% $NaHCO_3$.	0	45	0	0	0	+				Acidosis
Appropriate for Na, Cl and K replacement										
Darrow	104	120	36	0	0	(+)	+	20-80		Acidosis
Butler Talbot ...	22	30	15	5	50	+			100-150	Acidosis
Butler Talbot ...	22	30	15	5	100	+			100-150	Acidosis
NaCl KCl	137	102	36	0	0	(+)	+	20-80		Alkalosis
Appropriate for Parenteral Feeding										
Hydrolysate of Caseine	33	50	7	29	50	+	(+)		25-50	Nutrition
Appropriate for Shock										
Whole Blood ...	32	80	4			+		5-30		Shock
Plasma	80	200	10			+		5-40		Shock

* All solutions are used to replace water and provide for expenditure according to the categories indicated in the table.

(+) indicates that the solution should be modified by dilution or that there are serious drawbacks to this method of administration. The subcutaneous injection of 5 per cent. solution of glucose is irritating locally and immobilizes water and electrolyte for several hours. A mixture of one part 5 per cent. glucose and one part physiological saline or equivalent has few of these objections. Molar sodium lactate should be diluted to one seventh molar, if injected subcutaneously, or to less than one third molar, if injected intravenously. The solutions containing porassium that are designed for subcutaneous administration (Darrow's solution or the mixture of NaCl and KCl) should be diluted one part to 2 or 3 parts of 5 or 10 per cent. glucose if injected intravenously. While solutions of amino acids or proteins hydrolysates have been injected subcutaneously in a 3 per cent. solution, they are irritating locally.

The table shows the analysis of one type of enzyme hydrolysate of caseine and these values do not apply to other preparations. Solutions are available that contain practically no sodium and potassium. If the electrolyte content is critical, the analysis of the particular solution used should be consulted. Only the electrolyte content of the plasma was estimated in the case of whole blood, since the electrolyte of the cells is not immediately available to the body as a whole.

TABLE II

SUITABLE MAINTENANCE REQUIREMENTS PER 100 CALORIES METABOLIZED

	H_2O	*Protein Amino Acids*	*Glucose*	*NaCl*	*KCl*
Gm.	90-150	2.5	22	0.06-0.12	0.07-0.14
mM.				1-2	1-2

Table II shows the estimated requirements, when all fluids must be administered parenterally, and when there are no abnormal losses and no unusual amount of sweat. Under these circumstances the expenditure of sodium, potassium and chloride is small, and the fluids administered should not contain more than about 10 ml of physiological saline. Twenty ml per 100 calories metabolized of a mixture of equal parts physiological saline and isotonic potassium chloride (4.5 gm. NaCl and 5.5 gm. KCl per liter) meets the expenditure of Na, K and Cl. It will be seen that the caloric requirement cannot be supplied except by injecting about 150 ml of 15 per cent. glucose or 220 ml of 10 per cent. solution. A fifteen per cent solution is irritating to the veins and may produce thrombosis. Two hundred and twenty ml per 100 calories is a high fluid intake, and while it may be used, it is seldom desirable. Fortunately it is seldom necessary to prescribe full calories, since the consumption of a moderate amount of tissue fat is of little moment except that it delays the recovery of body protein. The use of homogenized suspensions of fat is being carried out successfully but still is experimental. If the use of intravenous fat becomes generally available, complete parenteral feeding will be theoretically possible. It is usually advisable to add one of the intravenous preparations of vitamins when prolonged parenteral therapy is being carried out.

In most examples of severe dehydration, shock is likely to develop. The circulatory failure accompanying loss of extracellular water and electrolytes is treated most effectively by replacing these deficits, but transfusions of blood and to a lesser extent, plasma, improve the results. When potassium solutions are going to be given to patients suffering from severe dehydration or shock, it is important to start the treatment with the intravenous injection of 10 to 20 ml of saline or a mixture of sodium chloride and sodium lactate. This procedure is indicated, because the concentration of potassium in serum is likely to be slightly high despite a large intracellular deficit of potassium. Salt solutions will improve the circulation and renal function so as to minimize the dangers of potassium intoxication. However, it is seldom necessary to delay the injection of the solution containing potassium more than an hour. Since the potassium-containing solution is injected slowly, the rate can be diminished, if renal function remains impaired.

In the authors' experience it is seldom necessary in severe acidosis due to infantile diarrhea to give more sodium bicarbonate or lactate than is contained in Darrow's solution. Since this condition is accompanied by as great losses of electrolyte as are met in any other conditions, this solution should be equally effective in other types of severe acidosis due to electrolyte depletion. If it seems necessary to give sodium bicarbonate or lactate, the dose is indicated in the table. It should be remembered that acidosis usually is accompanied by deficits of potassium as well as sodium and that the administration of potassium makes it unnecessary to give large doses of sodium bicarbonate to restore the serum concentrations of bicarbonate.

The deficits of extracellular electrolyte are unlikely to be greater than one third of the normal extracellular contents or 9 mM of chloride or 12 mM of sodium per kilogram of body weight. The deficit of these ions may be replaced rapidly by intravenous or subcutaneous injections. The deficit of potassium is unlikely to be greater than 17 mM per kilogram of body weight. This deficit cannot be restored rapidly because the injection of potassium at a rapid rate and in too large amounts may produce potassium intoxication. Furthermore, the cells do not seem to be able to repair the deficiency of intracellular potassium very rapidly. The authors believe that the optimal dose that is safe and efficiently utilized is 3 mM of potassium (0.22 gms. of KCl) per kilogram per day. One to two mEq of potassium per kilogram per day usually is sufficient to produce potassium retention and prevent serious decrease in serum potassium concentration. The injection of the dose for one day should be at a rate that requires 4 hours or more for the total amount since this assures that there is time for equal distribution of potassium throughout body fluids. When there is oliguria owing to shock or dehydration, the concentration of potassium in serum may be high. In order to minimize the dangers of potassium intoxication, intravenous injection of about 20 ml per kilogram of a solution containing sodium chloride or sodium chloride and sodium lactate at physiological strength should precede the use of solutions containing potassium. This will improve the circulation and start renal excretion so that it is safe to inject the solution containing potassium. This procedure need not delay starting the potassium therapy by more than an hour. In cases with high electrolyte concentrations in serum it is advisable to use a salt mixture diluted about half with 5 per cent. glucose or only 5 per cent. glucose. It usually takes 4 to 6 days to replace a large deficit of potassium.

In alkalosis physiological saline is effective unless there are large deficits of potassium. Theoretically the mixture of sodium and potassium chloride is more appropriate in most cases and has been proved to be more effective in cases of alkalosis resulting from prolonged vomiting or as a result of post-operative suction.

The treatment of marked oliguria and anuria as a result of intrinsic renal disease was discussed briefly in connection with shock. Coller and associates have pointed out that, for 1 to 3 days after operations, the kidneys fail to respond to certain renal loads that have been a part of post-operative care in many hospitals. The kidneys fail to excrete sodium and water adequately. For this reason the water and electrolyte expenditure of post-operative patients is temporarily low, and the fluids prescribed should be correspondingly reduced. However, if there is shock or if deficits of water and electrolyte develop, the intake of salt solutions should be higher. The best method of treating post-operative shock is by transfusions, preferably by giving blood at the time of operations according to the blood losses. Since patients with deficits of water and electrolyte do not withstand operations well, such deficiencies always should be replaced before operations.

BIBLIOGRAPHY

1. DARROW, D. C.: The relation of tissue composition to problems of water and electrolyte balance, New England Jour. Med., 1945, CCXXXIII, 97.
2. DARROW, D. C., SCHWARTZ, R., IANNUCCI, J. F. and COVILLE, F.: The relation of serum bicarbonate to muscle composition, Jour. Clin. Invest., 1948, XXVII, 198.
3. HARRISON, H. E.: The sodium content of bone and other calcified material, Jour. Biol. Chem., 1937, CXX, 457.
4. HEPPEL, L. A.: Electrolytes of the muscle and liver in potassium depleted rats, Am. Jour. Physiol., 1939, CXXVII, 385.
5. MILLER, H. C., and DARROW, D. C.: Relation of muscle electrolyte to alterations in the serum potassium and to toxic effects of injected potassium, Am. Jour. Physiol., 1940, CXXX, 747.
6. FERREBEE, J. W., PARKER, D., CARNES, W. H., GERITY, M. K., ATCHLEY, D. W. and LOEB, R. F.: Certain effects of desoxycorticosterone; development of "diabetes insipidus" and replacement of muscle potassium by sodium, Am. Jour. Physiol., 1941, CXXXV, 230.
7. DARROW, D. C. and MILLER, H. C.: The production of cardiac lesions by repeated injections of desoxycorticosterone acetate, Jour. Clin. Invest., 1942, XXI, 601.
8. MUNTWYLER, E., GRIFFEN, G. E., SAMUELSON, G. S. and GRIFFITH, L. E.: Relation of the electrolyte compositions of serum to skeletal muscle, Federation Proceed., 1949, VIII, 231.
9. SINGER, R. B., and HASTINGS, A. B.: An improved method of estimation of the disturbances of the acid-base equilibrium of human blood, Medicine, 1948, XXVII, 223.
10. PETERS, J. P. and VAN SLYKE, D. D.: Quantitative Clinical Chemistry, 2nd edition, Williams and Wilkins Co., Baltimore, 1946.
11. DARROW, D. C., MARTIN DA SILVA, M. and STEVENSON, S. S.: Production of acidosis in premature infants by protein milk, Jour. Pediat., 1945, XXVII, 43.
12. HOFFMAN, W. S., GROSSMAN, A. and PARMELEE, A. H.: Electrolyte balance studies on premature infants on evaporated milk, Am. Jour. Dis. Child., 1949, LXXVII, 49.
13. HOFFMAN, W. S., PARMELEE, A. H. and GROSSMAN, A.: Mechanism of production of acidosis in premature infants by protein milk, Am. Jour. Dis. Child., 1948, LXXV, 637.
14. DARROW, D. C. and YANNET, H.: The changes in distribution of body water accompanying increase and decrease in extracellular electrolyte, Jour. Clin. Invest., 1935, XIV, 266.

15. McCANCE, R. A. V.: Experimental sodium chloride deficiency in man, Proceed Roy. Soc., London, Series B, 1936, CXIX, 245.
16. DANOWSKI, T. S., WINKLER, A. W. and ELKINTON, J. R.: The treatment of shock due to salt depletion: comparison of the hemodynamic effects of isotonic saline, hypertonic saline and isotonic glucose solutions, Jour. Clin. Invest., 1946, XXV, 130.
17. GILMAN, A.: Experimental sodium loss analogous to adrenal insufficiency: resulting water shift and sensitivity to hemorrhage, Am. Jour. Physiol., 1934, CVIII, 662.
18. YANNET, H. and DARROW, D. C.: The effect of depletion of extracellular electrolytes on the composition of muscle, heart and liver, Jour. Biol. Chem., 1940, CXXXV, 721.
19. WINKLER, A. W., DANOWSKI, T. S. and ELKINTON, J. R.: The rôle of colloid and saline in treatment of shock, Jour. Clin. Invest., 1946, XXV, 220.
20. RAPAPORT, S.: Hyperosmolarity and hyperelectrolytemia in pathologic conditions of childhood, Am. Jour. Dis. Child., 1947, LXXIV, 682.
21. TOBLER, L.: Über Veränderungen des Mineralstoffbestand des Säuglingsköpers bei acuten und chronischen Gewichtsverlusten, Jahrbuch f. Kinderheilk., 1911, LXXIII, 566.
22. YANNET, H.: The effect of alkalosis on the relationship between serum calcium to protein in vivo, Jour. Biol. Chem., 1941, CXXXVII, 409.
23. DARROW, D. C., PRATT, E. L., FLETT, J., Jr., GAMBLE, A. H. and WIESE, H. F.: Disturbances in water and electrolyte in infantile diarrhea., Pediatrics, 1949, III, 129.
24. SCHMIDT, C.: Characteristic der epidemischen Cholera gegenüber verwandten Transudationenanomalien, Leipzig und Mitan, 1850.
25. HWANG, KEH-WEI and MOA, ING-CHI.: Pa-pin (transient paralysis) complicating Asiatic cholera, Am. Jour. Med. Sci., 1947, CCXV, 153.
26. HARRISON, H. E., TOMPSETT, R. R. and BARR, D. P.: Serum potassium in two cases of sprue, Proceed. Soc. Exp. Biol. and Med., 1943, LIV, 315.
27. ATCHLEY, J. L., LOEB, R. F., RICHARDS, D. W. Jr., BENEDICT, E. M. and DRISCOLL, M. E.: On diabetic acidosis, a detailed study of electrolyte balance following withdrawal and establishment of insulin therapy, Jour. Clin. Invest., 1933, XII, 297.
28. HOLLER, J. W.: Potassium deficiency occurring during treatment of diabetic acidosis, Jour. Am. Med. Assoc., 1946, CXXXI, 1186.
29. NICHOLSON, W. N. and BRANNING, W. S.: Diabetic acidosis, Iour. Am. Med. Assoc., 1947, CXXXIV, 1292.

30. GREENMAN, L., MATUR, F. M., GOW, R. C., PETERS, J. H. and DANOWSKI, T. S.: Some observations on the development of hypokaliemia during therapy of diabetic acidosis in juvenile and young adult subjects, Jour. Clin. Invest., 1949, XXVIII, 409.
31. FRANKS, M., FERRIS, R. F., KAPLAN, N. O. and MEYERS, G. B.: Metabolic studies in diabetic coma. I. The effect of early administration of dextrose, Arch. Int. Med., 1947, LXXX, 739.
32. BROWN, M. R., CURRENS, J. H. and MARCHAND, J. F.: Muscular paralysis and electrocardiographic abnormalities resulting from potassium loss in chronic nephritis, Jour. Am. Med. Assoc., 1944, CXXIV, 545.
33. MUDGE, G. H. and VISLOCKY, K.: Electrolyte changes in human striated muscle in acidosis and alkalosis, Jour. Clin. Invest., 1949, XXVIII, 482.
34. MARCHAND, J. F. and FINCH, C. A.: Fatal spontaneous potassium intoxication in patients with uremia, Arch. Int. Med., 1944, LXXIII, 384.
35. FLYNN, J. M.: Clinical syndrome of potassium intoxication, Am. Jour. Med., 1946, I, 337.
36. KEITH, N. M.: Clinical intoxication with potassium: its occurrence in severe renal insufficiency, Am. Jour. Med. Sci., 1949, CCXVII, 1.
37. DURLACHER, S. H., DARROW, D. C. and WINTERNITZ, M. C.: Effect of depletion of potassium on the survival after nephrectomy or ureteral ligation, Am. Jour. Physiol., 1942, CXXXVI, 577.
38. WINKLER, A. W., HOFF, H. and SMITH, P. K.: Toxicity of orally administered potassium salts in renal insufficiency, Jour. Clin. Invest., 1941, XX, 119.
39. BLALOCK, A.: Experimental shock, Arch. Surg., 1931, XXII, 310, 314 and 398.
40. FOX, C. L. and BAER, H.: Redistribution of potassium, sodium and water in burns and trauma and its relation to phenomena of shock, Am. Jour. Physiol., 1947, CLI, 155.
41. CRISMON, J. M. and FUHRMAN, F. A.: Distribution of sodium and water in muscle following cold injury, Science, 1946, CIV, 408.
42. DANOWSKI, T. S., GREENMAN, L., PETERS, J. H., GOW, R. and MATUR, F.: Metabolic studies of infants recovering from vomiting, Jour. Clin. Invest., 1949, XXVIII, 777.
43. BURNETT, C. H., BURROWS, B. A., COMMONS, R. R. and TOWERY, B. T.: Studies of alkalosis. II. Electrolyte abnormalities in alkalosis resulting from pyloric obstruction, Jour. Clin. Invest., 1950, XXIX, 175.
44. KENNEDY, T. J., WINKLEY, J. H. and DUNNING, J. H.: Gastric alkalosis with hypokaliemia, Am. Jour. Med. 1946, VI, 790.

45. BENNET, S., NADLER, C. S., GAZES, P. C. and LANNING, M.: The effect of vomiting due to intestinal obstruction on serum potassium, Am. Jour. Med., 1949, VI, 712.
46. RANDALL, H. T., HABIF, D. U., LOCKWOOD, J. S. and WERNER, S. C.: Potassium deficiency in surgical patients, Surgery, 1949, XXVI, 341.
47. PEARSON, O. H. and ELIEL, L. P. Postoperative alkalosis and potassium deficiency, New Eng. Jour. Med., 1950, CCXLIII, 471.
48. McQUARRIE, I., JOHNSON, R. M. and ZIEGLER, M. R.: Plasma and electrolyte disturbance in a patient with hyperadrenocortical syndrome contrasted with that found in Addison's disease, Endocrinology, 1937, I, 762.
49. WILLSON, D. M., POWER, M. H. and KEPLER, E. J.: Alkalosis and low potassium in a case of Cushing's syndrome, Jour. Clin. Invest., 1940, XIX, 701.
50. KEPLER, E. J., SPRAGUE, R. G., CLAGETT, O. T., POWER, M. H., MASON, H. L. and ROGERS, H. M.: Adrenal tumor associated with Cushing's syndrome, Jour. Clin. Endocrinol., 1948, VIII, 499.
51. NEWBURGH, L. H. and JOHNSTON, N. W.: The insensible loss of water, Physiol. Reviews, 1942, XXII, 1.
52. GAMBLE, J. L.: Physiological information from studies on the life raft ration, Harvey Lectures, Series, XLII, 247.
53. GAMBLE, J. L. and BUTLER, A.: Measurement of renal water requirement, Transact. Assoc. Am. Physicians, 1944, LVIII, 157.
54. COOKE, R. E., PRATT, E. L. and DARROW, D. C.: The metabolic response of infants to heat stress, Yale Jour. Biol. and Med., 1950, XXII, 227.
55. MACEY, I. G.: Nutrition and Chemical Growth, C. C. Thomas, Springfield, Illinois, 1946.
56. BURCH, G. E.: Rate of water and heat loss from the respiratory tract of normal subjects in a subtropical climate, Arch. Int. Med., 1945, LXXVI, 308.
57. ADOLPH and ASSOCIATES: Physiology of man in the desert, Interscience Publishers, New York, 1947.
58. MOREIRA, M., JOHNSON, R. C., FORBES, A. P. and CONSALAZIO, F.: Adrenal cortex in work in heat, Am. Jour. Physiol., 1945, CXLIII, 169.
59. CONN, J. W.: The electrolyte composition of sweat, clinical implication as an index of adrenal cortical function, Arch. Int. Med. 1949, LXXXIII, 416.

60. GAMBLE, J. L.: Extracellular fluid: extracellular fluid and its vicissitudes. Renal defense of extracellular fluid: control of acid base excretion and factors of water expenditure, Bull. Johns Hopkins Hosp., 1937, LXI, 151 and 174.
61. GILMAN, A. and COWGILL, G. R.: Osmotic relation between blood and gastric juice, Am. Jour. Physiol., 1933, CIII, 143.
62. GAMBLE, J. L. and ROSS, S. G.: The factors in dehydration following pyloric obstruction, Jour. Clin. Invest., 1925, I, 403.
63. DARROW, D. C. and CARY, M. K.: A clinical and chemical study of non-diabetic ketosis with acidosis, Jour. Pediat., 1935, VI, 676.
64. GAMBLE, J. L. and ROSS, S. G.: Body fluid changes due to continued loss of external secretion of the pancreas, Jour. Exp. Med., 1928, XLVIII, 859.
65. GAMBLE, J. L., FAHEY, K. R., APPLETON, J. E. and MacLACHLAN, E. A.: Congenital alkalosis with diarrhea, Jour. Pediat., 1945, XXV, 509.
66. DARROW, D. C.: Congenital alkalosis with diarrhea, Jour. Pediat., 1945, XXV, 519.
67. GARDNER, L. I., MacLACHLAN, E. A., TERRY, M. L. and BUTLER, A. M.: Chloride diarrhea and systemic alkalosis in potassium deficiency, Federation Proceed., 1949, VIII, 201.
68. ALBRIGHT, F.: Personal communication.
69. OGDEN, E.: Extrarenal sequel to experimental renal hypertension, Bull. New York Acad. Med., 1947, XXIII, 643.
70. STARLING, E. H.: Fluid of the Body, Herter Lecture, W. T. Keener and Co., Chicago, 1909.
71. LANDIS, E. M., BROWN, E., FANTEUX, M. and WISE, C.: Control of the venous pressure in relation to cardiac "competence", blood pressure and exercise, Jour. Clin. Invest., 1946, XXV, 237.
72. WESSON, L. G., Jr., ANSLOW, W. P., Jr. and SMITH, H.: The excretion of strong electrolytes, Bull. New York Acad. Med., 1948, XXIV, 586.
73. VERNEY, E. B.: The antidiuretic hormone and the factors which determine its release, Proceed. Roy. Soc., Series B, 1947, CXXXV, 25.
74. KENDALL, E. C.: Influence of the adrenal cortex on the metabolism of water and electrolytes, Vitamines and Hormones 6, 1950, VI, 277.
75. LEAF, A., COUTER, W. T. and NEWBURGH, L. H.: Evidence that renal sodium excretion by normal human subjects is regulated by adrenal cortical activity, Jour. Clin. Invest., 1949, XXVIII, 1067.
76. BRADLEY, S. E. and BLAKE, W. D.: Pathogenesis of renal dysfunction during congestive heart failure, Am. Jour. Med., 1949, VI, 470.

77. PITTS, R. F.: Renal excretion of acids, Federation Proceed, 1948, VII, 418.
78. PITTS, R. F. and LOTSPEICH, W. G.: Bicarbonate and renal regulation of acid-base balance, Am. Jour. Physiol., 1946, CXLVII, 138.
79. MENAKER, W.: Buffer equilibria and reabsorption in the production of urinary acidity, Am. Jour. Physiol., 1948, CLIV, 174.
80. PITTS, R. F., AYER, J. L. and SCHIESS, W. A.: Renal regulation of acid-base balance in man. III. Reabsorption of bicarbonate, Jour. Clin. Invest., 1949, XXVIII, 32.
81. SARTORIUS, O. W., ROEMMELT, J. C. and PITTS, R. F.: IV. The nature of the renal compensation to ammonium chloride acidosis, Jour. Clin. Invest., 1949, XXVIII, 423.
82. BERLINER, R. W. and KENNEDY, T. J., Jr.: Renal tubular secretion of potassium in the normal dog, Proceed. Soc. Exp. Biol. and Med., 1948, LXVII, 545.
83. ELKINTON, J. R. and WINKLER, A. W.: Transfer of intracellular potassium in experimental dehydration, Jour. Clin. Invest., 1944, XXIII, 93.
84. VAN SLYKE, K. K. and EVANS, I.: The paradox of aciduria in the presence of alkalosis caused by hypochloremia, Ann. Surg., 1947, CXXVI, 545.
85. WARING, A. J., KAJDI, L. and TAPPAN, U.: A congenital defect in water metabolism, Am. Jour. Dis. Child, 1945, LXIX, 323.
86. DANCIS, J., BIRMINGHAM, J. R. and LESLIE, S. H.: Congenital diabetes insipidus resistant to treatment with pitressin, Am. Jour. Dis. Child., 1948, LXXV, 316.
87. WILLIAMS, R. R.: Nephrogenic diabetes insipidus occurring in males and transmitted by females, Jour. Clin. Invest., 1946, XXV, 937.
88. WARKANY, J. and MITCHELL, A. G.: Diabetes insipidus. A critical review of the etiology, diagnosis and treatment, with a report of four cases, Am. Jour. Dis. Child., 1939, LVII, 603.
89. BLUMGART, H. L.: Antidiuretic effect of pituitary extract applied intranasally in a case of diabetes insipidus, Arch. Int. Med., 1922, XXIX, 508.
90. LOEB, R. F.: The adrenal cortex and electrolyte behavior, Bull. New York Acad. Med., 1942, XVIII, 263.
91. HARRISON, H. E. and DARROW, D. C.: The distribution of body water and electrolytes in adrenal insufficiency, Jour. Clin. Invest., 1938, XVII, 77.
92. HARRISON, H. E. and DARROW, D. C.: Renal function in experimental adrenal insufficiency, Am. Jour. Physiol., 1939, CXXV, 631.

93. GAUNT, R., BIRNIE, J. H. and EVERSOLE, W. J.: Adrenal cortex and water metabolism, Physiol. Reviews, 1949, XXIX, 281.
94. ROBINSON, F. J., POWER, M. H. and KEPLER, E. J.: Two new procedures to assist in the recognition and exclusion of Addison's disease, Proceed., Staff Meet. Mayo Clinic, 1941, XVI, 577.
95. KNOWLTON, A. I., LOEB, E. N., STOERK, H. C. and SIEGAL, H. C.: Desoxycorticosterone acetate; potentiation of its action by sodium chloride, Jour. Exp. Med., 1947, LXXXV, 187.
96. WILDER, R. M., KENDALL, E. C., SNELL, A. M., KEPLER, E. J., RYNEARSON, E. H. and ADAMS, M.: Intake of potassium, important consideration in Addison's disease; metabolic study, Arch. Int. Med., 1937, LIX, 367.
97. GRACE, W. J. and BARR, D. P.: Complications of alkalosis, Am. Jour. Med., 1948, IV, 331.
98. KIRSNER, J. B. and PALMER, W. L.: Alkalosis complicating the Sippy treatment of peptic ulcer. Analysis of 135 episodes, Arch. Int. Med., 1942, LXIX, 789.
99. BURNETT, C. H., BURROWS, B. A. and COMMONS, R. R.: Studies of alkalosis. I. Renal function during and following alkalosis resulting from pyloric obstruction, Jour. Clin. Invest., 1950, XXIX, 169.
100. BORST, J. G. G.: The maintenance of adequate cardiac output by regulation of the urinary excretion of water and sodium chloride; an essential factor in the genesis of edema, Acta Med. Scandinav., 1948, CXXX, Supplement 207.
101. COOPER, D. R., IOB, V. and COLLER, F. A.: Response to parenteral glucose of normal kidneys and kidneys of post-operative patients, Ann. Surg., 1949, CXXIX, 1.
102. COLLER, F. A., IOB, V., VAUGHAN, H. H., KALDER, N. B. and MOYER, C. A.: Translocation of fluid produced by the intravenous administration of isotonic salt solutions in man post-operatively, Ann. Surg., 1945, CXXII, 663.
103. CROOK, C. B., IOB, V. and COLLER, F. A.: Correction of blood loss during surgical operations, Surg. Gyn. and Obstet., 1946, LXXXII, 417.
104. VAN SLYKE, D. D.: The effects of shock on the kidney, Ann. Int. Med., 1948, XXVIII, 701.
105. MACGRAITH, G.: Renal syndrome of wide distribution induced possibly by renal anoxia, Lancet, 1945, II, 293.
106. PRATT, E. L.: Treatment of anuria. Management of patient with intrarenal lesions, Am. Jour. Dis. Child., 1948, LXXVI, 14.

107. LUCTSCHER, J. A., Jr. and BLACKMAN, S. S., Jr.: Severe injury to the kidneys and brain following sulfathiazole administration: high serum sodium and chloride and persistent cerebral damage, Ann. Int. Med., 1943, XVIII, 741.

108. ALBRIGHT, F., CONSALAZIO, W. V., COOMBS, F. S., SULKOWITZ, H. W. and TALBOT, J.: Metabolic studies and therapy in a case of nephrocalcinosis with rickets and dwarfism, Bull. Johns Hopkins Hosp., 1940, LXVI, 7.

109. BUTLER, A. M., WILSON, J. L. and FARBER, S.: Dehydration and acidosis with calcification of renal tubules, Jour. Pediat., 1936, VIII, 489.

110. TARAIL, R.: Relation of the abnormalities in concentration of serum potassium to electrocardiographic disturbances, Am. Jour. Med., 1948, V, 828.

111. NADLER, C. S., BELLET, S. and LANNING, M.: Influence of serum potassium and other electrolytes on the electrocardiogram in diabetic acidosis, Am. Jour. Med., 1948, V, 838.

112. FRENKEL, M., GROEN, J. and WILLABRANDS, A. F.: Low serum potassium level during recovery from diabetic coma, Arch. Int. Med., 1947, LXXX, 728.

January 1, 1952

Lightning Source UK Ltd.
Milton Keynes UK
UKHW030321081118
331792UK00011BA/2280/P

9 780483 502